Introduction to the US Food System

Public Health, Environment, and Equity

Roni Neff, Editor

Johns Hopkins Center for a Livable Future

JB JOSSEY-BASS™
A Wiley Brand

Cover design by Wiley
Fruit image © littleny | Thinkstock
Crop Duster image © Brian Brown | Thinkstock
Sky image © Brian Brown | Thinkstock
Wheat Field image © Brian Brown | Thinkstock
Multicultural hands holding fresh potatoes image © Dougal Waters | Getty

Published by Jossey-Bass
A Wiley Brand
One Montgomery Street, Suite 1200, San Francisco, CA 94104-4594—www.josseybass.com

Jossey-Bass books and products are available through most bookstores. To contact Jossey-Bass directly call our Customer Care Department within the U.S. at 800-956-7739, outside the U.S. at 317-572-3986, or fax 317-572-4002.

Wiley publishes in a variety of print and electronic formats and by print-on-demand. Some material included with standard print versions of this book may not be included in e-books or in print-on-demand. If this book refers to media such as a CD or DVD that is not included in the version you purchased, you may download this material at http://booksupport.wiley.com. For more information about Wiley products, visit www.wiley.com.

Library of Congress Cataloging-in-Publication Data
Introduction to the US food system : public health, environment, and equity / Roni Neff, editor.
  p. ; cm.
 Includes bibliographical references and index.
  ISBN 978-1-118-06338-5 (paperback)—ISBN 978-1-118-91306-2 (pdf)—ISBN 978-1-118-91305-5 (epub)
 I. Neff, Roni, 1967- editor.
 [DNLM: 1. Food supply—United States. 2. Environment—United States. 3. Food Industry—United States. 4. Nutritional Physiological Phenomena—United States. 5. Public Health—United States. WA 695]
 RA601
 363.80973—dc23
                                                                                        2014015934

Printed in the United States of America
FIRST EDITION

PB Printing SKY10033587_030222

Contents

List of Figures and Tables

Figures

Tables

Dedication

Bob Lawrence
Bob Lawrence founded the Center for a Livable Future in 1996 and led its development into the thriving interdisciplinary academic center it is today. We all owe so much to his mentorship, vision, and personal example. As this book goes to press, Bob has announced his retirement; we will miss him greatly.

• • •

Helaine and Sid Lerner
The Lerners have been dedicated advocates for measures to improve our food system and supporters of the Center for a Livable Future's mission since its inception.

• • •

Andy Pasternack
Andy Pasternack of Jossey-Bass reached out initially about developing this book and stewarded its initial phases with kindness, thought, and patience. Sadly, he passed away before the book was completed.

• • •

Educators and students of the food system
Finally, the book is dedicated to the educators and students who will read it. Your enthusiasm for creating a better food system inspires us all. We hope this book gives you the tools you need to make it happen!

Introduction

This textbook provides an overview of the US food system, with particular focus on the food system's interrelationships with public health, the environment, equity, and society. Through eighteen chapters and seventy-four focus and perspective boxes, authored altogether by one hundred and six food system experts, this book brings together information and perspectives reflecting the breadth of issues and ideas important to understanding today's US food system and to shaping its future. The readings highlight issues of public health, ecological impact, and implications for communities, equity and society more broadly; they address as well supply, demand, cost, stakeholder interests, history, power, politics and policy, ethics, and culture.

Student interest in the food system has grown dramatically since the new millennium, and academic courses and programs addressing the food system have proliferated. This book is intended to address the need for textbook material covering broad food system issues, and focusing on the food system's relationship with the public's health more specifically. Our aims are for the book to provide a resource to educators from a variety of disciplines, support their efforts to meet growing student demand for course work on food system topics, engage students, stimulate critical thinking, and, overall, to help students better understand our food system.

The book is a project of the Johns Hopkins Center for a Livable Future (CLF), an academic center founded in 1996 with the mission to "examine the complex interrelationships among diet, food production, environment and human health, to advance an ecological perspective in reducing threats to the health of the public, and to promote policies that protect health, the global environment and the ability to sustain life for future generations." Figure I.1 presents the concept model that frames our activities (www.jhsph.edu/research/centers-and-institutes/johns-hopkins-center-for-a-livable-future/about). Based at the Johns Hopkins Bloomberg School of Public Health, the CLF engages in research, education, policy, practice, and communications activities on diverse issues at the intersection of food systems and public health. This book advances the CLF's educational mission and builds on our experience as an interdisciplinary, food-system–focused academic center within a school of public health and within the Johns Hopkins University. The book reflects input from many CLF faculty members, staff, CLF-Lerner Fellows, research assistants, and colleagues across the public health school and the university, as well as many external colleagues.

This textbook is designed for use in food-system courses taught in many types of departments or schools, for example, public health, nutrition, environment, policy, planning, geography, nursing, business, and sociology, as well as in interdepartmental offerings. We expect it will be used in introductory courses at the advanced undergraduate and graduate levels. The book's chapters cover the core content of the food system and are presented with enough explanations to make it useful for those with little background in the food system, and it also shares the complexities stimulating to those with more knowledge and experience. The focus and perspective boxes add depth and fodder to enrich discussions

FIGURE I.1 Center for a Livable Future Concept Model

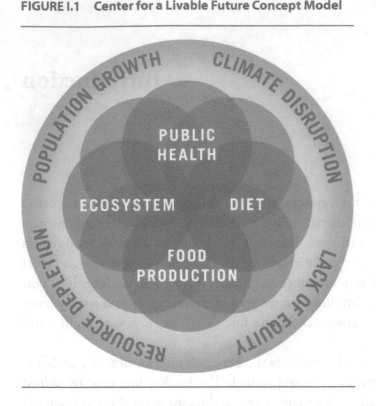

and assignments. We also intend for the book to be useful to those outside of academia seeking a solid introduction to food-system issues.

For many students, learning about food systems goes beyond the academic. This book and its associated discussion questions and online instructional activities present content and exercises that engage students personally and professionally. Students are encouraged to leave the classroom and computer to supplement their learning in the real world—at the table, in the store, at farms or gardens, and in sites throughout their communities. Additionally, through sometimes provocative content, the book pushes students to think critically and to question popular assumptions—as well as the ideas put forward by the authors.

While challenging students, the activities and discussion questions also target most of the core competency areas for public health—all of which have relevance for other fields as well: analytical and assessment skills, policy development and program planning skills, communication skills, cultural competency skills, community dimensions of practice skills, ethical analysis skills, and leadership and systems thinking skills (Council on Linkages Between Academia and Public Health Practice, 2010).

Another strength of the book is the diversity of the chapter and focus and perspective authors, many of whom are leaders in their fields. The contributors approach their material from within a variety of disciplinary perspectives and languages. In some chapters, public health is emphasized throughout, in others, the authors approach the topic from their own lenses and encourage students to connect the information back to public health, environment, equity, and systems issues. This diversity of approaches can help strengthen students' understanding and can provide a foundation to help them interface with the range of food-system stakeholders and approaches.

This textbook aims to be comprehensive in the sense of addressing the major food-system topics, but it cannot possibly be comprehensive in the sense of covering every process, project, idea, and issue, not only because of the sheer number of these but also because this is a vibrant and growing field. Additionally, although the US food system is intimately intertwined with global food systems, this book would be many times longer if it sought to do justice to global issues as well as domestic ones.

WHAT'S INSIDE

What is the best way to organize a textbook about a system? By definition, all the parts interact and overlap. Figure I.2 provides a simplified visual organizing framework indicating primary ways in which the chapter content interrelates. Activities, drivers, and outcomes are numbered to reflect chapters in this book. Selected examples are shown for each category in the outer ring. We will return to this

FIGURE I.2 Textbook Concept Model

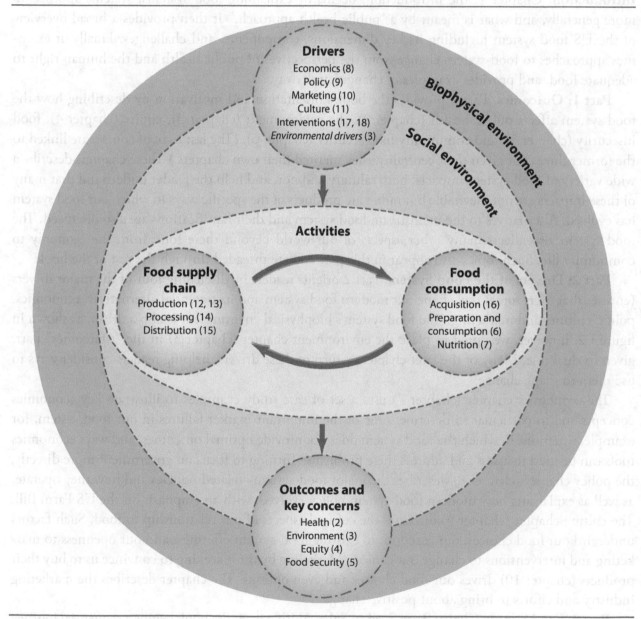

Note: Numbers refer to Chapters

model in each section overview, highlighting the section's connection to the whole. Throughout the chapters, and the focus and perspective features, we have sought to minimize repetition, referring the reader to discussion elsewhere in the book. Nonetheless, some repetition is necessary in order to provide appropriate overviews within the context of particular chapters, and different authors often approach topics from quite different angles.

PARTS

Introduction. Chapter 1, the introduction, begins by explaining food systems, systems approaches more generally, and what is meant by a "public health approach." It then provides a broad overview of the US food system including its key dimensions, components, and challenges. Finally, it examines approaches to food-system change from the perspectives of public health and the human right to adequate food, and provides examples of changes underway.

Part 1: Outcomes. Part 1 provides the book's orientation and motivation by describing how the food system affects public health (chapter 2), the environment (chapter 3), equity (chapter 4), food insecurity (chapter 5), and community food security (chapter 6). (The last two, of course, are linked to the former three, but given their centrality, they merited their own chapters.) These chapters describe a wide variety of food-system impacts, both salutary and not, and help the reader understand that many of these impacts are not inevitable but rather are products of the specific ways in which our food system has evolved. Alternatives to the mainstream food system and their ramifications are also discussed. The food system also affects many other aspects of our world beyond these four, from the economy to community life. Such topics also appear in this part and are threaded through the rest of the book.

Part 2: Drivers of the Food System. Part 2 orients readers by discussing four of the major drivers (entities that exert force) that shape our modern food system and its potential alternatives: economics, policy, culture, and marketing. The food system's biophysical environment is also a driver, as shown in figure I.2, however, we opted to place the environment chapter (chapter 3) in the "Outcomes" part, given its dual role. Many of the later chapters return to these drivers, helping readers consider ways to use them to shape change.

The economics chapter (chapter 7) uses a set of case study examples to illustrate key economics concepts and in particular to describe some of the important market failures in our food system, for example, situations in which the food system does not provide optimal outcomes, and ways economics tools can be used to assess and address these problems. Turning to focus on government more directly, the policy chapter (chapter 8) describes the major food-system–related policies and how they operate, as well as explaining how modern food-system policy evolved, with an emphasis on the US Farm Bill. The culture chapter (chapter 9) discusses the cultural aspects of our relationship to food. Such factors undergird our food choices, our reactions to existing food-system offerings, and our openness to marketing and interventions to change our choices. Marketing by those seeking to convince us to buy their products (chapter 10) drives our food choices and even options. The chapter describes the marketing industry and efforts to bring about positive change.

Part 3: Food Supply Chain: from Seed to Sales. With part 3, the book begins a sequential journey through the major activities in the food chain up to the point when food enters consumers' hands.

Chapters provide overviews of crop production (chapter 11), food animal production (chapter 12), food processing and packaging (chapter 13), and food distribution (chapter 14). The chapters describe sector history, structure, and operations, including discussion of policy, economic, and industry drivers, as well as impacts on public health, environment, and equity.

Part 4: Food in Communities and on Tables. Part 4 continues along the food chain with four chapters discussing what we eat and what happens when food reaches our tables and communities. We begin with an overview of the contours of current US diets (chapter 15), covering not only the "what" but also the "when" and "where," and some of the population diversity in diets—"who." The nutrition chapter (chapter 16) then explains what happens to this food inside our bodies, what we "ought" to be eating from a health standpoint and why. This nuts-and-bolts overview discusses key macronutrients and micronutrients as well as total diet and whole food approaches, and introduces the reader to the field of public health nutrition. The food environments chapter (chapter 17) reviews literature on how food availability within various environments affects our eating behaviors and how environments could be changed to help make the healthy choice (broadly defined) the easy choice. The preceding chapters have made clear that our current food system is profoundly unhealthy for people and the planet. Although some changes in our diets will occur naturally as the food system's problems lead to changed costs and incentives, it is not always clear that those changes will come in the desired time frame or will lead us in the desired direction. Chapter 18 focuses on interventions to change eating behaviors in desired directions. This concluding chapter provides a review of important theories that can guide intervention development and then provides example interventions targeting change from the individual to societal levels.

FOCUS AND PERSPECTIVES FEATURES

The book's main chapters are complemented and in some cases balanced by focus and perspectives features authored by experts in research, policy, and practice. The focus features are intended to provide additional interest and to help bring food-system issues alive for readers. They include articles digging deeper into topics of interest, case study examples, tables, and graphics. Perspectives pieces present analyses or viewpoints rooted in evidence (including lived experience in some cases). These are used to demonstrate some of the existing views among those working on food-system issues. We expect readers will disagree with some, many will make them think, some will inspire them, and some might even make them angry. In some cases the distinction is subjective between what should be categorized as a focus or perspective, and you might disagree with our choices. Note that because of page limits and the desire to present a variety of ideas and content, we did not attempt to balance each piece with a counterargument from a different author. **We emphasize that the perspectives present their authors' views, not those of the chapter authors or editor**.

Together, these chapters and the focus and perspectives features present a broad view of today's US food system in all its complexity (figures I.3 to I.10). They highlight the challenges we face and provide reasons to be hopeful as well. The textbook also provides opportunities for students to examine the food system's (nay, the world's) stickiest problems and think critically about solutions.

FIGURE I.3   Child's Poster about Healthy Food Placed on City Buses

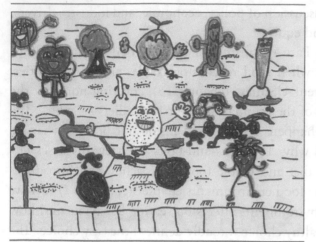

Source: Shydi Griffin, Baltimore City.

FIGURE I.4   Seniors Choosing Vegetables

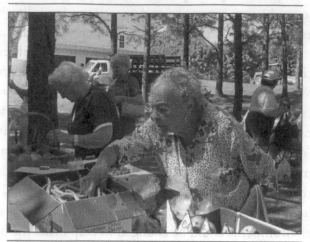

Source: Local Food Hub.

FIGURE I.5   Cows at Albright Farm

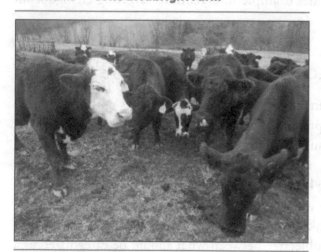

Source: Mia Cellucci, CLF.

FIGURE I.6   Students Eating Lunch

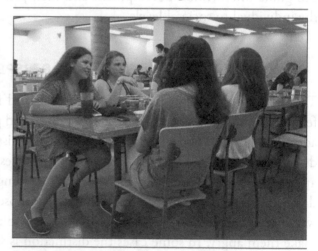

Source: Johns Hopkins, Diversity Leadership Council

FIGURE I.7   Lunchables

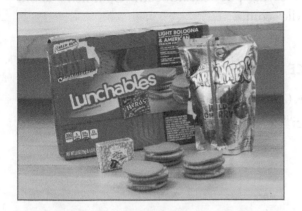

Source: Michael Milli, CLS.

FIGURE I.8   Baby Eating Spaghetti

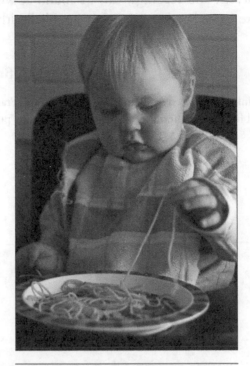

Source: istockphoto.

FIGURE I.9   Green Buffers, Clean Water

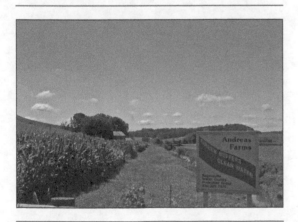

Source: USDA.

FIGURE I.10   Man with Carrots

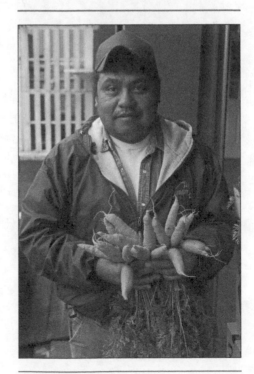

Source: Local Food Hub.

An instructor's supplement is available at www.wiley.com/go/neff. Additional materials, such as videos, podcasts, and readings, can be found at www.josseybasspublichealth.com. Comments about this book are invited and can be sent to publichealth@wiley.com.

REFERENCE

Council on Linkages Between Academia and Public Health Practice. (2010). *Core competencies for public health professionals*. Retrieved from www.phf.org/resourcestools/pages/core_public_health_competencies.aspx

Acknowledgments

This book is a project of the Johns Hopkins Center for a Livable Future (CLF). We would like to thank the board and staff of the GRACE Communications Foundation for their help and encouragement.

The book builds on CLF's legacy of contribution and is a direct extension of its mission. It was developed with the collective effort and expertise of many on staff. In particular, thanks go to Pam Rhubart Berg for her extensive help with graphics and the online supplement, Brent Kim for many and varied contributions, Christine Grillo for rewrites and edits, Shawn McKenzie for ongoing support and wisdom, and Bob Lawrence for oversight and mentorship. Thanks also to other CLF staff members including Amanda Behrens, Dave Love, Jillian Fry, Leo Horrigan, Bob Martin, Shawnel McLendon, Mike Milli, Keeve Nachman, Anne Palmer, Joci Raynor, Allison Righter, Angela Smith, and Chris Stevens.

We have been so fortunate to work with the experts who provided the content for the book. In particular, we thank the chapter authors for choosing to contribute their time to develop and edit their chapters and supplementary materials. Much appreciation also goes to the focus and perspective authors, particularly those who developed new content for the book.

We owe much gratitude to the center's talented student research assistants and CLF-Lerner Fellows, in particular, Patti Truant, Susie DiMauro, and Kate Johnson, who served at different times as my "right hand" on the project. Others who contributed substantial effort include Ruthie Burrows, Karina Christiansen, Linnea Laestadius, Kathryn Rees, David Robinson, and Faith Tandoc.

We would like to thank proposal reviewers Molly Anderson, Frank J. Chaloupka, Kate Clancy, Hugh Joseph, Leslie Mikkelsen, Marion Nestle, Tasha Peart, and Angie Tagtow, who provided valuable feedback on the original book proposal. Jill K. Clark, Ardyth Harris Gillespie, and Hugh Joseph provided thoughtful and constructive comments on the complete draft manuscript. Feedback from these reviewers convened by Jossey-Bass was invaluable in improving the manuscript. Thanks also to Kate Clancy, Jessica Goldberger, Fred Kirschenmann, Jeffrey O'Hara, and Mary Story for review of particular content and for their helpful suggestions.

For many years, CLF had considered developing a textbook. The spark that got this project started came when Andy Pasternack of Jossey-Bass reached out to me. In turn, his interest in developing a food system and public health textbook was sparked by a conversation with food system leader Angie Tagtow. Seth Schwartz of Jossey-Bass was a wonderful steward for this project. He was responsive and patient as I figured out how to edit and format a book and provided wisdom to guide the project throughout. Justin Frahm and Susan Geraghty were supportive and helpful in the production phases.

Personally, I thank my husband, John McGready, and sons, Micah and Emmet, for their support, for taking on extra roles during crunch times, and for keeping me laughing. And, I thank my parents, Joanne and Martin Neff, for their ongoing support and encouragement.

—Roni Neff, editor, on behalf of the Johns Hopkins
Center for a Livable Future

About the Editor

Roni Neff is an assistant professor in the Johns Hopkins Bloomberg School of Public Health, Department of Environmental Health Sciences, with a joint appointment in Health Policy and Management. She directs the Food System Sustainability and Public Health program at the Johns Hopkins Center for a Livable Future (CLF), where she has worked since 2006.

Roni has worked in food systems and in public health research, policy, and practice throughout her career. She has played a significant role in advancing the public health voice in food and agriculture policy and research, including through research, speaking engagements, and leadership work with the American Public Health Association. Her academic interests include food waste, food and agriculture policy, and food system workers.

She teaches two courses, "Baltimore Food Systems: A Case Study in Urban Food Environments" and "Food System Sustainability Practicum," and lectures frequently in other classes and around the country. She has been recognized for excellence in teaching annually since developing the Baltimore class and received the Faculty Excellence in Service-Learning Award from Johns Hopkins' SOURCE program in 2014.

She received her PhD from the Johns Hopkins Bloomberg School of Public Health, MS from the Harvard School of Public Health, and AB from Brown University.

Author Affiliations

Patricia Allen, PhD, chair and professor, Department of Food Systems & Society, Marylhurst University, Marylhurst, Oregon

Julian M. Alston, PhD, professor, Department of Agricultural and Resource Economics; director Robert Mondavi Institute Center for Wine Economics, University of California, Davis

Alice Ammerman, DrPH, RD, director, Center for Health Promotion and Disease Prevention; professor, Department of Nutrition, Gillings School of Global Public Health and School of Medicine, University of North Carolina at Chapel Hill

Andrea S. Anater, PhD, MPH, MA, public health nutrition researcher, RTI International, Research Triangle Park, North Carolina

Molly D. Anderson, PhD, Partridge Chair in Food and Sustainable Agriculture Systems, College of the Atlantic, Bar Harbor, Maine

Anne Barnhill, PhD, assistant professor, Department of Medical Ethics and Health Policy, University of Pennsylvania, Philadelphia

Fedele Bauccio, chief executive officer and cofounder, Bon Appétit Management Company

Amanda Behrens, MS, MPH, senior program officer, Center for a Livable Future, Johns Hopkins Bloomberg School of Public Health, Baltimore

Renata Bertazzi Levy, PhD, associate researcher, Department of Preventive Medicine, Faculty of Medicine, University of São Paulo Medical School; researcher, Center for Epidemiological Studies in Health and Nutrition, School of Public Health, University of São Paulo

Aaron Bobrow-Strain, PhD, associate professor, Politics Department, Whitman College, Walla Walla, Washington

Rebecca L. Boehm, doctoral candidate, Department of Food and Nutrition Policy, Tufts Friedman School of Nutrition Science and Policy, Boston

Amanda B. Breen, PhD, MPH, assistant professor of psychology, Neumann University, Aston, Pennsylvania

Michael Buchenau, executive director, Denver Urban Gardens

Larissa Calancie, doctoral candidate, Gillings School of Global Public Health and the Center for Health Promotion and Disease Prevention, University of North Carolina at Chapel Hill

Geoffrey Cannon, senior visiting research scholar, Centre for Epidemiological Studies in Health and Nutrition, School of Public Health, University of São Paulo

Sean B. Cash, PhD, associate professor, Department of Food and Nutrition Policy, Tufts Friedman School of Nutrition Science and Policy, Boston

George A. Cavender, PhD, research assistant professor, The Food Processing Center, University of Nebraska, Lincoln

Sarah Chard, PhD, associate professor, Department of Sociology and Anthropology, University of Maryland Baltimore County, Baltimore

Wei-Ting Chen, MA, doctoral candidate, Department of Sociology, Johns Hopkins University, Baltimore

Mariana Chilton, PhD, MPH, associate professor, Department of Health Management and Policy, Drexel University School of Public Health, Philadelphia

Kate Clancy, PhD, senior fellow, MISA, visiting scholar, Center for a Livable Future, Johns Hopkins Bloomberg School of Public Health, Baltimore

Rafael Moreira Claro, PhD, professor, Department of Nutrition, Federal University of Minas Gerais (UFMG), Belo Horizonte, Brazil; researcher, Center for Epidemiological Studies in Health and Nutrition, School of Public Health, University of São Paulo

Megan Clayton, CLF-Lerner Fellow, doctoral candidate, Department of Health, Behavior and Society, Johns Hopkins Bloomberg School of Public Health, Baltimore

Fergus M. Clydesdale, PhD, distinguished professor, Department of Food Science, University of Massachusetts Amherst and director of the Food Science and Policy Alliance, Amherst, Massachusetts

Melissa Cunningham Kay, MS, MPH, RD, doctoral student, Gillings School of Global Public Health and School of Medicine, University of North Carolina at Chapel Hill

Meghan F. Davis, DVM, MPH, PhD, assistant professor, Department of Environmental Health Sciences, Johns Hopkins Bloomberg School of Public Health, Baltimore

Molly DeMarco, PhD, MPH, research scientist, Center for Health Promotion & Disease Prevention, instructor, Department of Nutrition, Gillings School of Global Public Health and School of Medicine, University of North Carolina at Chapel Hill

Larissa S. Drescher, PhD, Marketing and Consumer Research, TUM Business School, Technische Universität München, Germany

John Fisk, PhD, director, Wallace Center, Winrock International, Arlington, Virginia

Charles A. Francis, PhD, professor of agronomy, University of Nebraska—Lincoln

Julia Freedgood, managing director, farmland and community initiatives, American Farmland Trust, Northampton, MA

Susanne Freidberg, PhD, professor of geography, Dartmouth College, Hanover, New Hampshire

Tianna Gaines-Turner, Witnesses to Hunger Participant, Philadelphia

Ashley N. Gearhardt, PhD, assistant professor of psychology, University of Michigan, Ann Arbor

Joel Gittelsohn, MS, PhD, professor, Department of International Health, Johns Hopkins Bloomberg School of Public Health, Baltimore

Alan M. Goldberg, PhD, professor of toxicology, chairman of the board, Center for Alternatives to Animal Testing, Bloomberg School of Public Health; principal, Global Food Ethics Project, Bloomberg School of Public Health, Johns Hopkins University, Baltimore

Miguel I. Gómez, PhD; Ruth and William Morgan Assistant Professor of Applied Economics and Management, Charles H. Dyson School of Applied Economics and Management, Cornell University, Ithaca, New York

Dana Gunders, MS, staff scientist in food and agriculture, Natural Resources Defense Council, San Francisco

Doug Gurian-Sherman, PhD, director of sustainable agriculture and senior scientist, Center for Food Safety, Washington, DC

Julie Guthman, PhD, professor, Division of Social Sciences, University of California, Santa Cruz

James Hale, PhD candidate, Colorado State University, Department of Sociology, Fort Collins

Devon J. Hall Sr., program manager, Rural Empowerment Association for Community Help (REACH), Warsaw, North Carolina

Michael W. Hamm, PhD, C.S. Mott Professor of Sustainable Agriculture and director, Center for Regional Food Systems, Michigan State University, East Lansing

Ross A. Hammond, PhD, senior fellow, Economic Studies Program director, Center on Social Dynamics and Policy, The Brookings Institution, Washington, DC

Jennifer C. E. Hartle, DrPH, MHS, CIH, Stanford Prevention Research Center, Stanford University School of Medicine, Stanford, California; former CLF-Lerner Fellow

Heather Hartline-Grafton, DrPH, RD, senior nutrition policy and research analyst, Food Research and Action Center, Washington, DC

Wenonah Hauter, executive director, Food & Water Watch, Washington, DC

Corinna Hawkes, PhD, head of policy and public affairs, World Cancer Research Fund International, London

Michael Heller, grass farmer, Claggett Farm, Chesapeake Bay Foundation, Upper Marlboro, Maryland

Leo Horrigan, MHS, food system correspondent, Center for a Livable Future, Johns Hopkins Bloomberg School of Public Health, Baltimore

Laura Jackson, PhD, director, Tallgrass Prairie Center, professor of Biology, University of Northern Iowa, Cedar Falls

Michael F. Jacobson, PhD, executive director, Center for Science in the Public Interest, Washington, DC

Saru Jayaraman, co-founder and co-director, Restaurant Opportunities Centers United; director, Food Labor Research Center, University of California, Berkeley; and author, *Behind the Kitchen Door* (Cornell University Press, 2013)

Katherine Abowd Johnson, MS, CLF-Lerner Fellow; doctoral candidate, Department of Health, Behavior and Society, Johns Hopkins Bloomberg School of Public Health, Baltimore

Brent F. Kim, MHS, project officer, Center for a Livable Future, Johns Hopkins Bloomberg School of Public Health, Baltimore

Frederick Kirschenmann, PhD, distinguished fellow and former director, Leopold Center for Sustainable Agriculture, Iowa State University, Ames; president, Stone Barns Center for Food and Agriculture, Pocantico Hills, New York

Linnea Laestadius, PhD, MPP, assistant professor, Department of Public Health Policy & Administration, Joseph J. Zilber School of Public Health, University of Wisconsin-Milwaukee; former CLF-Lerner Fellow

Anna Lappé, co-founder, Small Planet Institute and Small Planet Fund; director, Real Food Media Project, Oakland, CA; author, *Diet for a Hot Planet: The Climate Crisis at the End of Your Fork and What You can Do about It*

Frances Moore Lappé, Small Planet Institute, Cambridge, Massachusetts

Robert S. Lawrence, MD, director, Center for a Livable Future, professor, Department of Environmental Health Sciences, Johns Hopkins Bloomberg School of Public Health, Baltimore

Jill S. Litt, PhD, associate professor, Department of Environmental & Occupational Health, University of Colorado School of Public Health, Aurora

David C. Love, PhD, MSPH, project director Public Health and Sustainable Aquaculture Project, Center for a Livable Future, assistant scientist, Department of Environmental Health Sciences, Johns Hopkins Bloomberg School of Public Health, Baltimore

Luke H. MacDonald, PhD, assistant scientist, Department of Environmental Health Sciences, Johns Hopkins Bloomberg School of Public Health, assistant director, Johns Hopkins University Global Water Program, Baltimore

Robert P. Martin, director, Food System Policy, Center for a Livable Future, Johns Hopkins Bloomberg School of Public Health, Baltimore

Shawn E. McKenzie, MPH, associate director, Center for a Livable Future, Johns Hopkins Bloomberg School of Public Health, Baltimore

Edward W. McLaughlin, Robert G. Tobin Professor of Marketing; director, undergraduate program, Dyson School of Applied Economics and Management, Cornell University, Ithaca, New York

Carlos Augusto Monteiro, MD, PhD, professor of nutrition and public health and head, Center for Epidemiological Studies in Health and Nutrition, School of Public Health, University of São Paulo

Carole Morison, farmer-agricultural consultant, Bird's Eye View Farm, Pokomoke City, Maryland

Alanna Moshfegh, research leader, Food Surveys Research Group, Agricultural Research Service, United States Department of Agriculture, Beltsville, Maryland

Michael Moss, investigative reporter, *New York Times;* author, *Salt, Sugar, Fat: How the Food Giants Hooked Us*

Jean-Claude Moubarac, PhD, postdoctoral research fellow at Center for Epidemiological Studies in Health and Nutrition, School of Public Health, University of São Paulo

Mark Muller, director, Food and Justice Program, Institute for Agriculture and Trade Policy, Minneapolis

Keeve E. Nachman, PhD, MHS, assistant professor, Departments of Environmental Health Sciences and Health Policy and Management; program director, Food Production and Public Health, Center for a Livable Future, assistant scientist, Department of Environmental Health Sciences, Baltimore

Michael Newbury, PhD, professor of American studies and English and American literatures, Fletcher D. Proctor Professor of American History, Middlebury College, Middlebury, Vermont

Anne M. Palmer, MAIA, program director, Food Communities and Public Health, Center for a Livable Future, Johns Hopkins Bloomberg School of Public Health, Baltimore

Courtney A. Pinard, PhD, research scientist, Gretchen Swanson Center for Nutrition; assistant professor, Department of Health Promotion, Social & Behavioral Health, College of Public Health, University of Nebraska Medical Center, Omaha

Richard Pirog, PhD, senior academic specialist and senior associate director, Center for Regional Food Systems, Michigan State University, East Lansing

Jennifer L. Pomeranz, JD, MPH, assistant professor, Department of Public Health, Temple University, College of Health Professions and Social Work, Philadelphia

Janet E. Poppendieck, PhD, policy director, New York City Food Policy Center at Hunter College, New York.

Rebecca M. Puhl, PhD, deputy director of research, Yale University Rudd Center for Food Policy & Obesity, New Haven, Connecticut

Jenny Rabinowich, MPH, deputy country director for programs, Last Mile Health, Tiyatien Health, Liberia

LaDonna Sanders-Redmond, founder, lead organizer, Campaign for Food Justice Now, Minneapolis

Bradley J. Rickard, PhD, assistant professor, Charles H. Dyson School of Applied Economics and Management, Cornell University, Ithaca, New York

Allison Righter, MSPH, RD, program officer, Center for a Livable Future, Johns Hopkins Bloomberg School of Public Health, Baltimore

Wayne Roberts, PhD, food policy analyst and writer, Toronto

Bernard E. Rollin, PhD, University Distinguished Professor; professor of philosophy, animal sciences, and biomedical sciences; university bioethicist, Department of Philosophy, Colorado State University, Fort Collins

Erin G. Roth, senior ethnographer, Center for Aging Studies, University of Maryland, Baltimore County, Baltimore

Lainie Rutkow, PhD, JD, MPH, assistant professor, Department of Health Policy and Management, Johns Hopkins Bloomberg School of Public Health, Baltimore

Kristin S. Schafer, MA, policy and communications director, Pesticide Action Network, Oakland, California

Kellogg J. Schwab, PhD, professor, Department of Environmental Health Sciences, Johns Hopkins Bloomberg School of Public Health, Baltimore

Adam Sheingate, PhD, associate professor, Department of Political Science, Johns Hopkins University, Baltimore

Jared Simon, MPH, MBA, director of marketing, Hain Celestial, Lake Success, New York

Angela Smith, MA, project advisor, Center for a Livable Future, Johns Hopkins Bloomberg School of Public Health, Oronoco, Minnesota

Teresa M. Smith, MS, graduate research assistant, doctoral candidate, Department of Health Promotion, Social & Behavioral Health, College of Public Health, University of Nebraska Medical Center; consultant, Gretchen Swanson Center for Nutrition, Omaha

Anim Steel, executive director, Real Food Generation Challenge

Angie Tagtow, MS, RD, LD, director, USDA Center for Nutrition Policy and Promotion; co-founder, Iowa Food Systems Council; owner, Environmental Nutrition Solutions, LLC

Linden Thayer, doctoral student, Gillings School of Global Public Health and School of Medicine, Center for Health Promotion and Disease Prevention, University of North Carolina at Chapel Hill

Patricia L. Truant, MPH, CLF-Lerner Fellow; doctoral candidate, Department of Health Policy & Management, Johns Hopkins Bloomberg School of Public Health, Baltimore

Moises Velasquez, journalist and author, *An Epidemic of Absence: A New Way of Understanding Allergies and Autoimmune Diseases*. Berkeley, California

David Wallinga, MD, MPA, director and founder, Healthy Food Action, Minneapolis.

Jennifer L. Wilkins, PhD, RD, senior associate extension officer and lecturer, Division of Nutritional Sciences, Cornell University, Ithaca, New York

D'Ann L. Williams, DrPH, MS, research associate, Department of Environmental Health Sciences, Johns Hopkins Bloomberg School of Public Health, Baltimore; former CLF-Lerner Fellow

Mark Winne, senior advisor, Center for a Livable Future, Johns Hopkins Bloomberg School of Public Health, Baltimore

Derek Yach, MBChB MPH, executive director, The Vitality Institute; past senior vice president, PepsiCo for Global Health and Agriculture Policy, New York

Amy L. Yaroch, PhD, executive director, Gretchen Swanson Center for Nutrition; professor, Department of Health Promotion, Social & Behavioral Health, College of Public Health, University of Nebraska Medical Center, Omaha

Lisa R. Young, PhD, RD, adjunct professor, Department of Nutrition, Food Studies, and Public Health, New York University; author, *The Portion Teller Plan*

About the Center for a Livable Future

Founded in 1996, the Johns Hopkins Center for a Livable Future (CLF) is an interdisciplinary academic center dedicated to conducting research on the public health implications of our food system, educating a wide range of students, and advocating for evidence-based policy reform. The center is based within the Bloomberg School of Public Health, and collaborates with faculty members, staff, and students throughout Johns Hopkins University—and beyond.

CLF's core program areas apply a public health lens to issues surrounding: food production, food communities, food system sustainability, and food system policy. The center's education initiatives include the CLF-Lerner Fellows Program, which was awarded 133 doctoral fellowships to 62 individuals since 2003; "Teaching the Food System," a free, downloadable curriculum and set of resources for educators; a certificate program in "Food System, Environment, and Public Health" offering graduate students specialized knowledge and understanding of the relevance of the food system to many different competencies in public health; online courses available at the Bloomberg School, Coursera; and more.

The CLF explores the interrelationships among health, environment, diet, and food production—and works to improve those systems to ensure food security for present and future generations. In a livable future, all systems that sustain us operate in balance to support human and ecosystem health, equity, and resilience.

Chapter 1

Food Systems

Roni A. Neff and Robert S. Lawrence

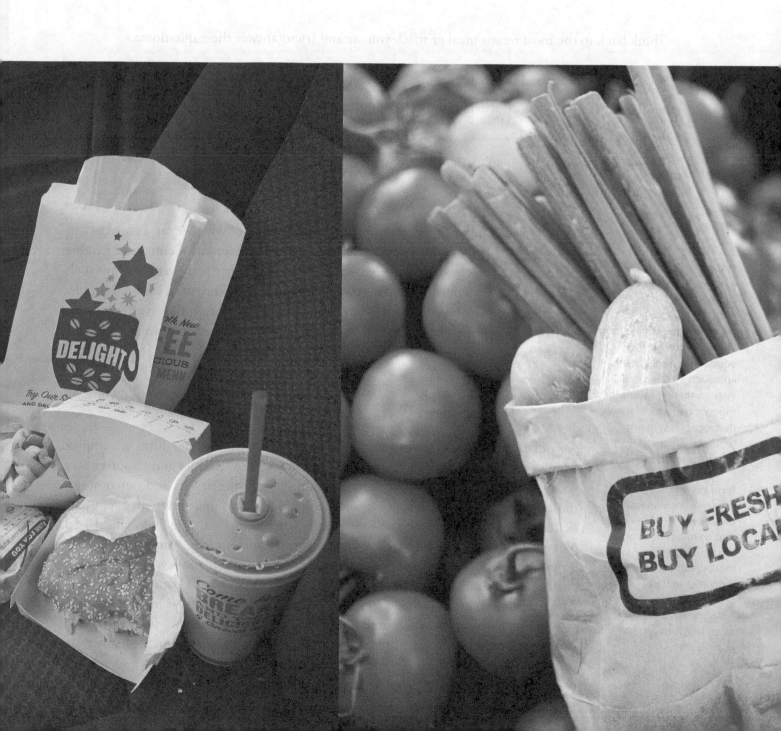

Learning Objectives

- Explain a systems approach to food systems.

- Describe a public health approach to assessing food systems.

- Provide a broad overview of the US food system, including its key dimensions, components, and challenges.

- Discuss different approaches to food system change, including public health and human rights, and provide examples of changes underway.

Think back to the most recent meal or snack you ate and try to answer these questions:

- Where did the food originate, how was it processed, and how did it get to you?

- How much did it cost, where did the money go, and why?

- How healthy was it?

- How did producing it affect the environment? Workers? Animals?

- Why did you choose it?

Most of us can answer a few of these questions for some of what we eat. Few of us can answer all of them for everything we eat. We at the Johns Hopkins Center for a Livable Future created this textbook to help students of the food system answer questions such as these, not only in relation to their own meals but also for the entire US food supply. To understand the breadth of relevant issues and the opportunities to affect public health, the environment, equity, and other outcomes, we need to examine the food system as a system—complex, diverse, global, and interconnected.

THE FOOD SYSTEM AS A SYSTEM

system
A network of interacting components that together form a complex whole, though they are influenced by factors outside their boundaries; also, systems approach, systems thinking, systems theory: approaches, thought patterns, or theory that focus on systems; typically contrasted with linear approaches

food system
A system encompassing all the activities and resources that go into producing, distributing, and consuming food; the drivers and outcomes of those processes; and all the relationships and feedback loops between system components

A **system** is a network of interacting components that together form a complex whole. The **food system** is a system encompassing all the activities and resources that go into producing, distributing, and consuming food; the drivers and outcomes of those processes; and, the extensive and complex relationships between system participants and components. The food system's functional parts include land-based parts (e.g., agriculture, farmland preservation); environment (e.g., water, soil, energy); economy (e.g., distribution, processing, retail); education; policy; social justice; health; and food cultures (Peemoeller, nd). Although a system's components themselves are important, it is the relationships among components that make a system a system. To give a simplified example, what we eat affects what is produced, which in turn affects what we will eat. Studying systems focuses our attention on the many ways these relationships may play out—including considering cascades of effects, unintended consequences, feedback loops, and the most strategic and practical ways to intervene for change.

Factors outside a system's boundaries, such as in the social or biophysical environment, also influence change within systems (and vice versa). For example, the food system is driven in part by food system policies. These are part of the system, but also lie within the social environment. The system is also driven by policies that lie primarily outside of the food system's boundaries, such as immigration laws. The food system can be analyzed using categories including scale, production type, governance, drivers (e.g., population and climate change), food security, and supply chains (Clancy, 2011).

Is there one food system? In some ways, yes—it's all connected. In other ways, we can understand this grand system as a network of interconnected **subsystems** (or systems that are components of a broader system) existing at different scales from local to global, and across geography and time. There are food systems in Baltimore and Annapolis, and a food system in the state of Maryland that encompasses both. All of these interact in different ways with each other, with the US food system, and with food systems around the world that send us products and shape the food prices experienced by consumers from Baltimore to Bangkok. That's why in this book you will sometimes see the term, *food system*, and sometimes *food systems*. Figure 1.1 provides a concept model of the food system (Nourish, 2012).

subsystems
A system that is also a component of a broader system (e.g., the food production system is a subsystem of the food system)

The model depicts multiple interacting systems: biological, economic, social, and political. In the biological system, components including biodiversity, land use, and climate change interact to create or destroy nutrients, which feed into agriculture (chapters 11, 12). Agriculture also uses additional **inputs**, or resources, including water, soil, energy, and sunlight, as well as chemicals, labor, and know-how. From agriculture comes food, which travels through an economic system (chapter 7) from wholesaling and food processing (chapter 13) to a distribution system including transport and stores, restaurants and farmers markets (chapter 14), and from there into the social or demand system. That system comprises the many environments in which we live (chapter 17) and make food choices (chapters 15, 16), and the factors that drive such choices, including culture (chapter 9), marketing (chapter 10), and behavior change interventions (chapter 18). Coming out of the demand system are money, which travels back up through the economic system, and varying levels of civic engagement, which plays into the political system affecting food (chapter 8). This graphic depicts waste as the main output of the system, and indeed it is an important one, as described in focus 15.3. Other important outputs not depicted include effects such as health (chapter 2), environmental quality (chapter 3), equity (chapter 4), food security (chapter 5), and community food security (chapter 6.)

inputs
Resources and materials entering a production system, such as feed, drugs, energy, water, and labor

Imagine that the static diagram shown in figure 1.1 is animated, with flows of inputs and outputs moving constantly back and forth across every arrow. Each piece, whether small or large, is separately animated with its own internal logic: every farmer, every farm, every aquifer for irrigation, every crop, every distribution truck and driver, each policy maker making policy that shapes those activities, and so on. Turn on the switch and let it roll, change, and evolve—that's a food system.

Systems approaches developed originally in the field of engineering. Although many food system analyses and activities, and most of what you will read about in this textbook, take place in the "real" world, formal systems approaches seek to model the complex reality of food systems using software, as described in focus 1.1 and box 1 in the online supplement. Once created, such models enable analysts to input varying conditions and thus to gain insights into how the impacts may play out. By contrast,

FIGURE 1.1   The Food System

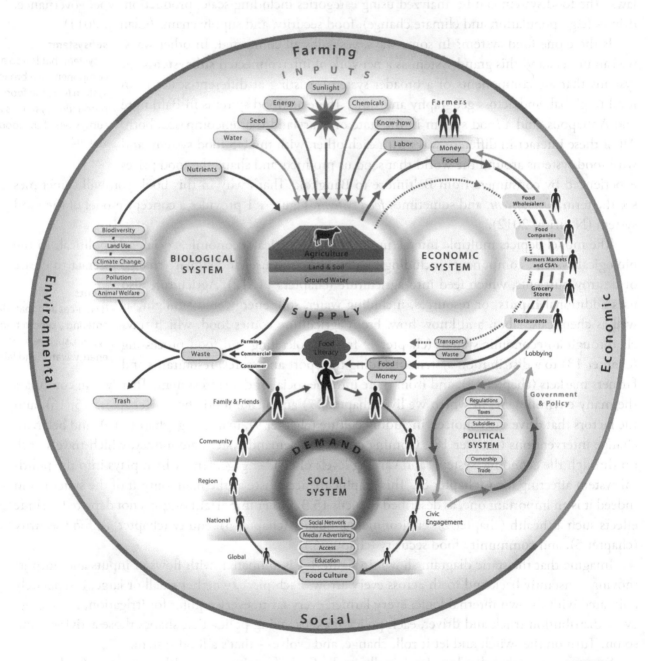

Nourish Food System Map

What's Your Relationship to Food? Look Closer.

systems thinking (or systems approaches) take a more conceptual approach to understanding and working with complexity. There is increasing recognition of the benefits of a systems approach for advancing the quality of public health activities. Focus 1.2 provides further examples of the utility of a systems approach to food.

FOCUS 1.1. COMPLEX ADAPTIVE SYSTEMS
Ross A. Hammond

The food system is a classic example of a complex adaptive system (CAS)—a system composed of many different actors at many different levels of scale, interacting with each other in subtle or nonlinear ways that strongly influence the overall behavior of the system. Actors can be people but also larger social units, such as firms and governments, and smaller biological units, such as cells and genes. The CAS perspective has proved enlightening in the study of food systems and other economic, political, social, physical, and biological systems (Axelrod, 1997; Hammond & Dube, 2012; Holland, 1992; Miller & Page, 2002) because it can help researchers to analyze, model, and anticipate interactions between system actors and overall system dynamics. CASs share many general properties, including the following:

- *Individuality*: Each level is composed of autonomous actors who adapt their behavior individually. Change within CASs is often driven by decentralized, local interactions of these individual parts.

- *Heterogeneity*: Substantial diversity among actors at each level—in goals, rules, adaptive repertoire, and constraints—can shape dynamics of a CAS in important ways.

- *Interdependence*: CASs usually contain many interdependent interacting pieces, connected across different levels, often with feedback.

- *Emergence*: CASs are often characterized by emergent, unexpected phenomena—patterns of collective behavior that form in the system are difficult to predict from separate understanding of each individual element.

- *Tipping*: CASs are also often characterized by "tipping." Nonlinearity means that the impacts caused by small changes can seem hugely out of proportion. The system may spend long periods in a state of relative stability, yet be easily tipped to another state by a disturbance that pushes it across a threshold.

Complexity can be a significant challenge for policy makers and for intervention design. The interconnected dynamics of a complex system may lead policy efforts to overlook potential synergies, and successful interventions in a single area may be counteracted by responses elsewhere in the system. Policies that do not take into account the full set of actors and their responses can even backfire dramatically, as illustrated by the Lake Victoria catastrophe (Fuggle, 2001; Murray, 1989). In 1960, a nonnative species of fish (the Nile perch) was introduced into Lake Victoria, with the policy goal of improving the health and wealth of the communities surrounding the lake in Kenya, Tanzania, and Uganda through this new protein source. But the policy did not take into account the other actors in the system—specifically, the other organisms forming the lake's complex ecosystems. Although the perch initially appeared a success, its introduction set off a chain reaction. The perch wiped out the native cichlid species of fish, which were crucial in controlling a species of snail living in the lake. The snails flourished and with them the larvae of schistosomes, to whom they play host. Schistosomes are the cause of the often-fatal disease of schistosomiasis or bilharzia in humans, and their exploding numbers created a public health and economic crisis. Thus, the original policy goal (improving health) backfired because the adaptive reaction of another set of actors in the system was not anticipated.

(Continued)

(Continued)

Other characteristics of complex systems also pose policy design challenges. Nonlinearity makes prediction difficult—multiple forces shape the future and their effects do not aggregate simply. Heterogeneity means that any given intervention may not work equally well across all contexts or subgroups. Decentralized dynamics can be a challenge because many conventional policy levers and interventions are centralized or top-down.

Despite its challenges, complexity can also be a source of opportunity for policy makers and intervention designers. For example, nonlinearity means that near the right thresholds, even small interventions can have big impacts on the system, tipping it to a new state. Understanding heterogeneity in a system can also create an opportunity because it enables interventions to be closely targeted for maximum impact.

Systems can be studied qualitatively, via systems mapping or systems thinking, but quantitative systems modeling techniques that have proven useful in other topic areas are also increasingly being applied to the study of food systems. For example, one methodology is **agent-based computational modeling (ABM)**. In ABM, complex dynamics are modeled by constructing "artificial societies" on computers. Every actor (or "agent") is individually represented and placed in a spatial context, with specified initial conditions and a set of rules governing interactions with others and their environment. The models grow macro-level patterns and trends from the bottom up (Epstein, 2006), enabling consideration of multiple (and multilevel) mechanisms. The generated macro-level patterns can be directly compared with data to calibrate the model.

agent-based computational modeling (ABM)
A quantitative systems modeling technique in which complex dynamics are modeled by constructing "artificial societies" on computers

ABM and other complex systems modeling techniques represent a promising avenue for future study of the rich and complex dynamics of food systems and for the design of effective interventions and policies to address outcomes they drive—from obesity and malnutrition through economic development.

Source: Adapted from Hammond (2009).

FOCUS 1.2. FOOD IN THE FOOD SYSTEM
Michael W. Hamm and Richard Pirog

FIGURE 1.2   Industrial Cattle Production Facility

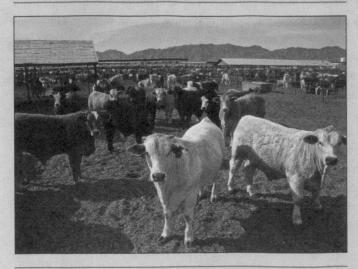

Source: USDA.

Most people go to the supermarket, a restaurant, or a drive-through and buy their food with little thought to what it took moving that food from the farm to our mouths. To illustrate the benefits of taking a system perspective, let's look at putting two food items on our table: a hamburger and fresh apples.

A system needs to be in place for a hamburger to appear on your plate. The beef calves are typically raised on a combination of rangeland and pasture and corn- or soybean-based feeds on the farm or ranch and then on a corn- or soybean-based feed at the finishing facility (figure 1.2). Calves are typically raised to nine hundred pounds on farms or ranches and then sent to finishing facilities for the final three hundred pounds.

At the processing facility the final meat products are produced, then shipped in refrigerated or freezer trucks or trains to a distribution center. They may go through several more distribution points before arriving at the point of purchase.

This system of raising, finishing, slaughtering, and distributing beef has evolved with "efficiency" in mind—how little can be spent to put a hamburger on your plate? Efficiency only increases up to a certain scale, but reaching that scale of maximum efficiency mandates fairly large numbers of animals flowing through the system simultaneously.

This is relevant when considering beef produced in different ways—for example, pasture-finished and close to where we live. It's not simply a matter of a farmer appearing at the farmers market with a chest full of hamburger or buying pasture-raised, local beef at the supermarket. A farmer raising small numbers of beef cattle must find a USDA- or state-certified processing facility (many state certification programs have been eliminated because of cost). These are often distant from the farmer and at a scale that won't accept a few cows at a time. In addition, the per-animal processing cost is higher and the farmer's time is greater due to small volume. Thus, consumer cost is higher—for many prohibitively so. If a goal were to increase the availability of "local, pasture-finished beef" it would require at least four things: a reasonably accessible processor, sufficient volume for the processor over the entire year, a sufficient price to make it worthwhile for the farmer, and distribution to the point of purchase. A lot needs to be in place to move an animal product from the farm to your fork—different system scales do not necessarily have interchangeable components.

A very different example is fresh apples on our table. Their availability in the marketplace year round is partially through diverse harvest times in various regions across the country and world as well as our ability to preserve these apples via postharvest treatment. At harvest, apples are often waxed and stored in controlled-atmosphere rooms (basically low-oxygen environments) to retard spoilage. This can either be on a farm, at a packer-shipper facility, or at a distribution facility. Apples in the marketplace can travel a circuitous route that starts at the orchard and typically goes through storage, packing, shipping, several distributors, and finally a store's produce section (figure 1.3). Because apples are a perennial tree fruit, the farmer has several years of invested activity

FIGURE 1.3   Uniform Apples in Grocery Store

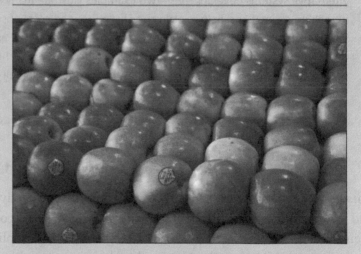

Source: Chichacha via Flickr Commons. https://www.flickr.com/photos/10673045@N04/2387957261/in/photolist-4D1UuV-4R5YRW.

and cost before the trees bear fruit. A catastrophic weather event (such as a hard freeze soon after fruit set) can destroy or severely limit the harvest for a year. Most apples in the marketplace are grown on large farms within a system built for large volumes—making apples relatively cheap and efficient to produce.

Michigan is useful as an example because it blends large-scale and small-scale production. Until the new millennium, Michigan apples largely went to juice and sauce processors. With the juice market collapse as offshore apple concentrate hit the market (China now supplies about two-thirds of our domestic apple juice), farmers needed a new strategy. This involved change at multiple points including planting new apple varieties, building controlled-atmosphere storage, and developing supply chains and markets. On the smaller scale the system is no less complicated, but often undeveloped. A small-scale farmer can sell fresh apples directly in season at, for example, a farmers market (figure 1.4). But to sell over an extended season (beyond three

(Continued)

(Continued)

FIGURE 1.4   Farmers Market Apples

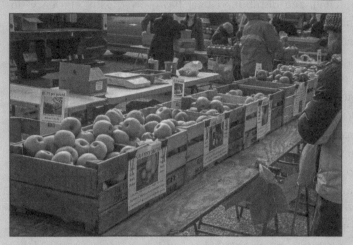

Source: CLF.

months from harvest), a storage facility (controlled-atmosphere refrigeration) is necessary or the apples will go soft and rot. To sell wholesale to a grocery store, two things are usually necessary—aggregation from multiple farms and distribution. This requires a system parallel to that designed to handle large volumes. The farmer can sell directly to these stores, but often there are scale limitations because of buyer needs.

Thus a complicated set of relationships, infrastructure, information, and technology exists for the vast majority of food found in the marketplace. In some cases, strategies to aggregate smaller farms' products and channel them into the existing system for large-scale distribution are evolving (see focus 6.1), whereas in others a system that parallels the existing one needs development. Issues of efficiency, profitability, accessibility, and affordability arise as these parallel or alternative systems develop. These two examples illustrate many interacting system factors for consideration in making change and help explain the challenges and costs of supplying food through alternative systems. Policies and regulations at varying levels of government as well as in the private sector tend to reinforce the dominant system and make alternatives difficult to develop. Without appreciating and approaching multiple points across this system and the policies that support or inhibit alternative development, it is unlikely that long-lasting change will occur.

PUBLIC HEALTH

This book examines food systems by applying the perspectives of many disciplines and using diverse lenses. Chapter focus and perspective contributors write from their own points of reference. From among the many disciplines present, this book contains a particular emphasis on public health approaches to understanding and addressing the food system, including health, environment, and social equity viewpoints. What does that mean?

Public health is "the science and art of preventing disease, prolonging life and promoting … health … through organized community efforts" (Winslow, 1920, p. 30). And **health**, as defined by the World Health Organization, is "a state of complete physical, mental and social well-being and not merely the absence of disease or infirmity" (World Health Organization [WHO], 1946).

A public health approach emphasizes **primary prevention**—looking to root causes and trying to stop harmful exposures before they happen, rather than focusing on addressing the consequences—although it does that, too. Additionally, a

public health
"The science and art of preventing disease, prolonging life and promoting … health … through organized community efforts" (Winslow, 1920, p. 30)

health
"A state of complete physical, mental and social well-being and not merely the absence of disease or infirmity" (World Health Organization, 1946)

primary prevention
Approach that addresses root causes and tries to stop harmful exposures before they happen; secondary prevention involves treating early stage conditions to prevent worsening; tertiary prevention involves mitigating the effects of disease

public health approach means stepping back and focusing on a **population-based approach**. The field commonly looks to **social determinants of health**, **structural determinants of health**, and **environmental determinants of health**. When public health does focus at the individual level, the emphasis is often on interventions with the potential to target many people's individual risk factors simultaneously. At the same time, because it focuses on populations, public health also emphasizes a need to target efforts to those within populations who experience **health disparities** and populations marginalized by poverty, discrimination, or environmental injustice. Additionally, public health approaches are applied, evidence-based, and multidisciplinary. Although traditionally public health emphasized a linear method of understanding problems (*x* causes *y*), both qualitative and systems approaches have lately attracted much interest. Today systems thinking and leadership is one of the field's eight core competencies for professionals (Council on Linkages Between Academia and Public Health Practice, 2010).

Public health professionals have long worked on food system issues from a variety of angles. Perhaps most popular have been research and interventions addressing obesity, food marketing, **healthy food** access, food safety, nutrition, and food insecurity. Additionally, lines of work have focused on the public health implications of **industrial food animal production (IFAP)**, occupational health, and impacts of pesticides and other chemicals used in food production and processing, among others. Most recently, a movement within public health has sought to address food system issues more broadly and systemically, including engaging in community food security and in food and agriculture planning and policy efforts. All of these topics are addressed in this book. In addition, a public health lens is applied to other food system topics that have received less attention. Focus 1.3 presents a public health vision for a healthy, sustainable food system.

THE US FOOD SYSTEM: AN OVERVIEW

The writer, Wendell Berry said, "Eaters … must understand that eating takes place inescapably in the world, that it is inescapably an agricultural act, and how we eat determines, to a considerable extent, how the world is used" (Berry, 1990, p. 149). Our food system shapes our world (see figure 1.5). The US food system, serving a population of 314 million, sells more than $1.8 trillion in goods and services each year and produces nine billion animals (Food Chain Workers Alliance, 2012; US Department of Agriculture [USDA] National Agricultural Statistics Service, 2012). This system, which affects and is affected by the global food system, is responsible for the following:

- 80 percent of consumptive water use (USDA Economic Research Service, 2012a)

- 51 percent of US land use (USDA Economic Research Service, 2012b)

population-based approach
Approach or intervention aimed at changing factors affecting the entire population

social determinants of health
Social and economic conditions that affect human health, such as where a person lives

structural determinants of health
Factors related to the economic, political, and social hierarchal issues (e.g., level of power and privilege) that affect health

environmental determinants of health
Factors in the biophysical environment, including the built environment, that affect health

health disparities
Differences in health status among groups of people based on factors such as socioeconomic status (SES), race, ethnicity, immigration status, environmental exposures, gender, education, disability, geographic location, or sexual orientation

FIGURE 1.5   Meatscape (Reflecting "How the World is Used")

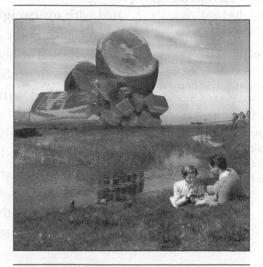

Source: Nicholas Lampert.

healthy food
"Foods that provide essential nutrients and energy to sustain growth, health and life while satiating hunger; usually fresh or minimally processed foods, naturally dense in nutrients, that when eaten in moderation and in combination with other foods, sustain growth, repair and maintain vital processes, promote longevity, reduce disease, and strengthen and maintain the body and its functions. Healthy foods do not contain ingredients that contribute to disease or impede recovery when consumed at normal levels" (as defined by the University of Washington Center for Public Health Nutrition, 2008)

industrial food animal production (IFAP)
An approach to meat, dairy, and egg production characterized by specialized operations designed for a high rate of production, large numbers of animals confined at high density, large quantities of localized animal waste, and substantial inputs of financial capital, fossil fuel, feed, pharmaceuticals, and indirect inputs embodied in feed (e.g., fuel and freshwater)

overweight
Adults are considered overweight if their body mass index (BMI) is 25.0 or higher, that is, if they are 10 to 20 percent heavier than what is considered a healthy weight range for someone of their height

- 16 percent of energy use (Canning, Charles, Huang, Polenske, & Waters, 2010)
- $1.139 trillion in consumer spending, or 9.8 percent of total personal income (USDA Economic Research Service, 2013)
- One-fifth of US private sector jobs (more than the health care sector!) (Food Chain Workers Alliance, 2012)
- Over 13 percent of US gross domestic product

Historically, most food in the United States and globally was produced with minimal nonhuman energy inputs and was consumed within a short distance of its production location. Significant change has been underway for more than one hundred years, but since World War II our food and agriculture system has undergone near total transformation. Today's food system is primarily industrial. An industrial system essentially treats a farm as a factory, using a set of inputs (seed, feed, pesticides, fertilizer, antibiotics, irrigation, fossil fuels) to create a set of outputs (product, waste, contamination) with an emphasis on specialization, standardization, and efficient throughput. The overall goal is to achieve the greatest possible yield at the lowest possible cost to the firm.

Food System Challenges

Our industrial food system is at the nexus of some of the most significant public health and environmental challenges we face today. Recent concerns about food safety range from melamine contamination of imported Chinese dairy products, to massive recalls of bacteria-contaminated ground turkey and peanut butter, to horsemeat in Irish hamburger and processed foods distributed throughout Europe, to arsenic in our rice and antibiotic residues in the shrimp we consume from southeast Asia. High obesity rates have focused attention on sugar-sweetened beverages, processed foods, and restaurant meals, and our national economic problems focus our attention (at least to an extent) on the nearly 15 percent of the population who are food insecure—including many of those who produce, process, and sell our food. Confronted by the enormity of the health problems associated with **overweight** and **obese** consumers, dire predictions are made of a health system—already the most expensive in the world—staggering under the need for more services. The health care system is further challenged by the crisis of antibiotic-resistant infections that has been linked in part to the misuse of antibiotics in animal agriculture. And farmers confront extreme weather events, such as droughts and floods, occurring with greater frequency, a broken farm policy with political gridlock in Washington, increasing concentration and near-monopoly control of everything from genetically modified seed to vertical integration of industrial food animal production and slaughter facilities, declining aquifers, community and worker exposures to contaminated air, water, and soil—and more.

Table 1.1 summarizes these and other challenges. Some of these derive from divorcing production from ecologic realities. Others represent unintended consequences of political and economic

TABLE 1.1 Key Food System Challenges

Public Health Challenges
- Food insecurity
- Food safety gaps
- Lack of healthy food access, affordability
- Obesity and diet-related disease
- Antibiotic resistance
- Chemical contaminants
- Lack of worker protection
- Soil, water, and air contamination
- Vulnerability to terrorism

Environmental (and Future Food Security) Challenges
- Climate change
- Soil depletion
- Water scarcity
- Peak oil and peak phosphorous
- Biodiversity loss
- Farmland loss
- Fisheries collapse

Additional Future Food Security Challenges
- Loss of small- and mid-sized farms
- Aging farmers
- Lack of food reserves
- Lack of planning for food security crises

Social Challenges
- Corporate concentration and monopoly control
- High, volatile food prices
- Challenging livelihoods of farmers and workers in the food system
- Policy gaps for genetically modified organisms
- Loss of rural community

developments or shifts in global trading patterns, and still others are the product of insufficient commitment to health promotion and equitable distribution of goods and services within society. These food system challenges are intertwined with other subsystems in the broader society; poverty, for example, is not a "food system problem" per se, and yet it indisputably contributes to many of the food system's most pressing problems. A systems perspective reminds us that the challenges, and the solutions we devise to address them, interact in complex ways. Enacting a living wage, for example, might reduce poverty and thus food insecurity; it could also lead to closure

obese
Adults are considered obese if their body mass index (BMI) is 30 or higher, that is, if they are over 20 percent heavier than what is considered a healthy weight range for someone of their height

of supermarkets, which operate on slim profit margins, and thus without additional intervention, might reduce food access in low-income neighborhoods.

As these threats accumulate, another concept from systems theory is useful as well: **resilience**, or a system's capacity to recover from disturbances. Disturbances that are sufficiently powerful versus a system's level of resilience can force the system across a threshold, precipitating major change and a new way of operating. Perspective 1.1 discusses resilience in more detail.

resilience
Ability to recover from perturbations

Perspective 1.1. When Your Boat Rocks, You Want Resilience Not Efficiency

Laura Jackson

Imagine being on a boat in calm seas and you are asked to bring a cup of soup to the captain. The task is an ordinary one and the only question is how fast should you walk without spilling the soup? Now imagine the same cup of soup, except that the boat is being tossed by huge waves. Walking speed is now no longer an issue. Instead you are looking for solid handholds, watching for the next wave to hit, keeping your knees flexed and your senses on high alert.

The first situation is an efficiency problem. The second situation is a resilience problem. Individuals, households, cities, businesses large and small, farmers, and even countries regularly provide for some level of resilience against all kinds of shocks. We buy house insurance, health insurance; wear seat belts and put money in savings; and get an education to increase our options in life. These measures cost money and time, yet we usually find the investment more than worthwhile. Better safe than sorry.

The resilience idea has taken off recently and is increasingly seen alongside or even replacing established concepts such as sustainability. *Resilience* is a good word that adds something new and useful to consider. What is the difference? In the context of agriculture, I think there are two big distinctions between *sustainability* and *resilience*.

First, there is the way things fail. Agricultural sustainability is about protecting nonrenewable resources: conserving what we have for future generations and renewing the health of soil and water to protect the future productivity (yield) of cropping systems. In contrast, according to authors Brian Walker and David Salt (2006), resilience thinking involves acknowledging the potential for a system-wide breakdown, a catastrophe. Like Humpty Dumpty, some systems can never be put back together again. In nature, we see countless examples of irreversible changes, such as lakes that go from crystal clear to perennially clouded with algae. Likewise, human civilizations (and their agricultural systems) can and do fail: the Roman Empire, Easter Island, the Mayans.

Second, there is the idea of the complex adaptive system. The idea of steady-state sustainability involves a relatively simple, closed agricultural system that behaves the same way, whether resources are abundant or scarce. The resilience idea applied to agriculture involves complex systems that adapt and change together, linking social and ecological processes. Soil, water, plants, livestock—the basic ecology of the food chain—are connected to transportation and processing infrastructure, the market economy, and human nutrition.

Resilience theory says that we could cross a threshold after which the agricultural system would transform itself into something completely different—and not necessarily in a good way. The threshold might be a very high price for diesel or phosphorus, rapid climate change, or a combination of factors. We don't know exactly where that threshold is in agriculture, just as we don't know when that next wave is going to hit the boat.

We have already experienced a radical shift in Iowa agriculture, a Humpty Dumpty–type moment. From the 1860s through the early 1950s, most Iowa farmers practiced a long crop rotation, with two to three years in small grains and pasture, followed by two to three years in row crops. It was integrated with livestock on the farm, cycled nutrients, managed weeds through rotation and tillage, and in the early years used on-farm energy for traction (oats-powered horses). One could say it was fairly resilient, at least for ninety years, weathering many changes in technology, crop breeding, and public policy. However, after World War II the sudden availability of inexpensive nitrogen fertilizer, first-generation broadleaf and grass herbicides, and favorable government policies precipitated a major transformation to the corn, beans, and concentrated livestock systems that we see today. Once the process was underway, there was no going back.

Is the current agricultural food system resilient? According to the research on resilience, efficiency has a dark side. Efficient, streamlined systems have eliminated unprofitable, redundant features. To translate to agriculture, there is no need to grow nitrogen-fixing alfalfa when fertilizer is cheap. Livestock can be raised more efficiently in a specialized operation. Regional differences in climate and infrastructure lead to "comparative advantage" so it simply does not pay to keep any cattle on grass in northern Iowa. However, redundancy can be a lifesaver if there is a sudden change in input costs, land prices, or climate. As the saying goes, "don't put all your eggs in one basket."

Resilience might be improved by investing in the know-how, tools, and infrastructure to produce different varieties or species of crops and livestock, reduce dependence on inputs, or find alternative markets. This is "inefficient" and certainly expensive under the current system. But similar to insurance, by the time we wish we carried some, it could be too late.

Other insurance policies that could provide some system resilience include the following:

- Growing perennial plants keeps roots in the ground and limits soil erosion in the event of a severe rain event. Fields of corn and soybeans are vulnerable from October through June.

- Keeping the groundwater clean and the creeks swimmable; investing in parks and privately owned natural areas will keep options open for future generations who may need to use the land in different ways. Areas that sacrifice their quality of life could miss out on economic opportunities.

- A diversity of people with a wide range of skills in a strong local community can help one another out in uncertain times, providing resilience. Who knows, they might let you borrow a piece of equipment.

- Commodity markets can internalize costs of greater soil and water conservation, passing on some of the responsibility of supporting clean water and ecosystem services to processors, retailers, and consumers.

Tremendous changes are ahead in energy, fertilizer, global commodities markets (both demand and supply), and most of all, climate. And those are just the known threats. Unfortunately, the market and government farm policies are largely discouraging resilience right now. The average farmer probably can't afford resilience. Likewise, most university and corporate agricultural research continues to pursue efficiency and optimization. With a laser focus on yield trend lines, will agriculture be able to flex its knees when that next wave hits?

This article was first published Spring 2001 in the quarterly newsletter of the Leopold Center for Sustainable Agriculture. More about the Leopold Center is available on the Web: www.leopold.iastate.edu. This Perspective reflects the viewpoint of the article author, not of the chapter authors.

Food System Benefits

Although it is clear that our food system is not healthy, it is also important to recognize the many positives that do derive, at least for now, even from our damaged and threatened food system. First, today's US food supply may be more plentiful and by some definitions inexpensive than at any time in history. The food from today's system provides most of us in the United States with enough nutrition to support our basic well-being and the energy to continue our life activities and even thrive (even if many people's diets are damaging over the long term, and even if they might thrive yet more by eating healthier diets). And, for those who do eat nutritious diets, their eating may not only be protective against illness but also can provide positive health benefits from energy to strength to a feeling of well-being—even if the foods were produced using environmentally or socially damaging methods. Further, our food often provides pleasure, comfort, and excitement. Food is at the core of most cultures and religions; it bonds friends, families, and, in some cases, communities together; and is also often a vehicle to help bridge cultures. As noted above, the food system provides livelihood to a fifth of the population. Agriculture preserves farmland, which, even when damaged, is in many ways preferable environmentally to development on that land because better practices can later restore soil quality and the ecosystem. Many of these benefits can be further strengthened and refined by efforts for food system reform.

The challenges across the food system call for comprehensive and coordinated responses from many sectors of society. What sorts of change are needed? The Kellogg Foundation has defined "good food" as food that is healthy, green, fair, and affordable. We would add to this list accessible and humanely produced. Most food falls somewhere on the spectrum between this ideal and the extreme of health, environmentally, and socially damaging production. Often, once a food meets criteria such as humaneness or healthiness, affordability suffers. Yet, as described in chapter 6; perspectives 4.5, 11.2, and 17.2, and focuses 6.1, 17.3, and 18.3; and elsewhere in this book, many efforts are underway to solve the simultaneous equations and produce truly good food. Beyond the qualities of the food itself, there is need for efforts to promote a healthier and more sustainable food *system*, encompassing all the food system activities, the policies and politics, the economic forces, the culture, and so on.

Focus 1.3 extends beyond the qualities of the food to present public health-oriented principles of a healthy, sustainable food system—endorsed by four major health-oriented professional associations.

◎ FOCUS 1.3. PRINCIPLES OF A HEALTHY, SUSTAINABLE FOOD SYSTEM

We, the American Public Health Association, the American Dietetic Association, the American Nurses Association, and the American Planning Association, support socially, economically, and ecologically sustainable food systems that promote health—the current and future health of individuals, communities, and the natural environment.

A healthy, sustainable food system is:

Health Promoting

- Supports the physical and mental health of all farmers, workers, and eaters

- Accounts for the public health impacts across the entire life cycle of how food is produced, processed, packaged, labeled, distributed, marketed, consumed, and disposed

Sustainable

- Conserves, protects, and regenerates natural resources, landscapes, and biodiversity

- Meets our current food and nutrition needs without compromising the ability of the system to meet the needs of future generations

Resilient

- Thrives in the face of challenges, such as unpredictable climate, increased pest resistance, and declining, increasingly expensive water and energy supplies

Diverse in

- Size and scale—includes a diverse range of food production, transformation, distribution, marketing, consumption, and disposal practices, occurring at diverse scales, from local and regional to national and global

- Geography—considers geographic differences in natural resources, climate, customs, and heritage

- Culture—appreciates and supports a diversity of cultures, sociodemographics, and lifestyles

- Choice—provides a variety of health-promoting food choices for all

Fair

- Supports fair and just communities and conditions for all farmers, workers, and eaters

- Provides equitable physical access to affordable food that is health promoting and culturally appropriate

Economically Balanced

- Provides economic opportunities that are balanced across geographic regions of the country and at different scales of activity, from local to global, for a diverse range of food system stakeholders

- Affords farmers and workers in all sectors of the system a living wage

Transparent

- Provides opportunities for farmers, workers, and eaters to gain the knowledge necessary to understand how food is produced, transformed, distributed, marketed, consumed, and disposed

- Empowers farmers, workers, and eaters to actively participate in decision making in all sectors of the system

A healthy, sustainable food system emphasizes, strengthens, and makes visible the interdependent and inseparable relationships between individual sectors (from production to waste disposal) and characteristics (health promoting, sustainable, resilient, diverse, fair, economically balanced, and transparent) of the system.

Source: American Public Health Association, American Dietetic Association, American Nurses Association, and American Planning Association. (2010).

These principles in many ways reflect the public health vision we as authors hold. We also complement that vision with one that places even more robustly the food system's people and their dignity at the center. The **human right to adequate food**, according to the United Nations, "is realized when every man, woman and child, alone or in community with others, has physical and economic access at all times to adequate food or means for its procurement" (United Nations Economic and Social Council, 1999). Although some imagine the right to be about a government obligation to provide food, in actuality, the core implication is that people should have the wherewithal to procure their own food. Additionally, the right requires that

human right to adequate food
Realized when every man, woman, and child, alone or in community with others, has physical and economic access at all times to adequate food or means for its procurement, according to the United Nations (United Nations Economic and Social Council, 1999)

FIGURE 1.6 Human Dignity: Workers Standing up for an Increase in the Minimum Wage

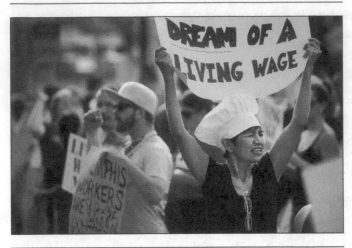

Source: Jim Weber, The Commercial Appeal.

governments respect and protect the right and facilitate food access (and if truly needed, provide food in order to fulfill the right). A rights framework makes these activities government's duty, not kindness or charity, and places human dignity at the center (see figure 1.6).

Another important aspect of this human rights approach is that it goes well beyond addressing hunger to encompassing food system goals such as those expressed in the "Healthy Sustainable Food System" statement. "Adequate" food is that which provides appropriate nutrients and calories, is safe from contamination, and is accessible, acceptable, and available to all people within a society and to future generations. The 1976 International Covenant on Economic, Social and Cultural Rights indicates that states are obligated to take measures "to improve methods of production, conservation and distribution of food by making full use of technical and scientific knowledge, by disseminating knowledge of the principles of nutrition and by developing or reforming agrarian systems in such a way as to achieve the most efficient development and utilization of natural resources" (United Nations General Assembly, 1976, p. 4).

Beyond the tenets of the right to food, another aspect of affirming the dignity of individuals is avoiding stigma around dietary choices, food insecurity, or obesity (as described in focus 18.1). It is easy to incorrectly infer information about someone's total diet based on small observations. Additionally, the food choices available to each of us are constrained by systemic factors well beyond our preferences. And, the factors we prioritize in decision making vary widely, such as from nutrition, environment, or animal welfare to taste, cost, convenience, or social status, each of which could lead to a different set of food choices. Even among those motivated to change their diets, it is notoriously difficult to do so, and particularly to maintain lasting change (Kolata, 2008). Broader changes in the food system can lead to new healthy defaults and norms that more readily facilitate individual changes.

As chapter, focus, and perspective authors describe throughout this book, positive change is afoot in every sector of our food system. Growing numbers of farms are transitioning to methods that use more **agroecology** principles (i.e., methods with benefits for the environment, health, and society), and even in mainstream industrial production some environmentally beneficial methods, such as **no-till farming** (planting crops without tilling the soil), are becoming widespread. The number of farmers markets bringing local produce to consumers multiplies annually. Growing consumer interest in health and in foods produced with reduced negative impact has created markets for these products and others. As demand changes, new institutions are being established, from farm-to-school programs and food hubs to aggregate food, to institutional composting facilities and to gleaning programs that gather and distribute unharvested food. More broadly, programs to address food insecurity increasingly seek to make available higher-quality food to those in need, through emergency feeding,

agroecology
The science and practice of applying ecological principles to agriculture to develop practices that work with nature to mimic natural processes and conserve ecological integrity; other labels for ecological approaches to agriculture include *ecological agriculture, agricultural ecology, sustainable agriculture, permaculture*

no-till farming
Planting crops directly into the residue of the former crop without plowing

school meals, and other programs, and to improve access to food assistance programs. Interventions are also proliferating to bring fresh food into underserved areas. There is also increasing attention to the experiences of workers within the food system and a newly vibrant movement of workers standing up for better treatment. One of the most active areas of engagement has been intervening to prevent and address obesity. Following several decades of incessant increases in rates of obesity, some studies have observed a leveling off (Ogden, Carroll, Kit, & Flegal, 2014). It is too early to know whether this trend will endure or to understand fully the contribution of healthier diets to the trend.

These changes have been driven in part by concern about the previously described threats—and in part by a groundswell of positive interest in food and a tremendous energy among everyday consumers to learn about food; eat "food with a story" and food they can trust; and appreciate high-quality, fresh, and well-prepared foods. As consumers get educated through these mainstream movements, many become motivated to support broader changes, whether addressing challenges in their communities or supporting the kinds of food production they would like to see expand. A growing food justice movement seeks to address the inequities throughout the food system and to bring new leadership to all of these efforts.

These changes are important and can contribute to positive evolution for public health, environment, and social equity. At the same time, these changes still remain but a small part of our overall food system. The vast majority of food production, processing, distribution, and consumption has yet to be significantly affected.

"Wicked Problems"

Sociologists use the term, **wicked problems** to describe problems for which stakeholders do not agree on the problem or its causes; each attempt to create a solution changes the problem; solutions are not right or wrong, just better or worse; solutions must be tailored to the situation; and they cannot be solved by people from any one discipline alone; multidisciplinary approaches are required (Kreuter, De Rosa, Howze, & Baldwin, 2004). Food system problems are indeed "wicked" (see figure 1.7)

As we look to supporting our current food system's capacity to feed the population and to addressing the system's public health, environmental, social equity, and food insecurity harms, the "wickedness" of these problems makes one's head spin. Even answers that initially seem obvious often turn out not to be. For example, it is widely presumed that ending farm commodity subsidies will address obesity. In fact, studies using evidence and modeling are remarkably consistent in finding that the impact on processed food prices and obesity will likely be negligible. Readers of this book will consider that evidence (chapter 7 and focus 7.2) and will have the opportunity to contemplate and review evidence germane to other critical questions, such as these:

wicked problems
Problems for which stakeholders do not agree on the problem or its causes; each attempt to create a solution changes the problem; solutions are not right or wrong, just better or worse; solutions must be tailored to the situation; and they cannot be solved by people from any one discipline alone; multidisciplinary approaches are required

- People often prefer foods that are not good for them or the environment. Given that, what, if anything, "should" we do to help improve diets?

- Is "good food" possible, when affordability is one of the criteria? And if not (for now), which should we prioritize: local, green, fair, affordable, or humane?

- How important are small community food security interventions given the vastness of food system problems?

- When current food insecurity is staring us in the face, how much money should we divert to costly conservation interventions that might help reduce future food insecurity?

FIGURE 1.7 Wicked Problems

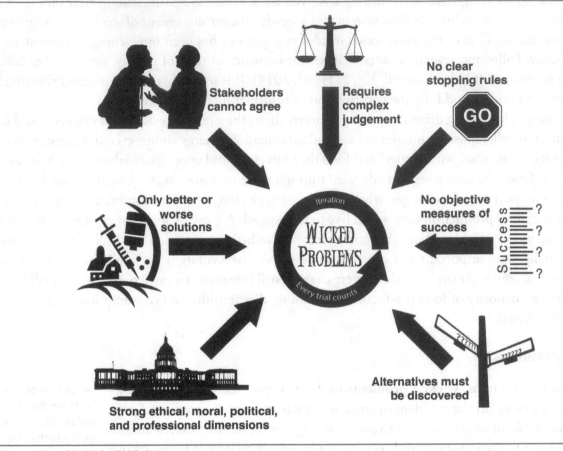

Source: Adapted by Michael Milli, CLF.

- Is it more efficient to source globally rather than locally or regionally?

- Is it elitist to seek out local and sustainable foods?

- Should all food system workers receive a living wage? Even if it leads potentially to higher food prices and possibly to some stores in low-income communities going out of business?

- Which comes first in changing the food system, supply or demand?

- People have raised "sky is falling" concerns about the food system since at least the time of Thomas Malthus. And the food supply has only increased since then. So is all this worry really necessary? Won't technology help us out?

- Why is it so hard for even motivated individuals to change their diets, especially for the long term?

- What role should corporations play in voluntarily improving the food they provide? What role should policy play in pressuring them?

Overall, we hope the readings in this book will stimulate ideas and energy for improving the food system, including the following:

- Reducing food system public health threats including diet-related disease, food-borne illness, and contaminant exposures for communities and workers

- Reducing food system environmental harms including damage to and overuse of resources and climate change

- Increasing the supply of and demand for foods that are healthy, green, fair, affordable, and humane

- Improving access to and affordability of healthy foods

- Supporting justice and social equity for all food system participants

- Strengthening local and regional food systems

- Ensuring the long-term availability of our food supply

- Encouraging enjoyment of food flavors and freshness while supporting food traditions, community, and conviviality

SUMMARY

The food system encompasses all the activities and resources that go into producing, distributing, and consuming food; the drivers and outcomes of those processes; and all the relationships and feedback loops between system components. When considering the food system, systems thinking is useful in understanding the complex and interactive networks of relationships engaged in bringing us our food and in gaining insights into processes and potential unintended consequences. The US food system occupies a central place in US society, economy, land and resource use, and employment. There are many positives in the mainstream food system (figures 1.8a–d) but also a host of serious problems and challenges. Approaches to food system reform that complement systems strategies include public health and the right to adequate food. The chapter concludes by highlighting some of the questions readers will consider as they proceed through this book.

KEY TERMS

Agent-based computational modeling (ABM)	Obese
Agroecology	Overweight
Environmental determinants of health	Population-based approach
Food system	Primary prevention
Health	Public health
Health disparities	Resilience
Healthy food	Social determinants of health
Human right to adequate food	Structural determinants of health
Industrial food animal production (IFAP)	Subsystems
Inputs	System
No-till farming	Wicked problems

FIGURE 1.8   Even with Its Limitations, Our Food System Provides for Us in Many Ways

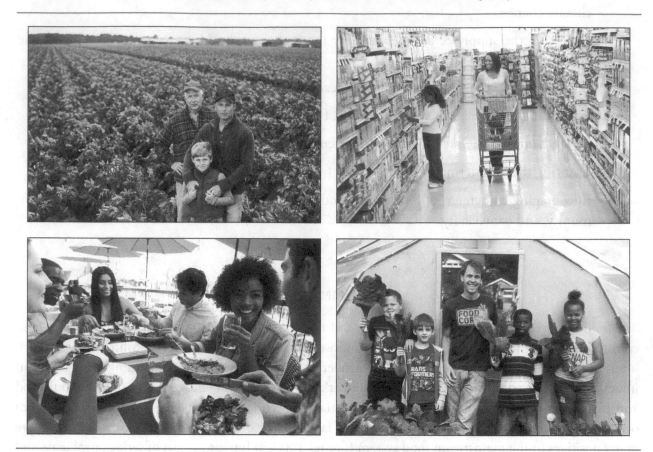

Sources: istockphoto 20863061, istockphoto 6218137, istockphoto 33603160, USDA-Robyn Wardell.

DISCUSSION QUESTIONS

1. Why should we study the food system? What is the benefit of a systems approach?

2. Poet Wendell Berry wrote, "A significant part of the pleasure of eating is in one's accurate consciousness of the lives and the world from which food comes." Is this true for you? For others?

3. Is "good food" possible, when affordability is one of the criteria? And if not (for now), which should we prioritize: local, green, fair, affordable, or humane?

4. How important are small community food security interventions given the vastness of food system problems?

5. When current food insecurity is staring us in the face, does it make sense to divert money to costly conservation interventions that might help reduce future food insecurity?

6. Is it more efficient to source globally?

7. Is it elitist to seek out local and sustainable foods or an alternative food system?

8. Should all food system workers receive a living wage? Even if it leads to higher food prices and the possibility that some stores in low-income communities go out of business?

9. Which comes first in changing the food system, supply or demand?

10. People have raised "sky is falling" concerns about the food system since at least the time of Thomas Malthus. And the food supply has only increased since then. So is all this worry really necessary? Won't technology help us out?

11. Why is it so hard for even motivated individuals to change their diets, especially for the long term?

12. What role should corporations play in voluntarily improving the food they provide?

REFERENCES

American Public Health Association, American Dietetic Association, American Nurses Association, and American Planning Association. (2010). *Principles of a healthy, sustainable food system*. Retrieved from www.planning.org/nationalcenters/health/pdf/HealthySustainableFoodSystemsPrinciples_2012May.pdf

Axelrod, R. (1997). *The complexity of cooperation: Agent-based models of competition and collaboration*. Princeton, NJ: Princeton University Press.

Berry, W. (1990). The pleasures of eating. *What are people for?* New York: North Point Press.

Canning, P., Charles, A., Huang, S., Polenske, K. R., & Waters, A. (2010). *Energy use in the U.S. food system* (No. ERR 94). Washington, DC: US Department of Agriculture Economic Research Service.

Clancy, K. (2011). *Food systems: Some history and theory*. Presentation, Center for a Livable Future. Retrieved from https://www.youtube.com/watch?v=wpN8joWQugs&feature=youtu.be

Council on Linkages Between Academia and Public Health Practice. (2010). *Core competencies for public health professionals*. Washington, DC: Public Health Foundation.

Epstein, J. M. (2006). Remarks on the foundations of agent-based generative social science. In L. Tesfatsion & K. L. Judd (Eds.), *Handbook of computational economics* (Vol. *2*). Amsterdam: Elsevier.

Food Chain Workers Alliance. (2012). *The hands that feed us*. Retrieved from http://foodchainworkers.org/wp-content/uploads/2012/06/Hands-That-Feed-Us-Report.pdf

Fuggle, R. F. (2001). *Lake Victoria: A case study of complex interrelationships*. Nairobi: UNEP.

Hammond, R. A. (2009). Complex systems modeling for obesity research. *Preventing Chronic Disease*, *6*(3). Retrieved from www.cdc.gov/pcd/issues/2009/jul/09_0017.htm

Hammond, R. A., & Dube, L. (2012). A systems science perspective and transdisciplinary models for food and nutrition security. *PNAS Early Edition, pp. 1–8*.

Holland, J. H. (1992). *Adaptation in natural and artificial systems*. Cambridge, MA: MIT Press.

Kolata, G. (2008). *Rethinking thin: The new science of weight loss—and the myths and realities of dieting*. New York: Farrar, Strauss & Giroux.

Kreuter, M. W., De Rosa, C., Howze, E. H., & Baldwin, G. T. (2004). Understanding wicked problems: A key to advancing environmental health promotion. *Health Education and Behavior*, *31*(4), 441–454.

Miller, J. H., & Page, S. E. (2002). *Complex adaptive systems: An introduction to computational models of social life*. Princeton, NJ: Princeton University Press.

Murray, J. D. (1989). *Mathematical biology*. Berlin: Springer-Verlag.

Nourish Food System Map, www.nourishlife.org. Copyright 2012 WorldLink, all rights reserved.

Ogden, C. L., Carroll, M. D., Kit, B. K., & Flegal, K. M. (2014). Prevalence of childhood and adult obesity in the United States, 2011–2012. *JAMA*, *311*(8), 806–814.

Peemoeller, L. (nd). *Food systems planning*. Retrieved from www.foodsystemsplanning.com/about

US Department of Agriculture Economic Research Service. (2012a). *Irrigation and water use*. Retrieved from www.ers.usda.gov/topics/farm-practices-management/irrigation-water-use.aspx#.UVg4dL_jtzo

US Department of Agriculture Economic Research Service. (2012b). *Land use, land value & tenure*. Retrieved from www.ers.usda.gov/topics/farm-economy/land-use,-land-value-tenure.aspx#.UU7E8lueCcw

US Department of Agriculture Economic Research Service. (2013). *Table 7—Food expenditures by families and individuals as a share of disposable personal income*. Retrieved from www.ers.usda.gov/data-products/food-expenditures.aspx#.UU4qwVueCcx

United Nations Economic and Social Council. (1999) *The right to adequate food*. Retrieved from www.srfood.org/images/stories/pdf/backgrounddocuments/2-eng-gcn12–1999–1.pdf

United Nations General Assembly. (1976). *International covenant on economic, social and cultural rights*. Retrieved from www.ohchr.org/EN/ProfessionalInterest/Pages/CESCR.aspx

University of Washington Center for Public Health Nutrition. (2008). Nutrition and physical activity plan, appendix G. Retrieved from http://depts.washington.edu/waaction/plan/append/g.html

US Department of Agriculture National Agricultural Statistics Service. (2012). *The census of agriculture*. Retrieved from www.agcensus.usda.gov

Walker, B., & Salt, D. (2006). *Resilience thinking: Sustaining ecosystems and people in a changing world*. Washington, DC: Island Press.

Winslow, C.E.A. (1920). The untilled fields of public health. *Science, 51*(1306), 23–33.

World Health Organization. (1946). *Preamble to the constitution of the world health organization*. New York: Author.

Outcomes

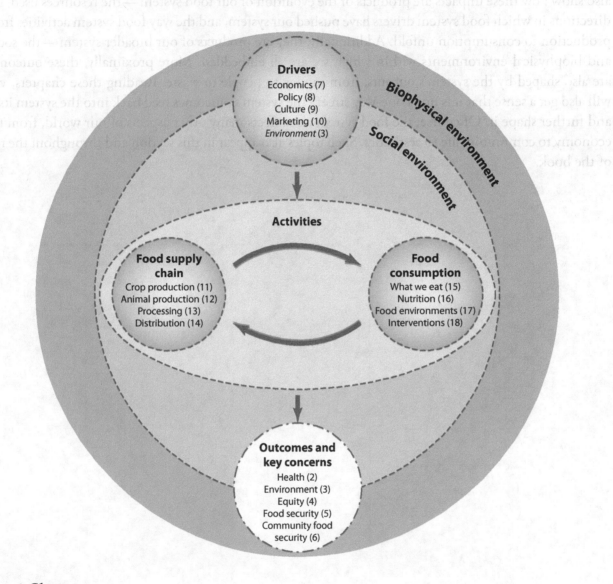

Part 1 Chapters

Part 1 focuses on some of the most important outcomes of the US food system: public health, environment, equity, food security, and community food security. Although these outcomes may be seen as the ultimate end goals of a functional food system, we start here because these themes are central to everything else that is covered in the book. These chapters orient you and provide the motivation for digging into the details of how the food system operates. Together, they describe a wide variety of positive and negative impacts deriving from the mainstream food system and alternatives. The chapters also show how these impacts are products of the evolution of our food system—the resources used, the directions in which food system drivers have pushed our system, and the way food system activities from production to consumption unfold. Additionally, they are products of our broader system—the social and biophysical environments within which we are all embedded. More proximally, these outcomes are also shaped by the system's outputs, from money to people to waste. Reading these chapters, you will also get a sense that it is not a one-way street. The system's outcomes feed back into the system itself and further shape it. Of course, the food system also affects many other aspects of our world, from the economy to community life to aesthetics. Such topics also appear in this section and throughout the rest of the book.

Chapter 2

Food System Public Health Effects

Brent F. Kim and Jennifer L. Wilkins

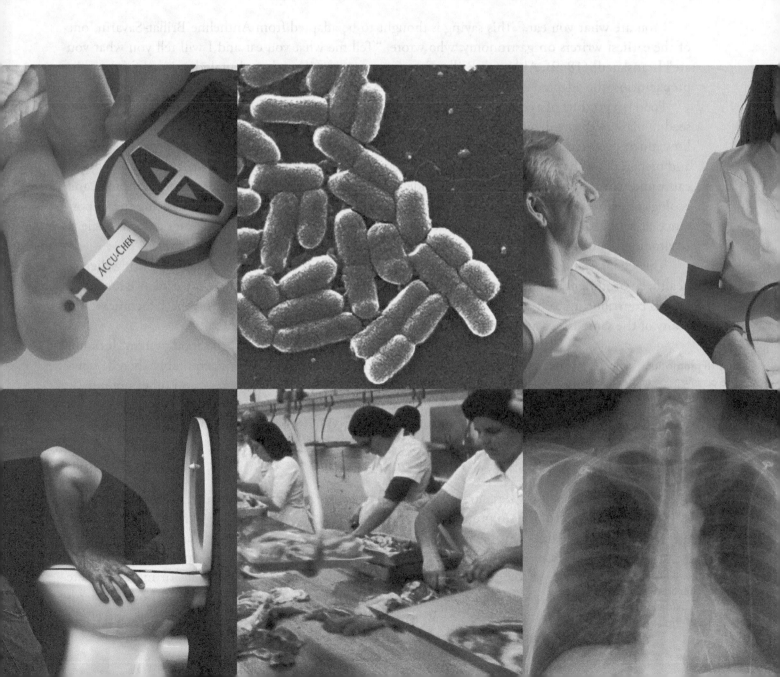

Learning Objectives

- Apply a holistic framework that considers the spectrum of beneficial and adverse health effects, and their contributing factors, across the whole food system.

- Describe major diet-related conditions, their health and economic impacts, and their dietary risk factors.

- Describe some of the occupational and environmental health risks associated with food and agricultural industries.

- Provide examples of potential chemical and microbial hazards in food, the health effects of foodborne contamination, and points where the food supply may be contaminated.

- Identify opportunities to protect and promote health through the food system.

"You are what you eat." This saying is thought to be adapted from Anthelme Brillat-Savarin, one of the earliest writers on gastronomy, who wrote, "Tell me what you eat and I will tell you what you are" [translated] (1842). Although Brillat-Savarin was emphasizing the cultural identity of food and its preparations, the adapted saying is often used to describe the health effects of one's diet.

Food is a product of a complex system involving people, infrastructure, resources, and activities from seed to plate to disposal, all of which influence, to a considerable degree, the public's health. What and how much people eat, as well as how, where, and what food is produced, processed, distributed, sold, and prepared, can have profound health effects, both beneficial and harmful. The relationships between cause and effect, however, are rarely fully understood and often involve complex social, economic, and ecological pathways. In this sense, we might say we are the *food system* we eat, emphasizing the importance of a holistic perspective—one that accounts for relationships among diet, agriculture, society, environment, and health.

This chapter summarizes the health effects associated with the food system, highlighting dietary health, environmental and occupational health, and food safety. We also explore the evidence for causal factors contributing to food system health effects. The focus here is primarily on the US context, but many of the same issues apply in other countries and regions.

health promotion
The optimization of the body's systems and building reserves against forces averse to good health; education and other activities aimed at promoting health

The burden of adverse health effects associated with the food system does not weigh evenly on all Americans, nor are the health benefits equitably shared. Low-income communities, communities of color, migrant workers, and other potentially disadvantaged populations face unique challenges in the food system; these are discussed at length in chapter 4 and referred to throughout this book.

DIETARY HEALTH

phytonutrients
Compounds in plant foods that have been associated with beneficial functions in the body (e.g., aiding nutrient absorption, inhibiting oxidation, improving cholesterol)

Food provides our bodies with nutrients for growth, maintenance, and repair, but the role of diet in promoting health extends far beyond supplying the basics for survival. Medical historian Henry E. Sigerist noted that "health is not simply the absence of disease: it is something positive, a joyful attitude toward life, and a cheerful acceptance of the responsibilities that life puts upon the individual." In more concrete terms, Breslow (1999) describes **health promotion** as optimizing the body's systems and building reserves against forces averse to good health. Diets higher in certain **phytonutrients**, for example, have been associated with enhanced cardiovascular,

FIGURE 2.1   Clinician's Prescription for Fruits and Vegetables

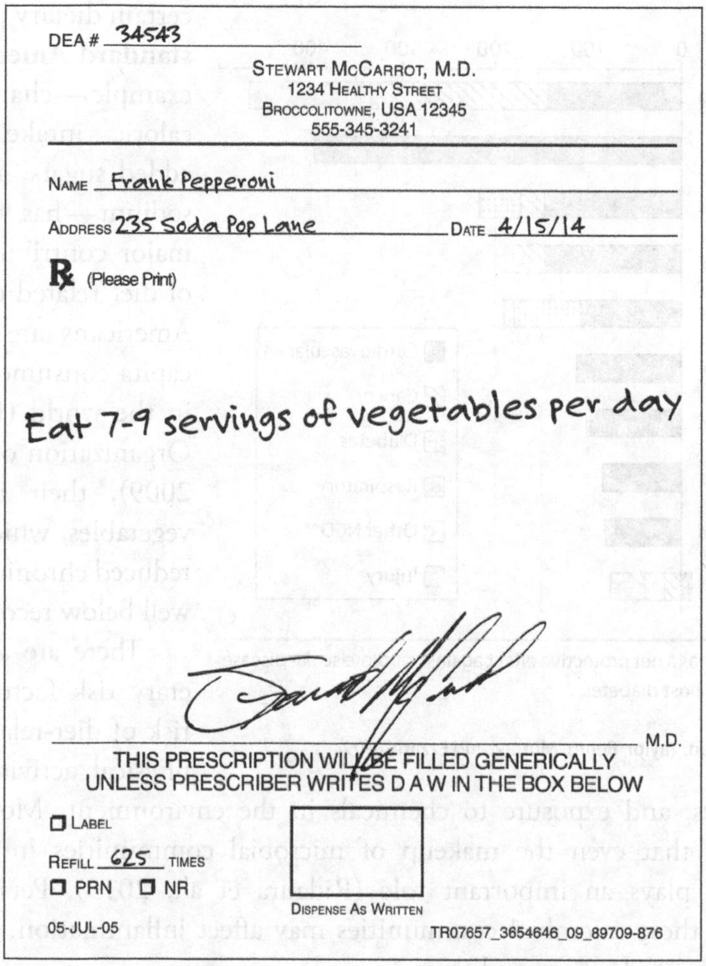

DEA # 34543

STEWART MCCARROT, M.D.
1234 HEALTHY STREET
BROCCOLITOWNE, USA 12345
555-345-3241

NAME Frank Pepperoni

ADDRESS 235 Soda Pop Lane   DATE 4/15/14

℞ (Please Print)

Eat 7-9 servings of vegetables per day

_____ M.D.

THIS PRESCRIPTION WILL BE FILLED GENERICALLY
UNLESS PRESCRIBER WRITES D A W IN THE BOX BELOW

☐ LABEL

REFILL 625 TIMES
☐ PRN   ☐ NR

DISPENSE AS WRITTEN

05-JUL-05   TR07657_3654646_09_89709-876

Source: Michael Milli, CLF.

cognitive, and immune function; improved bone and eye health; reduced inflammation; improved athletic performance; and other health-promoting benefits (Carkeet, Grann, Randolph, Venzon, & Izzy, 2012). In light of these benefits, some public health advocates are piloting fruit and vegetable prescription programs (figure 2.1).

During the twentieth century, longevity in the United States increased from less than fifty years to more than seventy-five. This unprecedented advancement, coupled with medical innovations to help manage the threat of disease, enabled the public health community to dedicate more resources to health promotion (Breslow, 1999). Preventing diet-related disease, however, remains a major focus. In 1971, A. R. Omran published his classic paper on the **epidemiologic transition,** a shift "whereby pandemics of infection are gradually displaced by degenerative and man-made diseases as the chief form of **morbidity** and primary cause of death" (Omran, 1971, p. 516). Cardiovascular disease, cancers, type 2 diabetes, obesity, and other preventable, diet-related diseases are now among the leading causes of death in the United States (figure 2.2). Accordingly, public health priorities in the United States and other developed countries shifted from infectious disease to these and other **chronic diseases.**

epidemiologic transition
A shift in the patterns of disease among a population, whereby infectious diseases are gradually surpassed by chronic illness as the primary cause of morbidity (illness) and death

morbidity
Illness or symptom; alternately, disease incidence rate

chronic diseases
Diseases that generally progress slowly and persist for many years

FIGURE 2.2   US Deaths (in Thousands) Attributable to Modifiable Risk Factors, by Disease, in 2005

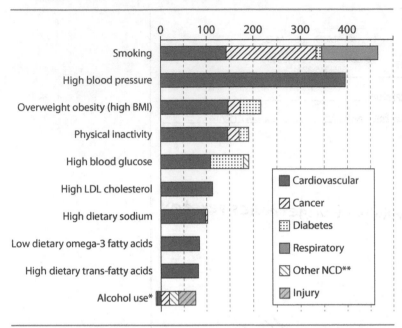

*Regular moderate alcohol use has a net protective effect against cardiovascular disease, and a small protective effect against diabetes.

**Noncommunicable diseases

Source: Danaei, Ding, Mozaffarian, Taylor, Rehm, Murray, and Ezzati (2009).

diet-related diseases
Diseases associated with certain dietary patterns

Standard American Diet (SAD)
Diet common to US citizens, characterized by excess caloric intake of refined grains, added sugars, added fats, meats, total calories, and sodium, and inadequate intake of fruits and vegetables

As their name implies, **diet-related diseases** are associated with certain dietary patterns. The so-called **standard American diet (SAD)**, for example—characterized by excess caloric intake of refined grains, added sugars, added fats, meat, and sodium—has been implicated as a major contributor to the prevalence of diet-related disease. And although Americans are among the top per capita consumers of animal products in the world (Food and Agriculture Organization of the United Nations, 2009), their intake of fruits and vegetables, which are associated with reduced chronic disease risks, remains well below recommended levels.

There are also numerous nondietary risk factors that influence the risk of diet-related disease, including physical activity levels, income, genetics, and exposure to chemicals in the environment. Mounting evidence suggests that even the makeup of microbial communities in the human digestive tract plays an important role (Ridaura et al., 2013). Perspective 2.1 describes how these microbial communities may affect inflammation, with implications for obesity and other conditions.

This section highlights several major diet-related diseases and their dietary risk factors. Although we focus on health and economic effects, the range of other human costs—including physical suffering and the emotional toll related to caring for and losing loved ones—is also extensive and defies our capacity to justly describe them here.

Perspective 2.1. Gut Bacteria, Diets and Inflammation
Moises Velasquez

Chronic, low-grade inflammation has long been recognized as a feature of metabolic syndrome, a cluster of dysfunctions that tends to precede full-blown diabetes and that also increases the risk of heart disease, stroke, certain cancers, and even dementia—the top killers of the developed world. The syndrome includes a combination of elevated blood sugar and high blood pressure, low "good" cholesterol, and an abdominal cavity filled with fat, often indicated by a "beer belly." But recently, doctors have begun to question whether chronic inflammation is more than just a symptom of metabolic syndrome: could it, in fact, be a major cause?

Here's the traditional understanding of metabolic syndrome: You ate too much refined food sopped in grease. Calories flooded your body. Usually, a hormone called insulin would help your cells absorb these calories for use. But the sheer overabundance of energy in this case overwhelms your cells. They stop responding to insulin. To compensate, your pancreas begins cranking out more insulin. When the pancreas finally collapses from exhaustion, you have diabetes. In addition, you develop resistance to another hormone called leptin, which signals satiety, or fullness. So you tend to overeat. Meanwhile, fat cells, which have become bloated and stressed as they try to store the excess calories, begin emitting a danger signal—low-grade inflammation.

But new research suggests another scenario: inflammation might not be a symptom, it could be a cause. According to this theory, it is the immune activation caused by lousy food that prompts insulin and leptin resistance. Sugar builds up in your blood. Insulin increases. Your liver and pancreas strain to keep up. All because the loudly blaring danger signal—the inflammation—hampers your cells' ability to respond to hormonal signals. Maybe the most dramatic evidence in support of this idea comes from experiments where scientists quash inflammation in animals. If you simply increase the number of white blood cells that alleviate inflammation—called regulatory T-cells—in obese mice with metabolic syndrome, the whole syndrome fades away.

Now, on the face of it, it seems odd that a little inflammation should have such a great impact on energy regulation. But consider: this is about apportioning a limited resource exactly where it's needed, when it's needed. When not under threat, the body uses energy for housekeeping and maintenance—and, if you're lucky, procreation, an optimistic, future-oriented activity. But when a threat arrives, you reprioritize. All that hormone-regulated activity declines to a bare minimum. Your body institutes a version of World War II rationing: troops (white blood cells) and resources (calories) are redirected toward the threat. Nonessential tasks shut down. Forget tomorrow. The priority is to preserve the self today.

This, some think, is the evolutionary reason for insulin resistance. Cells in the body stop absorbing sugar because the fuel is required—requisitioned, really—by armies of white blood cells. The problems arise when that emergency response, crucial to repelling pillagers in the short term, drags on indefinitely.

Where does the perceived threat come from—all that inflammation? Some ingested fats are directly inflammatory. And dumping a huge amount of calories into the bloodstream from any source, be it fat or sugar, may overwhelm and inflame cells. But another source of inflammation is hidden in plain sight, the one hundred trillion microbes inhabiting your gut (and on your skin and in your nose and mouth, happily coexisting with the ten trillion of your own cells). Junk food, it turns out, may not kill us entirely directly, but rather by prompting the collapse of an ancient and mutually beneficial symbiosis, and turning a once cooperative relationship adversarial.

We all carry a few pounds' worth of microbes in our gut, a complex ecosystem collectively called the microbiota. Most of our microbes inhabit the colon, the final loop of intestine, where they help us break down fibers, harvest calories, protect us from micro-marauders and, much, much more. What do we do for our microbes in return? Some scientists argue that mammals are really just mobile digestion chambers for bacteria. After all, your stool is roughly half living bacteria by weight.

Microbes naturally form communities, with different microbial communities reflecting different diets. In obese people, not only are anti-inflammatory microbes relatively scarce, microbial diversity in general is depleted, and community structure degraded. Microbes that, in ecological parlance, we might call weedy species, scurry around unimpeded.

We're already familiar with cavities. Tooth decay is as old as teeth, but it intensified with increased consumption of refined carbohydrates just before the industrial revolution. Previously, plaque microbes probably occupied the ecological niche of your mouth more peaceably. But dump a load of sugar on them, and certain species expand exponentially. Their by-product—acid—which, in normal amounts, protects you from foreign bacteria—now corrodes your teeth.

Something similar may occur with our gut microbes when they're exposed to the highly refined, sweet and greasy, junk-food diet. The very qualities that improve palatability and lengthen shelf life—high sugar content,

(Continued)

(Continued)

fats that resist turning rancid, and a lack of organic complexity—make refined foods toxic to your key microbes. This diet also changes gut permeability and alters the makeup of our microbial organ. Our "friendly" community of microbes becomes unfriendly, even downright pathogenic, leaking noxious byproducts where they don't belong. The bugs that bloom may act in their own self-interest. They want more of that sweet, fatty food on which they thrive.

Now, not everyone accepts that inflammation drives metabolic syndrome and obesity. And even among the idea's proponents, no one claims that all inflammation emanates from the microbiota. Moreover, if you accept that inflammation contributes to obesity, then you're obligated to consider all the many ways to become inflamed.

Whether inflammation drives obesity or just contributes, how much of it emanates from our microbiota, or even whether it causes weight gain, or results from it—these are still somewhat open questions. But it is clear that chronic, low-grade inflammation, wherever it comes from, is unhealthy.

Source: Condensed from Velasquez (2013). See hyperlinks in original for references. Moises Velasquez is the author of *An Epidemic of Absence: A New Way of Understanding Allergies and Autoimmune Diseases.*

Obesity

obese
Adults are considered obese if their body mass index (BMI) is 30 or higher, that is, if they are over 20 percent heavier than what is considered a healthy weight range for someone of their height

Adults are considered **obese** if they are over 20 percent heavier than what is considered a healthy weight range for someone of their height. These diagnostic criteria are meant to capture approximate levels of body fat. Obesity—and in particular, high levels of abdominal fat—exerts its burden of disease by increasing the risk of a range of other health outcomes, including insulin resistance, type 2 diabetes, high blood pressure, elevated blood cholesterol, coronary heart disease, various cancers, osteoarthritis, stroke, asthma, pregnancy complications, increased surgical risks (Pi-Sunyer, 2002), and premature death (Whitlock et al., 2009). Obesity can also impair quality of life through reduced mobility, bodily pain, poorer mental health (Fontaine & Barofsky, 2001), and social stigma (Puhl & Heuer, 2009).

Obesity in the United States has reached epidemic levels. Between 1980 and 2002, obesity prevalence among US adults doubled from 15 to 30 percent. By 2010, 36 percent of adults and 17 percent of children and adolescents were obese (see figure 2.3). Although recent data suggest obesity rates are leveling off, they remain unprecedentedly high.

Although it is generally true that consuming more calories than are expended leads to weight gain, the dietary risk factors for obesity are more nuanced and often

FIGURE 2.3   Obesity Prevalence among US Adults, Children, and Adolescents, 1960–2010

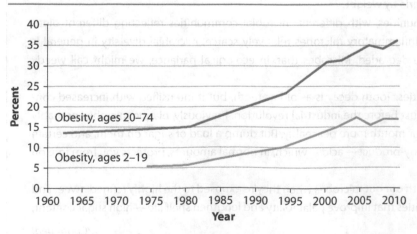

Data source: Fryar, Carroll, and Ogden (2012a, 2012b).

involve complex biological and behavioral pathways. Consuming foods with a high **energy density**, in particular, have been strongly associated with higher caloric intake and weight gain. Energy-dense foods are often highly palatable (they taste good) and are digested quickly. Because they have less volume, they may not trigger stretch receptors in the stomach that help signal **satiety**. For these reasons, it is easy to overconsume calories from energy-dense foods (Yao & Roberts, 2001). Sugar-sweetened beverages are also of particular concern, in part because they do not induce high levels of satiety and they provide a high number of calories in an easily and quickly ingested form (Malik, Willett, & Hu, 2013).

Obesity has also been associated with a wide range of other social, economic, and environmental risk factors that influence what and how much people eat (see chapter 17). Eating away from home, for example, such as at restaurants and fast food outlets, has been strongly associated with obesity. This is thought to be because of energy-dense offerings, large portion sizes, and consumers' tendency to underestimate the caloric content of menu items (Story, Kaphingst, Robinson-O'Brien, & Glanz, 2008).

The burden of health effects attributable to obesity raises the question of whether it should be considered a disease; the National Institutes of Health and American Medical Association have declared it as such. Although partly an issue of semantics—there are no formal criteria for what constitutes disease—clinicians have speculated that classifying obesity as a disease may draw more resources toward research and treatment, and therefore reduce stigma by acknowledging that it is not a problem of inadequate willpower (Frellick, 2013). See focus 18.1 for a discussion of obesity stigma and its impacts.

Cardiovascular Disease

Cardiovascular disease (CVD) refers to a group of disorders that affect the heart (**heart disease**) and blood vessels. Types of CVD include **coronary artery disease,** which can lead to heart attacks; and **cerebrovascular disease,** which can lead to strokes. These conditions commonly occur due to cholesterol and other fatty buildup on artery walls, hindering or blocking blood flow.

CVD is the leading cause of mortality in the United States, responsible for one in three deaths. An estimated one in three US adults (seventy-eight million) have **hypertension**, a condition that greatly increases the risk of heart attack and stroke (Go et al., 2013).

Dietary risk factors for CVD include high saturated fat intake, which has been associated with increased blood LDL ("bad") cholesterol levels, and high salt intake, which can lead to hypertension. A growing body of evidence suggests sugar—particularly sugar-sweetened beverages—may be a greater contributor to CVD than previously thought, in part through effects on the liver (Stanhope et al., 2011). Higher intake of red meat (beef, pork, and lamb), especially processed red meat, has been strongly associated with earlier death from CVD, possibly due to a combination of factors including salt and chemical preservatives in processed meat, saturated fat, and heme iron (Pan et al., 2012). Red meat's contribution to CVD may be explained in part by recent evidence indicating that bacteria in the human digestive tract play an intermediary role between intake of L-carnitine, a compound abundant in red meat, and increased CVD risk (Koeth et al., 2013).

energy density
Amount of calories provided by a food, relative to its mass or volume

satiety
Feeling of fullness

cardiovascular disease (CVD)
A group of diseases that affect the heart or blood vessels

heart disease
Disease affecting the heart, such as coronary artery disease and congestive heart failure

coronary artery disease
Disease involving reduced blood flow to the heart muscle

cerebrovascular disease
Disease affecting blood flow to the brain

hypertension
High blood pressure

Evidence is accumulating, meanwhile, that fruit and vegetable intake may protect against CVD. In one large-scale study, the risk of CVD was 28 percent lower for persons consuming five or more servings of fruits and vegetables per day compared with those eating less than 1.5 servings per day (Hung et al., 2004).

Type 2 Diabetes

Diabetes
A chronic health condition in which the body's cells do not adequately take in blood glucose

Type 2 diabetes
The most common form of diabetes; the body either resists the effects of insulin—a hormone that regulates the uptake of glucose into cells—or does not produce enough insulin to maintain a normal glucose level

prediabetes
A condition in which blood glucose levels are elevated, but not high enough to be classified as diabetes

Diabetes is a chronic condition in which cellular uptake of blood glucose is inadequate. Without careful management, persons with diabetes can have excess glucose accumulate in their blood. This can lead to fatigue, infection, sexual dysfunction, nerve and kidney damage, limb amputations, blindness, and other adverse outcomes. **Type 2 diabetes** is strongly linked to lifestyle factors, particularly diet and exercise.

Based on 2010 estimates, 8.3 percent (25.8 million) of US adults have diabetes, including diagnosed (18.8 million) and undiagnosed (7 million) cases. Nearly two million adults are newly diagnosed with diabetes each year. Type 2 diabetes is by far the most prevalent form of the disease, accounting for 90 to 95 percent of cases. Until recently, type 2 diabetes was almost exclusive to adults, but as more and more children are diagnosed with the condition, it is no longer accurate to refer to it as *adult-onset* diabetes. Taken together, diabetes and **prediabetes** affect over half (57 percent) of US adults (Centers for Disease Control and Prevention [CDC], 2011a).

Obesity is a leading risk factor for type 2 diabetes. Dietary risk factors include frequent consumption of red and processed meat (Micha, Michas, & Mozaffarian, 2012) and sugar-sweetened beverages (Malik, Popkin, Bray, Depres, Willett, & Hu, 2010). Some evidence also implicates unhealthy fats and foods that rapidly raise blood glucose (such as foods made with refined grains). Diets high in whole grains, fiber, magnesium, fruits and vegetables, nuts, and dairy, by contrast, may be protective against diabetes (Schulze & Hu, 2005).

Cancer

cancer
A group of diseases characterized by uncontrolled division of abnormal body cells

An estimated one in five Americans (21 percent) will die from a **cancer**. Four in ten Americans are expected to receive cancer diagnoses in their lifetimes (The President's Cancer Panel, 2010).

Dietary factors are thought to account for roughly one-third of cancers occurring in Western countries. The most clearly established diet-related risk factors are obesity and alcohol intake (Key, Allen, Spencer, & Travis, 2002). Evidence is mounting of strong links between red and processed meat intake and various cancers and earlier death from cancer (Pan et al., 2012).

Studies in the early 1990s suggested fruits and vegetables may have a protective effect against cancer; later, more rigorous studies found little or no association between overall fruit and vegetable intake and reduced cancer rates. Compounds commonly found in certain fruits and vegetables, however, such as lycopene (tomatoes) and folic acid (dark green leafy greens, and other vegetables), show promise in reducing the risk of certain cancers (Hung et al., 2004).

TABLE 2.1   Direct Medical Costs Associated with Diet-Related Disease in the United States

Disease	Direct Costs, in Billions USD	Year	Source
CVD	273	2010	Heidenreich et al. (2011)
Obesity	147	2008	Finkelstein, Trogdon, Cohen, and Dietz (2009)
Cancer	125	2010	Mariotto, Yabroff, Shao, Feuer, and Brown (2011)
Type 2 diabetes	113	2007	Huang, Basu, O'Grady, and Capretta (2009)

Economic Impacts of Diet-Related Disease

Diet-related diseases—coupled with longer life spans—are costly to the US health care system (see table 2.1). Cardiovascular disease alone accounts for 17 percent of direct US medical expenditures, and the cost is projected to triple by 2030. Because these diseases also have nondietary risk factors, not all of these costs can be attributed to what people eat.

The direct medical costs of these conditions are compounded by the costs of travel, lodging, lost earnings from missed work, and other indirect costs to patients and their family members, as well as the value of future income lost due to disability and premature death.

Food Insecurity

Although the problem of diet-related disease in the United States seems to be attributable, at least in part, to caloric excess, nearly one in seven US households suffers from **food insecurity**—a condition that can include hunger (in more extreme cases), as well as having to skip meals, compromise on nutrition, or rely on emergency food sources such as food banks, food pantries, and soup kitchens (Coleman-Jensen, Nord, Andrews, & Carlson, 2011). As chapter 5 describes at length, food insecurity contributes to developmental and mental health impacts, diet-related conditions including nutrient deficiencies, obesity, and type 2 diabetes, and other adverse health effects.

food insecurity
Having inadequate economic resources to enable consistent access to safe, adequate, and nutritious food to support an active and healthy life for all household members (low food security: reduced quality, variety, desirability of diet; very low food security: multiple indications of disrupted eating patterns and reduced food intake)

OCCUPATIONAL AND ENVIRONMENTAL HEALTH

Feeding the population of New York City would require an area of agricultural land roughly double the size of New York State, illustrating the need to produce large volumes of food and sometimes transport it long distances (Peters, Bills, Lembo, Wilkins, & Fick, 2008). Providing these needs requires a legion of food producers, processors, distributors, and retailers—constituting the **food supply chain**—who provide roughly 480,000 metric tons of food (including imports), or 3.4 pounds per citizen, each day, to US consumers (US Department of Agriculture Economic Research Service, 2013). In the United States, these enterprises collectively employ roughly one-fifth of the nation's private workforce (Food and Agriculture Organization of the United Nations, 2009; Food Chain Workers Alliance, 2012). The provision of food and livelihoods are pillars of a functioning society, but the value of these services arguably does not absolve food and agricultural industries of responsibility for a range of occupational and environmental health risks associated with their practices.

food supply chain
People, activities, and resources involved in getting food from farms, ranches, waters, and other sources to consumers; major stages include production, processing, distribution, retail

industrial food animal production (IFAP)
An approach to meat, dairy, and egg production characterized by specialized operations designed for a high rate of production, large numbers of animals confined at high density, large quantities of localized animal waste, and substantial inputs of financial capital, fossil fuel, feed, pharmaceuticals, and indirect inputs embodied in feed (e.g., fuel and freshwater)

pesticides
Natural or synthetic chemicals used with the intent of killing, repelling, or controlling populations of target organisms ("pests") that interfere with human interests; includes insecticides (targeted to insects), herbicides (targeted to plants), and fungicides (targeted to fungi)

Many food system workers face high risks of injury, infectious disease, and exposure to chemical contaminants. Furthermore, environmental hazards associated with food industries are not confined by property lines; nearby communities are often burdened by air, water, soil, and vector-borne threats to health. Concerns have been raised that production sites may also serve as the source of widespread disease outbreaks.

Some of these hazards are more commonly associated with industrialized operations that have come to dominate US food supply chains. Industrial crop production, for example, is characterized in part by large-scale, specialized, and mechanized farms that rely heavily on fossil fuels, pesticides, synthetic and mineral fertilizers, and other inputs. Similarly, **industrial food animal production (IFAP)** is characterized in part by specialized operations that confine large numbers of animals (and their waste) at high density, with heavy use of feed, pharmaceuticals, and other inputs. Chapters 11 and 12 describe these production methods in detail and provide insights into the types of practices that contribute to public health risks.

Pesticides

Pesticides include insecticides, herbicides, fungicides, and other natural and synthetic chemicals used with the intent of killing, repelling, or controlling populations of target organisms ("pests") (see figure 2.4). People may be exposed to pesticides through inhalation, direct skin contact, or ingestion (typically via contaminated food or water). Some pesticides pose low or negligible health risks; however, many have been associated with long-term adverse effects, including increased risks for certain cancers and disruption of the body's reproductive, immune, endocrine, and nervous systems (Horrigan, Walker, & Lawrence, 2002). As described in focus 2.1, some pesticides may also interfere with embryonic and fetal development and may be particularly harmful to children.

FIGURE 2.4 Worker Pouring Roundup for Use

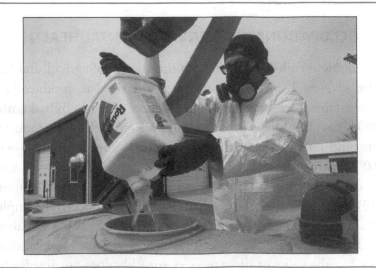

Source: Tim McCabe, USDA NRCS.

FOCUS 2.1. PESTICIDES AND CHILDREN'S HEALTH
Kristin S. Schafer

In a given day, children may absorb a wide range of potentially harmful pesticides from the food they eat, the water they drink, and the air they breathe. Public health experts point to dietary intake of pesticide residues as the primary form of children's exposure (Forman & Silverstein, 2012; National Research Council, 1993). Children of farmworkers are also at risk because they may receive especially high exposures, such as via air and residues on parents' clothing; occupational exposure is discussed in the main chapter text.

For young children, these exposures are occurring just as their bodies are at their most vulnerable. Additionally, because of their small size, a given dose will have a greater impact on a child than an adult. Scientific studies show that chronic exposures, even at very low levels, can cause a range of health harms.

Brain Architecture and Nervous System Harms

Public health experts have called the damage that chemicals are causing children's developing minds a "silent pandemic" (Grandjean & Landrigan, 2006, 2014), and scientists now point to a combination of genetic and environmental factors—including exposure to pesticides, which are known to harm nervous system development—to explain the rapid rise of developmental, learning, and behavioral disabilities (Landrigan, Lambertini, & Birnbaum, 2012; Szpir, 2006).

Recent studies leave little doubt that exposures to pesticides during fetal development, infancy, and childhood play a key role in compromising children's cognitive abilities. Prenatal exposure to low levels of neurotoxic pesticides, for example, has been shown to fundamentally alter brain architecture (Rauh, Perera, Horton, Whyatt, Bansal, & Hao, 2012; Selevan, Kimmel, & Mendola, 2000) and cause cognitive impairment including a significant (up to a seven-point) drop in IQ (Landrigan et al., 2012).

A recent comprehensive review of the science on health effects of pesticides by the Ontario College of Family Physicians (2012, p. 2) found exposure to pesticides in the womb to be "consistently associated with measurable deficits in child neurodevelopment." Evidence of neurodevelopmental harms linked to early life exposures is particularly strong for the class of pesticides known as organophosphates, including the widely used insecticide chlorpyrifos.

Cancer, Birth Defects, and More

Recent science also links pesticide exposure to a range of other childhood health harms, and many of these diseases and disorders are on the rise.

Childhood Cancers

A large number of recent studies link pesticide exposure to childhood leukemia, brain tumors, and neuroblastoma. Some evidence suggests pesticide exposure may also be associated with non-Hodgkin's lymphoma, Wilms' tumor, and Ewing's sarcoma. Many studies find in utero exposure and parental exposure before conception to be particularly important (Carozza Li, Elgethun, & Whitworth, 2008; Metayer & Buffler, 2008).

Birth Defects

Parents exposed to pesticides occupationally, from exposures in their community or by in-home pesticide use, may face increased risk of birth defects in their newborns. For example, several studies in agricultural areas correlate conception during peak pesticide spray season with increased birth defect risk (Winchester, Huskins, & Ying, 2009).

(Continued)

(Continued)

Timing of Puberty

Although the number of studies is relatively small, researchers have found some associations between pesticide exposure and pubertal effects. Most studies focus on in utero exposures to endocrine-disrupting pesticides that can interfere with the healthy development of the reproductive system—particularly if exposure occurs at certain times in the process (Biro, Greenspan, & Galvez, 2012). The majority of studies focus on precocious puberty in girls, but a few have also found links between pesticide exposure and changes in the timing of puberty among boys.

Obesity and Diabetes

So much new science exists about the links between obesity and environmental contaminants that a new term has emerged: *obesogen* (Holtcamp, 2012). Findings increasingly suggest that exposures to pesticides and other chemicals play a role by altering development in ways that raise the likelihood of obesity and related metabolic effects such as diabetes (Baillie-Hamilton, 2002).

Asthma

Many studies have explored the relative importance of common "respiratory irritants" in the home environment to triggering the onset of asthma, including cockroaches, dust mites, molds, and air pollutants. Many pesticides are considered respiratory irritants, and studies suggest that pesticide exposures may play a role in triggering asthma attacks, exacerbating symptoms, and heightening the overall risk of developing asthma (Hernández, Parrón, & Alarcón, 2011). Pesticides may also play a role in increasing asthma incidence by affecting the immune system, triggering either hypersensitivity or suppression of the immune response (Hernández et al., 2011).

For a more thorough review of the evidence linking pesticide exposure to children's health harms, see Pesticide Action Network's 2012 report, *A Generation in Jeopardy*, available online at www.panna.org/kids.

acute pesticide poisonings Any illness or health effects resulting from suspected or confirmed exposure to a pesticide within forty-eight hours

In the United States, the agricultural industry accounts for an estimated 75 percent of pesticide use. Among US agricultural workers, the majority of recent **acute pesticide poisonings** have resulted from pesticides drifting away from target areas, including toward agricultural workers involved in other activities. Workers can also be exposed by entering areas that were recently sprayed or by failing to follow safe usage guidelines. Acute poisonings have been implicated in short-term effects to skin, eyes, and nervous, gastrointestinal, respiratory, and cardiovascular systems, and may increase risks for chronic neurological, respiratory, and other health problems (Calvert et al., 2008). Pesticides may also drift into homes and schools, run off into nearby surface waters, or seep into ground water supplies. Once in the environment, some pesticides are known to persist and accumulate, contributing to long-term health and ecological harms.

Nitrates

Farmers may apply synthetic and mineral fertilizers, manure, and treated sewage sludge to crop fields. Without careful management, these practices can introduce excess nutrients into ground and surface waters, posing a range of public health harms. Nitrate contamination in drinking water, for example, has been linked to reproductive harms, diabetes, thyroid conditions, and certain cancers. Excess nutrients in surface waters may be linked to ecological feedback that negatively affects human health, including the proliferation of highly toxic marine micoorganisms. These and related concerns are discussed in chapters 3 and 12.

Pathogens

pathogens
Disease-causing organisms (e.g., *Staphylococcus aureus* [bacteria], *Influenza* [virus], and *Cryptosporidium* [parasite])

Poultry, hogs, cattle, and other animals raised for food harbor **pathogens** including certain bacteria, viruses, and parasites. As described in chapter 12, the conditions in IFAP operations present frequent opportunities for transmitting pathogens from animals to humans. In production and processing operations, for example, workers may be in contact with large volumes of animals, carcasses, and animal waste, and may spread these pathogens into their homes and communities. Animal waste applied to nearby land may run off into nearby surface waters and leach into groundwater, transporting pathogens (and chemical contaminants) along with it. Pathogens may be blown out of IFAP operations by ventilation systems, and carried downwind, and transported by flies and other vectors into surrounding communities (Graham et al., 2008).

Pathogen concerns are heightened by the rising prevalence of bacteria that are resistant to antibiotics, making infections more difficult and expensive to treat. In 2005, methicillin-resistant *Staphylococcus aureus*—a resistant strain of the bacteria commonly known as *staph*—was responsible for an estimated ninety-four thousand infections and over eighteen thousand deaths in the United States (Klevens et al., 2013). The evolution of antibiotic resistance is often attributed to the use of antibiotics in medicine; however, a growing body of evidence has implicated antibiotic use in IFAP as a major contributor to the proliferation and spread of resistant pathogens (see chapter 12).

Airborne Hazards from IFAP

People working in and near IFAP facilities are frequently exposed to airborne hazards such as gases emitted from animal waste, bacterial toxins, and airborne particulates. Adverse health effects among workers in indoor IFAP operations have been widely documented, including reduced lung function, bronchitis, and acute respiratory distress syndrome—a life-threatening condition that prevents the lungs from supplying the body with adequate oxygen. High rates of respiratory symptoms—as well as headaches, anxiety, depression, sleep disturbances, and other physiological and psychological effects—have also been documented among communities near IFAP operations (see chapter 12).

Injury Hazards

Injury rates among employees in major food production, processing, distribution, and retail industries are over 50 percent higher than the average for US private industries (see figure 2.5 and table 2.2). An estimated 20 percent of work-related fatalities occur in these industries, which employ only 15 percent of the private workforce. These rates are averaged across many types of businesses and conceal the fact that some food system occupations are much more severely affected. Chapter 12 and Focus 2.2 below, discuss injury hazards in greater depth.

FIGURE 2.5   Nearly One in Five Meat Processing Workers Is Injured Each Year

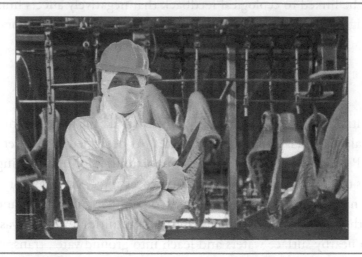

Source: Industrial butcher. Corespics Vof | Dreamstime.com.

TABLE 2.2   Work-Related Injuries and Fatalities Associated with Selected Food System Industries

Industry	Injuries per Hundred Full-time Workers, 2011	Fatalities, 2010*	Annual Average Employment (Thousands), 2011
Beer, wine, and distilled alcoholic beverage merchant wholesalers	7.2	12	164.3
Beverage manufacturing	7.0	5	169.2
Seafood product preparation and packaging	6.5	5	36.1
Animal production	6.4	153	163.6
Grocery and related products merchant wholesalers	5.7	26	717.9
Dairy product manufacturing	5.5	6	133.8
Crop production	5.1	323	413.8
Fruit and vegetable preserving and specialty food manufacturing	5.0	6	174.2
Animal slaughtering and processing	4.8	11	487.8
Bakeries	4.7	14	283.2
Support activities for agriculture and forestry	4.6	35	331.7
Sugar and confectionary product manufacturing	4.6	NR	66.7
Food and beverage stores	4.6	79	2,859.7
Other food manufacturing	4.5	5	166.4
Fishing, hunting, and trapping	3.8	37	8.6
Food service and drinking places	3.5	122	9,619.1
Grain and oilseed milling	3.0	5	59.2
All US private industries	3.3	4,206	107,654.2**

*Note that fatalities are counts rather than rates; industries with fewer employees typically have fewer deaths.
**Includes food system and non-food-related industries
NR = none reported
Source: Bureau of Labor Statistics (2013).

FOCUS 2.2. FOOD SYSTEM WORKERS AT RISK
Roni A. Neff and Megan L. Clayton

Food system workers experience exceptionally high injury, illness, and fatality rates, as well as challenges in protecting their rights. They are disproportionately minorities and immigrants who earn low wages with few benefits and work in jobs characterized by repetitive tasks, little decision making, and a lack of workplace power (Food and Agriculture Organization of the United Nations, 2009; Food Chain Workers Alliance, 2012).

Table 2.1 in the main text presents reported occupational injury and fatality rates for food system industries. High rates result from direct hazards: use of machinery, vehicles, and sharp tools; extreme temperatures; heavy objects; repetitive tasks; slippery surfaces; and pathogen and chemical exposures. These rates tell one part of the story; but nationally, only one-third to two-thirds of nonfatal occupational injuries are reported (Leigh, Marcin, & Miller, 2004) and reported occupational illnesses generally include only the most obviously work-related and short-latency conditions. This underreporting worsens injury and illness by limiting employers' incentives to improve conditions, diminishing government and public attention to the issue, and preventing appropriate targeting of interventions.

Inadequate Safety Interventions

In one survey of workers across food sectors, 52 percent reported that they did not receive health or safety training and 33 percent indicated that employers did not always provide necessary work equipment (Food Chain Workers Alliance, 2012). Many workers also face language and literacy barriers. Even when training and related resources are available, workers may not comprehend messages or labels, and may miss warnings in emergent situations.

Employers have few incentives to implement preventive interventions. Staffing at the US Occupational Safety and Health Administration (OSHA) is so low that the agency can inspect each workplace only once every 131 years on average. Further, the average fine for a "serious" violation was just $2,107 in FY 2011. Only eighty-four criminal cases have *ever* been prosecuted, despite hundreds of thousands of worker deaths since Congress created OSHA in the 1970s (AFL-CIO, 2012). Many employers find it cheaper to deal with the costs of injuries and illnesses (including in workers' compensation premiums, absenteeism, presenteeism [being at work but not fully present], turnover, and occasional enforcement) than to invest in prevention.

Rights in the Workplace

Workers are legally allowed to refuse tasks if they believe there is imminent danger. In a recent survey of food workers, however, nearly 12 percent reported being required to do something that put their safety at risk (Food and Agriculture Organization of the United Nations, 2009; Food Chain Workers Alliance, 2012). In meat process-ing industries, for example, production pressures create risks such as mandatory overtime, inadequate breaks, and production speeds faster than workers can safely handle. Across the food chain, workers report that asking for time off to deal with injury or illness can lead to employer threats or even termination (Food Chain Workers Alliance, 2012).

Policies that exempt workers from basic labor protections and lenient regulation limit workers' abilities to protect health and safety. This is especially true for farmworkers, who are exempt from rights to overtime pay and collective bargaining; and, altogether, few food workers are unionized.

When workers become injured or ill due to workplace exposures, most should be covered by workers' compensation—employer-funded and state-run insurance funds providing medical care and steady income to injured workers. In practice, however, many cases are never reported, and workers on small farms are exempt

(Continued)

(Continued)

(Arcury, Grzywacz, Sidebottom, & Wiggins, 2013). One Washington State study found that the farming-forestry-fishing sector had both the highest rate of reported injury and illness in the state and the second lowest workers' compensation claim filing rate (Fan, Bonauto, Foley, & Silverstein, 2006).

Child Labor, Slavery

Child labor and cases prosecuted by the US Department of Justice using laws forbidding peonage, indentured servitude and trafficking have been found in US agricultural and other food processing work (Lo & Jacobsen, 2011). An estimated 400,000 of the 1.4 to 3 million US migrant and seasonal farmworkers are children, some as young as six (Association of Farmworker Opportunity Programs, nd). Food and agricultural workers have been found in chains, housed in box trucks, and found to be victims of physical and sexual abuse (Lo & Jacobsen, 2011).

Conclusion

Consumers receive next to no information about the treatment of workers who produce, process, distribute, and sell their food. Some campaigns have started to change this, including the Coalition of Immokalee Workers' efforts to publicize conditions for tomato workers and efforts to promote fair trade products such as coffees, as well as new campaigns from the Restaurant Opportunities Centers United and Food Chain Workers Alliance. Some people avoid meat out of concern for animal and environmental welfare. Should worker welfare also play a role in our food choices?

FOOD SAFETY

food safety
Generally refers to the prevention of health risks associated with contaminated food

food-borne illnesses
Illness resulting from recent ingestion of contaminated food (e.g., with microbial pathogens or toxins)

The US food supply has been described as the safest in the world, but the accuracy of this claim depends on the criteria for "safe." It has been suggested that if standardized criteria were applied to an international ranking system, the United States would rank well on some **food safety** criteria (e.g., pesticide residues) but poorly on others (e.g., animal drug and hormone residues) (Wirt, 2004). Food supplies are susceptible to many types of contaminants. **Food-borne illnesses** are typically the result of recent exposure to bacterial, viral, or parasitic pathogens, or toxins produced by certain microorganisms. By contrast, exposure to chemical contaminants in food, such as pesticides and heavy metals, may contribute to long-term risks for chronic health problems, such as cancer. This section of the chapter explores both types of contaminants, exposure routes, and health impacts.

Food-borne Illness

Each year, about one in six Americans gets sick from contaminated food or beverages, resulting in roughly 130,000 hospitalizations and 3,000 deaths (CDC, 2011b). Approximately one thousand food-borne illness outbreaks are reported annually in the United States—such as the outbreak of *Salmonella* in 2010, linked to eggs, which sickened nearly two thousand people (CDC, 2010). Contaminated

TABLE 2.3 Selected Pathogens Commonly Responsible for Food-borne Illness in the United States, 2000–2008

Pathogen	Type	Estimated Annual Food-borne Illnesses		Estimated Annual Deaths from Food-borne Illness		Commonly Associated Foods
Norovirus	Virus	5,500,000	(58%)	150	(11%)	Salads, sandwiches
Salmonella spp.,*nontyphoidal	Bacteria	1,000,000	(11%)	380	(28%)	Eggs, meat
Clostridium perfringens	Bacteria	970,000	(10%)	26	(2%)	Beef, poultry, gravies
Campylobacter spp.	Bacteria	850,000	(9%)	76	(6%)	Poultry
Staphylococcus aureus	Bacteria	240,000	(3%)	6	(<1%)	Dairy, deli meats
E. coli spp.*	Bacteria	210,000	(2%)	21	(2%)	Ground beef, leafy greens
Toxoplasma gondii	Parasite	87,000	(1%)	330	(24%)	Meat
Vibrio spp.*	Bacteria	52,000	(1%)	48	(4%)	Seafood
Listeria monocytogenes	Bacteria	1,600	(<1%)	260	(19%)	Deli meats, produce
Total for thirty-one known pathogens		9,400,000		1,400		
Total for all known pathogens and unspecific agents		47,800,000		3,000		

Note: Figures rounded to two significant digits.
Species pluralis (spp.) is Latin for "multiple species."
**84 percent of food-borne illness cases had unidentified causes.
Source: Scallan et al. (2011).

food poses serious risks to those who are exposed, causing conditions such as fever, nausea, diarrhea, chronic illness, and, in some cases, death. Vulnerable populations—very young or old people or those with weakened immune systems—are at an increased risk of poorer health outcomes from food-borne illnesses. Antibiotic resistant strains of bacterial pathogens (see chapter 12) heighten these concerns. Table 2.3 describes some of the more common pathogens responsible for food-borne illness.

The food supply is susceptible to microbial contamination at multiple points along the supply chain:

Production As discussed in chapter 12, microbial contamination of food is often attributable to animal waste from IFAP operations. For example, if groundwater sources are contaminated with animal waste, and that water is used for irrigation, pathogens and other contaminants may be transferred to crops.

Processing The widespread nature of food-borne illness outbreaks is a consequence, at least in part, of processing plants sourcing raw materials from a large number of producers and distributing products over a broad geographic area. For example, if a shipment of spinach from one farm is contaminated with *E. coli* (as in the 2006 case of bagged spinach [CDC, 2006]) and gets mixed together with greens from other farms before being nationally distributed, the entire batch may become contaminated. As author Michael Pollan (2006) writes, "In effect, we're washing the whole nation's salad in one big sink." Similarly, an entire shipment of ground beef or poultry can be tainted by a single contaminated carcass.

FIGURE 2.6 *Salmonella*

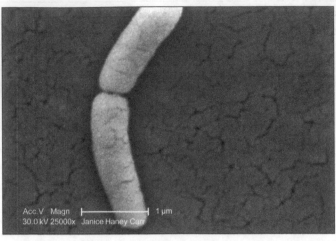

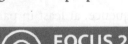

Source: CDC 10993, Janice Haney Carr.

Distribution Containers used to ship and store food present opportunities for contamination, particularly if they are not properly disinfected. Studies of tanker trucks used to transport dairy products, for example, have found populations of *Salmonella* (figure 2.6) and *Listeria* bacteria at levels high enough to pose health risks to consumers (Van Kessel, Karns, Gorski, McCluskey, & Perdue, 2004).

Retail and Preparation Contaminants can be introduced or spread by people who handle food in home and commercial kitchens. Food, utensils, and surfaces such as countertops and cutting boards are all susceptible to contamination by pathogens. Noroviruses—the most common known cause of food-borne illness—are typically spread this way. The symptoms of Norovirus infection—inflammation of the intestinal lining (**gastroenteritis**), vomiting, diarrhea, fever, and chills—are often misattributed to "stomach flu." Handwashing, disinfecting surfaces and utensils, avoiding cross-contamination with raw meat, and cooking food thoroughly can help prevent food-borne illness. In restaurants and other settings where workers handle food, offering paid sick days and ensuring access to sinks, soap, and running water are important preventive measures. Additionally, at all points along the supply chain, including distribution, retail, and home storage, perishable foods and ingredients must be stored under specific conditions—such as controlled temperatures—to inhibit the growth of pathogens.

gastroenteritis
Inflammation of the intestinal lining (e.g., as a result of *Norovirus* infection)

Chemical Contaminants in Food

Pesticide residues, heavy metals, and certain food preservatives and colorants are among the many chemicals found in the food supply that may pose health risks to consumers who ingest them. Chemical contaminants in food may be synthetic, such as bisphenol-A (see focus 2.3), or of natural origin, such as fungal toxins (e.g., aflatoxin) produced by molds that can infest agricultural products such as grains and nuts. Arsenic is an example of a chemical that is naturally occurring and used for industrial and agricultural purposes.

FOCUS 2.3. BISPHENOL-A: A UBIQUITOUS FOOD SYSTEM CONTAMINANT

Jennifer C. Hartle

endocrine disruption
Chemical interference with the body's endocrine system, which may result in adverse developmental, reproductive, neurological, and immune effects in humans and wildlife

Bisphenol-A (BPA), a synthetic chemical first approved for use in food packaging in the 1960s (US Food and Drug Administration [FDA], 2013), is now a pervasive contaminant of the food system because of its widespread application in food storage materials. The migration of BPA from packaging into food creates a public health concern because BPA can alter the body's hormonal actions (vom Saal et al., 2007). This phenomenon is called **endocrine disruption**.

Agencies regulating BPA in the United States currently place only limited restrictions on its use, maintaining the perspective that low-dose health effects seen in animal experiments have not been reliably reproduced (Environmental Protection Agency, 2013; FDA, 2013). Some countries recognize the potential harm of BPA with a **precautionary approach**, meaning they develop protective policies on a precautionary basis, even when there remains scientific uncertainty about the cause-and-effect relationship between exposures and health outcomes.

BPA is widely utilized because its chemical structure is well suited for use in manufacturing polycarbonate plastics, epoxy resins, and flexible polyvinyl chloride (PVC) products. In the food system, BPA can be found in plastic food delivery and storage materials. Epoxy resins made from BPA line the inside of canned foods, beverages, and glass jar lids. Plastic cling wrap is often made with PVC that contains BPA. BPA is also detectable in paperboard food containers as a result of thermal receipts with BPA color developer being introduced into the recycled paper stream (Ozaki, Yamaguchi, Fujita, Kuroda, & Endo, 2004). In the environment, BPA contamination can be measured in household dust, indoor and outdoor air (Wilson, Chuang, Morgan, Lordo, & Sheldon, 2007), in water polluted by runoff from landfills, and waste from water treatment plants (Kang, Kondo, & Katayama, 2006).

With so many contributing sources, BPA exposure in the human population is ubiquitous. BPA has been measured in the urine of 92.6 percent of the US population (Calafat, Ye, Wong, Reidy, & Needham, 2008). Dietary ingestion is the main contributor of BPA exposure, accounting for 99 percent of total exposure in preschoolers (Wilson et al., 2007) and 74 to 88 percent for children six to twelve years old (von Goetz, Wormuth, Scheringer, & Hungerbuhler, 2010). These exposures can be detected throughout the human body including in serum, urine, saliva, breast milk, semen, amniotic fluid, and follicular fluid (Vandenberg, Hauser, Marcus, Olea, & Welshons, 2007).

When humans ingest BPA, it is biotransformed in the liver into bisphenol-A-glucuronide, a highly water-soluble metabolite (by-product of digestion). This metabolite is then rapidly excreted by the kidneys with urine. By monitoring BPA doses administered to healthy adults from ingestion to excretion, evidence shows that BPA is completely cleared from the body in twenty-four hours (Volkel et al., 2002). There is concern that BPA metabolism may not be as efficient in vulnerable populations, such as fetuses, infants, and children, because their systems are still developing (Kang et al., 2006). Dermal (skin) absorption and inhalation of BPA, the main routes of exposure for occupational settings, are of concern because exposures from these pathways are able to circumvent the liver and enter the circulatory system directly (Vandenberg et al., 2007).

As an endocrine disruptor, BPA's estrogen-mimicking abilities may adversely affect reproductive development in both sexes. BPA exposure could be contributing to increases in rates of heart disease, diabetes, and obesity, as well as brain development issues, altered behaviors, and some cancers (Vandenberg et al., 2007; vom Saal et al., 2007). In the occupational setting, where exposures can be much higher than in the general population, BPA exposure could be affecting reproductive hormones (National Toxicology Program, 2008).

BPA is no longer approved for manufacturing polycarbonate baby bottles and toddler drinking cups in the United States; however, other food system uses and environmental releases remain unregulated. Figure 2.7 illustrates how the current regulatory structure allows BPA to contaminate the food system, consumer products, and the environment. This creates potential for human exposure, and, ultimately, possible adverse health effects. Many public health advocates believe there is sufficient evidence of BPA's harmfulness to support the adoption of a precautionary approach to protect public health while additional scientific evidence is being collected.

precautionary approach Approach based on the idea that if an activity raises significant threat of harm to human health or the environment, it should be stopped or slowed (e.g., precautionary measures should be taken) even if the cause-and-effect relationships are not fully established by scientific evidence; places the burden of proof that the activity is not harmful on the activity's proponent (e.g., a manufacturer); also precautionary principle

(Continued)

(Continued)

FIGURE 2.7   BPA Exposure Framework

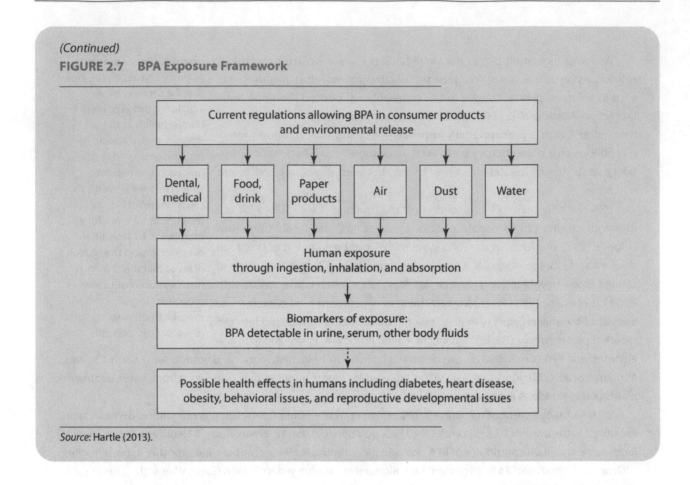

Source: Hartle (2013).

Dougherty (2000) estimated the levels at which typical US consumers ingest thirty-seven chemicals associated with adverse health effects. The study highlighted six chemicals of particular concern, primarily because of their effects on cancer risk and the estimated amounts at which Americans ingest them in food: chlordane, DDT, and dieldrin (pesticides); arsenic; and dioxins and polychlorinated biphenyls (industrial chemicals). Exposure to these six chemicals was predominantly attributable to seafood consumption—illustrating the potential for certain chemicals to contaminant marine environments, where they may persist and accumulate in the aquatic food chain even long after their use is discontinued (DDT, for example, was banned in the United States in the 1970s). Although greatly overshadowed by contributions from seafood, beef was a substantial contributor to dietary DDT, dieldrin, and dioxin intake, and rice was a substantial contributor to dietary arsenic intake.

There are many other chemicals that weren't on the top-six list for this study but that still pose public health concerns. Mercury, for example, is a heavy metal that can accumulate in fatty tissues. When people eat foods contaminated with mercury, such as tuna and other large predatory fish, the metal accumulates in their bodies and can cause brain and kidney problems later in life. Coal-fired power plants are the predominant anthropogenic source of mercury emissions. (Air emissions settle to earth and eventually enter the aquatic food chain.)

Fruits and vegetables were negligible in their contributions to the six particular chemicals highlighted in the aforementioned study. However, consumers may still wish to reduce their dietary pesticide exposure by washing produce well or choosing organic varieties—particularly for the items listed

TABLE 2.4 The Twelve Conventionally Grown Fruits and Vegetables Most Contaminated with Pesticides

1.	Apples
2.	Celery
3.	Cherry tomatoes
4.	Cucumbers
5.	Grapes
6.	Hot peppers
7.	Nectarines (imported)
8.	Peaches
9.	Potatoes
10.	Spinach
11.	Strawberries
12.	Sweet bell peppers

Note: Additionally, conventional kale, collard greens, and summer squash may contain pesticide residues of special concern.
Source: Environmental Working Group (2013).

in Table 2.4. Lu, Toepel, Irish, Fenske, Barr, and Bravo (2006) found that after children switched from conventional to organic produce, traces of several chemical pesticides in their urine dropped to undetectable levels. Eating conventionally grown produce is recommended over not eating fruits and vegetables at all, because the health benefits of diets rich in fruits and vegetables outweigh the risks of pesticide exposure. The child health effects of chronic exposure to pesticides are discussed in focus 2.1.

CONCLUSION

The food system intersects with health at all stages of the supply chain. As discussed in chapters throughout this book, citizens can leverage these relationships for a healthier food system, such as by advocating for government policies that mitigate food system harms and promote safer alternatives. Additionally, the combined effect of our dietary choices—"voting with our forks"—can send market signals that help transform food supply chains in ways that protect and promote health.

SUMMARY

Food production, processing, distribution, retail, and consumption play integral roles in promoting health and wellness, and also contribute to a range of public health harms. Certain compounds in fruits and vegetables, for example, play key roles in optimizing the body's systems and building reserves against forces averse to good health. The standard American diet, by contrast, has been implicated as a contributor to a range of chronic illness, including obesity, cardiovascular disease, type 2 diabetes, and various cancers. These conditions have reached epidemic proportions in the United States and exert a heavy public health and economic toll. Additionally, the industries involved in producing food and getting it onto US plates support populations by providing employment and an abundant food supply, but they also contribute to occupational and environmental health harms, including via exposures to chemical, microbial, and physical hazards. Preventive measures can be effective in reducing these risks.

KEY TERMS

Acute pesticide poisonings	Gastroenteritis
Cancer	Health promotion
Cardiovascular disease (CVD)	Heart disease
Cerebrovascular disease	Hypertension
Chronic diseases	Industrial food animal production (IFAP)
Coronary artery disease	Morbidity
Diabetes	Obese
Diet-related diseases	Pathogens
Endocrine disruption	Pesticides
Energy density	Phytonutrients
Epidemiologic transition	Precautionary approach (or principle)
Food-borne illnesses	Prediabetes
Food insecurity	Satiety
Food safety	Standard American Diet (SAD)
Food supply chain	Type 2 diabetes

DISCUSSION QUESTIONS

1. What are some indicators that could be used to measure the magnitude of different public health problems related to the food system? Discuss their strengths and limitations.

2. What has led to the rise in diet-related disease in the United States?

3. Which of the public health challenges associated with the food system receive the most attention in the media and why? Is the media's attention appropriately focused, and if not, how should its focus be shifted?

4. Efforts to enact policies intended to protect health (e.g., a soda tax) are often countered by arguments placing blame on nondietary factors (e.g., "soda is not the problem, it's lack of exercise"). Indeed, it is challenging to determine how much of a given health outcome is attributable to diet versus other risk factors. How should these arguments be addressed?

5. It has been argued that public health risks associated with an industrial food system are justified by the need to "feed the world." Do you agree? Why or why not? Is it possible to have a food system that produces abundantly and is widely protective of health?

6. What are the costs and benefits of taking a precautionary approach to regulation?

7. What does it mean for our food to be "safe"? How do we know when it is safe?

REFERENCES

AFL-CIO. (2012). *Death on the job*. Retrieved from www.aflcio.org/content/download/22781/259751/DOTJ2012 nobugFINAL.pdf

Arcury, T. A., Grzywacz, J. G., Sidebottom, J., & Wiggins, M. F. (2013). Overview of immigrant worker occupational health and safety for the agriculture, forestry, and fishing (AgFF) sector in the Southeastern United States. *American Journal of Industrial Medicine*, *56*(8), 911–924.

Association of Farmworker Opportunity Programs. (nd). *Children in the fields: Learn the facts*. Retrieved from http://afop.org/children-in-thefields/learn-the-facts/#AFOP_estimates

Baillie-Hamilton, P. F. (2002). Chemical toxins: A hypothesis to explain the global obesity epidemic. *Journal of Alternative and Complementary Medicine*, *8*, 185–192.

Biro, F. M., Greenspan, L. C., & Galvez, M. P. (2012). Puberty in girls in the 21st century. *Journal of Pediatric and Adolescent Gynecology*, *25*(5), 289–294.

Breslow, L. (1999). From disease prevention to health promotion. *Journal of the American Medical Association*, *281*(11), 1030–1033.

Brillat-Savarin, A. (1842). *Physiologie du gout, ou meditations de gastronomie transcendante*. Paris: Auguste Sautelet.

Bureau of Labor Statistics. (2013). *Injuries, illnesses, and fatalities*. Retrieved from www.bls.gov/iif

Calafat, A. M., Ye, X., Wong, L. Y., Reidy, J. A., & Needham, L. L. (2008). Exposure of the U.S. population to bisphenol-A and 4-tertiary-octylphenol: 2003–2004. *Environmental Health Perspectives*, *116*(1), 39–44.

Calvert, G. M., Karnik, Á. J., Mehler, L., Beckman, J., Morrissey, B., Sievert, J., … Moraga-Mchaley, S. (2008). Acute pesticide poisoning among agricultural workers in the United States, 1998–2005. *American Journal of Industrial Medicine*, *51*, 883–898.

Carkeet, C., Grann, K., Randolph, R. K., Venzon, D. S., & Izzy, S. M. (Eds.). (2012). *Phytochemicals: Health promotion and therapeutic potential*. Boca Raton, FL: CRC Press.

Carozza Li, B., Elgethun, K., & Whitworth, R. (2008). Risk of childhood cancers associated with residence in agriculturally intense areas in the United States. *Environmental Health Perspectives*, *116*(4), 559–565.

Centers for Disease Control and Prevention. (2006). *Multi-state outbreak of E. coli O157:H7 infections from spinach*. Retrieved from www.cdc.gov/ecoli/2006/september

Centers for Disease Control and Prevention. (2010). *Investigation update: Multistate outbreak of human salmonella enteritidis infections associated with shell eggs*. Retrieved from www.cdc.gov/salmonella/enteritidis

Centers for Disease Control and Prevention. (2011a). *National diabetes fact sheet: National estimates and general information on diabetes and prediabetes in the United States, 2011*. Atlanta, GA: Author.

Centers for Disease Control and Prevention. (2011b). Vital signs: Incidence and trends of infection with pathogens transmitted commonly through food—Foodborne diseases active surveillance network, 10 U.S. Sites, 1996–2010. *Morbidity and Mortality Weekly Report*, *60*(22), 749–755.

Coleman-Jensen, A., Nord, M., Andrews, M., & Carlson, S. (2011). Household food security in the United States in 2010. *Advances in Nutrition*, *2*, 153–154.

Danaei, G., Ding, E. L., Mozaffarian, D., Taylor, B., Rehm, J., Murray, C.J.L., & Ezzati, M. (2009). The preventable causes of death in the United States: Comparative risk assessment of dietary, lifestyle, and metabolic risk factors. *PLoS, Medicine 6*(4), e1000058.

Dougherty, C. (2000). Dietary exposures to food contaminants across the United States. *Environmental Research*, *84*(2), 170–185.

Environmental Protection Agency. (2013). *Bisphenol-A (BPA) action plan summary*. Retrieved from www.epa.gov/oppt/existingchemicals/pubs/actionplans/bpa.html

Environmental Working Group. (2013). *EWG's 2013 shopper's guide to pesticides in produce*. Retrieved from www.ewg.org/foodnews/summary.php

Fan, Z. J., Bonauto, D. K., Foley, M. P., & Silverstein, B. A. (2006). Underreporting of work-related injury or illness to workers' compensation: Individual and industry factors. *Journal of Occupational and Environmental Medicine*, *48*(9), 914–922.

Finkelstein, E. A., Trogdon, J. G., Cohen, J. W., & Dietz, W. (2009). Annual medical spending attributable to obesity: Payer-and service-specific estimates. *Health Affairs (Project Hope)*, *28*(5), w822–w831.

Fontaine, K. R., & Barofsky, I. (2001). Obesity and health-related quality of life. *Obesity Reviews*, *2*(3), 173–182.

Food and Agriculture Organization of the United Nations. (2009). *The state of food and agriculture: Livestock in the balance*. Rome: Author. Retrieved from www.fao.org/docrep/012/i0680e/i0680e.pdf

Food Chain Workers Alliance. (2012). *The hands that feed us: Challenges and opportunities for workers along the food chain*. Retrieved from http://foodchainworkers.org/wp-content/uploads/2012/06/Hands-That-Feed-Us-Report.pdf

Forman, J., & Silverstein, J. (2012). Organic foods: Health and environmental advantages and disadvantages. *Pediatrics*, *130*(5), e1406–e1410.

Frellick, M. (2013, July 9). Obesity as disease? Physicians debate the pros and cons of AMA decision. *Heartwire*. Chicago, IL. Retrieved from www.medscape.com/viewarticle/793302

Fryar, C. D., Carroll, M. D., & Ogden, C. L. (2012a). *Prevalence of overweight, obesity, and extreme obesity among adults: United States, trends 1960–1962 through 2009–2010*. NCHS Health E-stat. Retrieved from www.cdc.gov/nchs/data/hestat/obesity_adult_09_10/obesity_adult_09_10.htm

Fryar, C. D., Carroll, M. D., & Ogden, C. L. (2012b). *Prevalence of obesity among children and adolescents: United States, Trends 1963–1965 through 2009–2010*. NCHS Health E-stat. Retrieved from www.cdc.gov/nchs/data/hestat/obesity_child_09_10/obesity_child_09_10.htm

Go, A. S., Mozaffarian, D., Roger, V. L., Benjamin, E. J., Berry, J. D., Borden, W. B., ... Turner, M. B. (2013). Heart disease and stroke statistics—2013 update: A report from the American Heart Association. *Circulation*, *127*(1), e6–e245.

Graham, J. P., Leibler, J. H., Price, L. B., Otte, J. M., Pfeiffer, D. U., Tiensin, T., & Silbergeld, E. K. (2008). The animal-human interface and infectious disease in industrial food animal production: Rethinking biosecurity and biocontainment. *Public Health Reports*, *123*(3), 282–299.

Grandjean, P., & Landrigan, P. J. (2006). Developmental neurotoxicity of industrial chemicals. *Lancet*, *368*(9553), 2167–2178.

Grandjean, P., & Landrigan, P. J. (2014). Neurobehavioural effects of developmental toxicity. *Lancet Neurology*, *13*(3), 330–338.

Hartle, J. C. (2013). *Food system contributions to bisphenol-A exposures*. DrPH dissertation. Baltimore, MD: Johns Hopkins University.

Heidenreich, P. A., Trogdon, J. G., Khavjou, O. A., Butler, J., Dracup, K., Ezekowitz, M. D., ... Woo, Y. J. (2011). Forecasting the future of cardiovascular disease in the United States: A policy statement from the American Heart Association. *Circulation*, *123*(8), 933–944.

Hernández, A. F., Parrón, T., & Alarcón, R. (2011). Pesticides and asthma. *Current Opinion in Allergy and Clinical Immunology*, *11*, 90–96

Holtcamp, W. (2012). Obesogens: An environmental link to obesity. *Environmental Health Perspectives*, *120*(2), a62–a68.

Horrigan, L., Walker, P., & Lawrence, R. S. (2002). How sustainable agriculture can address the environmental and public health harms of industrial agriculture. *Environmental Health Perspectives*, *110*(5), 445–456.

Huang, E. S., Basu, A., O'Grady, M., & Capretta, J. C. (2009). Projecting the future diabetes population size and related costs for the U.S. *Diabetes Care*, *32*(12), 2225–2229.

Hung, H.-C., Joshipura, K. J., Jiang, R., Hu, F. B., Hunter, D., Smith-Warner, S. A., ... Willett, W. C. (2004). Fruit and vegetable intake and risk of major chronic disease. *Journal of the National Cancer Institute*, *96*(21), 1577–1584.

Kang, J. H., Kondo, F., & Katayama, Y. (2006). Human exposure to bisphenol A. *Toxicology*, *226*(2–3), 79–89.

Key, T. J., Allen, N. E., Spencer, E. A., & Travis, R. C. (2002). The effect of diet on risk of cancer. *Lancet*, *360*(9336), 861–868.

Klevens, R. M., Morrison, M. A., Nadle, J., Petit, S., Gershman, K., Ray, S., ... Fridkin, S. K. (2013). Invasive methicillin-resistant staphylococcus aureus infections in the United States, *298*(15), 1763–1771.

Koeth, R. A., Wang, Z., Levison, B. S., Buffa, J. A., Org, E., Sheehy, B. T., ... Hazen, S. L. (2013). Intestinal microbiota metabolism of l-carnitine, a nutrient in red meat, promotes atherosclerosis. *Nature Medicine*, *19*(April), 1–12.

Landrigan, P. J., Lambertini, L., & Birnbaum, L. S. (2012). A research strategy to discover the environmental causes of autism and neurodevelopmental disabilities. *Environmental Health Perspective*, *120*, a258–a260.

Leigh, J. P., Marcin, J. P., & Miller, T. R. (2004). An estimate of the US government's undercount of nonfatal occupational injuries. *Journal of Occupational and Environmental Medicine*, *46*(1), 10–18.

Lo, J., & Jacobson, A. (2011). Human rights from field to fork: Improving labor conditions for food sector workers by organizing across boundaries. *Race/Ethnicity: Multidisciplinary Global Contexts*, *5*(1), 61–82.

Lu, C., Toepel, K., Irish, R., Fenske, R. A., Barr, D. B., & Bravo, R. (2006). Organic diets significantly lower children's dietary exposure to organophosphorus pesticides. *Environmental Health Perspectives*, *114*(2), 260.

Malik, V. S., Popkin, B. M., Bray, G. A., Depres, J.-P., Willett, W. C., & Hu, F. B. (2010). Sugar-sweetened beverages and risk of metabolic syndrome and type 2 diabetes. *Diabetes Care*, *33*(11), 2477–2483.

Malik, V. S., Willett, W. C., & Hu, F. B. (2013). Global obesity: Trends, risk factors and policy implications. *Nature reviews. Endocrinology*, *9*(1), 13–27.

Mariotto, A. B., Yabroff, K. R., Shao, Y., Feuer, E. J., & Brown, M. L. (2011). Projections of the cost of cancer care in the United States: 2010–2020. *Journal of the National Cancer Institute*, *103*(2), 117–128.

Metayer, C., & Buffler, P. A. (2008). Residential exposures to pesticides and childhood leukaemia. *Radiation Protection Dosimetry*, *132*(2), 212–219.

Micha, R., Michas, G., & Mozaffarian, D. (2012). Unprocessed red and processed meats and risk of coronary artery disease and type 2 diabetes—An updated review of the evidence. *Current Atherosclerosis Reports*, *14*(6), 515–524.

National Research Council. (1993). *Pesticides in the diets of infants and children*. Washington, DC: National Academies Press.

National Toxicology Program. (2008). *NTP-CERHR monograph on the potential human reproductive and developmental effects of bisphenol-A*. Research Triangle Park, NC: Author.

Omran, A. R. (1971). The epidemiologic transition: A theory of the epidemiology of population change. *The Milbank Memorial Fund Quarterly*, *49*(4), 509–538.

Ozaki, A., Yamaguchi, Y., Fujita, T., Kuroda, K., & Endo, G. (2004). Chemical analysis and genotoxicological safety assessment of paper and paperboard used for food packaging. *Food and Chemical Toxicology*, *42*(8), 1323–1337.

Pan, A., Sun, Q., Bernstein, A. M., Schulze, M. B., Manson, J. E., Stampfer, M. J., ... Hu, F. B. (2012). Red meat consumption and mortality: Results from 2 prospective cohort studies. *Archives of Internal Medicine*, *172*(7), 555–563.

Peters, C. J., Bills, N. L., Lembo, A. J., Wilkins, J. L., & Fick, G. W. (2008). Mapping potential foodsheds in New York State: A spatial model for evaluating the capacity to localize food production. *Renewable Agriculture and Food Systems*, *24*(1), 72–84.

Pi-Sunyer, F. X. (2002). The obesity epidemic: pathophysiology and consequences of obesity. *Obesity Research*, *10*(Suppl. 2), 97S–104S.

Pollan, M. (2006). The vegetable-industrial complex. *New York Times*, October 15. Retrieved from www.nytimes.com/2006/10/15/magazine/15wwln_lede.html

Puhl, R. M., & Heuer, C. A. (2009). The stigma of obesity: A review and update. *Obesity*, *17*(5), 941–964.

Rauh, V. A., Perera, F. P., Horton, M. K., Whyatt, R. M., Bansal, R., Hao, X., et al. (2012). Brain anomalies in children exposed prenatally to a common organophosphate pesticide. *Proceedings of the National Academy of Sciences*, *109*(20), 7871–7876.

Ridaura, V. K., Faith, J. J., Rey, F. E., Cheng, J., Duncan, A. E., Kau, A. L., ... Gordon, J. I. (2013). Gut microbiota from twins discordant for obesity modulate metabolism in mice. *Science*, *341*(6150), 1241214.

Sanborn, M., Bassil, K., Vakil, C., Kerr, K., & Ragan, K. (2012). *Systematic review of pesticide health effects*. Toronto: Ontario College of Family Physicians.

Scallan, E., Hoekstra, R. M., Angulo, F. J., Tauxe, R. V., Widdowson, M.-A., Roy, S. L., ... Griffin, P. M. (2011). Foodborne illness acquired in the United States—Major pathogens. *Emerging Infectious Diseases*, *17*(1), 7–15.

Schulze, M. B., & Hu, F. B. (2005). Primary prevention of diabetes: What can be done and how much can be prevented? *Annual Review of Public Health*, *26*, 445–467.

Selevan, S. G., Kimmel, C. A., & Mendola, P. (2000) Identifying critical windows of exposure for children's health. *Environmental Health Perspectives*, *108*(Suppl. 3), 451–455.

Stanhope, K. L., Bremer, A. A., Medici, V., Nakajima, K., Ito, Y., Nakano, T., … Havel, P. J. (2011). Consumption of fructose and high fructose corn syrup increase postprandial triglycerides, LDL-cholesterol, and apolipoprotein-B in young men and women. *The Journal of Clinical Endocrinology and Metabolism*, *96*(10), E1596–E1605.

Story, M., Kaphingst, K. M., Robinson-O'Brien, R., & Glanz, K. (2008). Creating healthy food and eating environments: Policy and environmental approaches. *Annual Review of Public Health*, *29*, 253–272.

Szpir M. (2006). Tracing the origins of autism: A spectrum of new studies. *Environmental Health Perspectives*, *114*, A412–A418.

The President's Cancer Panel. (2010). *Reducing environmental cancer risk: What we can do now*. Washington, DC: National Cancer Institute.

US Department of Agriculture Economic Research Service. (2013). *Loss-adjusted food availability documentation*. Retrieved from www.ers.usda.gov/data-products/food-availability-(per-capita)-data-system/loss-adjusted-food-availability-documentation.aspx#.UoZ_99LhLTp

US Food and Drug Administration. (2013). *Bisphenol A (BPA): Use in food contact application*. Retrieved from www.fda.gov/NewsEvents/PublicHealthFocus/ucm064437.htm

Vandenberg, L. N., Hauser, R., Marcus, M., Olea, N., & Welshons, W. V. (2007). Human exposure to bisphenol-A (BPA). *Reproductive Toxicology*, *24*(2), 139–177.

Van Kessel, J., Karns, J., Gorski, L., McCluskey, B., & Perdue, M. (2004). Prevalence of *salmonellae*, *listeria* monocytogenes, and fecal coliforms in bulk tank milk on US dairies. *Journal of Dairy Science*, *87*(9), 2822–2830.

Velasquez, M. Are happy gut bacteria key to weight loss? *Mother Jones*, April 22, 2013

Volkel, W., Colnot, T., Csanady, G. A., Filser, J. G., & Dekant, W. (2002). Metabolism and kinetics of bisphenol-A in humans at low doses following oral administration. *Chemical Research in Toxicology*, *15*(10), 1281–1287.

vom Saal, F. S., Akingbemi, B. T., Belcher, S. M., Birnbaum, L. S., Crain, D. A., Eriksen, M., et al. (2007). Chapel Hill bisphenol A expert panel consensus statement: Integration of mechanisms, effects in animals and potential to impact human health at current levels of exposure. *Reproductive Toxicology*, *24*(2), 131–138.

von Goetz, N., Wormuth, M., Scheringer, M., & Hungerbuhler, K. (2010). Bisphenol-A: How the most relevant exposure sources contribute to total consumer exposure. *Risk Analysis*, *30*(3), 473–487.

Whitlock, G., Lewington, S., Sherliker, P., Clarke, R., Emberson, J., Halsey, J., … Peto, R. (2009). Body-mass index and cause-specific mortality in 900,000 adults: Collaborative analyses of 57 prospective studies. *Lancet*, *373*(March), 1083–1096.

Wilson, N. K., Chuang, J. C., Morgan, M. K., Lordo, R. A., & Sheldon, L. S. (2007). An observational study of the potential exposures of preschool children to pentachlorophenol, bisphenol-A, and nonylphenol at home and daycare. *Environmental Research*, *103*(1), 9–20.

Winchester, P. D., Huskins, J., & Ying, J. (2009). Agrichemicals in surface water and birth defects in the United States. *Acta Paediatrica*, *98*, 664–669.

Wirt, K. (2004). *Another myth: American agriculture yields world's "cheapest, safest" food*. CropChoice.com. Retrieved from www.cropchoice.com/leadstry1af8.html?recid=2501

Yao, M., & Roberts, S. B. (2001). Dietary energy density and weight regulation. *Nutrition Reviews*, *59*(8 Pt. 1), 247–258.

Chapter 3

Ecological Threats to and from Food Systems

Molly D. Anderson

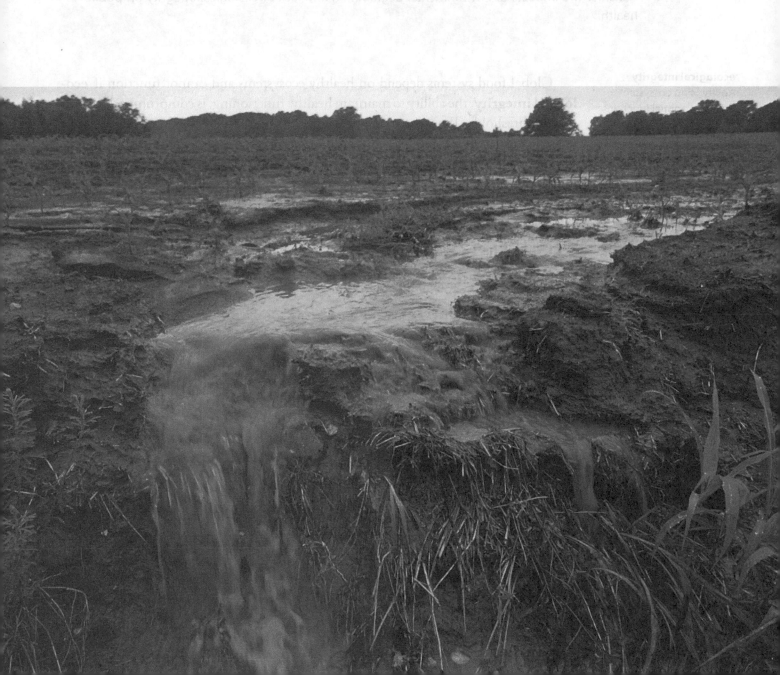

Learning Objectives

- Understand why food production capacity depends on ecological integrity.

- Describe how food systems have affected the status of land, oceans, freshwater, genetic diversity, energy resources, and ecosystem services.

- Compare the environmental impacts of industrialized, agroecological, and small-scale traditional systems.

- Be aware of some leading ways to assess the ecological integrity of food systems.

- Understand the importance of and be able to give examples of policies that can ameliorate ecological threats.

- Gain insight into consumer attitudes toward sustainably produced foods.

- Consider the impacts of environmental degradation and lack of ecological integrity on public health.

ecological integrity
Ability of an ecosystem to maintain normal functions

ecosystem services
Benefits that humans derive from ecosystems

provisioning services
A type of ecosystem service; direct provision from ecosystems of goods (e.g., food, medicine, timber, fiber, biofuels) valuable to humans

regulating services
A type of ecosystem service; control of the rate and extent of natural processes (e.g., water filtration, waste decomposition, climate regulation, crop pollination, regulation of some human diseases)

supporting services
A type of ecosystem service; functions provided by ecosystems that are necessary for the provision of all other ecosystem services (e.g., the cycling of nutrients through an ecosystem and breakdown of waste)

Global food systems depend on healthy ecosystems and cannot function if **ecological integrity**, the ability to maintain healthy functioning, is compromised beyond certain thresholds. The capacity to produce food is one of many food- and agriculture-related **ecosystem services** (benefits from ecosystems, often critical for human life). There are four types of ecosystem services (Millennium Ecosystem Assessment, 2005):

- **Provisioning services**—direct provision of goods (e.g., food, medicine, timber, fiber, biofuels)

- **Regulating services**—control of the rate and extent of natural processes (e.g., water filtration, waste decomposition, climate regulation, crop pollination, regulation of some human diseases)

- **Supporting services**—functions necessary for the provision of all other ecosystem services (e.g., the cycling of nutrients through an ecosystem, photosynthesis, soil formation)

- **Cultural services**—psychological and emotional benefits from human relations with ecosystems (e.g., recreational, aesthetic, and spiritual experiences)

An estimated 60 percent of the ecosystem services that support life on earth are being degraded or used unsustainably, with many of these changes caused in part by current and past management of land for food, fiber, and timber (Millennium Ecosystem Assessment, 2005). Humans enjoy these services freely now and often do not recognize their value, but replacing them will be prohibitively costly or impossible. For example, several species (e.g., bees, wasps, bats, lizards) pollinate crop plants as part of their life cycles. Bee pollination directly or indirectly benefits about one mouthful in three of the US diet, and honeybees are responsible for more than $15 billion in increased crop value each year (US Department of Agriculture Agricultural

Research Service, 2012), although, as will be discussed, their populations are threatened (figure 3.1). Ecosystem services are frequently externalized benefits of agriculture, that is, their value is not included in the direct or indirect costs of production. Tegtmeier and Duffy (2004) estimated that biodiversity and benefits to human health of selected ecosystem services in US agriculture were $5.7 to $16.9 billion per year in 2002. Of these estimates, the value of the selected ecosystem services to crop production was estimated to be $4,969 to $16,151 million per year; and livestock production benefited from ecosystem services worth $714 to $739 million per year.

FIGURE 3.1 Bee Pollination Directly or Indirectly Benefits about One Mouthful in Three of the US Diet

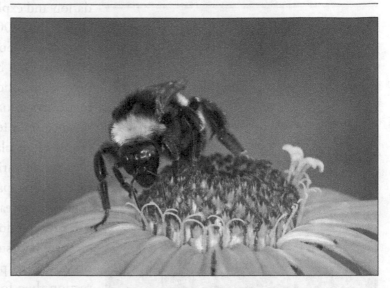

Source: John Flannery via Flickr Creative Commons. (2013). Bee on Zinnea. https://www.flicker.com/photos/drphotomoto/9417297659/

This chapter begins with an overview of the current status of major resources (soil, freshwater, oceans, genetic diversity, energy) and ecosystem services necessary for food production. The next section addresses the most important processes through which human practices in the food system are threatening ecological integrity. The chapter concludes by discussing the feasibility of changing food system practices to more sustainable options and of the socioeconomic trade-offs involved in such changes. It also suggests policy approaches to move the global food system toward greater use of sustainable practices. As you read this chapter, consider the potential public health and food security implications of the described ecological challenges. Where do the food security threats described in this chapter rank compared to the more direct public health threats described in chapter 2?

cultural services
A type of ecosystem service; psychological and emotional benefits from human relations with ecosystems (e.g., recreational, aesthetic, and spiritual experiences)

STATUS OF NATURAL RESOURCES AND ECOSYSTEM SERVICES ESSENTIAL TO FOOD SYSTEMS

Global food production and the productivity of most commodity crops (such as maize [corn], rice, and soybeans) have risen dramatically since the middle of the twentieth century. For example, average maize yields in the United States increased from about 25 bushels (bu) per acre, between the earliest records in the 1860s until the 1930s, to 136 bu per acre in 2002 (Kucharik & Ramankutty, 2005). These yield increases were due to technological changes such as advances in plant genetics and machinery, increased reliance on irrigation and agrochemicals to enhance soil nutrient status and resistance to pests, and a relatively benign climate. Similar yield increases were achieved in several other crops.

Although yield and productivity increases since the 1930s have been impressive, environmental costs have been significant. Food production practices have degraded or used up natural resources worldwide; in some places, degradation is severe enough that food production is no longer possible.

FIGURE 3.2 **Soybean Monoculture Crop Being Sprayed by Crop Duster**

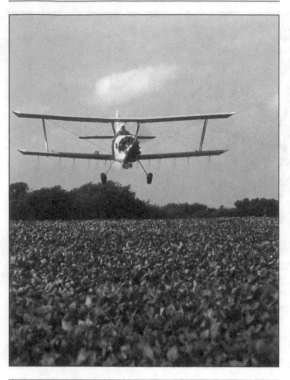

Source: Ken Hammond.

Industrialized agricultural and fishing systems have been responsible for the most serious environmental degradation and exploitation (McIntyre, Herren, Wakhungu, & Watson, 2009; United Nations Department of Economic and Social Affairs, 2011). These systems are characterized by mechanization, usually powered by petroleum, and use of large and sophisticated equipment; irrigation to ensure a consistent supply of water; reliance on a few commercial animal or fish species or crops, often planted in **monocultures** (large plantings of a single variety of a single crop) (see, for example, figure 3.2); separation of cropping and livestock production; widespread use of synthetic pesticides and fertilizers; and a predominant drive toward economic efficiency at current costs of inputs. The environmental impacts of these food production practices are described in this section then followed by a section on new or emerging ecological threats to food systems. Focus 3.1 provides an overview of ways to measure and monitor ecosystem health.

monocultures
Large plantings of a single variety of a single crop

 FOCUS 3.1. ASSESSING ECOLOGICAL INTEGRITY OF FOOD SYSTEMS

Molly D. Anderson

Assessing and monitoring the health of ecosystems have become increasingly important with increased pressure on resources from a rapidly growing population and changed consumption patterns. Some of the most widely used methods are ecological footprinting, life-cycle analysis, and the use of indicators. **Ecological footprinting** calculates the amount of land and other resources "consumed" by the lifestyles of people in different countries. Footprint analyses show that consumption of global resources exceeded available **biocapacity** (the area of productive land and water available to produce resources or absorb carbon dioxide waste, given current management practices) sometime in the late 1970s. By 2006, global consumption exceeded capacity by 44 percent. The United States had the largest total ecological footprint of any country in the world and the second largest ecological footprint per capita (after the United Arab Emirates) in 2006 (Global Footprint Network, 2010).

ecological footprinting
A measure of human demand on ecosystems, typically expressed in hectares of biologically productive land

biocapacity
The area of productive land and water available to produce resources or absorb carbon dioxide waste, given current management practices

Life-cycle assessments create estimates of the total environmental and social costs associated with a product, either by summing impacts at each stage of the food system (e.g., input production and supply, food production, processing, distribution, retailing and storage, consumption, waste disposal) or by tallying the costs to each industry sector involved in creating that product. They sometimes show counterintuitive results, such as that processing packaging and household storage and consumption of food in the United States each use as much or more energy as the production stage (see figure 3.3) (Canning, Charles, Huang, & Polenske, 2010; Heller & Keolian, 2000). They help show where reforms are most needed in the food system to reduce energy or resource use.

Indicators also can provide good information about ecological integrity. Indicators are defined in many different ways, but they are generally some form of data showing movement toward or away from a target, such as the amount of sediment in a stream, the prevalence of childhood food insecurity, or the rate of soil **erosion**. Their value depends on the data being tracked, the implicit goals of the project, its embedded assumptions, how widely the indicators are used, and who uses them. A few indicator sets, often those with substantial food industry backing, show that the efficiency of US agriculture is increasing steadily and environmental costs are declining (e.g., Keystone Center, 2012). However, most reports based on comprehensive indicators show major areas of concern in depletion of essential resources, environmental degradation, and externalization of environmental costs onto other countries and future generations within the United States (e.g., Food and Agriculture Organization [FAO], 2011a; Heinz Center, 2008; McIntyre et al., 2009; United Nations Environment Programme, 2007).

Farmers and food businesses increasingly participate in **standard systems** or sets of production criteria that farmers or business must meet to provide buyers (a business or the end consumer) a guarantee of qualities that are important to them. Standards often include indicators of social sustainability or ecological integrity. The US Department of Agriculture administers the US organic agriculture standard; many other standards of food qualities are in use. Figure 3.4, for example, presents a sampling of the many labels used to connote aspects of sustainability. Standard systems vary widely in their performance criteria, implementation protocols, and credibility.

FIGURE 3.3   Energy Expended in Producing and Delivering One Food Calorie in the United States

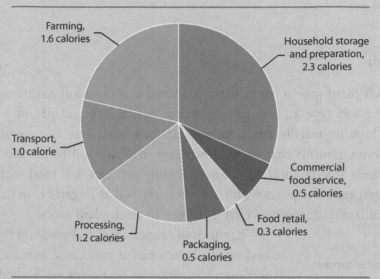

Source: Heinberg and Bomford (2009).

erosion
Washing or blowing away of topsoil

FIGURE 3.4   Sustainability Labels

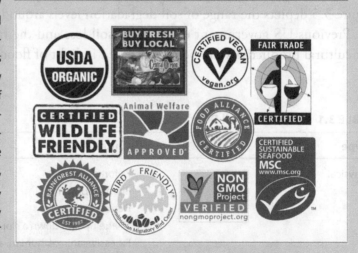

standard systems
Sets of production criteria that farmers or businesses meet to provide buyers (another business or the end consumer) with a guarantee of qualities important to them

There is a clear need to shift to more sustainable agricultural practices (Reganold et al., 2011), but exactly what these constitute is contentious. The final section of this chapter describes different systems of agriculture with lower environmental impacts and how policies might encourage a shift toward such systems.

Soil

Each plant grown for human or animal consumption has its own range of tolerable conditions—an ideal soil type and range of nutrient availability and pH in which it can thrive. The best soils for agriculture usually are deep, well-drained, and close to neutral in acidity. Good topsoil teems with microorganisms that break down crop residue. Soil forms slowly as rock breaks up and dissolves, a process aided by soil organisms, creating particles that bind with decaying biomass to form larger soil aggregates. The pores within and between soil aggregates help to retain moisture for biological growth, facilitate drainage, and enable oxygen to reach plant roots.

soil fertility
Capacity of soil to support plant growth; affected by microbial activity, contamination, organic matter, soil type, and other factors

When topsoil erodes, this ideal medium for plant growth is displaced from fields to end up in places where it may cause damage. Moreover, substances in the soil such as fertilizer, manure, and pesticides are flushed into waterways, where they too may cause damage, as will be described. Overgrazing by livestock, inappropriate irrigation, and soil contamination have also decimated **soil fertility** in many parts of the world, leaving barren or salt-riddled land that can no longer produce crops (see table 3.1).

According to the Food and Agriculture Organization, around 25 percent of the earth's land is classified as severely degraded and another 8 percent as somewhat degraded (FAO, 2011b). Figure 3.5 depicts the range of soil degradation levels around the world.

Previous US government estimates of soil loss and the rates that can be sustained without losing agricultural productivity are being reassessed in light of flood data from the early twenty-first century.

TABLE 3.1   Causes of Soil Degradation

Type	Causes
Physical	Deforestation
	Biomass burning
	Denudation
	Tillage up and down a slope
	Excessive animal, human, and vehicular traffic
	Uncontrolled grazing
Chemical	Excessive irrigation with poor quality water
	Lack of adequate drainage
	No, little, or excessive use of inorganic fertilizers
	Land application of industrial and urban wastes
Biological	Removal and burning of residues
	No or little use of biosolids (e.g., manure, mulch)
	Monoculture without growing cover crops in the rotation cycle
	Excessive tillage

Source: Lal, Iivari, and Kimble (2003, p.12).

According to a 2010 study by the US Geological Survey, erosion in Iowa—the center of America's breadbasket—averaged 5.2 tons of eroded soil per acre per year, slightly higher than the estimated rate at which soil can be lost without reducing productivity. Yet 2008 flood events in Iowa triggered erosion rates twelve times the sustainable loss rate in affected areas (Cox, Hug, & Bruzelius, 2011).

In addition to soil erosion and contamination, another major threat to the availability of soil for producing food is development, particularly when it occurs near to population centers and on high-quality soils. Focus 3.2 provides an overview of this threat and some approaches to addressing it.

FIGURE 3.5   Soil Degradation around the World

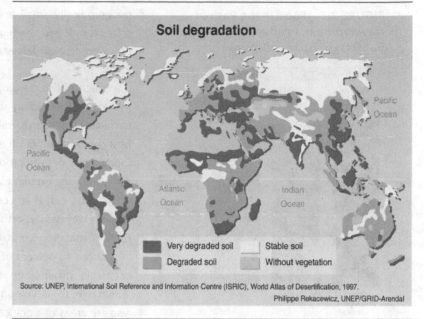

Source: UNEP, International Soil Reference and Information Centre (ISRIC), World Atlas of Desertification, 1997.

Philippe Rekacewicz, UNEP/GRID-Arendal

Source: UNEP.

FOCUS 3.2. FARMLAND PROTECTION
Julia Freedgood

Between 1982 and 2010, 24 million acres of farmland (as much land as Indiana and Rhode Island combined) were developed into shopping malls, subdivisions, and other urban land uses (US Department of Agriculture Natural Resources Conservation Service, 2013). Farmland is ideal for development because it typically is open, flat, and well drained—and typically less expensive than competing urban and suburban land uses. Figure 3.6 illustrates farmland conversion from 1982 to 2007. States shown in the darkest gray developed more than a million acres. The

FIGURE 3.6   Farmland Conversion from 1982–2007. Every state lost agricultural land.

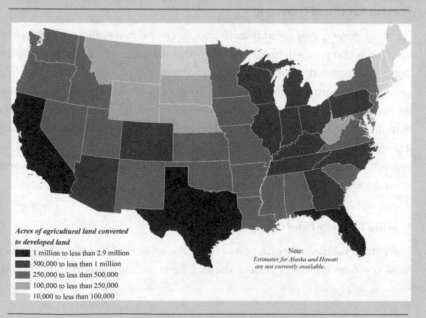

Acres of agricultural land converted to developed land
- 1 million to less than 2.9 million
- 500,000 to less than 1 million
- 250,000 to less than 500,000
- 100,000 to less than 250,000
- 10,000 to less than 100,000

Note: Estimates for Alaska and Hawaii are not currently available.

Note: Estimates for Alaska and Hawaii are not currently available.
Source: American Farmland Trust (2010).

(Continued)

(Continued)

FIGURE 3.7   Food in the Path of Development, Produced in Counties Subject to Urban Influences

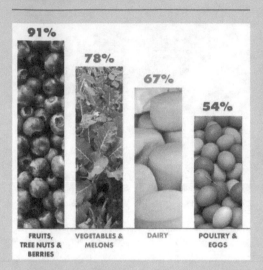

| FRUITS, TREE NUTS & BERRIES | VEGETABLES & MELONS | DAIRY | POULTRY & EGGS |

Note: Percentage, by market value, produced.
Source: AFT (2009).

geographically small and densely populated Northeastern states developed the highest percentages of their farmland, for example, New Jersey at 27 percent (Dempsey & Ferguson, 2010).

Much of this development took place on the best quality cropland, including about fourteen million acres of prime farmland (American Farmland Trust, 2010). Prime soils have the best combination of physical and chemical characteristics for food and other farm production, and the best combination of soil properties, growing season, and water supply to produce continued yields in an economically and environmentally sustainable way (US Department of Agriculture Natural Resources Conservation Service, 2012).

About 40 percent of the value of agricultural production occurs in urban-edge counties, where farmland is most vulnerable to development (RCA Appraisal, 2011). These also are areas of significant food production (see figure 3.7). Developing this land threatens domestic food security; the United States already needs another thirteen million acres of fruit and vegetable production to meet recommended dietary requirements (Buzby, Wells, & Vocke, 2006) and therefore has become a net importer for the first time in its history (Johnson, 2014).

What Is Farmland Protection?

Farmland protection denotes public and private efforts to ensure land remains available for agricultural production. There are three main approaches.

Prevent Farmland Conversion

Planning, zoning, and smart growth policies can promote efficient development patterns to reduce farmland loss by directing growth toward population centers and community infrastructure, and by encouraging higher density, compact development patterns. Urban, regional, and other forms of planning involve dynamic processes to help communities envision their future to create better choices for how people work and live. Comprehensive or master plans identify areas where a community wants to encourage growth, preservation, and other community needs including farmland protection. Most communities use zoning to implement these plans. Zoning regulates land uses and lot sizes, building height, signage, setbacks, parking, and other things. Agricultural protection zoning designates areas where farming is the primary land use and discourages other land uses in those areas.

Provide Tax Relief and Other Incentives

Every state has passed legislation to offset the impacts of suburban land values on agricultural property taxes. Most common are either current use or differential assessments to tax farmland at its value for farming, not its full market value, which is usually development. Right-to-farm laws are intended to protect farmers from nuisance suits and overly restrictive local regulations. Most are enacted at the state level, but local governments also pass laws to strengthen and clarify state laws and to educate residents about normal agricultural activities. Agricultural district laws help stabilize the land base and support the business of farming using incentives to entice farmers voluntarily to enroll and create designated areas where agriculture is encouraged and protected. Nineteen agricultural district programs have been created in sixteen states (American Farmland Trust, 2012).

Permanently Protect Farmland

Agricultural conservation easements are the primary permanent farmland protection tool. They are voluntary deed restrictions property owners can donate or sell to protect productive agricultural land. Twenty-eight states and at least ninety-one local governments have independently funded programs to purchase agricultural conservation easements, and 119 private land trusts have protected farm and ranch land, mostly with donated easements. The federal Farm and Ranch Lands Protection Program provides matching funds to qualified public and private programs. These efforts have jointly saved at least five million acres of farm and ranch land (American Farmland Trust, 2013). Other approaches involve the private marketplace. Mitigation policies require developers to permanently protect an equivalent or greater amount of farmland when they convert agricultural land to other uses, and transfer of development rights (TDR) programs shift development from farmland (sending areas) to designated growth zones (receiving areas).

Conclusion

The urbanization that drove farmland conversion in the twentieth century will accelerate in the twenty-first century. For the first time in history, half of the world's population is now believed to live in urban areas (United Nations Population Division, 2008). With 70 percent of the earth's nine billion people potentially living in urban areas by 2050, even with dramatic technological advances, agricultural land will become increasingly critical to food security in the United States and around the world. As Lester Brown, founder and president of the Earth Policy Institute, stated, "In this era of tightening world food supplies, the ability to grow food is fast becoming a new form of geopolitical leverage. Food is the new oil. Land is the new gold" (2012).

Freshwater

Freshwater is surprisingly scarce on earth, yet essential for crop growth as well as human consumption, livestock production, and industrial use. Most of the earth's surface is covered with water, but only about 2.5 percent is freshwater and only 0.77 percent is held in **aquifers** (underground water storage), soil, lakes, rivers, swamps, plants, and the atmosphere (Postel, Daily, & Ehrlich, 1996). Agriculture accounts for more than 70 percent of freshwater usage worldwide (UN World Water Assessment Program, 2014); in some western US states, up to 90 percent of freshwater goes into agriculture (US Department of Agriculture Economic Research Service, 2012). Focus 3.3 explores the concept of "virtual water"—the water that travels the globe, embodied in the food we eat.

aquifers
Underground water basins

FOCUS 3.3. VIRTUAL WATER AND FOOD SYSTEMS
Luke H. MacDonald and Kellogg J. Schwab

It takes water to grow food. This simple concept leads to surprising insights when taking a systems approach. First, it is surprising just how much water is needed to grow food. Although drinking water may readily come to mind when we think of water shortages, water consumed for drinking is a small, almost insignificant portion of our overall water use. The volume of water used for agriculture far outweighs all other human water uses combined. As noted in the main text, over 70 percent of human water withdrawals are for food production. This fact clearly links water security to food security.

To give an idea of what this means for one person, let's start by examining water requirements for typical vegetarians. One kilogram of wheat usually requires over 1 m³ of water and produces 3,500 kilocalories (Hoekstra & Hung, 2003; Zehnder, Yang, & Schertenleib, 2003). Under reasonable water efficiency assumptions, a vegetarian diet consisting mainly of wheat requires 360 m³ (95,040 gallons) per year for food for one person, as compared to just 1 to 3 m³ (264 to 792 gallons) per year in drinking water (Zehnder et al., 2003). As you can see, agricultural water demand is much, much greater than demand for other water uses, even for vegetarians.

Moving up the trophic ladder from plants to animals, water requirements increase four to ten times in terms of water used per unit mass of food and water per unit energy of food (Zehnder et al., 2003). Cows drink water and eat grain that, in turn, requires water to grow. Viewed in this way, one kilogram (2.2 lbs) of beef requires about 5 m³ (1,320 gallons) of water and contains 2,000 kilocalories on average in the United States (Zehnder, 1997), which precipitously drops the energy yield to water-used ratio from 3,500 kilocalories per m³ (13.3 kilocalories per gallon) of water for wheat to 400 kilocalories per m³ (1.5 kilocalories per gallon) of water for beef.

A second insight is that not all water is equal. Because water is distributed unevenly, areas with high rainfall require little irrigation, and other areas rely exclusively on irrigation. Irrigation, whether pumped from the ground or diverted from surface flows, requires resources and energy. Following the principle that not all water is equal, hydrologists and agronomists classify green water versus blue water. Green water is the main water source for rain-fed agriculture: water in soil. Blue water requires human intervention to contribute to agriculture: water in surface water bodies and aquifers (Hoekstra et al., 2012).

A third insight is that the same food item requires different amounts of green and blue water depending on where and when it grew. Above, we used a single figure of 1 kg wheat per m³ (0.008 lbs per gallon) of water, but in truth water productivity varies regionally. In North America and Western Europe, the water productivity of wheat is generally more than 1 kg per m³ (0.008 lbs per gallon), but it is below 0.6 kg per m³ (0.005 lbs per gallon) in much of Africa and Central Asia (Hoekstra & Hung, 2003, 2005). The amount of water needed to grow food varies depending on sunlight, temperature, soil, farming technology, water efficiency, and other factors. Thus, the water content embedded in strawberries from different countries, for example, in your local supermarket can dramatically vary.

The study of virtual water ties together these three insights into a systems approach to better understand water flow through the food trade. One can simply add the embedded green and blue water volumes in food items while examining agricultural imports and exports to understand the flow of water in global food trade.

Something startling emerges from this analysis: just ten countries account for 94 percent of all net virtual food-water exports, and the majority of countries, especially poor countries, are net importers of virtual food water (Liu, Zehnder, & Yang, 2009). (Net virtual food-water-exporting countries are not necessarily the same as net food-exporting countries.) Top virtual food-water exporters include, in order of volume,

United States, Canada, Argentina, France, and Australia. Depending on this limited number of food-water exporters may make the world increasingly vulnerable to interlinked water and food security threats (Hoekstra et al., 2012).

Another important finding is that green water dominates the global food trade, accounting for about 94.4 percent of the virtual water trade (Liu et al., 2009). This suggests that water-scarce regions import food water from water-rich regions rather than invest in developing blue water infrastructure for agriculture. Hence, the global food trade becomes a balancing force to economically redistribute water in the context of unevenly distributed water resources. Looking forward, future food security depends on sustainable water management based on an understanding of virtual water flows to create balanced use of limited water resources.

Although freshwater is continuously recycled through evaporation and condensation as rain, it may be so degraded after agricultural use that it cannot be reused easily and cost-effectively. Water running off or leaching through agricultural soils is often contaminated with salts, nutrients, pesticides, or sediment. Agriculture is responsible for most of the contamination of groundwater and surface water. Table 3.2 describes ways agricultural activities affect water quality (Ongley, 1996).

siltation
Accumulation of soil particles in bodies of water

salinization
A process in which salts accumulate in upper layers of soil, often from improper irrigation techniques, although sometimes because of naturally occurring concentrations of salt

TABLE 3.2   Major Agricultural Impacts on Water Quality

Agricultural Activity	Possible Impacts	
	Surface Water	Groundwater
Tillage and plowing	Transport of sediments carrying phosphorus and pesticides; **siltation** of river beds and loss of habitat, spawning ground for fish	NA
Fertilization	Runoff of nutrients, especially phosphorus, leading to eutrophication, causing taste and odor in public water supply, excess algae growth leading to fish kills	Nitrate leaching to groundwater
Spreading manure, raising animals in feedlots	Soil and water contamination through runoff of pathogens and metals from manure spread in excess or leaking from storage tanks and potential eutrophication through runoff of phosphorus and nitrogen	Contamination of groundwater, especially by nitrogen and pathogens
Pesticide application	Contamination of surface water and public health impacts from eating fish from affected areas; pesticides carried as dust over long distances contaminate aquatic systems thousands of miles away	Human health problems from contaminated wells
Irrigation	Runoff of salts leading to **salinization** of surface water; runoff of fertilizers and pesticides to surface waters with ecological damage	Contamination with salts and nutrients (especially nitrate)
Aquaculture	Release of pesticides, feed ingredients such as antibiotics, and high levels of nutrients to surface water and groundwater through feed and feces, leading to contamination and eutrophication	Contamination with pesticides, nutrients, and pharmaceuticals

Source: After Ongley (1996).

wetlands
Marshy areas where water remains close to the surface for all or most of the year

runoff
The flow of water from rain, irrigation water, and other sources over land; often carries topsoil and contaminants into bodies of water

Furthermore, agriculture is responsible for the most loss of **wetlands** (marshy areas where water remains close to the surface) in the United States. Wetlands are important because they absorb **runoff** (surface-water flow) and help prevent flooding of adjacent land, provide habitat and breeding areas for birds and other wildlife, and help to protect water quality (US Environmental Protection Agency [US EPA], 2001). Half of the wetlands in the United States have been drained, with the most intensive losses occurring between the mid-1950s and mid-1970s, decreasing since then (US EPA, 2012).

In many large rivers of the world, only 5 percent of former water volume remains in-stream because of withdrawals for irrigation (FAO, 2011b). In the southwest United States, the Colorado River no longer reaches the sea year-round, and many large lakes have shrunk. Sediment from eroding soils is filling reservoirs, reducing hydropower and water supply. Groundwater is being pumped intensively, often exceeding the ability of aquifers to recharge. The Ogallala Aquifer under the US Great Plains has been pumped so intensively that the water table has fallen and residents, crops, livestock, and meat-processing plants are hurting for water. Aquifers are becoming increasingly polluted and contaminated by saltwater intrusion in some coastal areas (United Nations Department of Economic and Social Affairs, 2011).

Oceans

Ocean health is vital to food production: in 2009, fish accounted for 16.6 percent of the world population's intake of animal protein and 6.5 percent of all protein consumed. Globally, fish provided about three billion people with almost 20 percent of their intake of animal protein and 4.3 billion people with about 15 percent of the animal protein they consumed. About 64 percent of fish harvested in 2011 came from the oceans; most of the remainder was raised by inland aquaculture (FAO, 2012).

fish stocks
Amounts of commercially desirable fish

Overexploitation
Excessive harvesting of a population (e.g., fish) such that the population cannot recover to its previous size

In 2009, only 12.7 percent of world **fish stocks** (amounts of commercially desirable fish) were estimated to be not fully exploited; all other fish stocks were fully exploited, overexploited, depleted, or recovering (FAO, 2012). Depletion of fish stocks occurs when fish cannot be harvested at the same rates they have been harvested previously because of reduced populations. **Overexploitation** results in lower yields than the biological and ecological potential of a fishery. Overexploited fisheries need strict management plans limiting fishing to restore their full productivity. Beyond overfishing, the health of oceans is threatened by contamination with plastic trash and; oversupply of nutrients, pesticides, and sediment; acidification; and dilution from melting ice caps and glaciers, which pour freshwater into the adjacent ocean.

aquaculture
Farm-raising fish, crustaceans, shellfish, or aquatic plants, either inland in tanks or ponds, or in enclosures in lakes, rivers, or oceans

Farm-raising fish or **aquaculture** is a growing industry and helps replace fish supplies that are no longer available from wild capture. From 1980 to 2010, world aquaculture production expanded by almost twelve times, at an average annual rate of 8.8 percent (FAO, 2012). However, aquaculture as commonly practiced has many environmental costs, including increased pressure on marine fisheries to supply fishmeal to feed farmed fish, waste that overloads local water capacity to absorb it, and disease transmission to wild fish populations (McIntyre et al., 2009). (See focus 12.1.)

Genetic Diversity

Two kinds of genetic diversity are critical to agriculture: **wild (natural) biodiversity** (the genetic diversity of ecosystems not managed by humans) and **agrobiodiversity**, the genetic diversity of domesticated crops and animal species. Natural biodiversity is important because it contributes to the nutritional value of human diets, in addition to providing invaluable ecosystem services.

Agriculture has been responsible for the loss of valuable ecosystem services from biodiversity. For example, annually in the United States, pesticide applications lead to costs of $409.8 million through loss of honeybees and pollination, plus $666.8 million through loss of beneficial predators (Tegtmeier & Duffy, 2004; 2002 dollars). Habitat loss by conversion to cropland or grazing land is one of the top five global threats to biodiversity (FAO, 2010). Logging virgin forest in the tropics has the largest impacts per acre due to high **species richness** (number of species per unit of area) in the tropics. But agriculture is also responsible for biodiversity loss in temperate zones, such as in much of the United States. For example, taking land that has been set aside for conservation and converting it to crops in response to rising crop prices also destroys valuable habitat.

Agrobiodiversity is the legacy of centuries of seed and livestock selection by farmers. As changing climatic and pest conditions demand changing agricultural practices, agrobiodiversity is the source for traits that might be bred into edible species, such as drought, pest, and flood resistance.

Energy

Agriculture, livestock production, and fishing use energy to convert the solar energy captured by plants, including some that humans cannot digest directly, into nutrient-dense forms usable by humans. Currently every stage of industrialized food systems relies heavily on petroleum, consuming far more calories in production, processing, distribution, and other activities than are produced for eventual human consumption. Dependence on petroleum can increase food prices because food and oil prices are tightly linked (FAO, 2011a; Heinberg, 2012) (see figure 3.8). Reliance on fossil fuels reduces the **resilience** of food systems (ability to recover from perturbations, adapt so as to reduce harm from future perturbations, or learn to avoid perturbations). This is because the supply of

wild (natural) biodiversity
The genetic diversity of ecosystems not managed by humans

agrobiodiversity
Genetic diversity of domesticated plants and animals

species richness
Number of species per unit of area

FIGURE 3.8   Links between Energy Prices and Food Prices

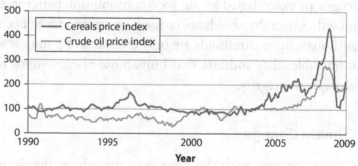

Note: The y-axis is price index (2004 baseline = 100).
Source: FAO (2011).

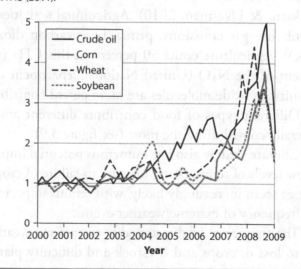

Note: The y-axis is price index (2000 price = 1).
Source: Heinberg and Bomford, (2009).

resilience
Ability to recover from perturbations, adapt so as to reduce harm from future perturbations, or learn to avoid perturbations

fossil fuels is controlled by factors well outside the food system and their price is volatile. Further, burning fossil fuels is the foremost contributor to climate change, the most serious perturbation facing most food systems. Food systems will not be able to continue their heavy dependence on petroleum, but there is no ready substitute for fossil fuels in current food system applications.

Biofuel production (ethanol and biodiesel) has surged as an alternative to supplement fossil fuels, but land conversion from food crops to biofuel has led to rising food prices, increased marginalization of poor farmers on poor land, and worsening food security (High-Level Panel of Experts, 2013; Lagi, Bar-Yam, Bertrand, & Bar-Yam, 2011).

PROCESSES THROUGH WHICH ECOLOGICAL HEALTH IS THREATENED

anthropogenic
Human-caused

Threats to ecological health are intimately interrelated and influenced by human behavior. For example, changing consumption patterns within nations have assumed global significance with growing population pressure on resources; and **anthropogenic** (human-caused) climate change is responsible for a cascade of other threats. This section addresses four ecological threats to food systems that are new, newly acknowledged as problematic, or have become much more serious during the twenty-first century. Climate change, anthropogenic changes to the nitrogen cycle, and erosion of biodiversity may have exceeded "planetary boundaries," or critical thresholds that represent unacceptable environmental change (Rockström et al., 2009); these challenges are exacerbated by our food consumption patterns, especially when they interact with population growth. Once thresholds are crossed, reversing a trend becomes much more difficult or even impossible. Although these thresholds are only estimates of points at which global environmental change becomes intractable, they indicate that human use of ecosystems is seriously out of balance with protection of ecological integrity.

Climate Change

Climate change, with the specters of drought or floods, more extreme weather events, and increasing temperatures, is the most well-known anthropogenic contributor to environmental change (Ingram, Ericksen, & Liverman, 2010). Agricultural activities account for about 30 percent of anthropogenic greenhouse gas emissions, primarily as carbon dioxide (CO_2), methane (CH_4), and nitrous oxide (N_2O). Agriculture emits 50 percent of this CH_4 (with half of that coming from livestock) and 70 percent of the N_2O (United Nations Department of Economic and Social Affairs, 2011). Methane and nitrous oxide molecules are more potent contributors to climate change than carbon dioxide.

Different types of food contribute different amounts of greenhouse gases, with meat and dairy generally contributing the most (see figure 3.9).

Climate change also has numerous potential impacts on agriculture, ranging from increasing yields at low levels of temperature increase to failure of crop growth at higher levels. Higher levels of climate change seem increasingly likely, with serious impacts on crop productivity, freshwater availability, and the frequency of extreme weather events.

The frequency of disasters due to extreme weather events has quintupled since the 1970s, leading to loss of crops and livestock and difficulty planning for future production. By far, most of this increase can be accounted for by the greater incidence of hydro-meteorological disasters (for example, floods, storms, droughts, and extreme temperatures) associated with climate change (see figure 3.10). Developing countries tend to suffer more from the adverse consequences of natural hazards given multiple vulnerabilities associated with lower levels of development and inadequate resources, which constrain their efforts to build better and more resilient infrastructure and implement adequate disaster risk management strategies (United Nations Department of Economic and Social Affairs, 2011). Poor populations in the United States also suffer disproportionately from natural hazards, as evidenced during Hurricane Katrina in 2005 and its aftermath.

Another consequence of climate change on food systems is ocean acidification, which occurs as the oceans absorb excess carbon dioxide produced through greenhouse gases. About 30 to 40 percent of the anthropogenic carbon dioxide in the atmosphere dissolves into oceans, rivers, and lakes (Feely et al., 2004). As the ocean becomes more acidic, it is no longer a hospitable environment for creatures that deposit calcium, such as corals and shellfish, and plankton, which make up the base of the ocean's food chain.

Climate change also is predicted to enable the spread into temperate zones of livestock and plant diseases previously restricted to tropical and subtropical climates, and to put greater pest pressure on crops in the United States. Although increasing the cost of crop and livestock production, some of these diseases are likely to have direct impacts on human health as well.

FIGURE 3.9 Lifecycle Greenhouse Gas Emissions from Common Proteins and Vegetables

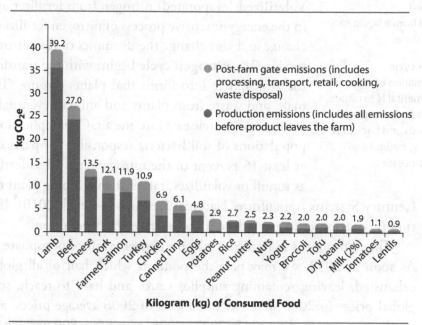

Legend:
● Post-farm gate emissions (includes processing, transport, retail, cooking, waste disposal)
● Production emissions (includes all emissions before product leaves the farm)

Kilogram (kg) of Consumed Food

Source: Environmental Working Group (2011).

FIGURE 3.10 Extreme Weather Events and Corn Yields

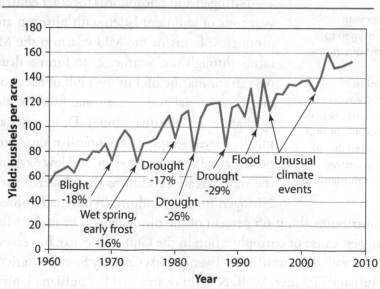

Source: US Global Climate Change Research Program (2009).

Disruption of the Nitrogen Cycle and Nutrient Limitations

volatilized
Changed from a liquid to a gaseous state

nitrogen cycle
Transformation of nitrogen from elemental N to nitrate, nitrite, and other nitrogen compounds and back to N, affected by natural and human processes

legumes
Members of the pea family of plants (*Leguminaceae*)

dead zone
Area of water with insufficient oxygen to support most organisms

eutrophication
Abnormal increases in nutrient levels (particularly nitrogen and phosphorus) in waterways, often due to runoff from excessive application of nutrients to crops

Volatilized (evaporated) nitrogen from fertilizer applied to soil and fossil fuels used in the energy-intensive process of nitrogen fertilizer production contribute to climate change and also change the dynamics of the nitrogen cycle, an important ecosystem service. The **nitrogen cycle** begins with the transformation of elemental nitrogen in the atmosphere into forms that plants can use. These plants are consumed by animals, and waste from plants and animals eventually decompose into inert forms of nitrogen or are released into the air. Overapplication of nitrogen fertilizers can reduce populations of soil bacteria responsible for parts of the nitrogen cycle. In addition, at least 15 percent of the nitrogen applied as fertilizer is lost from agricultural land as runoff or volatilizes, rather than reaching plant roots (Committee on Twenty-First Century Systems Agriculture, National Research Council, 2010). In addition to being wasteful, such runoff contributes to groundwater and surface water pollution.

The phosphorus in fertilizers is also a concern; mined phosphate supplies are being used up rapidly. As soon as 2033, we may pass the point at which half of all globally available supplies have been exhausted, leaving remaining supplies scarce and hard to reach, so that prices rise steadily. Average global prices in 2010 were twice the level of 2006 average prices, and when demand for phosphorus fertilizer outstripped supply in 2007–2008, prices rose 800 percent (Soil Association, 2010). Nitrogen and phosphorus are the two most common limiting nutrients for plant growth. Although nitrogen can be supplied to plants by growing **legumes** (members of the pea family of plants) that extract nitrogen from the atmosphere and turn it into forms usable by other plants, there is no ready substitute for mined phosphorus.

Nitrogen and phosphorus together contribute to a different set of problems. Each year tons of sediment laden with nitrogen and phosphorus run off the prodigiously productive farms in the Midwest into the Mississippi River, joined by runoff from farms through the Southeast, to form a **dead zone** (area of water with inadequate oxygen for marine life) in the Gulf of Mexico, one of the United States' most important commercial and recreational fisheries. Between 2005 and 2011, this zone averaged about 6,700 square miles. Dead zones are caused by **eutrophication** (excessive nutrient levels) supporting intensive algae growth. The bacteria that feed on decomposing algae consume oxygen, and low oxygen levels and reduced sunlight penetrating the water create conditions that threaten survival of fish and other aquatic animals. Nitrogen from agriculture (synthetic fertilizer, manure, and soluble nitrogen in soil) contributes about 65 percent of the nitrogen load from the Mississippi River Basin and constitutes the biggest cause of eutrophication in the Gulf of Mexico; but excess phosphorus is an important contributor as well (Committee on Twenty-First Century Systems Agriculture, National Research Council 2010; Hufnagl-Eichiner, Wolf, & Drinkwater, 2011; Louisiana Universities Marine Consortium, 2012) (see figure 3.11).

Erosion of Agrobiodiversity

Although people consume about 7,000 plant species, only 150 of these are commercially important. About 103 species account for 90 percent of the world's food crops; and rice, wheat, and maize account for about 60 percent of the calories and 56 percent of the protein people derive from plants (Thrupp,

1997). About 20 percent of farm animal breeds have been brought close to extinction by market forces that demand only the most productive livestock, and approximately one breed is being lost each month (FAO, 2006). Human reliance on a small proportion of all plants that can be consumed, and within that number on a small number of varieties of each plant, is because of choices made during the industrialization of agriculture and not necessarily because the selected species and varieties are the most nutritious or the hardiest (or the tastiest!). Allowing agrobiodiversity to diminish dramatically reduces the options for crop and livestock species that can thrive under future conditions (FAO, 2010).

FIGURE 3.11   Gulf of Mexico Dead Zone

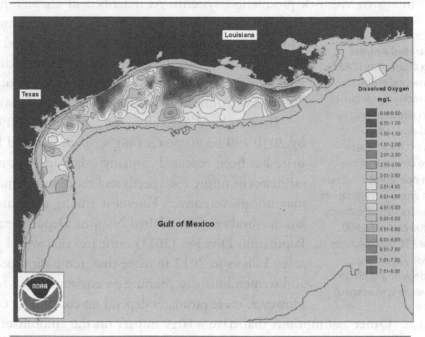

Source: NOAA.

Food Consumption Patterns and Interactions with Population Growth

Shifts in global food consumption patterns are another emerging ecological threat, exacerbated by rapid population growth since the 1990s. Growth in consumption of livestock products per capita outpaced growth in consumption of other major food groups between the 1960s and end of the century. Since the early 1960s, consumption of milk per capita in the developing countries has almost doubled, meat consumption more than tripled, and egg consumption increased by a factor of five (FAO, 2009b). The United States was second only to Luxembourg in 2007 in terms of meat consumption per capita (FAO data reported in *Economist* Online, 2012). US meat consumption, however, dropped by 10 percent between 2007 and 2012, so Americans are

FIGURE 3.12   US Meat and Poultry Availability per Capita

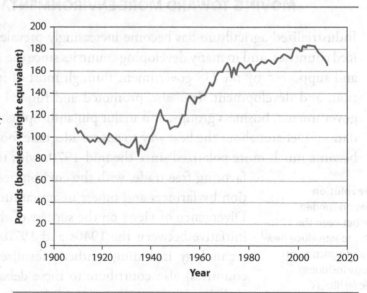

Source: Earth Policy Institute (2012).

eating less meat (see figure 3.12) (Plumer, 2012). Even with this decline, US meat consumption is considerably above meat consumption in most other countries.

Increased demand for meat in industrialized and developing countries is being met largely through intensive livestock production systems. As described in chapter 12, whereas grass-fed livestock systems are relatively benign, the public health, social, and environmental costs of raising livestock in concentrated animal feeding operations (**CAFOs**) include difficulties managing massive amounts of animal waste, water contamination, odor, loss of property values in neighboring communities, and costs of growing and transporting grain for feed (FAO, 2006; Pew Commission on Industrial Farm Animal Production, 2009).

Concentrated Animal Feeding Operatins (CAFOs) Environmental Protection Agency category for large facility in which animals are confined and fed or maintained for at least forty-five days out of the year, the operation does not produce crops or vegetation, and it meets size thresholds (e.g., 1,000 cattle, 10,000 swine, or 125,000 chickens may classify as a "large CAFO," depending on how animal waste is managed)

The Food and Agriculture Organization (2009a) has predicted that food demand by 2050 will be 70 percent higher than demand between 2005 and 2007; this estimate has been repeated in many other analyses of future food demands. However, estimates of future food needs and economic demand rely on many assumptions that may not prove correct. Foremost among these are assumptions about future population numbers. The United Nations Department of Economic and Social Affairs, Population Division (2011) estimates that world population will increase from over seven billion in 2012 to more than ten billion people by 2050. Such a surge would add tremendously to pressure on environmental resources used for food production. However, these estimates depend on continuing current population policies.

Other assumptions that have a large impact on the amount of food that future populations will need include projected diet, particularly protein sources, production practices, proportion of food crops dedicated to biofuel production, and political will sufficient to distribute food more equitably. Efforts to reduce food waste can further change the equation by freeing up resources and reallocating food to those in need (see focus 15.3). Given these uncertainties, a prudent future path entails protection of natural resources necessary for food production—and restoration, wherever possible, of degraded resources.

MOVING TOWARD MORE ENVIRONMENTALLY SUSTAINABLE PRACTICES

Industrialized agriculture has become increasingly prevalent in the United States, in other industrialized countries, and in many developing countries since the 1930s. Industrialized agriculture is promoted and supported by the US government through most of its funding for agricultural research, innovation, and development. It is also promoted and funded by several other relatively wealthy national governments, business groups, and major philanthropists including the Bill and Melinda Gates Foundation. Debates about the best way to ensure adequate food production today and into the future have become much more polarized since the mid-1970s with the emergence of neoliberal political agendas favoring free trade, with the environmental movement, and with broader participation by farmers and others in agricultural research (Sumberg & Thompson, 2012). Divergence of views on the success of the **Green Revolution** (a foundation-funded initiative between the 1940s and 1970s to introduce new hybrids and agricultural technology including synthetic fertilizers, pesticides, and irrigation to developing countries) also contribute to these debates. Food price volatility since 2007–2008 and climate change have raised the stakes of decisions about the kinds of agriculture systems in which to invest. Alternatives with lower environmental impacts are important to ameliorate the food security threats and other ecological problems reviewed in this chapter.

Green Revolution A foundation-funded initiative between the 1940s and 1970s to introduce new hybrids and agricultural technology including synthetic fertilizers, pesticides, and irrigation to developing countries, primarily in Latin America and Asia

Alternative Agricultural Production Systems

Many different agricultural systems are used in the United States and worldwide. To put these into perspective, traditional small-scale cropping and fishing for **subsistence** (only family needs and not sale) are responsible for at least 70 percent of global food production. There are 1.5 billion peasants working on 380 million farms, 800 million peasants growing food in urban gardens, 410 million people gathering food products from forests and grasslands, 190 million **pastoralists** (traditional livestock herders), and over 100 million peasant fishers, making up almost half of the world's population (ETC Group, 2009). Their practices are not always environmentally sound. They may deplete resources in limited geographical areas, but the small scale of their operations restrict environmental damage to smaller areas than those affected by industrialized cropping and fishing, which are designed to manage and harvest up to hundreds of acres of land or ocean in a similar way, and to extract as much crop or fish yield as possible from a given area. In addition, traditional cropping, fishing, and herding practices have been developed by communities dependent on a resource base for decades, if not centuries. This community base often encourages producers to consider factors beyond short-term efficiency, such as stability of family welfare and stability of food production during years of bad weather.

Another approach to farming practices is **agroecology**, which draws from both traditional and modern practices, and emphasizes working with nature to mimic natural processes and conserve ecological integrity. Agroecological practices include **organic farming** (a farming system developed in the middle of the twentieth century that eschews use of synthetic pesticides and fertilizers and emphasizes building soil quality); **polycultures** (planting multiple crops close together in ways that maximize beneficial interactions between species); **agroforestry** (tree species combined with crops or grazing); **crop rotations** (sequencing different crops on the same field) and **biological controls** (using natural predators or diseases to control pests). Agroecology also entails greater efficiency of water and nutrient use; enhancement of soil fertility with manure and **green manure** (legumes that fix nitrogen); and various integrated cropping systems such as mixed farming with crops and livestock and **integrated pest management** (a system of controlling pests using least toxic pesticides applied only when necessary to avoid economic loss).

Although many agroecological practices are also used in industrialized systems, the focus of agroecological systems is on local control over inputs and markets and on multifunctionality, or production over time of numerous benefits, rather than industrialized agriculture's emphasis on economic efficiency at today's prices for inputs and products, using inputs from wherever they can be obtained most cheaply, and selling in the highest global markets. Agroecological practices require good knowledge of environmental constraints and attributes, and they often need more labor than industrialized agriculture, but they can have high productivity and yields close to those achieved in industrialized systems, without many of their environmental costs (Badgley et al., 2007; McIntyre et al., 2009; Pretty, 2008; Tilman, Cassman, Matson, Naylor, & Polasky, 2002; Tomich et al., 2011). Perspective 3.1 presents one farmer's view of what sustainable farming means.

subsistence
Growing food solely for household use (in contrast to commercial sales)

pastoralists
Traditional livestock herders

agroecology
The science and practice of applying ecological principles to agriculture to develop practices that work with nature to mimic natural processes and conserve ecological integrity; other labels for ecological approaches to agriculture include *ecological agriculture, agricultural ecology, sustainable agriculture, permaculture*

organic farming
Farming system that eschews use of synthetic pesticides and fertilizers and emphasizes building soil quality

polycultures
Planting multiple crops close together in ways that maximize beneficial interactions between species

agroforestry
Combining tree production with crops or grazing; the latter is sometimes called *silvopastoralism*

crop rotations
Sequencing different crops on the same field to use nutrients effectively and avoid pest outbreaks

biological controls
Use of natural predators or diseases to control pests

green manure
Legumes that fix nitrogen

integrated pest management
A system of controlling pests using least toxic pesticides applied only when necessary to avoid economic loss

Perspective 3.1. A Farmer's Thoughts on Defining Sustainable Farming

Michael Heller

I operate a 285-acre farm in Upper Marlboro, Maryland, and produce grass-fed beef, organic vegetables (with a 275-member CSA [community-supported agriculture]), and native trees and shrubs to be used for riparian habitat restoration. I'm often asked by visitors, "Just what is sustainable farming?" There are many possible ways to answer. Here are a few.

Sometimes I'll recount a gentle Zen story about a man galloping wildly on a horse. As he is passing a crowd of people someone shouts to him, "Where are you going?" After a brief hesitation the man shakes his head and says, "I don't know. You'll have to ask the horse." Thinking of today's food system, the man on the horse might well represent a farmer or a consumer. The horse would represent industrial agriculture or our runaway food system in which a head of lettuce, grown in the Salinas Valley of California and shipped here to Maryland, requires about thirty-six times as much fossil fuel energy in transport as it provides in food energy when it arrives (Halweil, 2002). Sustainable farming is putting reins on the horse and into the hands of farmers and consumers, where we (together) shape our own food system.

Sustainable farming is also the process of decision making on the farm. What are the filters that a farmer uses to make decisions?—because these filters shape the farm. I consider the following to be equally important criteria when making decisions about farming activities or marketing on the farm: "Is it financially sound?" "Does it build soil quality?" "How does it affect water quality and the environment?" "Does it strengthen our community?" I consider our community to include our customers, our neighbors, and the farm, including all of us who live and work on the farm, our animals, and the wildlife. An additional key filter is "Will it strengthen or weaken our ability to be able to make our own decisions on the farm?" I have made this last item a conscious part of our criteria after visiting my friend David, who runs a poultry farm in Somerset County, Maryland.

I was asking David numerous questions. "How much feed do you give the chickens?" His answer, "Whatever the company tells me." "When do you clean out the bedding in the poultry house?" His answer, "Whenever the company tells me." Finally, after one of my questions David said, "Michael, you have to understand. On my farm the only decision I get to make is what time of day I walk through the houses to pick up dead birds." He has eliminated any concerns about being able to sell what he grows—the company brings the birds and the company comes and takes them away. But he has given up nearly total control of decision making on his farm. Selling directly from our farm to our customers gives us, and our customers, control of this part of the food system.

Sustainable farming is working with ecological processes—that is, using cover crops, crop rotations, and beneficial insects—rather than fighting them with herbicides, insecticides, and chemical fertilizers. For example, our pastures have tremendous plant diversity and include many plants that most livestock farmers and agriculture specialists would call weeds (lamb's quarters, dandelion, pigweed, and so forth). Why spray to kill these "weeds" that have higher nutrition values than alfalfa according to laboratory tests? (Alfalfa is usually considered the standard of excellence for livestock feeds.) I can confirm that my cows enthusiastically agree with the lab findings as they chomp down on these beneficial plants.

Another aspect of sustainable farming is building soil quality on farms. Every handful of healthy soil contains billions of living organisms—protozoa, nematodes, bacteria, fungi, algae, and others. All these critters are working for the farmer to contribute to the soil's ability to supply nutrients to grow healthy plants, but these critters have got to eat, too. Farmers can add food to the soils by using cover crops, grazing animals on pastures, and mulching; alternatively, farmers can deplete soils by only harvesting crops and using fertilizers to grow more crops for harvest. Building soils (supporting and encouraging the "mini-livestock" in the soil) is the best long-term way to protect water quality and fortunately for everyone, it is also the best way to enhance long-term profitability.

When defining sustainability it is important to consider local food systems — but it is necessary also to take a global view. Occasionally people who come visit my farm say, "I love the way you farm, but we couldn't feed the world this way. So is it really sustainable?" This gets my dander up because large-scale industrial agriculture has successfully convinced many people that it is the high-input (fertilizers, pesticides, and diesel fuel) model that can feed the world. To understand sustainability from a more global perspective it is important to know that it has been estimated that the industrial food chain uses 70 percent of agricultural resources to provide 30 percent of the world's food, whereas local sustainable farms worldwide produce the remaining 70 percent using only 30 percent of the resources (ETC Group, 2013). This seems hard to believe, but just using an example contrasting two farms here in Maryland it appears reasonable. I have a friend who is a very good farmer who produces ten thousand acres of grain on the Eastern Shore. From his ten thousand acres of production not one pound of grain goes directly to feed a person, but rather gets transported to feed hogs, chickens, cows, or turned into ethanol. Contrast this with our farm in Upper Marlboro, where we produce grass-fed beef (on marginal, hilly lands) and organic vegetables (on flatter, better farmland) that provide a significant portion of the food that directly feeds more than three hundred families. We know the families that eat the food we grow, and the vegetables and meat go directly from our farm to their tables (with virtually no waste because of transportation and spoilage). So understanding global food sustainability requires a deeper understanding of how food is raised and how it gets transported to each person's dinner table. Buying food from local farmers in this country really helps support global sustainability by strengthening local farming over large-scale industrial agriculture.

Yogi Berra, the gifted Yankee catcher who had a way of inadvertently coining curiously clever aphorisms, once ruefully said, "The future ain't what it used to be." With that sentiment, he could have been a farmer. There is certainly a common perception about farmers that they are always complaining and pining for the past, back when things were better. However, I recently attended a two-day sustainable farming meeting with hundreds of farmers. Although I didn't hear a single complaint, most in attendance would have agreed that "the future ain't what it used to be" — in a good way! The talk was of exciting opportunities — new ideas and farming practices and the growing consumer interest in healthy, local foods. The average age of farmers in Maryland is fifty-nine years old (NASS, 2014), but at this sustainable farming conference the average age was decades younger. And so sustainable farming (this is a truism!) is also having the farmers to farm, now and in the future.

Many agricultural practices to reduce specific types of environmental degradation are well known but not used consistently by farmers. For example, soil erosion can be minimized with **cover cropping** (planting crops aimed at preventing erosion, building soil fertility, and suppressing weeds when soil would otherwise be vacant), **no-till farming** (planting crops directly into the residue of the former crop without plowing), **strip cropping** (planting crops with different structural characteristics in rows to minimize wind erosion), plowing on the contour of the slope to avoid runoff between rows, and polycultures. Agricultural practices to protect biodiversity include maintaining **buffer zones** of vegetation along streams and rivers; reducing or eliminating toxic pesticides to reduce death of nontarget species; and planting **hedgerows** (dense hedges between fields or along streams) and polycultures to provide nesting sites, food, and shelter for wildlife. Practices to reduce crop pests and maintain soil health include rotations and use of **beneficial insects** that eat pests.

Researchers at Iowa State University (Davis, Hill, Chase, Johanns, & Liebman, 2012) demonstrated that more diverse three-crop and four-crop rotations equaled or

cover cropping
Planting crops aimed at preventing erosion, building soil fertility, and suppressing weeds when soil would otherwise be vacant

no-till farming
Planting crops directly into the residue of the former crop without plowing

strip cropping
Planting crops with different structural characteristics in rows to minimize wind erosion

buffer zones
Strips of vegetation along streams and rivers that prevent stream bank erosion and may provide habitat for wildlife species

hedgerows
Dense hedges between fields or along streams

beneficial insects
Insects that eat crop pests or provide other ecosystem services, such as pollination

greenwashing
Exaggerated claims of environmental benefits

exceeded the performance of conventional maize-soybean rotations in terms of grain yields, mass of harvested products, and profit, and still suppressed weeds effectively with lower synthetic pesticide use, reducing freshwater toxicity by a factor of two. Longer-term rotations like these were once more common in Iowa, but they are relatively rare now because agricultural policies and markets favor production of maize and soybeans and not the additional crops included in longer rotations.

Agricultural Policies

How can policy encourage a shift toward agroecological practices? Most governmental agricultural conservation efforts in the United States focus on voluntary programs, although a body of environmental legislation primarily enacted in the 1970s (e.g., the Clean Water Act, restrictions on draining wetlands and plowing up perennial grassland) sets limits on what farmers can do with their land. The success of voluntary programs depends on the willingness of producers and other businesses to participate. Political and economic macro-scale factors, such as global demand for biofuels or commodity crops, have powerful impacts on producers' decisions to enroll in or abandon conservation programs (Stuart & Gillon, 2012). Many farmers and food companies are unwilling or financially unable to adopt practices that reduce short-term profits, even if they might enhance stability of global food systems and improve ecological integrity. Another concern with voluntary programs is that without independent verification, some may engage in **greenwashing** (exaggerated claims of environmental benefits).

Overall, current voluntary approaches are not adequate, as can be seen from trends in resource degradation. Climate change and other current threats point to a tremendous need for greater resilience in the food system. Supplementing voluntary approaches with a strong regulatory framework would have greater impact, but regulatory approaches are politically difficult to implement given resistance from those benefiting from a weak regulatory system. Regardless of the type of policy, environmental goals and thresholds for severe damage to environmental resources must be determined in order to set appropriate policies. Without such goals and limits, current agricultural and environmental trends indicate that more critical resource-use thresholds will be surpassed.

As described in chapters 7 and 8, many policy tools exist to influence individual and societal practices, including payment for ecosystem services (which creates a market for ecosystem services in addition to food, fiber, fuel, and other farm products so that farmers can be compensated for protecting ecosystem services); regulation and fines for environmental degradation, using the "polluter pays" principle (in which the onus to clean up a polluted site is on the person or company responsible for the pollution and benefiting in some way from it); and financial support to convert farming systems to organic or other agroecological practices with lower environmental costs but perhaps lower yields, particularly in the first years of conversion.

Specific policies must be implemented at the system level with attention to impacts at multiple geographic scales and beyond the primary area of interest to minimize harmful side effects and maximize beneficial changes throughout the food system. Examples of such systemwide approaches are encouragement of local food systems and local food procurement by schools and other institutions. As policies are implemented, the time scales needed for transitions should be accommodated. For example, infrastructure to support local or regional farming takes time to be rebuilt; US policies since the mid-twentieth century have encouraged the loss of diverse and decentralized infrastructure for farming areas.

Policy is one way to stimulate change. There are many others, from economics to psychology to culture. Agricultural decisions are strongly affected by demand, so consumer demand for foods produced in environmentally sustainable ways is a critical driver of change. Perspective 3.2 provides a snapshot of US consumer perceptions of such foods.

Perspective 3.2. Consumer Perceptions of Environmentally Sustainable Foods

A nationally representative survey of US consumers included questions on the environmental sustainability of food choices. Findings presented in figures 3.13 and 3.14 show that a majority of consumers think about the sustainability of their diets. Many also make efforts to reduce the environmental impacts of their diet, such as buying local or organic food and purchasing products in recyclable packaging.

FIGURE 3.13   How Much Consumers Think about Food Sustainability

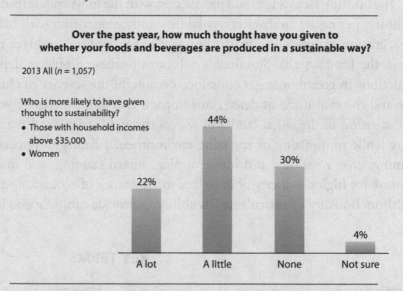

Over the past year, how much thought have you given to whether your foods and beverages are produced in a sustainable way?

2013 All (n = 1,057)

Who is more likely to have given thought to sustainability?
• Those with household incomes above $35,000
• Women

A lot	22%
A little	44%
None	30%
Not sure	4%

FIGURE 3.14   Environmental Sustainability-Related Actions Consumers Take

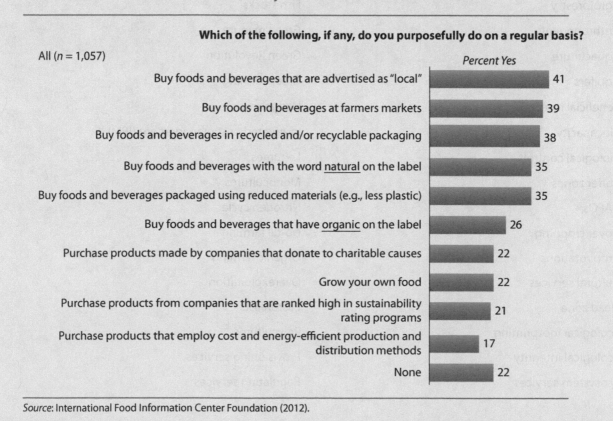

Which of the following, if any, do you purposefully do on a regular basis?

All (n = 1,057)

Percent Yes

Buy foods and beverages that are advertised as "local"	41
Buy foods and beverages at farmers markets	39
Buy foods and beverages in recycled and/or recyclable packaging	38
Buy foods and beverages with the word <u>natural</u> on the label	35
Buy foods and beverages packaged using reduced materials (e.g., less plastic)	35
Buy foods and beverages that have <u>organic</u> on the label	26
Purchase products made by companies that donate to charitable causes	22
Grow your own food	22
Purchase products from companies that are ranked high in sustainability rating programs	21
Purchase products that employ cost and energy-efficient production and distribution methods	17
None	22

Source: International Food Information Center Foundation (2012).

SUMMARY

Although industrialized agriculture and fishing have increased total food production and productivity, they have led to decreased ecological integrity and they threaten future food production capacity. Given the many ways reduced food security affects physical and mental health (see chapter 5), not to mention the ways hunger could play out in global conflict and migration, these ecological issues are public health issues of the highest order. Even beyond food security, losses of ecosystem services will have many costly real-world implications for human health and society.

The limiting factors for food production with the most widespread consequences are climate change, declining per capita freshwater availability and competition with other uses, overexploitation of fisheries, erosion of agrobiodiversity, shortages of phosphorus, and lack of a ready substitute for fossil fuel use in the food system. Sustainable solutions to these problems depend first on immediate dramatic reductions in greenhouse gas emissions because of the severity of climate change's impacts on agriculture and the multitude of deleterious impacts that climate change will bring. Another important step is restoration of degraded land and waters through agricultural practices that maintain high productivity while minimizing or reversing environmental damage. Agroecological practices such as organic farming, crop rotations, and intercropping, mixed farming, and integrated water management show promise for high productivity as well as maintenance of ecological integrity. Such practices respect the multifunctionality of agriculture, its ability to provide multiple goods and services simultaneously.

KEY TERMS

Agrobiodiversity

Agroecology

Agroforestry

Anthropogenic

Aquaculture

Aquifers

Beneficial insects

Biocapacity

Biological controls

Buffer zones

CAFOs

Cover cropping

Crop rotations

Cultural services

Dead zone

Ecological footprinting

Ecological integrity

Ecosystem services

Erosion

Eutrophication

Fish stocks

Green manure

Green Revolution

Greenwashing

Hedgerows

Integrated pest management (IPM)

Legumes

Monocultures

Nitrogen cycle

No-till farming

Organic farming

Overexploitation

Pastoralists

Polycultures

Provisioning services

Regulating services

Resilience	Strip cropping
Runoff	Subsistence
Salinization	Supporting services
Siltation	Volatilized
Soil fertility	Wetlands
Species richness	Wild (natural) biodiversity
Standard systems	

DISCUSSION QUESTIONS

1. In what ways does industrialized farming affect ecological integrity?

2. Do agriculture and fishing face a black-and-white choice between high yields and environmental conservation? Explain your answer.

3. Why are voluntary conservation measures generally insufficient on their own to maintain ecological integrity?

4. The concept of ecosystem services is gaining increasing recognition. What are some of the most important ecosystem services provided by agriculture? To what extent do you think a threatened loss of ecosystem services can drive change in policy and practice? Why?

5. This chapter describes numerous converging threats that together may take a substantial toll on future food security in the United States and globally. Are there still reasons to be hopeful? If so, what are they? Should "hopeful" be a goal?

6. What do you see as the most promising ways you yourself could engage to promote a more environmentally sustainable food system?

7. Farmer Michael Heller endorses a broad definition of sustainable farming going well beyond environmental impacts. To what extent do you agree or disagree with this definition?

REFERENCES

American Farmland Trust. (2010). *2007 NRI: Changes in land cover/use analysis*. Retrieved from www.farmlandinfo.org/2007-national-resources-inventory-changes-land-coveruse

American Farmland Trust. (2012). *Farmland information center fact sheet: Agricultural district programs*. Retrieved from www.farmlandinfo.org/agricultural-district-programs

American Farmland Trust. (2013). *A nationwide survey of land trusts that protect farm and ranch land*. Retrieved from www.farmlandinfo.org/nationwide-survey-land-trusts-protect-farm-and-ranch-land

Badgley, C., Moghtader, J., Quintero, E., Zakem, E., Chappell, M. J., Avilés-Vázquez, K., Samulon, A., & Perfecto, I. (2007). Organic agriculture and the global food supply. *Renewable Agriculture and Food Systems, 22*(2), 86–108.

Brown, L. (2012). *Full planet, empty plates: The new geopolitics of food scarcity*. New York: W. W. Norton.

Buzby, J. C., Wells, H. F., & Vocke, G. (2006). *Possible implications for U.S. agriculture from adoption of select dietary guidelines* (No. ERR-31). Washington, DC: US Department of Agriculture Economic Research Service. Retrieved from www.ers.usda.gov/publications/err-economic-research-report/err31.aspx

Canning, P., Charles, A., Huang, S., & Polenske, K. R. (2010). *Energy use in the U.S. food system* (No. ERR-94). Washington, DC: US Department of Agriculture Economic Research Service.

Committee on Twenty-First Century Systems Agriculture, National Research Council. (2010). *Toward sustainable agricultural systems in the 21st century*. Washington, DC: National Academies Press.

Cox, C., Hug, A., & Bruzelius, N. (2011). *Losing ground*. San Francisco: Environmental Working Group.

Davis, A. S., Hill, J. D., Chase, C. A., Johanns, A. M., & Liebman, M. (2012). Increasing cropping system diversity balances productivity, profitability and environmental health. *PLOS ONE*, *7*(1), e47149.

Dempsey, J., & Ferguson, K. (2010). Farmland by the numbers. *American Farmland*, Fall/Winter, 12–17.

Earth Policy Institute. (2012). *Peak meat: US consumption falling*. Retrieved from www.earth-policy.org/data_highlights/2012/highlights25

Economist Online. (2012). *Kings of the carnivores*. Retrieved from www.economist.com/blogs/graphicdetail/2012/04/daily-chart-17

Environmental Working Group. (2011). *Meat-eaters guide to climate change and health*. Retrieved from www.ewg.org/meateatersguide/a-meat-eaters-guide-to-climate-change-health-what-you-eat-matters

ETC Group. (2009). *Who will feed us? Questions for the food and climate crises*. Issue Communique #102. Retrieved from www.etcgroup.org/content/who-will-feed-us

ETC Group. (2013). Putting the cartel before the horse. Retrieved from www.etcgroup.org/content/new-report-putting-cartel-horse%E2%80%A6and-farm-seeds-soil-peasants

Feely, R. A., Sabine, C. L., Lee, K., Berelson, W., Kleypas, J., Fabry, V. J., & Miller, F. J. (2004). Impact of anthropogenic CO_2 on the $CaCO_3$ system in the oceans. *Science*, *305*(5682), 362–366.

Food and Agriculture Organization. (2006). *Livestock's long shadow: Environmental issues and options*. Rome: Author.

Food and Agriculture Organization. (2009a). *High level expert forum—How to feed the world in 2050*. Rome: Author.

Food and Agriculture Organization. (2009b). *The state of food and agriculture: Livestock in the balance*. Rome: Author.

Food and Agriculture Organization. (2010). *Global biodiversity outlook 3*. Rome: Author.

Food and Agriculture Organization. (2011a). *Energy smart food for people and climate*. Rome: Author.

Food and Agriculture Organization. (2011b). *State of land and water resources for agriculture*. Rome: Author.

Food and Agriculture Organization. (2012). State of the world's fisheries and aquaculture 2012. Rome: Author.

Global Footprint Network. (2010). *Ecological wealth of nations: Earth's biocapacity as a new framework for international cooperation*. San Francisco: Author.

Halweil, B. (2002). *Home grown: The case for local food in a global market*. Worldwatch Paper 163. Washington, DC: Worldwatch Institute.

Heinberg, R. (2012). Soaring oil and food prices threaten food supply. *UNCTAD Trade and Environment Review 2011/2012*. Retrieved from www.postcarbon.org/article/619300-soaring-oil-and-food-prices-threaten

Heinberg, R., & Bomford, M. (2009). *The food and farming transition: Toward a post carbon food system*. Post Carbon Institute. Available at www.postcarbon.org/report/41306-the-food-and-farming-transition-toward

H. John Heinz III Center for Science, Economics and the Environment (Heinz Center). (2008). *The state of the nation's ecosystems 2008: Measuring the lands, waters, and living resources of the United States*. Washington, DC: Island Press.

Heller, M. C., & Keolian, G. A. (2000). *Life cycle-based sustainability indicators for assessment of the U.S. food system* (Report No. CSS00–04). Ann Arbor: Center for Sustainable Systems, University of Michigan.

High Level Panel of Experts. (2013). *Biofuels and food security*. Rome: High Level Panel of Experts on Food Security and Nutrition of the Committee on World Food Security.

Hoekstra, A. Y., & Hung, P. Q. (2003). Virtual water trade. In *Proceedings of the International Expert Meeting on Virtual Water Trade's Value of Water Research Report* (Series No. 12). Delft: UNESCO-IHE.

Hoekstra, A. Y., & Hung, P. Q. (2005). Globalisation of water resources: International virtual water flows in relation to crop trade. *Global Environmental Change*, *15*, 45–56. Retrieved from www.waterfootprint.org/Reports/Hoekstra_Hung_%282005%29.pdf

Hoekstra, A. Y., et al. (2012). Global monthly water scarcity: Blue water footprints versus blue water availability. *PLOS ONE, 7*(2), e32688.

Hufnagl-Eichiner, S., Wolf, S. A., & Drinkwater, L. E. (2011). Assessing social-ecological coupling: Agriculture and hypoxia in the Gulf of Mexico. *Global Environmental Change, 21*(2), 530–539.

Ingram, J., Ericksen, P., & Liverman, D. (2010). *Food security and global environmental change.* London: Earthscan.

International Food Information Center Foundation. (2012). *Food and health survey.* Retrieved from www.foodinsight.org/Content/5519/IFICF_2012_FoodHealthSurvey.pdf

Johnson, R. (2014). *The U.S. trade situation for fruits and vegetables.* Congressional Research Service. Retrieved from www.fas.org/sgp/crs/misc/RL34468.pdf

Keystone Center. (2012). *Environmental and socioeconomic indicators for measuring outcomes of on-farm agricultural production in the United States.* Field to Market, Keystone Alliance for Sustainable Agriculture. Retrieved from www.fieldtomarket.org/report

Kucharik, C. J., & Ramankutty, N. (2005). Trends and variability in U.S. corn yield over the twentieth century. *Earth Interactions, 9*, 1–29.

Lagi, M., Bar-Yam, Y., Bertrand, K. Z., & Bar-Yam, Y. (2011, September 21). *The food crises: A quantitative model of food prices including speculators and ethanol conversion.* arXiv:1109.4859. Cambridge, MA: New England Complex Systems Institute.

Lal, R., Iivari, T., & Kimble, J. M. (2003). *Soil degradation in the United States: Extent, severity and trends* (p. 12). Boca Raton, FL: CRC Press.

Liu, J., Zehnder, A. J. B., & Yang, H., (2009). Global consumptive water use for crop production: The importance of green water and virtual water. *Water Resources Research, 45*(5), W05428.

Louisiana Universities Marine Consortium. (2012). *News.* Retrieved from www.gulfhypoxia.net

Maryland Department of Agriculture. (2014). A quick look at Maryland agriculture. Retrieved from mda.maryland.gov/Documents/ag.../AgBrief_Agriculture.pdf

McIntyre, B. D., Herren, H. R., Wakhungu, J., & Watson, R. T. (Eds.). (2009). *North America and Europe (NAE) report.* International Assessment of Agricultural Knowledge, Science and Technology for Development. Washington, DC: Island Press.

Millennium Ecosystem Assessment. (2005). *Ecosystems and human well-being: Synthesis.* Washington, DC: Island Press.

National Agricultural Statistics Service. (2014). *2013 state agriculture overview: Maryland.* Retrieved from www.nass.usda.gov/Quick_Stats/Ag_Overview/stateOverview.php?state=MARYLAND

Ongley, E. D. (1996). *Control of water pollution from agriculture.* FAO Irrigation and Drainage Paper 55. Rome: Food and Agriculture Organization.

Pew Commission on Industrial Farm Animal Production. (2009). *Putting meat on the table: Industrial farm animal production in America.* Philadelphia and Baltimore, Pew Charitable Trusts and Johns Hopkins University Bloomberg School of Public Health.

Plumer, B. (2012). Americans are eating less and less meat [*Washington Post* Wonkblog]. Retrieved from www.washingtonpost.com/blogs/ezra-klein/post/americans-are-eating-less-and-less-meat/2012/01/11/gIQANUvmqP_blog.html

Postel, S. L., Daily, G. C., & Ehrlich, P. R. (1996). Human appropriation of renewable freshwater. *Science, 271*(5250), 785–788.

Pretty, J. (2008). Agricultural sustainability: Concepts, principles and evidence. *Philosophical Transactions of the Royal Society B, 363*, 447–465.

Reganold, J. P., Jackson-Smith, D., Batie, S. S., Harwood, R. R., Kornegay, J. L., Bucks, D., Flora, C. B., Hanson, J. C., Jury, W. A., Meyer, D., Schumacher, A. Jr., Sehmsdorf, H., Shennan, C., Thrupp, L. A., & Willis, P. (2011). Transforming U.S. agriculture. *Science, 332*, 670–671.

Rockström, J., Steffen, W., Noone, K., Persson, Å, Chapin III, F. S., Lambin, E. F., Lenton, T. M., Scheffer, M., Folke, C., Schellnhuber, H. J., Nykvist, B., de Wit, C. A., Hughes, T., van der Leeuw, S., Rodhe, H., Sörlin, S., Snyder, P. K., Costanza, R., Svedin, U., Falkenmark, M., Karlberg, L., Corell, R. W., Fabry, V. J., Hansen, J., Walker, B., Liverman, D., Richardson, K., Crutzen, P., & Foley, J. A. (2009). A safe operating space for humanity. *Nature, 461*, 472–475.

Soil Association. (2010). *A rock and a hard place*. Bristol, UK: Author.

Stuart, D., & Gillon, S. (2012). Scaling up to address new challenges to conservation on US farmland. *Land Use Policy*, *7*(3), 223–236.

Sumberg, J., & Thompson, J. (Eds.). (2012). *Contested agronomy: Agricultural research in a changing world*. Abingdon, Oxford, UK: Routledge.

Tegtmeier, E. M., & Duffy, M. D. (2004). External costs of agricultural production in the United States. *International Journal of Agricultural Sustainability*, *2*(1), 1–20.

Thrupp, L. A. (1997). *Linking biodiversity and agriculture: Challenges for food security*. Washington, DC: World Resources Institute.

Tilman, D., Cassman, K. G., Matson, P. A., Naylor, R., & Polasky, S. (2002). Agricultural sustainability and intensive production practices. *Nature, 418*, 671–677.

Tomich, T. P., Brodt, S., Ferris, H., Galt, R., Horwath, W. R., Kebreab, E., Leveau, J., Liptzin, D., Lubell, M., Merel, P., Michelmore, R., Rosenstock, T., Scow, K., Six, J., Williams, N., & Yang, L. (2011). Agroecology: A review from a global-change perspective. *Annual Review of Environment and Resources, 36*, 15.1–15.30.

UN Department of Economic and Social Affairs. (2011). *World economic and social survey 2011: The great green technological transformation*. New York: United Nations.

UN Department of Economic and Social Affairs, Population Division. (2011). *World population prospects: The 2010 revision, highlights and advance tables* (Working Paper No. ESA/P/WP). New York: United Nations.

UN Environment Programme. (2007). *Global environmental outlook (GEO-4): Environment for development*. Valleta, Malta: Progress Press.

UN Environment Programme. (2014). *Water and energy. Volume 1, The United Nations world water development report 2014*. Retrieved from http://unesdoc.unesco.org/images/0022/002257/225741e.pdf

UN Population Division. (2008). *An overview of urbanization, internal migration, population distribution and development in the world* (UN/POP/EGM/-URB/2008/01). Retrieved from www.un.org/esa/population/meetings/EGM_PopDist/P01_UNPopDiv.pdf

UN World Water Assessment Programme. (2014). *The United Nations World Water Development Report 2014: Water and Energy*. UNESCO.

US Department of Agriculture Agricultural Research Service. (2012). *Honey bees colony and collapse disorder*. Retrieved from www.ars.usda.gov/News/docs.htm?docid=15572

US Department of Agriculture Economic Research Service. (2012). *Overview: Irrigation and water use*. Retrieved from www.ers.usda.gov/topics/farm-practices-management/irrigation-water-use.aspx

US Department of Agriculture Natural Resources Conservation Service. (2013). *National soil survey handbook, title 430-IV*. Retrieved from www.nrcs.usda.gov/wps/portal/nrcs/detail/soils/survey/?cid=nrcs142p2_054242

US Department of Agriculture, Natural Resources Conservation Service. (2014). *RCA Appraisal: Soil and Water Resources Conservation Act*. Retrieved from http://www.nrcs.usda.gov/Internet/FSE_DOCUMENTS//stelprdb1044939.pdf

US Department of Agriculture, Natural Resources Conservation Service Center for Survey Statistics and Methodology, Iowa State University. (2013). *Summary report: 2010 national resources inventory*. Washington, DC.

US Environmental Protection Agency. (2001). *Functions and values of wetlands* [Fact Sheet] (EPA 843-F-01–002c). Retrieved from http://water.epa.gov/type/wetlands/outreach/upload/functions-values.pdf

US Environmental Protection Agency. (2012). *Wetlands—Status and trends*. Retrieved from http://water.epa.gov/type/wetlands/vital_status.cfm

US Global Climate Change Research Program. (2009). *Global climate change impacts in the U.S*. Retrieved from www.epa.gov/climatechange/impacts-adaptation/agriculture.html

Zehnder, A. J. (1997). Is water the first resource to control demographic development? *Proceedings of the Forum Engelberg, Food and Water: A Question of Survival* (pp. 85–98). Zurich: vdf, Hochschulverlag AG an der ETH Zurich.

Zehnder, A. J. B., Yang, H., & Schertenleib, R. (2003). Water issues: The need for action at different levels. *Aquatic Sciences—Research Across Boundaries, 65*(1), 1–20.

Chapter 4

The Food System and Health Inequities

Roni A. Neff, Anne M. Palmer, Shawn E. McKenzie, and Robert S. Lawrence

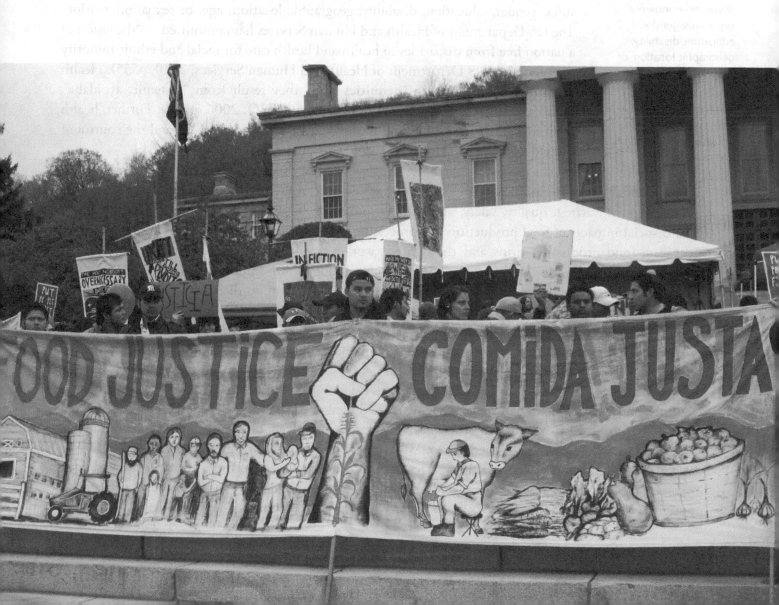

Learning Objectives

- Define health inequities and health disparities.

- Discuss root causes of food system–related health inequities.

- Discuss how inequities play out in the food system generally, in community food systems, and in community and occupational settings.

- Discuss potential equity-related pitfalls affecting well-meaning efforts to improve food systems.

- Provide examples of interventions to address inequities in each of these areas.

health disparities
Differences in health status among groups of people based on factors such as socio-economic status (SES), race, ethnicity, immigration status, environmental exposures, gender, education, disability, geographic location, or sexual orientation

health inequities
Health disparities resulting from systemic, avoidable, unfair, and unjust practices and policies

Today's food system generates and exacerbates health disparities and health inequities in US society and globally. **Health disparities** refer to differences in health status—for example, in life expectancy, health-related quality of life, obesity, diet-related disease, or asthma—between groups of people based on factors such as socioeconomic status (SES), race, ethnicity, immigration status, environmental exposures, gender, education, disability, geographic location, age, or sexual orientation. The US Department of Health and Human Services has committed to "the vision of a nation free from disparities in health and health care for racial and ethnic minority populations" (US Department of Health and Human Services, 2010, p. 35). Health disparities become **health inequities** when they result from "systemic, avoidable, unfair and unjust" practices and policies (NACCHO, 2006, p. 11). Further, health inequities "are sustained over time and generations and [are] beyond the control of individuals" (NACCHO, 2006, p. 11).

Health inequities in the food system are deeply linked to inequities throughout society, such as in individual and neighborhood socioeconomic status, race, and sex. They play out as inequities in food supply, nutrient quality, safety, affordability, and access; and in inequities in the environmental and social impacts of food production and processing. Additionally, they play out as power inequities among food production firms and the farmers, workers, and consumers affected directly by their decisions—and indirectly through disproportionate budgets for interest group activities. (These inequities are addressed in chapter 8.) Changes to the food system, as discussed in this chapter, can address food system inequities only to a certain point. True change requires altering the underlying social forces. As the National Association of City and County Health Officials (NACCHO, 2006, vii) writes, "Addressing the root causes of inequities in the distribution of disease and illness might seem like a luxury. But it is not."

The need to address both root causes and food system inequities begins with the fact that they are unjust and violate the human right to adequate food (described in chapter 1). Some in society benefit from healthful, high-quality, easy-to-access food and are relatively unexposed to the environmental health and social harms of the food system, whereas others are not so fortunate and suffer economically, socially, and via diminished health. The resultant health inequities are found in obesity rates, food insecurity, and occupational illness, and take their toll not only directly but also indirectly through stigma, financial impacts, time costs, and more. Food system inequities additionally affect the entire

Modified from Neff, Palmer, McKenzie, and Lawrence, (2009).

society, reducing the food system's overall quality, bringing down population health and well-being, and contributing to increased health and social costs. For the most part, the inequities described in this chapter are not affecting small, marginal populations. More than half the infants in the United States receive WIC, for example, and over half of the babies currently born are not white (US Census Bureau, 2012; US Department of Agriculture Food and Nutrition Service, 2013). Perspective 4.5 at the end of this chapter provides an extended discussion of the social benefits that can derive from jointly addressing food, health, and inequity.

HEALTH INEQUITIES AND FOOD SYSTEMS IN THE UNITED STATES

There are numerous substantial inequities in health outcomes across demographic groups in the United States. One example is life expectancy at birth, a common benchmark for comparing the health of populations. An African American male born in 2011 was expected to live until age seventy-two, more than four fewer years than a white male born that year, and six fewer than an African American female (Centers for Disease Control and Prevention [CDC], 2013). Geography is an even stronger proxy for inequity. Figure 4.1 shows the twenty-year gap in life expectancy at birth across Baltimore neighborhoods, from the highest (Roland Park, 83) to the lowest (Hollins Market, 63), which matches the life expectancy of Haiti.

FIGURE 4.1   Life Expectancy at Birth, 2011

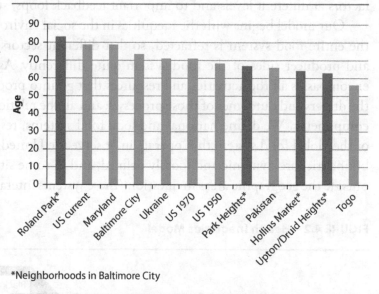

*Neighborhoods in Baltimore City

Source: Baltimore City Health Department and World Health Organization.

Strong evidence ties diet quality (Kirkpatrick, Dodd, Reedy, & Krebs-Smith, 2012; Wang, & Chen, 2011) and obesity and diet-related disease (Ogden, Lamb, Carroll, & Flegal, 2010a, 2010b; Wang & Beydoun, 2007) to racial-ethnic and socioeconomic disparities, although the relationships can be complex and can differ by gender and other factors. Nationally African Americans die from stroke (age-adjusted) at 141 percent of the rate of whites; of heart disease at 127 percent; and of diabetes at 204 percent (National Center for Health Statistics, 2012).

Food security inequities further shape health inequities. The United Nations has defined food security as a situation whereby "all people, at all times, have physical, social and economic access to sufficient, safe and nutritious food that meets their dietary needs and food preferences for an active and healthy life" (Food and Agriculture Organization, 2009, p. 1). Populations differ in ability to access healthy foods (foods that provide essential nutrients and support health), as described in chapters 5 and 17. Approximately 25 percent of African American and 26 percent of Hispanic households were classified as food insecure in 2011, nearly double the national percentage (US Department of Agriculture Economic Research Service, 2013). In the United States, food insecurity is also highly correlated with obesity, thus exacerbating the health harm and stigma (Dinour, Bergen, & Yeh, 2007). Food system impacts on health inequities also go beyond the "eating" pathway. Low-income, minority, and immigrant communities suffer from high exposure to occupational (Lipscomb, Loomis, McDonald, Argue,

& Wing, 2006) and community (Donham, Wing, Osterberg, & Flora, 2007) health threats associated with food production and processing methods, (as described in chapter 2).

Inequities: An Ecological Approach

In contemporary US society and within professional and research communities, diet has primarily been considered at the individual level, and interventions to improve diets and related health outcomes have largely targeted individual knowledge, attitudes, and behaviors (Huang & Glass, 2008). That approach is inadequate because individual-level choices are constrained by factors within the social, physical, and macro-level environments. Figure 4.2 illustrates how food systems influence health and contribute to health inequities. The model uses a systems framework directing attention to the interrelatedness of factors at different levels and to important feedback loops, such as in supply and demand.

Our model begins with the inequities in the social environment depicted as a prism, through which the entire food system is refracted, so that different sectors of society experience both the consumer and producer sides of the food system quite differently. As described in chapter 1, the food system encompasses all the activities and resources that go into producing, distributing, and consuming food; the drivers and outcomes of those processes; and all the relationships and feedback loops between system components. We define national and local food systems, respectively, as those segments or subsystems of the global food system that operate in or serve the United States or local areas. In either case, system boundaries are dynamic and loosely defined, and in some situations include activities taking place well outside the geographic areas in question. These systems interact with one another and with other parts of

FIGURE 4.2 Health Inequities Model

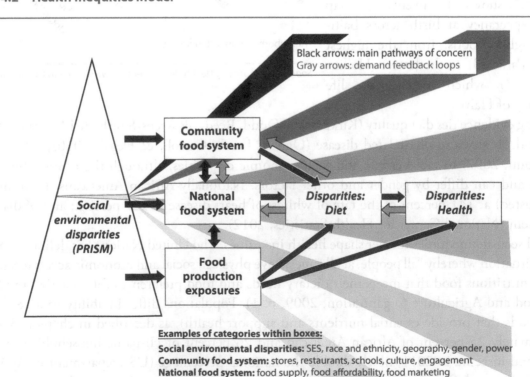

Black arrows: main pathways of concern
Gray arrows: demand feedback loops

Examples of categories within boxes:
Social environmental disparities: SES, race and ethnicity, geography, gender, power
Community food system: stores, restaurants, schools, culture, engagement
National food system: food supply, food affordability, food marketing
Food production exposures: community and occupational hazards
Diet disparities: disparities in affordability, access, consumption of healthy diet
Health disparities: disparities in rates of disease, injury, mortality, well-being

the food system and other social factors to contribute to inequities in diet, which in turn create health inequities. The model also shows how social inequities contribute to what we term *food production exposures*, or environmental and occupational exposures to food production hazards, and it shows how these hazards contribute directly to health inequities. This chapter dedicates less time to this pathway, which is discussed at greater length in chapters 2, 11, and 12. At the bottom of figure 4.2 are examples of categories within each of the model's main boxes.

Through feedback loops (relationships in which one thing affects another, which in turn affects the first), shown in gray, inequities in individual and community likelihood of obtaining high-quality food can affect the extent to which such foods are made available either in certain communities or society-wide. For example, some storekeepers report reluctance to stock healthier food choices, citing one reason as the perceived low demand for those foods in their communities (Gittelsohn et al., 2008).

Individual food choices, the psychosocial factors that influence choice, and environmental and occupational exposures of course vary within and between communities. Demographics are not destinies. The factors described previously, however, may contribute to aggregate-level inequities.

The model shows potential sites for intervention, located at each arrow. Interventions to change the relationship between food systems and health use two broad types of strategies: **population-based approaches** (aimed at changing factors affecting the entire population) and **targeted approaches** (aimed at changing the food system exposures or food demand within specific sectors of the population). Note that although a "rising tide may lift all boats," and population-based public health interventions may improve conditions for all, they can simultaneously *increase* health disparities. Efforts using new information or technologies may especially have this paradoxical effect. As human rights advocate, anthropologist, and physician Paul Farmer observed, the group that starts out healthier is often better educated with more resources, and is therefore more likely to use new technology or information more rapidly and effectively, thus experiencing a greater gain in health status than those with poorer health, less education, and fewer resources (Farmer, 2001). Similarly, perspective 4.1 presents Julie Guthman's argument that those who already believe in the message of the food movement and those who are already slim may be most open to adopting its encouraged practices. Figure 4.3 dramatizes the concept. It contrasts a population-based intervention—which may improve outcomes across the board but have the strongest effect on those most likely to engage with it, thus ironically increasing the disparity—with a targeted intervention, which may improve outcomes for the targeted population but have little effect on others.

population-based approach
Approach or intervention aimed at changing factors affecting the entire population

targeted approach
Approach to intervention that targets activities to a specific segment of the population

FIGURE 4.3 Population-Based Interventions May Increase Health Disparities

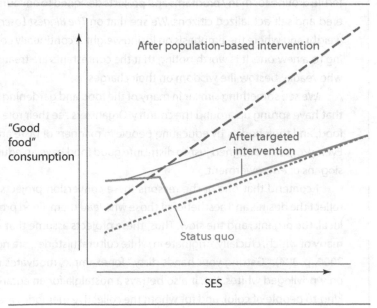

Perspective 4.1. Foodies on a Mission
Julie Guthman

In recent years, organizations devoted to food justice have proliferated, bolstered by the many high school and college students, mostly white and privileged, who want to volunteer or intern with such organizations. Much of this work involves bringing fresh fruits and vegetables and other healthy food into communities of color, sometimes explicitly in the hope of combating obesity. I've worked with many such students, and several have returned from internships to tell stories about how little the food or the mode of food delivery resonated with people in the community. In one memorable thesis, my student reported on a conversation with her African American neighbor. My student had mentioned that she worked for the organization that brought a truck of organic fruits and vegetables to her neighborhood. Her neighbor's response to why she did not shop from the truck (which was convenient and sold at below-market prices) was, "Because they don't sell no food! All they got is birdseed." She went on to exclaim, "Who are they to tell me how to eat? I don't want that stuff. It's not food. I need to be able to feed my family." When my student asked her what she would like the truck to offer, the neighbor said, "You know, what normal grocery stores have."

My point in telling this story is not to suggest how such projects could be more effective in reaching their target constituency—although they could. Instead, I want to bring into focus the civilizing mission in the alternative-food movement. By *civilizing mission*, I mean to connote the early colonial encounters between Europe and others. When confronted with different ways of life, Europe saw lack and tried to convert these others to the ways of Europeans, most obviously in the realm of religion but also in government, art, and everyday manners. Today, missionary work still involves civilizing, improving, and even providing charity to the "downtrodden," but rarely addressing the source of inequality. Missionary work, thus, often entails *bringing* individual improvement rather than *supporting* collective action. And, of course, the missionary's life is the one that neophytes are expected to emulate.

Countless historical examples exist of the tendency to teach people about food in relation to other social ends. For instance, in the Progressive Era, white middle-class reformers, primarily women, sought to acculturate newly arrived European immigrants to Anglo Protestant American diets, dress, drinking habits, and manners in the name of Americanization (Levenstein, 1988). Today's concern with health and responsibility has provided fertile ground for many programs and projects designed to encourage weight loss and to produce more empowered and self-actualized citizens. We see that on *The Biggest Loser*, where fat people compete to lose the most weight and where the emphasis on losing weight is continually coupled with putting one's life in order or aspiring to a new one. It is worth noting that the contestants are treated paternalistically by the hard-body trainers, who readily bestow life wisdom on their charges.

We see something similar in many of the food and gardening programs for both children and at-risk adults that have sprung up around the country. Organizers see their role as changing peoples' relationships to nature, food, and their bodies by educating people in manners of taste and norms of civil eating (Hayes-Conroy, 2009). Even programs designed just to distribute good food have an educational quality to them and occasionally use slogans of empowerment.

I contend that one of the reasons these conversion projects have the character they do is because they reflect the desires and aesthetics of those who lead them. Food project advocates extol food associated with the local, the organic, and the slow. Thus, these projects assume that particular ideals, aesthetics, and experiences, many of which, crucially, originate in white cultural histories, are normal, and widely shared (Kobayashi & Peake, 2000, p. 394). "Getting your hands dirty," for example, motivates many a farm and gardening activist, and not only privileged whites. Yet, it also betrays a nostalgia for an agrarian past that in the United States was far less kind to people of color, and for whom the collective memories are not good ones.

What missionaries often don't recognize is that their messages speak mainly to the almost or already converted. The audience for local, organic food, like the kind written about by Michael Pollan, tends to be those who already have a stake in good eating and status. I have come across many of Pollan's fans in classrooms, speaking engagements, and public forums. For the most part, they are white, educated, urbane, and thin—and are already quite convinced of alternative food's goodness. In a funny way, even Michael Pollan knows this. *In Defense of Food* (2008) is full of appeals to "us." In other words, it's not so much that the discourse of good food convinces its subjects; rather, subjects who are ready to believe it choose the discourse. Think about it: if you eat the Pollan diet, will it make you thin? Or is it that because you are thin, you are more likely to read about and eat the Pollan diet?

Source: Excerpt from *Weighing In* (Guthman, 2011).

ELABORATING THE PATHWAYS

In the following sections, we elaborate on three sets of pathways from social environment inequities to inequities in diet and health through the national food system, the local food system, and food production and processing exposures.

National Food System

Our nation's food system presents the entire population with a food supply in which less healthy foods tend to be more affordable than healthier ones, and in which consumers are strongly encouraged to buy these less healthy products, as described elsewhere in this textbook. Refracting through the lens of inequities highlights ways that food system risk factors for poor diet are exacerbated for those with low SES and for minorities. In the following sections we describe how three aspects of the food system may contribute to inequities: food supply, affordability, and marketing. Given the complexity of the food system, it is impossible to know exactly how food system reform would actually affect inequities. As was described in focus 1.1, a systems modeler might develop and manipulate an "artificial society" to help illustrate possible impacts of different scenarios. Although we cannot do that here, we instead share evidence-based ideas regarding selected cases. As you read these, consider whether you agree or whether alternate scenarios seem plausible to you.

Food Supply   Factors in the macro-environment, such as policy and economics, affect what food is produced and production methods. Food system policy is driven by financial and political power in the food system, which is based significantly on economic power and tilts toward agribusiness and food processing lobbies (Hauter, 2012). One US policy goal has been to reduce prices and increase supply of key commodity crops including corn and soybeans, which benefits such lobbies (chapter 8) and may contribute—indirectly—to the ubiquity of processed foods and relatively low-cost meats (Wallinga, Schoonover, & Muller, 2009). Although some food consumers have more alternatives, those with lower incomes, ethnic minorities, the less educated, and those from inner cities or rural backgrounds may be especially likely to have their available and likely food options dominated by the mainstream and less healthy offerings, as described in chapter 17. This is because of a combination of physical and economic access barriers, as well as marketing and cultural factors. What if the economic and legal incentives for food production, manufacturing, marketing, and sales were shifted to *promote* a healthier food supply overall, and if the mainstream food supply was then healthier and produced more sustainably? We speculate that prices, access, and social norms would likely change, and that impacts might be most apparent among communities that consume the most mainstream and heavily marketed food and foods that are made most affordable through the current food system policy. (Although, note that as a population-level intervention, this *could*, as discussed previously, increase the disparity even as it improves conditions for all.)

Food Affordability The second way that broad food system factors can affect health inequities is through the pathway of food affordability. Differentials in the ability to afford healthy food may affect diet-related disease disparities, and differentials in the ability to afford food altogether contribute to disparities in a variety of physical and mental health, and child development outcomes, as described in chapter 5. In the following sections we describe how the food system may contribute to those differentials, including via relative food prices, food assistance, and overall food prices.

Relative Food Prices Consumers describe price as a key factor in food purchasing decisions, and price elasticity (the extent to which price changes affect demand) may be greater the more limited the household budget (Powell & Chaloupka, 2009). Cost is significantly more important among those with lower income and among the nonwhite compared to higher-income and white respondents (Glanz, Basil, Maibach, Goldberg, & Snyder, 1998; Leibtag & Kaufman, 2003).

Those with low incomes must typically spend greater percentages of their incomes to purchase food than do others, although they spend less money overall. Many studies, dating at least to the 1960s, have examined the question of whether "the poor pay more" for the *same* food basket. A 1997 review article and more recent studies (Chung & Myers, 1999; Kaufman, MacDonald, Lutz, & Smallwood, 1997; Talukdar, 2008) find that the poor do pay more than others, although the differentials are small.

FIGURE 4.4 **Cheeseburgers versus Salad: The Importance of Price (poster reflecting quote from focus group participant)**

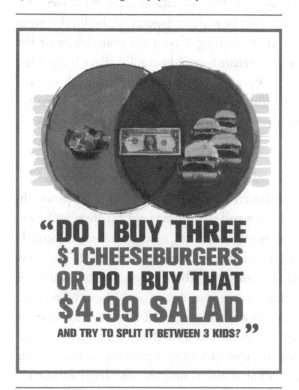

Source: Aviva Paley, CLF.

Another (2008) study found slightly lower prices in lower-income areas (Andreyeva, Blumenthal, Schwartz, Long, & Brownell, 2008). The evidence is mixed regarding whether accounting for suburban, urban, or rural status and store type (smaller and non-chain stores cannot obtain the economies of scale of larger stores) (Fellowes, 2006) would wash out any "poor pay more" price differential. The results may vary geographically.

Nutrient-dense foods such as fruits and vegetables are often more costly than more energy-dense foods with high sugar and fat content. Studies do suggest it is possible to eat a nutrient-rich diet at comparable cost to an energy-dense one (Ervin, Wang, Wright, & Kennedy-Stephenson, 2004; Lipsky, 2009; Reed, Frazã, & Itskowitz, 2004), and indeed, on a per meal basis healthier foods can be less expensive and more filling than preprepared alternatives. Regardless, nutrient-dense foods are often *perceived* as more expensive and that can affect choices (figure 4.4 reflects a quote from a focus group participant in Baltimore). Adding to the potential cost differential is the reality that perishable foods do not last as long as processed foods, so buying them can mean more money lost to waste (Zachary, Palmer, Beckham, & Surkan, 2013). Shifting to more nutrient-dense foods may also require new knowledge and time for food preparation, as well as departures from flavor preference, familiarity and cultural and social norms.

How do we make healthy diets affordable for all? Powell and Chaloupka (2009) reviewed the literature and found that decreasing the price of healthy products tends to be more effective than increasing the price of unhealthy products in addressing obesity and overweight. Their review states that larger price changes in particular had "a measurable effect" on weight, especially among youth, those with low SES, and those at particular risk for overweight. A US Department of Agriculture (USDA) study concluded that if prices of fruits and vegetables were subsidized by 10 percent, fruit consumption among low-income Americans would rise by 2.1 to 5.2 percent and vegetables by 2.1 to 4.9 percent—a substantial rise, though still leaving consumption well below the USDA's recommended dietary allowance (Dong & Bin, 2009). Taxing unhealthy foods and beverages is regressive as it disproportionally burdens those with lower SES, who spend a higher proportion of their income on food than wealthier individuals. Although some find the regressiveness unacceptable, others argue that the benefits of these regressive taxes for those with lower incomes outweigh the cost (a somewhat similar debate is presented in perspectives 5.2 and 5.3). Much more research is needed on the public health and disparity impacts of varying price strategies for different foods, in different contexts, and for different consumer groups.

In the discussion of price, the fungibility of time and money deserves mention. "Time poverty" helps explain why some people on low budgets choose to buy more expensive preprepared foods, versus cooking from scratch (Rose, 2007). Further innovation is needed to identify ways the food system can reduce the time cost of healthy foods and keep prices low, including through prepackaged items, funds to families to purchase cooking equipment, and recipe sharing.

Truly making food equitably affordable in our society would require righting income inequalities and enabling all people to earn adequate livelihoods to provide for their families. Instead, we provide food assistance and emergency food programs. As described extensively in chapter 5, these programs are reasonably successful in preventing outright hunger, but they do not reach all who might need them and do not provide enough to eliminate food insecurity. Further, foods provided directly, such as through schools and food pantries, are often energy-dense processed foods, although there are increasing efforts to incorporate fresh produce into the offerings. These programs have some elements aimed at preserving client dignity, but most could do more in this regard.

Overall Food Prices Another pathway from the food system to price to inequities is through long-term influences on domestic and global food prices. The US food supply and its prices are shaped by factors including social and economic conditions, agricultural and trade policies, production technologies, and environmental conditions (OECD-FAO, 2012; Trostle, 2008). Converging ecological crises of climate change, and of water, soil, and fossil fuel depletion, may contribute to long-term reductions in agricultural supply and substantial price volatility, as described in chapter 3. Even such seemingly unrelated factors as biofuel production and commodity speculation in financial markets are shown to have had important impacts on supply and prices (OECD-FAO, 2012). These price and supply effects have also led to instability and at times, price shocks that may be expected to hit hardest for consumers with low incomes—and for agricultural producers and low-SES rural communities.

Although price and supply influences may reduce food affordability over the short term, over the middle and longer term it is *possible* that these threats and resultant dislocations or incentives could lead to impacts that make healthy, local, sustainably produced food options more available. For example, high petroleum prices could eventually motivate at least a partial relocalization of food production and a turn toward lower-energy food production, processing, and distribution methods (Neff et al., 2009). New "green" investments in response to resource shortages and climate change could enable and incentivize further shifts. If food supply is a challenge, land may become more valued for growing crops for direct human consumption rather than animal feed, and meat could become less affordable. As food prices rise, garden food production could increase as well (Garden Writers Association Foundation, 2013; Horovitz, 2009), although it must be recognized that growing one's own food takes time, water, usable soil or space, skills and training, and startup resources. In sum, these shifts *could* eventually contribute to making the healthy and sustainable choice more the affordable choice, and thus more equitably accessible across the socioeconomic spectrum.

Food and Beverage Marketing   A third way that broad food system factors can affect health inequities is through inequities in food and beverage marketing (see chapter 10 for more on marketing). Audience segmentation in content and placement is a basic tenet of marketing. When this practice is effective in promoting unhealthy foods more in some communities than others, however, it can lead to behaviors and norms that exacerbate health disparities (Grier & Kumanyika, 2008). Studies have found that inequities in placement of outdoor food and beverage marketing may contribute to obesity and behaviors that increase risk for obesity, (Lesser, Zimmerman, & Cohen, 2013; Yancey et al., 2009) that more food commercials aired during shows popular with African American audiences than others, and that the distribution of items advertised was more heavily skewed toward unhealthy food (Henderson & Kelly, 2005; Tirodkar & Jain, 2003). Additionally, low-income children tend to watch more television and have greater media exposure—and thus more exposure to food commercials—than their higher-income counterparts (Grier & Kumanyika, 2008). When the US Federal Trade Commission compelled forty-four major food companies to provide food marketing data, only half stated that they did not target advertising based on gender, race, and ethnicity. Many of the remaining companies do; numerous examples are provided in the report (Federal Trade Commission, 2008). Few interventions and policies are specifically developed to reduce differential food marketing by race or ethnicity. Possible approaches include regulation, marketing guidelines and voluntary limits, zoning changes, counter-advertising, "shaming" the advertisers publicly, media literacy education, and even legal challenges on civil rights and human right to food or right to health grounds.

Community Food System

A broad body of literature identifies residential segregation in the United States and documents neighborhood-level inequities across many health outcomes. Refracting these inequities through the lens of food highlights dramatic differences in healthy food availability and in oversupply of less healthy foods across neighborhoods. Chapter 17 reviews literature on inequities in **food environments** (all aspects of our physical and nonphysical surroundings that may influence our diets) and their associated health impacts in depth, and describes interventions. Here we provide a basic overview of the evidence linking a set of community food environments to dietary disparities. Additionally, a community's food system affects health and inequities through numerous pathways beyond its physical environment, and we briefly comment on those as well.

food environments
All aspects of our surroundings that may influence our diets, including physical locations and marketing, media, and online exposures

Community Food Environments   Our lives are embedded within multiple food environments that shape the foods we find most available, affordable, and appealing. In the following, we briefly describe evidence regarding how three of these (retail, restaurants, and schools) may affect health disparities and associated interventions.

Retail Most studies have found that predominantly minority, low-income, and rural communities are particularly likely to have low access to supermarkets, chain supermarkets, and stores selling fresh foods. Corner stores (see figure 4.5) and other sites in low-income areas, by contrast, tend to offer an abundance of processed foods and few fresh items. Proximity to healthy food sources is particularly important for those without their own transportation and for those in far-flung rural areas. Neighborhood crime levels can also be a concern, affecting safety and limiting the shopping options some consumers are willing to use. Even when they have access, minority and low income consumers may avoid stores or farmers markets if they do not feel comfortable there. Interventions to address these access inequities include financing new supermarkets; initiatives to improve environments within existing stores; efforts to transport produce, farm-fresh goods and supermarkets to underserved areas; opening farmers markets in underserved areas; and efforts to transport underserved consumers to supermarkets and farmers markets.

FIGURE 4.5   Corner Store

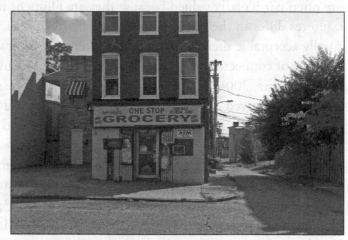

Source: Ruth Burrows, CLF.

Restaurants Larson, Story, and Nelson (2009) observed overall that most US studies find more fast food restaurants in low-income and minority areas, and full-service restaurants in wealthier areas, although results are not consistent (Larson et al., 2009; Powell, Chaloupka, & Bao, 2007). Further, the literature generally shows that consuming higher amounts of restaurant food, especially fast food, is associated with obesity and weight gain. (Although fast food restaurants are often singled out, offerings in full-service restaurants are also commonly high in calories, fat, sugar, and salt.) Findings are mixed regarding the impact of *geographic proximity* to restaurants; living nearby does not equate with eating the food (Larson et al., 2009; Powell et al., 2007). Given these mixed findings and the difficulty of intervening, beyond a few zoning interventions there have been few efforts to address differential restaurant exposure.

Schools Although school food environments are well documented to be associated with unhealthy consumption, as shown in chapter 17, the *disparities* in these impacts may be expected to stem from two areas: differential use of school food due to poverty and differential school district acceptance of food-related activities such as vending and food industry sponsorship of school activities like athletics. Accordingly, addressing health disparities via school food environments means first addressing school meal programs. Second, it can mean changing district regulations regarding accepted practices in vending and sponsorship. Finally, it means targeting food education programs to schools or areas with many low-income or minority children and engaging in culturally appropriate strategies. It is important to recognize that some of the most effective and progressive interventions addressing food in schools also involve the most substantial and costly change, and thus can be challenging or unaffordable for many schools—especially in poor neighborhoods. To avoid increasing inequities among schools, across-the-board implementation (following pilot projects) within districts should be recommended (Allen & Guthman, 2006) and funding should be made available to low-income school districts.

Nonphysical Aspects of the Community Food System The mix of cultures within a community may also be seen as part its food system. Culture may affect food consumption via preferences, openness to trying new foods, food preparation knowledge, and comfort levels regarding new or different cooking methods and ingredients. Further, as cultures interact with poverty, higher-fat foods and meats are often particularly valued because they are filling or have cultural and personal history significance. Cultures differ in their attitudes toward obesity as well, contributing potentially to differences in culturally acceptable dietary patterns and ultimately to health problems. Food may also be considered as a means of connecting to or holding onto cultural identity and distinguishing oneself from the mainstream (James, 2004). Foods promoted as "healthy" are sometimes viewed as foreign to a given culture or can be perceived as culturally inappropriate (James, 2004), whereas culturally aligned comfort foods may be seen as a way to provide something positive and culturally significant to children in the face of poverty and stress (Kaufman & Karpati, 2007). On the flip side, acculturation to US society has been found to predict numerous unhealthy behaviors across multiple immigrant and ethnic groups. In terms of diet, those with greater acculturation tend to consume more processed food with increased fats and sugars (Gordon-Larsen, Harris, Ward, & Popkin, 2003; Unger, Reynolds, Shakib, Spruijt-Metz, Sun, & Johnson, 2004). Of course, cultures are not static. Many cultures have experienced significant shifts based on information about health impacts of certain preferred foods (Prynne, Paul, Mishra, Greenberg, & Wadsworth, 2005).

A community's food system is composed of many elements beyond its physical environment and culture, and these play into the distribution of diets and health. Most direct, of course, is the distribution of income in a community; we discuss price and affordability and environmental and occupational exposures within a community's food system in the next section. Another important factor is the community's level of engagement to improve its food system and to address inequities, including level of programming and policy efforts, resources devoted to them, and community-based engagement and leadership. Another is a community's food-related emergency planning and response capacity, which affect the ways it is able to support residents' food needs in case of emergency events, including ensuring food gets to the most vulnerable. Additionally, a community's human and physical resources and its policy structure and economic incentives affect the food that can be produced, processed, and distributed locally. As described in chapter 16, locally produced foods may promote health for reasons including their appeal, which leads to increased produce consumption; and because of the **cultivars** of fruits and vegetables used. Local foods additionally may strengthen communities and provide jobs. As perspective 4.2 notes, though, it takes effort to use them to promote equity.

cultivars
Plant varieties produced by breeding

Perspective 4.2. Realizing Justice in Local Food Systems
Patricia Allen

No one can deny that local food is good food. To the extent that people are trying to solve problems of tastelessness, processed foods, and the numbing sameness of the food-procurement experience, local food systems can provide solutions. For other food system issues, particularly those involving social justice, the role of food system localization is less clear. This perspective raises questions about the congruence of local food systems and social justice through the lenses of demography, democracy, and geography.

Demography

In the local food movement there is a sense that, because people live together in a locality and encounter each other, they will make better, more equitable decisions that prioritize the common good. Although this is a beautiful vision, localities also contain wide demographic ranges and social relationships of power and privilege. At both global and local scales, those who benefit—and those who do not—are arranged along familiar lines of class, ethnicity, and gender. For example, nearly all local food campaigns and many of those involved in direct marketing prioritize supporting farmers, although to date there has been little discussion of other food system workers. Yet workers and owners in the food system have interests that are not necessarily consonant. In addition, an emphasis on farmers over farmworkers contains inadvertent racial inflections because most farm owners are white, and most farmworkers are people of color.

One of the most-cited benefits of local food systems is that of supporting the local community and keeping food dollars close to home. However, in addition to the disparities embedded in the local community, small-scale institutions are not always more equitable. Small, direct markets, for example, serve those with the ability to pay, just like all markets do. Many people working on direct marketing initiatives such as farmers markets and CSAs are working to garner extra-market sources of income (such as public subsidies or private grants) to support those without the means to pay market prices. These subsidies are necessary to ameliorate the inherent inequalities of market-based economic forms.

Demographic disparities, such as those of race, gender, and class, may be inadvertently reproduced in food system localization efforts between and within regions unless we make particular efforts to not do so. It is at the local level that completely new economic forms that prioritize equity can be imagined, piloted, and evaluated. Institutional food-purchasing programs can include social justice criteria in their operating principles and purchasing standards, and labeling schemes including social justice criteria can be implemented.

Democracy

Participatory democracy is a necessary condition for developing social equity in the food system at local and extra-local levels. Democratic control of the food system may be more likely in smaller geographic scales because of face-to-face interaction and awareness of how the food system affects people in the region. But people in groups can also pursue the paths of least resistance, choosing and pursuing priorities and topics that are "normal" and noncontroversial in order to facilitate congenial discussions.

Whereas more personal relationships may increase caring and compassion, it is also the case that people with few economic options or great dependency may be more reluctant to speak freely or raise issues that may offend their neighbors or employers. Social relations of power and privilege also determine who is allowed to be part of the conversation and shape who has the authority to speak and whose contributions are considered worthwhile.

For those working on local food projects, special efforts need to be made to include those who have been materially or discursively marginalized. This is easier said than done, of course. Often projects have limited budgets and limited time. In addition, people who have been historically excluded may not have the time, energy, transportation, and money to participate in local food-planning meetings or may have different agendas than local food organizers.

Geography

Most definitions of local food systems use physical definitions. Often they are based on a distance radius—30, 50, and 150 miles. Others suggest political boundaries such as the county or biological delimitations such as the watershed. What all of these definitions have in common is a sense that local is geographically determined and that proximity is important.

(Continued)

(Continued)

But what about people in other parts of the world who might be less resource-endowed or who have been historically impoverished? Although local food movements cannot be held responsible for rectifying injustices of the past, neither is it clear how physical geography is a defensible arbiter for boundaries of caring, action, or understanding. Local food movements can partner with other regions to address inequality and the policies that create and foster it, developing solidarity and expanding the scope of effective engagement.

Conclusion

For local food systems to play a role in increasing social equity, those of us working on local food systems must place our efforts in context and have clear goals. This involves (1) increasing understanding of the economic, political, and cultural forces that have configured the current agrifood system and (2) analyzing and reflecting on which local food system priorities and activities move in the direction of, rather than away from, social justice.

Local food systems create possibilities for seeing the real people, social relations, and conditions involved in the food system, leading people to think critically about the food system and, potentially, increasing social justice. We need to contextualize the local, understanding that place and community have been shaped by historical inequalities and work as we can to rectify those inequalities.

Source: Excerpted from Allen (2010).

Food Production and Processing Exposures

Finally, outside the eating pathway in the food system, exposures associated with agriculture and food-processing methods can directly affect health, as described in chapters 2, 12, and 13. Many rural communities are directly involved in or proximal to agriculture and food production and processing operations; studies have documented environmental injustice in the siting of industrial food animal production (IFAP) facilities, including disproportionate frequency in areas with high proportions of low-income and African American residents (Donham et al., 2007; Mirabelli, Wing, Marshall, & Wilcosky, 2006; Wilson, Howell, Wing, & Sobset, 2002; Wing, Cole, & Grant, 2000). As described in chapter 12, there is a growing body of research on the public health impacts of living near IFAP facilities, particularly regarding associations with respiratory conditions, mental health concerns (Donham et al., 2007), and risk of acquiring MRSA (methicillin-resistant *Staphylococcus Aureus*) infection (Casey et al., 2013).

Workers engaged in food production, processing, distribution, warehousing, and other aspects of the US food system report exceptionally high rates of occupational injury, illnesses, and fatality, as illustrated in focus 2.2. It is additionally a cruel irony that because of the low wages in many food system jobs, workers providing our food often struggle to afford or access healthy foods for themselves and their families, as described in perspective 4.3 and figure 4.6.

Perspective 4.3. The People Who Touch Your Food
Saru Jayaraman

> I was a server for fifteen years and raised four kids on a server's wages plus tips. Depending on other people to tip you … can be the most stressful part of being a server. There were many nights that I didn't even make enough to pay my babysitter … What most people don't realize is that servers don't make the minimum wage like most people. —Rita, Indian Rock Beach, Florida

There are nearly twenty million workers in the food system, the nation's largest private sector employer (Bureau of Labor Statistics [BLS], 2010). More than half of these workers—more than ten million people—work in the restaurant industry (Restaurant Opportunities Center United [ROC], 2010). Fifty-seven percent of Americans eat out at a restaurant at least once per week (Rasmussen Reports, 2013), supporting the restaurant industry's continued growth in the midst of the recent economic crises (BLS, 2010).

Unfortunately, despite its growth and potential, the restaurant industry provides largely poverty-wage jobs. In 2010, seven of the ten lowest-paid occupations were restaurant occupations (BLS, 2010), and over half of all restaurant workers earned less than the federal poverty line (US Department of Health and Human Services, 2011). Sadly, this results in food servers using food stamps at twice the rate of other US workers, meaning that many cannot put food on their own tables (ROC, 2010).

A major cause of low wages in the industry is the fact that the minimum wage for workers who earn tips has remained stuck at $2.13 per hour for the last twenty-one years, thanks to lobbying by the National Restaurant Association (NRA) (Liddle, 1996). The NRA claims that raising wages would force restaurants to raise menu prices exorbitantly. In fact, the 2012 Congressional minimum wage increase proposal would not increase the cost of food by more than ten cents per day for the average American household (Food Labor Research Center …, 2012).

Low wages tell only part of the story. Ninety percent of restaurant workers surveyed nationwide in 2010 reported not having access to paid sick days or health benefits through their employers. Not surprisingly, two-thirds of workers surveyed reported cooking and serving food while sick (ROC, 2010)—a risk to them and to food consumers. Workers also reported pervasive nonpayment of wages and misappropriation of tips.

There are some livable wage jobs in the industry, but unfortunately, immigrants, workers of color, and women often cannot access these jobs. Discrimination and other barriers have resulted in a $4 wage gap between white workers and workers of color (ROC, 2012a). Gender segregation also persists; in a recent study men held 79 percent of observed dining room management positions, and women held only 21 percent (ROC, 2012b).

To address these challenges, I cofounded the Restaurant Opportunities Center (ROC) after 9/11 together with workers displaced from the World Trade Center. ROC has grown into a national restaurant workers' organization with thirteen thousand members in thirty-two cities nationwide. ROC has opened two cooperative restaurants called COLORS, partnered with responsible restaurateurs, published almost twenty reports based on thousands of surveys, and won several workplace justice and policy victories (figure 4.6 shows workers protesting). The 2012 Congressional minimum wage bill included the first significant increase for tipped workers in twenty years.

(Continued)

(Continued)

FIGURE 4.6   Restaurant Opportunities Center Protest

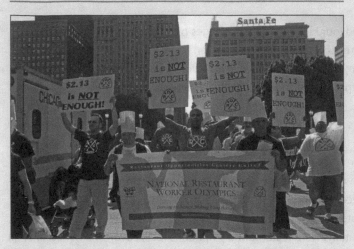

Source: ROC.

To build a groundswell of support to win this legislation, we launched a multiyear multimedia campaign to engage diners. In observing the success of consumer engagement in moving restaurants to provide locally sourced, organic menu items, especially after the release of pivotal books such as Eric Schlosser's *Fast Food Nation* and Michael Pollan's *Omnivore's Dilemma*, we created a National Diners' Guide and smartphone app (available on our website, www.rocunited.org) to give eaters information and tools to voice their values. We also released a book and series of films called *Behind the Kitchen Door*, with a foreword by Eric Schlosser. We created The Welcome Table (www.TheWelcomeTable.org), which is organizing eaters to voice the groundswell. In all of these ways, we are mobilizing workers, employers, and diners to improve the lives of those who touch our food.

Health inequities derive not only from geography and working roles, but also from the power imbalances between agribusiness and processing firms, and farmers, workers, and communities. For instance, as described in perspective 4.4, the vertically integrated poultry industry constrains farmer control over operations in multiple ways, with health and social impacts for the farmers (as well as other workers—and chickens.)

Perspective 4.4. Contract Chicken Farming
Carole Morison

As a farmer, I raised chickens under contract for twenty-three years with a multinational company. Once in the business, I learned that farmers have no control over the method of raising chickens.

The chicken industry is vertically integrated, whereby chicken companies own everything from embryo to market shelf. Companies provide the chicks, feed, medications, fuel, and any other items associated with raising the chickens. They contract with farmers to raise their chickens to a marketable age. The company determines the type of housing, equipment, the breed and quality of chicks, and what is in the feed.

Farmers (also known as *growers* or *producers*) enter the business believing they will make a decent living, but contract chicken farming is expensive. Chicken housing alone can put farmers in debt by millions. In 2012, the average cost of one chicken house was estimated at $380,000. On average, farms have at least eight chicken houses, which each can hold up to thirty-six thousand birds. Larger farms can have ten to twenty chicken houses and there are "mega farms" with twenty to thirty houses. Farmers are also left with the burden of disposing of manure and dead chickens.

New farmers must enter non-negotiable contracts with chicken companies. On a regular basis, companies demand upgrades to housing and equipment, which further adds to the debt. Farmers struggle to keep up because pay is so low. Companies give farmers the choice either to make the requested changes or the contract will be terminated. Most comply with the demands. Noncompliance often leads to bankruptcy. In my experience from talking with farmers, fear of financial ruin is the main reason farmers stay in contract industrial chicken farming. Most have mortgaged the family farm and homestead to get into the business.

Farmers are paid by a complicated formula of costs to raise the flock versus pounds of meat moved off the farm. Companies may deliver unhealthy chicks to one farm, and others receive healthy chicks. Receiving a flock of unhealthy chicks puts the farm at a disadvantage from the beginning, and no matter how hard a farmer tries, the farm will not do well on that flock. Many farmers believe that a company can and will manipulate how well individual farms will do.

Company personnel visit farms regularly to ensure that farmers are following company policy. I found it disheartening to hear that chicks needed to be culled (killed) because they weren't uniform in size or were not growing as fast as others. No chance is given for chicks not fitting the mold. This costs the farmer because the cost of the chick plus the feed it ate is deducted from their final pay.

The best interest of the chickens became a growing concern for me. Industry uses confinement housing to raise chickens, controlling every aspect of growing them. Most chicken houses today have solid walls, which keep out sunlight and only allow for fresh air through fans (tunnel ventilation). The companies claim this method provides a better environment and protects the chickens from outside elements. Another justification is that confinement enables chickens to grow faster by minimizing their activity, which keeps energy use down and translates into less feed used.

It's a dark and dreary life for the chickens. Lighting is dim to keep them docile. Movement consists of getting up to eat and drink and then plopping down again. Dust, feces, and ammonia build up as they lay on litter (pine shavings) saturated with manure from continual intense production inside the house, flock after flock.

Industrial chickens have been engineered to have large breasts and to grow fast. They grow from newly hatched chicks to 5- to 5 1/2-pound chickens in less than seven weeks. The chicks are cute, yellow, and fuzzy when they arrive on the farm. As they grow, it becomes obvious that their bones and organs cannot keep up. Many die from heart attacks and can only walk a few steps before they plop down from exhaustion. Over the years I became immune to watching this until I finally reached a point of asking myself, "how did I get this way"?

In addition to the financial pressures and frustrations with industry methods, farmers also face health concerns due to the dust-laden houses and to additives in the company feed. Concerns over the heavy use of antibiotics in the chicken feed have arisen because of the emergence of antibiotic-resistant bacteria. Arsenic is another concern because farmers are exposed through direct contact with the feed or through breathing the dust. Many farmers have unknowingly worked in environments that have the potential for severe health consequences. Feed formula is considered a trade secret and there is no legal mandate for companies to reveal the contents so farmers can learn what they are being exposed to.

The US chicken industry produced nine billion chickens in 2011 (National Chicken Council, 2012). Each chicken produces an average of three pounds of manure. Although the company owns the chickens, the farmers are left to dispose of their waste simply because the industry says so. Commonly, they spread it on farm fields as fertilizer. However, only a certain amount of manure can be safely applied on land before excess nutrients are not absorbed.

(Continued)

(Continued)

FIGURE 4.7   Carole Morison on her current farm

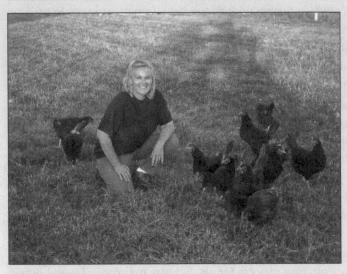

Source: Carole Morison

The chicken industry sets up shop mostly in poor, rural areas across the country and becomes the only game in town for farmers, workers, and communities. Through this knowledge, coupled with excessive wealth and power, the industry exerts undue control over politics. Change will come only when communities and farmers speak with a collective voice. I publicly took a stand and walked away from the industry in the movie *Food, Inc.* It was scary at the time, however, in doing so I learned that there is another way to be a farmer and enjoy what I do. My farm has transitioned to a pastured egg farm raising Animal Welfare Approved certified hens on a vegetarian diet (figure 4.7). They are able to roam freely and behave like chickens.

A 2012 report on working conditions for food chain workers presents information about the people on the front lines harvesting, processing, and serving our food. Figures 4.8a and 4.8b share some of the key findings. For example, just 13.5 percent of food chain workers earned a living wage, while over 30 percent experienced marginal, low or very low food security. One-third indicated having suffered wage theft just in the previous week. More than half (57 percent) had suffered injury or a health problem on the job, yet most workers (83 percent) did not receive health insurance from their employers, and 58 percent had no health insurance from any source.

FIGURE 4.8a   Charts from the Hands That Feed Us

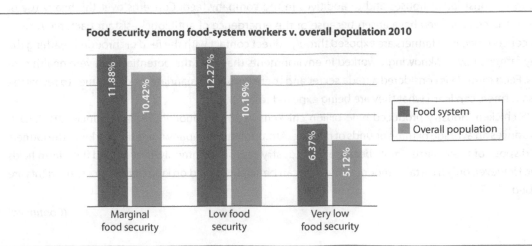

Source: Bureau of Labor Statistics, Occupational Employment Statistics, (2010)

FIGURE 4.8b   Wages and Working Conditions for Food Chain Workers

WAGES	
MEDIAN WAGE $9.65	
%	WAGE SEGMENT
23%	Subminimum wage
37.6%	Poverty wage
25.8%	Low wage
13.5%	Living wage

HOURS WORKED	
40%	Worked more than 40 hours per week
11%	Worked more than 60 hours per week at 2 or more employers

ACCESS TO BENEFITS	
79%	Do not have paid sick days or do not know if they do
83%	Do not receive health insurance from employer
58%	Do not have any health care coverage at all
53%	Have worked when sick
35%	Used emergency room for primary care

LACK OF MOBILITY	
32%	Did not receive any training by employer when employment began
74%	No ongoing job training by employer
75%	Never had opportunity to apply for better job
81%	Never received a promotion

EMPLOYMENT LAW VIOLATIONS	
36%	Experienced wage theft in the previous week
$35.48	Average weekly wage theft
12%	Observed minors working in workplace

BREAKS	
30%	Did not always receive lunch break
40%	Did not always receive 10-minute break

HEALTH AND SAFETY	
52%	Did not receive health and safety training from employer
32.7%	Did not receive proper equipment to do their job
11.7%	Did something that put their own safety at risk
57.2%	Suffered injury or health problem on the job

Source: Food Chain Workers Alliance Survey Data, (2012)

Perspective 4.5. Food, Equity, and Health: Making the Connections in Public Health Practice

Wayne Roberts

Extensive evidence accumulated over decades shows that economic inequality has a damaging impact on everyone's health—rich and poor alike. Inequality is not a win-lose game, where the rich win and the poor lose. On the contrary, inequity is a lose-lose game due to the stress and wear and tear that flow from the loss of

(Continued)

(Continued)

important, if intangible, supports to health and well-being—such as social trust, cohesion, belonging, common cause, mutual support, and public safety (Pickett & Wilkinson, 2011).

Evidence shows that wealthy people living in an inequitable economy don't enjoy as many healthy and active years of life as people who are wealthy or poor in a more equitable economy. People on low income in Sweden, for example, generally enjoy better health than wealthy people in Britain, just as the poor in Japan on average live longer and healthier lives than both the poor and wealthy of the United States (Pickett & Wilkinson, 2011, World Health Organization, 2013). This is a critical point for public health advocacy: equity improves health outcomes for everyone.

Prevention and treatment strategies for chronic health disorders that cause almost two-thirds of the world's approximately sixty million deaths each year should include a suite of measures that foster equity. Food system measures fostering equity deserve particular attention, if only because so many chronic health disorders—heart disease, diabetes, and certain cancers come immediately to mind—can be traced back to either food or agricultural products.

I got my chance to bring food and equity issues together in health campaigns when I worked from 2000 to 2010 for the Toronto Food Policy Council, which is often regarded as an international leader in municipal strategies for linking food with equity. It's not hard to find opportunities to work on food and equity issues together. Almost all food security challenges have an equity angle lurking in the background, just as most equity challenges have food repercussions. Healthy food and equitable food systems are means and ends to each other. For example, high rates of obesity in underserved and low-income neighborhoods are best understood through combined equity and food and nutrition lenses. A lack of affordable, welcoming, and quality food outlets can be remedied through public health partnerships with city planners, neighborhood organizations, food security organizations, and a variety of entrepreneurial food providers, including co-ops, healthy corner grocers, and supermarkets. As neighbors work on such projects, they become an empowered community, which in turn combines work on improving diets with increased support networks and rising confidence in the future—all of which contribute to an improved public health scene.

Both understanding and interventions are better managed when equity and food considerations are integrated. Amartya Sen won a Nobel Prize in economics for showing that famines were not caused by lack of food (which might sound a bit like saying poverty is not caused by lack of money), but by lack of equity and human rights (Sen, 1999). Likewise, to put a face on the billion people around the world who experience chronic hunger and food insecurity, most are children, women, and members of racially or ethnically marginalized groups.

Groups facing equity problems frequently face converging challenges with food access. People who suffer from discrimination, for example, more commonly live on lower incomes in underserved communities. Economizing on food might lead to a false economy for health, because fruits and vegetables are commonly more expensive per calorie than are less nutritious and less protective but more filling starch-based foods. Equally important to health and well-being, though less tangible and therefore more difficult to measure, are inequities leading to disrespect for a group's food culture. In Toronto, one of the world's most multicultural cities, dominant groups have long shamed and mocked foods eaten by people who are deemed inferior. Germans were called krauts because of sauerkraut, French were called frogs because of the foraging that produced their unique cuisine. Immigrant areas where southern and eastern Europeans lived when they first came to North America were often referred to in disparaging terms such as "garlic hill." Children of newcomers, already stressed by being in new cultures where people speak different languages, often have to deal with people who make fun of the food they bring from home or have to cope with institutions that don't offer dietary options—such as halal, kosher, or vegetarian—that respect their religious beliefs. Food literacy programs that uphold the worth of diverse cuisines, many of which are more supportive of physical health and environmental sustainability than the standard Anglo-American diet, present an obvious health promotion opportunity to link health benefits from food and equity.

My Toronto experience also taught me to address the mental health repercussions of food inequities. The very phrase *food security* is quite expressive of emotional anxieties, as well as physical hunger linked to food deprivation. As Toronto pediatrician and public health researcher, Dr. Catherine Mah, notes, when a family only has food for five days, they are nervous all week, not just hungry during the weekend. She believes that childhood food insecurity is so strongly associated with lifelong episodes of low self-worth and depression that she is campaigning for questions such as "did you ever experience hunger or food insecurity as a child?" to become standard questions in medical interviews (Roberts, 2012).

The rich interactions people have with food provide a wealth of opportunities for public health intervention. I worked in Toronto on community economic development projects that fostered a "quadruple win"—with benefits for human health, job creation, community cohesion, and a more resilient environment. Think of a transportation policy that makes it easy to shop for food by walking, biking, or taking public transit. A well-designed transit strategy will simultaneously lower air pollution from traffic jams, reduce traffic jams and associated "car rage" caused by congestion, increase healthy physical activities such as walking and cycling, improve public safety as a result of busier and friendlier streets, and create more easily accessed jobs for people without cars.

Such a widening circle of benefits invites public health leaders to initiate new approaches to partnerships based on a "whole-of-government–whole-of-society" approach. This can overcome the silos of narrow departments that miss overarching opportunities. Both equity and food will benefit from such broad-based government innovations, as will the economy and environment.

The public health renewal that comes from weaving healthy food and equity programming is based on a new way of appreciating the value of food. Instead of focusing on ways to reduce the cost of food, hoping to make more good food affordable and accessible, we can focus on ways to invest in increasing the value-added opportunities of food. The costly burden of chronic disease, to be hard-headed and crassly economic about it, is the "**opportunity cost**" of not investing in food-security programs that nourish people with safe, nutritious, and culturally appropriate food enjoyed in settings that foster dignity and belonging. From an economic standpoint, linking food and equity programs also highlights the logical argument that good food costs little compared to the medical and workplace productivity savings from preventing diseases caused by malnutrition.

opportunity cost
What one must give up in order to get something else

Investments in food-health-equity programs also yield multiple benefits that go far beyond savings in health care costs and reduction in absenteeism. School meals improve school attendance, especially for girls in the Global South, and the improved literacy from school attendance provides lifelong economic opportunities (Murphy, 2007). When money for government programs is tight or when lack of social empathy hinders investment in social programs, it helps to make a hardheaded case for spending on health that pays off in "human capital" (the economic value carried within a person's mind and body) and "social capital" (the economic benefits of a society that is more inclusive, trusting, and collaborative).

Food and meals fulfill essential biological needs for physical health, psychological well-being, and spiritual flourishing. Understanding food-equity-health links flows from this appreciation of food, which reclaims the full potential of both food and people. The ability of food and food environments to fuel human agency and empowerment, at the personal and community levels, bodes well for a dynamic relationship between healing professions and communities.

CONCLUSION

This chapter has described broad inequities in food supply, affordability, and access in nutrition and in food system hazardous exposures. We have discussed how these inequities are linked to longstanding social inequities and policies, practices, and structures within the food system. Some of the relationships are well supported by evidence; others are more speculative at this time. The chapter also describes policy and programmatic interventions that may address and reduce health inequities; perspective 4.5 provides further discussion of interventions that unite food, health, and equity.

Effective progress will depend partly on a broader recognition of the breadth of food system factors that contribute to these inequities. Community-engaged and participatory approaches are essential in the search for and development of effective solutions that will not be experienced as punitive, stigmatizing, unrealistic, or missing key components—and also to make sure the right questions are asked. Better still are approaches driven *by* community members. There is a great need to build leadership capacity among affected communities, and for others to cede space for their leadership. Population strategies should be balanced with efforts specifically targeted at removing barriers that create and perpetuate disparities. Food system and public health advocates must also join forces with those working to address underlying social inequities based primarily outside the food system. In all these areas, this chapter indicates a need for more evidence and evaluation, more innovation, more scaling up and policy change, and more action.

SUMMARY

Health disparities become health inequities when they result from "systemic, avoidable, unfair and unjust" practices and policies (NACCHO, 2006, p. 11) Health inequities in the food system are deeply linked to inequities throughout society and are damaging to everyone in society. Health inequities are promoted by factors in the national food system such as food supply, food affordability, and marketing; factors in the community food system, such as food access; social and cultural factors; and community and occupational exposures within the food production system. Community food system contributions to health inequities include neighborhood variation in both healthy and less-healthy food availability and cultural differences in food preferences. Communities near food production and processing facilities and workers throughout the food system face differential exposures by race and class that also contribute to health inequities. Finally, there are important inequities deriving from power imbalances between food industry firms and farmers, workers, and communities. Key to addressing inequities is building leadership among those most harmed and for others working in partnership with them to develop responses reflecting their concerns and interests.

KEY TERMS

Cultivars

Food environments

Health disparities

Health inequities

Opportunity cost

Population-based approach

Targeted approach

DISCUSSION QUESTIONS

1. Each of us is advantaged in some ways and disadvantaged in some ways. How have your own advantages and disadvantages affected your food choices or other food system experiences?

2. Many believe that truly addressing inequities in the food system requires going beyond food to address inequities in society. Yet, those social inequities are difficult to change for many reasons. Where would you focus your energies?

3. The authors note that in some cases their discussion of how our food system affects inequalities is speculative (particularly due to a lack of evidence on pathways from broad national and international food system forces to health inequities). Do you agree with their speculations? Why or why not?

4. Julie Guthman's piece, "Foodies on a Mission," is provocative. What you think of her view of a "civilizing mission in the alternative-food movement"?

5. How do you react to her conclusion, "If you eat the Pollan diet, will it make you thin? Or is it that because you are thin, you are more likely to read about and eat the Pollan diet?"

6. The chapter authors write that it is possible that over the middle and longer term, food system environmental threats might contribute to making the healthy and sustainable choice the affordable choice. Do you agree or disagree?

7. Patricia Allen writes, "Although local food movements cannot be held responsible for rectifying injustices of the past, neither is it clear how physical geography is a defensible arbiter for boundaries of caring, action, or understanding." Do you think we should have some special responsibility to those who are more local to us?

8. We know the food system has many inequities. Wayne Roberts describes evidence indicating that inequities harm everyone. Can you think of concrete ways inequities harm those on the privileged side?

9. Who controls the food system? Why does it matter?

REFERENCES

Allen, P. (2010). Realizing justice in local food systems. *Cambridge Journal of Regions, Economy and Society*, pp. 1–14.

Allen, P., & Guthman, J. (2006). From "old school" to "farm-to-school": Neoliberalization from the ground up. *Agriculture and Human Values*, 23, 401–415.

Andreyeva, T., Blumenthal, D. M., Schwartz, M. B., Long, M. W., & Brownell, K. D. (2008). Availability and prices of foods across stores and neighborhoods: The case of New Haven, Connecticut. *Health Affairs*, 27(5), 1381–1388.

Bureau of Labor Statistics. (2010, May). *Occupational employment statistics, national cross-industry estimates*. Retrieved from bls.gov/pub/special.requests/oes/oesm10nat.zip

Casey, J., Curriero, F. C., Cosgrove, S. E., Nachman, K. E., & Schwartz, B. S. (2013). High-density livestock operations, crop field application of manure, and risk of community-associated methicillin-resistant *Staphylococcus Aureus* infection in Pennsylvania. *JAMA*, 173(21), 1980–1990.

Centers for Disease Control and Prevention. (2013). *Table A: Deaths, age-adjusted death rates, and life expectancy at birth, by race and sex; and infant deaths and mortality rates, by race: United States, final 2010 and preliminary 2011*. Retrieved from www.cdc.gov/nchs/data/nvsr/nvsr61/nvsr61_06.pdf

Chung, C., & Myers, S. L. (1999). Do the poor pay more for food? An analysis of grocery store availability and food price disparities. *Journal of Consumer Affairs, 33*(2), 276–296.

Dinour, L. M., Bergen, D., & Yeh, M. C. (2007). The food insecurity–obesity paradox: A review of the literature and the role food stamps may play. *Journal of the American Dietetic Association, 107,* 2071–2076.

Dong, D., & Bin, B. H. (2009). *Fruit and vegetable consumption by low-income Americans: Would a price reduction make a difference?* (No. ERR-70). Washington, DC: US Department of Agriculture Economic Research Service.

Donham, K. J., Wing, S., Osterberg, D., & Flora, J. L. (2007). Community health and socioeconomic issues surrounding concentrated animal feeding operations. *Environmental Health Perspective, 115,* 317–320.

Ervin, R. B., Wang, C. Y., Wright, J. D., & Kennedy-Stephenson, J. (2004). Dietary intake of selected minerals for the United States population: 1999–2000. *Advance Data, 341.*

Farmer, P. (2001). *Pathologies of power: Structural violence and the materiality of the social.* Baltimore: Johns Hopkins University: The Eighth Annual Sidney W. Mintz Lecture in Anthropology.

Federal Trade Commission. (2008). *Marketing food to children and adolescents: A review of industry expenditures, activities, and self-regulation: A report to congress.* Washington, DC: Author.

Fellowes, M. (2006). *From poverty, opportunity: Putting the market to work for lower income families.* Washington, DC: The Brookings Institution.

Food and Agriculture Organization. (2009). *Declaration of the world summit on food security.* Rome: Author.

Food Labor Research Center, University of California, Berkeley Food Chain Workers Alliance, & Restaurant Opportunities Centers United. (2012). *Dime a day: The impact of the Miller/Harkin minimum wage proposal on the price of food* (p. 1). Retrieved from http://rocunited.org/dime-a-day-the-impact-of-millerharkin-minimum-wage-proposal-on-the-price-of-food

Garden Writers Association Foundation. (2013). *Gardening trend surveys: Gardening with edibles continues to expand.* Shallowater, TX: Author.

Gittelsohn, J., Franceschini, M.C.T., Rasooly, I. R., Ries, A. V., Ho, L. S., Pavlovich, W., … Frick, K. D. (2008). Understanding the food environment in a low-income urban setting: Implications for food store interventions. *Journal of Hunger & Environmental Nutrition, 2*(2), 33.

Glanz, K., Basil, M., Maibach, E., Goldberg, J., & Snyder, D. (1998). Why Americans eat what they do: Taste, nutrition, cost, convenience, and weight control concerns as influences on food consumption. *Journal of the American Dietetic Association, 98*(10), 1118–1126.

Gordon-Larsen, P., Harris, K. M., Ward, D. S., & Popkin, B. M. (2003). Acculturation and overweight-related behaviors among Hispanic immigrants to the US: The national longitudinal study of adolescent health. *Social Science and Medicine, 57,* 2023–2034.

Grier, S. A., & Kumanyika, S. K. (2008). The context for choice: Health implications of targeted food and beverage marketing to African Americans. *American Journal of Public Health, 98*(9), 1616–1629.

Guthman, J. (2011). *Weighing in: Obesity, food justice, and the limits of capitalism.* Berkeley: University of California Press.

Hauter, W. (2012). *Foodopoly: The battle over the future of food and farming in America.* New York: New Press.

Hayes-Conroy, J. (2009). *Visceral reactions: Alternative food and social difference in American and Canadian Schools.* PhD dissertation. State College: Pennsylvania State University.

Henderson, V. R., & Kelly, B. (2005). Food advertising in the age of obesity: Content analysis of food advertising on general market and African American television. *Journal of Nutrition Education and Behavior, 37*(4), 191–196.

Horovitz, B. (2009). Recession grows interest in seeds, vegetable gardening. *USA Today,* February 20.

Huang, T. T., & Glass, T. A. (2008). Transforming research strategies for understanding and preventing obesity. *Journal of the American Medical Association, 300*(15), 1811–1813.

James, D.C.S. (2004). Factors influencing food choices, dietary intake, and nutrition-related attitudes among African Americans: Application of a culturally sensitive model. *Ethnicity and Health, 9*(4), 349–367.

Kaufman, L., & Karpati, A. (2007). Understanding the sociocultural roots of childhood obesity: Food practices among Latino families of Bushwick, Brooklyn. *Social Science & Medicine, 64*(11), 2177–2188.

Kaufman, P., MacDonald, J., Lutz, S., & Smallwood, D. (1997). *Do the poor pay more for food? Item selection and price differences affect low income household food costs* (No. 759). Washington, DC: US Department of Agriculture Economic Research Service.

Kirkpatrick, S. I., Dodd, K. W., Reedy, J., & Krebs-Smith, S. M. (2012, May). Income and race/ethnicity are associated with adherence to food-based dietary guidance among US adults and children. *Journal of the Academy of Nutrition and Dietetics, 112*(5), 624–635.

Kobayashi, A., & Peake, L. (2000). Racism out of place: Thoughts on whiteness and an anti-racist geography in the new millennium. *Annals of the Association of American Geographers, 90*(2), 392–403.

Larson, N. I., Story, M. T., & Nelson, M. C. (2009). Neighborhood environments: Disparities in access to healthy foods in the U.S. *American Journal of Preventive Medicine, 36*(1), 74–81.

Leibtag, E. S., & Kaufman, P. R. (2003). *Exploring food purchase behavior of low income households*. Washington, DC: US Department of Agriculture Economic Research Service.

Lesser, L. I., Zimmerman, F. J., & Cohen, D. A. (2013) Outdoor advertising, obesity, and soda consumption: a cross-sectional study. *BMC Public Health, 13*(20).

Levenstein, H. A. (1988). *Revolution at the table: The transformation of the American diet*. New York: Oxford University Press.

Liddle, A. (1996, June 24). Associations urge Senate to retain wage provisions. *Nation's Restaurant News*. Retrieved from http://findarticles.com/p/articles/mi_m3190/is_n25_v30/ai_18440459

Lipscomb, H. J., Loomis, D., McDonald, M. A., Argue, R. A., & Wing, S. (2006). A conceptual model of work and health disparities in the United States. *International Journal of Health Services, 36*(1), 25–50.

Lipsky, L. M. (2009). Are energy-dense foods really cheaper? Reexamining the relation between food price and energy density *American Journal of Clinical Nutrition, 90*(5), 1397–1401. doi:10.3945/ajcn.2008.27384

Mirabelli, M. C., Wing, S., Marshall, S. W., & Wilcosky, T. C. (2006). Race, poverty, and potential exposure of middle-school students to air emissions from confined swine feeding operations. *Environmental Health Perspectives, 114*(4), 591–596.

Murphy, J. (2007). Breakfast and learning: An updated review. *Current Nutrition and Food Science, 3*, 3–36.

NACCHO. (2006). *Tackling health inequities through public health practice: A handbook for action*. Washington, DC: Author. Retrieved from www.naccho.org/topics/justice/upload/NACCHO_Handbook_hyperlinks_000.pdf

National Center for Health Statistics. (2012). *Health, United States, 2012*. Table 20. Retrieved from www.cdc.gov/nchs/hus/black.htm

National Chicken Council. (2012). *Broiler chicken industry key facts*. Retrieved from www.nationalchickencouncil.org/about-the-industry/statistics/broiler-chicken-industry-key-facts

Neff, R. A., Palmer, A. M., McKenzie, S. E., & Lawrence, R. S. (2009). Food systems & public health disparities. *Journal of Hunger & Environmental Nutrition, 4*(3–4), 282–314.

OECD-FAO. (2012). *OECD-FAO agricultural outlook 2012–2021*. Available from www.oecd-ilibrary.org/agriculture-and-food/oecd-fao-agricultural-outlook-2012_agr_outlook-2012-en

Ogden, C. L., Lamb, M. M., Carroll, M. D., & Flegal, K. M. (2010a). Obesity and socioeconomic status in adults: United States, 2005–2008. *NCHS Data Brief, 50*, 1–8.

Ogden, C. L., Lamb, M. M., Carroll, M. D., & Flegal, K. M. (2010b). Obesity and socioeconomic status in children and adolescents: United States, 2005–2008. *NCHS Data Brief, 51*, 1–8.

Pickett, K., & Wilkinson, R. (2011). *The spirit level*. Fairfield: Bloomsbury.

Pollan, M. (2006). *The omnivore's dilemma: A natural history of four meals*. New York: Penguin.

Pollan, M. (2008). *In defense of food: An eater's manifesto*. New York: Penguin.

Powell, L. M., & Chaloupka, F. J. (2009). Food prices and obesity: Evidence and policy implications for taxes and subsidies. *Milbank Quarterly, 87*(1), 229–257.

Powell, L. M., Chaloupka, F. J., & Bao, Y. (2007). The availability of fast-food and full-service restaurants in the United States: Associations with neighborhood characteristics. *American Journal of Preventive Medicine, 33*(4, Suppl. 1), S240–S245.

Prynne, C. J., Paul, A. A., Mishra, G. D., Greenberg, D. C., & Wadsworth, M.E.J. (2005). Changes in intake of key nutrients over 17 years during adult life of a British birth cohort. *British Journal of Nutrition, 94*, 368–376.

Rasmussen Reports. (2013, January 28). *57% dine out at least once a week*. Retrieved from www.rasmussenreports.com/public_content/lifestyle/general_lifestyle/january_2013/57_dine_out_at_least_once_a_week

Reed, J., Frazão, E., & Itskowitz, R. (2004). *How much do Americans pay for fruits and vegetables?* (No. 790). Washington, DC: US Department of Agriculture Economic Research Service.

Restaurant Opportunities Centers United. (2010). *Serving while sick: High risks and low benefits for the nation's restaurant workforce, and their impact on the consumer* (pp. 11–13). Retrieved from http://rocunited.org/wp-content/uploads/2013/04/reports_serving-while-sick_full.pdf

Restaurant Opportunities Centers United. (2012a). *Blacks in the restaurant industry brief*. Retrieved from http://rocunited.org/wp-content/uploads/2013/04/reports_blacks-in-the-industry_brief.pdf

Restaurant Opportunities Centers United. (2012b). *Tipped over the edge: Gender inequality in the nation's restaurant industry* (p. 19). Retrieved from http://rocunited.org/wp-content/uploads/2012/02/ROC_GenderInequity_F1–1.pdf

Roberts, W. (2012). Food insecurity: Uncomfortable food truths. *Crosscurrents, 15*(3), 16–19.

Rose, D. (2007). Food stamps, the thrifty food plan, and meal preparation: The importance of the time dimension for US nutrition policy. *Journal of Nutrition Education and Behavior, 39*, 226–232.

Schlosser, E. (2001). *Fast food nation: The dark side of the all-American meal*. Boston: Houghton-Mifflin.

Sen, A. (1999). *Development as freedom*. New York: Random House.

Talukdar, D. (2008). Cost of being poor: Retail price and consumer price search differences across inner-city and suburban neighborhoods. *Journal of Consumer Research, 35*(3), 457–471.

Tirodkar, M. A., & Jain, A. (2003). Food messages on African American television shows. *American Journal of Public Health, 93*(3), 439–441.

Trostle, R. (2008). *Global agricultural supply and demand: Factors contributing to the recent increase in food commodity prices*. Retrieved from www.ers.usda.gov/publications/wrs-international-agriculture-and-trade-outlook/wrs-0801.aspx#.UyIxjYWAnTU

Unger, J. B., Reynolds, K., Shakib, S., Spruijt-Metz, D., Sun, P., & Johnson, C. A. (2004). Acculturation, physical activity, and fast-food consumption among Asian American and Hispanic adolescents. *Journal of Community Health, 29*(6), 467–481.

US Census Bureau. (2010). *Current population survey, 2010*. Washington, DC: Author.

US Census Bureau. (2012). *Most children younger than age 1 are minorities, Census Bureau reports*. Retrieved from www.census.gov/newsroom/releases/archives/population/cb12–90.html

US Department of Agriculture Economic Research Service. (2013). *Food security in the U.S.: Key statistics & graphics*. Retrieved from www.ers.usda.gov/topics/food-nutrition-assistance/food-security-in-the-us/key-statistics-graphics.aspx

US Department of Agriculture Food and Nutrition Service. (2013). *About WIC: WIC at a Glance*. Retrieved from www.fns.usda.gov/wic/about-wic-wic-glance

US Department of Health and Human Services. (2010). *HHS action plan to reduce racial and ethnic health disparities* (No. 2013). Washington, DC: Author.

US Department of Health and Human Services. (2011). HHS Poverty Guidelines. *Federal Register, 76*(13), 36737–36738.

Wallinga, D., Schoonover, H., & Muller, M. (2009). Considering the contributions of U.S. agricultural policy to the obesity epidemic: Overview and opportunities. *Journal of Hunger & Environmental Nutrition, 4*(1), 3–19.

Wang, Y., & Beydoun, M. A. (2007). The obesity epidemic in the United States—Gender, age, socioeconomic, racial/ethnic, and geographic characteristics: A systematic review and meta-regression analysis. *Epidemiologic Reviews, 29*(1), 6–28.

Wang, Y., & Chen, X. (2011). How much of racial/ethnic disparities in dietary intakes, exercise, and weight status can be explained by nutrition- and health-related psychosocial factors and socioeconomic status among US adults? *Journal of the American Dietetic Association, 111*(12), 1904–1911.

Wilson, S. M., Howell, F., Wing, S., & Sobset, M. (2002). Environmental injustice and the Mississippi hog industry. *Environmental Health Perspectives, 110*, 195–201.

Wing, S., Cole, D., & Grant, G. (2000). Environmental injustice in North Carolina's hog industry. *Environmental Health Perspectives, 108*(3), 225–231.

World Health Organization. (2013). *Life expectancy by country.* Retrieved from http://apps.who.int/gho/data/node.main .688.

Yancey, A. K., Cole, B. L., Brown, R., Williams, J. D., Hillier, A., Kline, R. S., … McCarthy, W. J. (2009). A cross-sectional prevalence study of ethnically targeted and general audience outdoor obesity-related advertising. *Milbank Quarterly, 87*(1), 155–184.

Zachary, D. A., Palmer, A. M., Beckham, S. W., & Surkan, P. J. (2013). A framework for understanding grocery purchasing in a low-income urban environment. *Qualitative Health Research, 23*(5), 665.

Chapter 5

Public Health Implications of Household Food Insecurity

Mariana Chilton, Amanda Breen, and Jenny Rabinowich

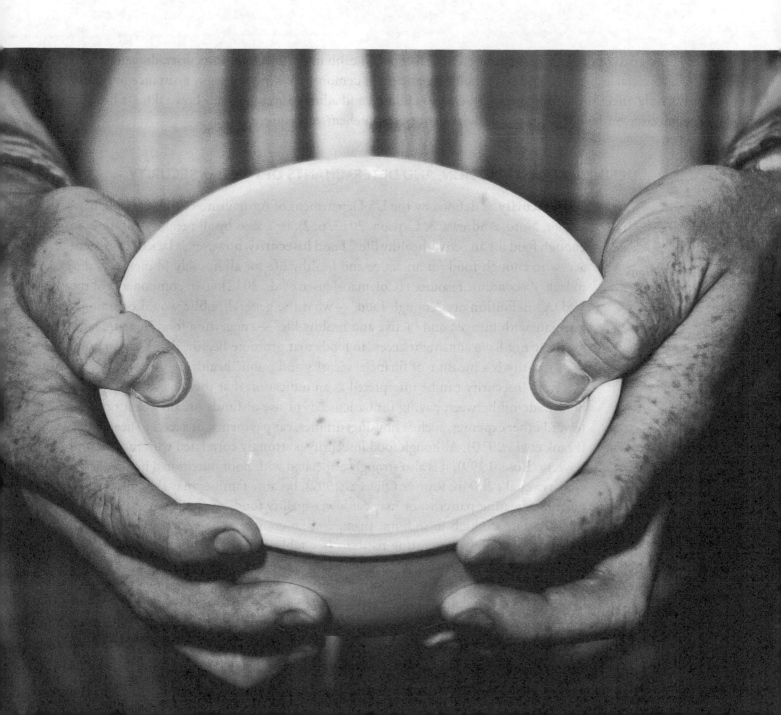

Learning Objectives

- Define and use household food insecurity terminology.

- Describe disparities in food insecurity by racial and ethnic differences and household characteristics.

- Identify mechanisms through which food insecurity is related to poor physical and mental health for children and adults.

- Recognize and understand key nutrition assistance programs, the policies that structure them, and some of the relevant politics.

- Identify and explore solutions to household food insecurity.

The goals of this chapter are to describe the public health impacts of food insecurity, drawing attention to racial and ethnic and household disparities, to demonstrate how nutrition assistance programs positively affect the health and well-being of children and adults, and to explain how taking a broader perspective on food insecurity can help identify comprehensive solutions.

DEFINITION, DISTRIBUTION, AND DETERMINANTS OF FOOD INSECURITY

food security
"Access by all people at all times to enough food for an active, healthy life" (Coleman-Jensen, Nord, Andrews, & Carlson, 2012, p. 2)

food insecurity
Having inadequate economic resources to enable consistent access to safe, adequate, and nutritious food to support an active and healthy life for all household members (low food security: reduced quality, variety, desirability of diet; very low food security: multiple indications of disrupted eating patterns and reduced food intake)

Food security, as defined by the US Department of Agriculture (USDA), (Coleman-Jensen, Nord, Andrews, & Carlson, 2012, p. 2), is "access by all people at all times to enough food for an active, healthy life." **Food insecurity**, however, is lack of consistent access to enough food for an active and healthy life for all household members due to lack of economic resources (Coleman-Jensen et al., 2012). Two components of the USDA's definition are "enough food"—what the general public would commonly associate with hunger, and "active and healthy life"—suggesting food-insecure families may not have consistent access to foods that promote health. By its very nature, food security is a measure of financial security and public health.

Food insecurity can be interpreted as an indication that there has been a household trade-off between paying for basic needs or use of funds usually spent on food toward other expenses, such as housing, utilities, car payments, or access to health care (Frank et al., 2010). Although food insecurity is strongly correlated with income and poverty (Rose, 1999), it is also strongly associated with poor nutritional intake (Bhattacharya et al., 2004b; Rose & Oliveira, 1997), because families may skip meals, have disordered eating patterns, or may eat lower-quality foods or foods that have longer shelf life but are high in sodium, sugar, and fat content. The very measure of food insecurity captures these eating patterns (see table 5.1). In addition, trade-offs that families make, such as paying for heat or for medicine (see figure 5.1) by reducing money spent on food, or getting behind on rent in order to have enough money to pay for meals, have strong negative health consequences for children and adults (Cutts et al., 2011; Frank et al., 2010; Jeng et al., 2010).

Current strategies to address food insecurity include government food assistance programs, private food donations, and efforts to encourage healthy food access. There is no nationally relevant, systematic

TABLE 5.1   Categorizations of Food Security Status as Measured by the USDA

Level	Category	Subcategory as Redefined in 2007	Description
Household	Food security	N/A	Zero to two reported indications of food access problems or limitations among adults or children in household; little or no indication of changes in diets or food intake
	Food insecurity	Low food security *(Formerly food insecurity without hunger*)* Worried food would run out Food bought did not last Could not afford balanced meal Cut size of meal or skipped meal	Reports of reduced quality, variety, or desirability of diet among adults or children in the household; little or no indication of reduced food intake
		Very low food security *(Formerly food insecurity with hunger*)* Cut or skipped meal Ate less than felt should Hungry but did not eat Lost weight Did not eat whole day Did not eat whole day, three-plus months	Reports of multiple indications of disrupted eating patterns and reduced food intake among adults or children in the household
Child	Food security	N/A	No reported indications of food-access problems or limitations among children (household may be food insecure)
	Food insecurity	Low food security *(Formerly food insecurity without hunger*)*	Reports of reduced quality, variety, or desirability of diet of children; little or no indication of reduced food intake of children
		Very low food security *(Formerly food insecurity with hunger)*	Reports of multiple indications of disrupted eating patterns and reduced food intake of children

*In 2007 the USDA Economic Research Service (ERS) announced a change in the terminology of food security, because the measure was deemed inadequate to truly gauge the experience of "hunger" by a report published by the National Academies of Science in 2006 (National Research Council, 2006; Nord et al., 2007).

plan to end food insecurity. Meanwhile, disparities and the prevalence of food insecurity have gone primarily unchanged up until 2008, when the rates increased drastically during the Great Recession.

Distribution, Disparities, and Key Determinants

The USDA Economic Research Service (ERS) eighteen-item survey, the **Household Food Security Survey Module (HFSSM),** is considered the gold standard measure of severity and depth of food insecurity in the United States (see table 5.1). Using this module, each year the USDA releases national and statewide food insecurity rates based on data from the Current Population Survey. Researchers working with specific populations also use the HFSSM to investigate the relationship between food insecurity and outcomes such as low birth weight, child development, anemia, suicidal ideation, social isolation, depression, diabetes, and obesity. In 2011, more than fifty million people (16.4 percent) in the United States lived in food insecure households,

Household Food Security Survey Module (HFSSM) Eighteen-item survey from the US Department of Agriculture Economic Research Service that is considered the gold standard measure of severity and depth of food insecurity in the United States

FIGURE 5.1   Some Families Reduce Their Spending on Food in Order to Pay for Their Medicines

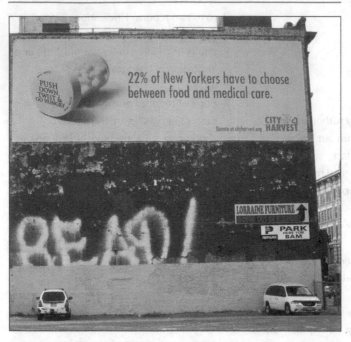

Source: Kevin Dooley, Read. Creative Commons https://www.flickr.com/photos/pagedooley/5926270312/

including approximately 16.7 million children (22.4 percent), according to the USDA (Coleman-Jensen et al., 2012). Before the recession, the food insecurity rates hovered around 12 percent of the US population without much change since the USDA ERS began measurement in 1995 (Coleman-Jensen et al., 2012).

Rates at the national and state levels may obscure stark racial, ethnic, gender, and age disparities, as can be seen from the USDA's 2011 data. For instance, 36.8 percent of female-headed households were food insecure relative to 14.9 percent of all US households. Households with children under the age of six are also more likely to be food insecure than others, with nearly 22 percent of such households affected. Additionally, more than 25 percent of African American households and 26 percent of Hispanic households were food insecure (Coleman-Jensen et al., 2012). Rates among American Indians and immigrant populations are harder to document and vary regionally. Among American Indians counted in national surveys, the prevalence rate before the recession was at 23 percent (Gundersen, 2008), but reports on specific Indian nations and communities show prevalence rates as high as 40 percent to 45 percent (Bauer et al., 2012, Mullany et al., 2012). Latino immigrants from Mexico and Central America have reported food insecurity at rates ranging from 28 percent to over 82 percent (Chilton et al., 2009; Quandt, Shoaf, Tapia, Hernandez-Pelletier, Clark, & Arcury, 2006; Sharkey, Dean, & Johnson, 2011). Such variability in rates depends on the sampling technique, the location and occupations of immigrants, and the variability in time spent in the United States.

The enduring nature of disparities in food insecurity rates among marginalized populations is cause for reexamining the programs aimed at addressing hunger in the United States, especially when the health consequences can be so devastating.

Health Consequences and Correlates of Food Insecurity

Food insecurity costs the country $167.5 billion dollars a year in health care, educational attainment, criminal justice, and emergency food assistance (Shepard, Setren, & Cooper, 2011). In the following sections, we describe how the health impacts of food insecurity reach far beyond nutrition-related diseases to have a profound effect on social and emotional health. In all of the studies we describe, researchers controlled for income and other indicators of socioeconomic status, demonstrating that over and above what we might expect from differences in income, marital status, and eligibility for subsidized health care, food insecurity has long-lasting negative effects on the US population.

Food Insecurity among Adults   According to the USDA, nearly 8.4 percent of households with elderly people were food insecure in 2011. Low-income and vulnerable seniors have difficulty meeting their proper nutrient intakes, and food insecurity exacerbates nutritional deficiencies (Coleman-Jensen et al., 2012). Neighborhood conditions such as walkability were also associated with food insecurity among elders (Chung, Gallo, Giunta, Canavan, Parikh, & Fahs, 2011). For working-age adults, food insecurity is associated with poor nutritional intake, which, in turn, negatively affects self-reported health (Rose, 1999). Food insecurity in adults is a risk factor for hypoglycemia, inadequate diabetes self-management, and the need to make trade-offs such as paying for medical care or prescriptions instead of food, which negatively affects a variety of health conditions (Seligman, Davis, Schillinger, & Wolf, 2010).

Researchers have associated food insecurity with obesity among women but not among men, and for children, the evidence is inconsistent and varying by age, race, ethnicity, and socioeconomic status (Institute of Medicine, 2001; Jones & Frongillo, 2007; Olson & Strawderman, 2008). The reasons for the rise in overweight and obesity in the United States are multifactorial and complex. Among the general public, the press, and policy makers, there is an overriding concern that household food insecurity and overweight and obesity can be reported simultaneously by the same individual. The Institute of Medicine recently considered the state of this research, finding that the primary link between obesity and food insecurity appears to be poor economic conditions. According to the USDA, among food-insecure families, food quality is more commonly compromised than quantity (Nord, Andrews, & Carlson, 2002). Without adequate resources for food, families must make decisions to maximize the amount of calories, satiety, and taste, and energy-dense foods are often cheaper and more filling than healthier foods, though the evidence is mixed (Drewnowski & Darmon, 2005) (see figure 5.2).

The connection between overweight and poverty may further be explained by variability in proximal access to fresh produce, lean meat, and low-fat purchasing options, and high geographic access to less healthy options, as described in chapter 17. Some researchers have also suggested that obesity may be an adaptive response to episodic food insufficiency (Alaimo, Olson, Frongillo, & Briefel, 2001b; Dietz, 1995), exacerbated by the monthly SNAP distribution cycle. As researchers move forward to identify potential linkages beyond nutrition and food intake, they are focusing on other significant factors, such as the extreme stress of insecure food access, which may be associated with disordered eating habits that create metabolic disorder and exacerbate overweight. Stress can further be associated with other risk factors

FIGURE 5.2 Restaurant

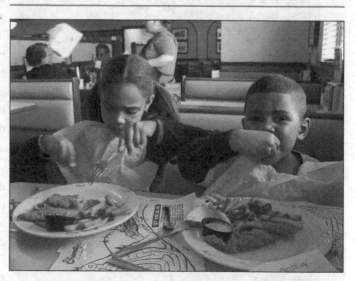

"My daughter, she loves this restaurant. And I told her, 'I don't have a lot of money, but when I get some money, I'll take you.' … This food isn't healthy, but it's the only place I can afford to take my kids."—Photo and voice by Taina P., Witnesses to Hunger Boston.

for obesity, including sleep deprivation and impact on hormonal risk factors (Barbosa-da-Silva, Fraulob-Aquino, Lopes, Mandarim-de-Lacerda, & Aguila, 2012; Olson, Bove, & Miller, 2007; Scarpellini & Tack, 2012).

Food insecurity affects health far beyond the obvious link with nutrition-related diseases. Researchers investigating food insecurity among women found that food insecurity is strongly associated with social isolation, depression, and anxiety (Melchior et al., 2009). In turn, these conditions affect women's ability to care for and raise their children effectively, to complete their educations, and to earn a living wage. After controlling for poverty and other factors, Tarasuk found that social isolation among women experiencing the most severe form of household food insecurity was 5.81 times greater than social isolation reported by women who were in food-secure households (Tarasuk, 2001b). Social isolation indicates less social support and greater risk for depression. Hamelin, Beaudry, and Habicht (2002) reported excess stress and anxiety among food-insecure families. Others have found high levels of depression and exposure to violence among food-insecure women (Chilton & Booth, 2007). Difficult life exposures can also increase the risk of food insecurity. For example, homeless and low-income mothers who experienced sexual assault in childhood were over four times more likely to have household-level food insecurity than women who had not been abused (Wehler et al., 2004).

Perspective 5.1 describes the Witnesses to Hunger Program, which we initiated to provide a window into some of the intersecting struggles and impacts experienced by people who are food insecure. Other photos interspersed through this chapter also come from that program.

Perspective 5.1. Witnesses to Hunger: Participation by Those Who Know Poverty and Hunger Firsthand
Tianna Gaines-Turner and Jenny Rabinowich

FIGURE 5.3   Breakfast

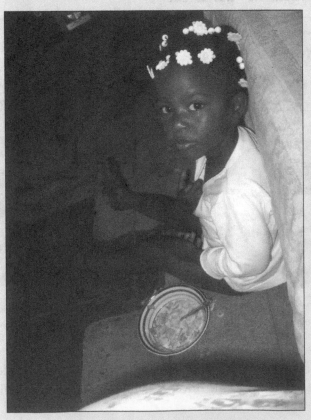

"With the money food stamps provide, I was able to feed her breakfast that morning. Without it what would she have eaten? I wanted to show that with the help she was able to eat breakfast that morning. She had cereal. She had milk. She didn't have to go without."—Photo and voice by Crystal S., Witnesses to Hunger Philadelphia.

In the Witnesses to Hunger program, mothers of young children use cameras to document their experiences with hunger and poverty. The program, hosted by the Center for Hunger-Free Communities at Drexel University School of Public Health, is rooted in the understanding that the true experts on food insecurity are those who have personal experience struggling with hunger, and that these experts need to be at the table when decisions are made on policies and programs that affect their lives.

In addition to showing the world about direct experiences with food and hunger, the photographers depict struggles with housing and homelessness, utilities being shut off, and a strong desire for better education and opportunity (see figures 5.3–5.6). They perceive these struggles as being intertwined with hunger. The women of Witnesses to Hunger have shown remarkable strength and courage to open up about some of the most trying parts of their lives. They have displayed their photos and spoken at the US Senate, at the US House of Representatives, and at multiple state capitol buildings. They speak out about the changes they want to see and are taking an active role in breaking the cycle of hunger and poverty.

FIGURE 5.4   Deep Freezer

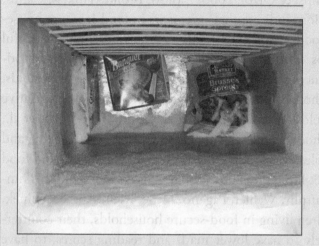

"That's the deep freezer now. It's empty. It's just those two items in that one little box. How is this supposed to feed a family of six?"—Photo and voice by Bonita C., Witnesses to Hunger Boston.

FIGURE 5.5   My Neighbor's Kitchen

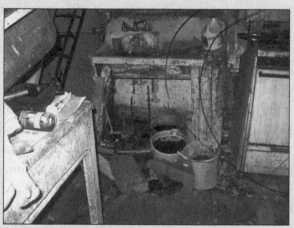

"You never know what goes on behind closed doors. Some people need to know exactly how we're living being single moms, being that we're on our own and we don't have that many opportunities. When something breaks, we may not be able to fix it because we have limited income. It's really hard to try to get everything fixed. How would my neighbor actually try to work with something like that? Being in a situation like that, your kids can stay hungry."—Photo and voice by Barbara I., Witnesses to Hunger Philadelphia.

FIGURE 5.6   Number 9,584

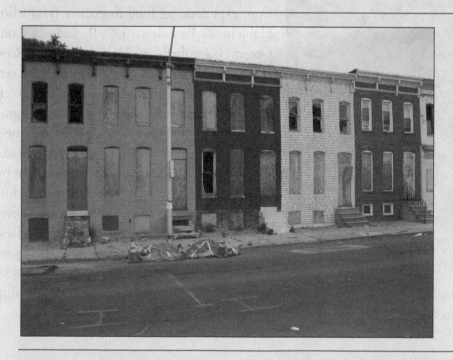

"We have all these houses. Why can't we fix up these houses? Our homeless rate would go down. The Section 8 list, the housing list, would not be ten thousand strong. I got my housing letter. I'm number 9,584 on the waiting list. That's where I am. Why I am nine thousand something and there are all these houses in Baltimore city that are vacant, not just in this area, but throughout the whole city? Why can't we go and fix these houses up?"—Photo and voice by Shaunte B., Witnesses to Hunger Baltimore.

Witnesses to Hunger has expanded to sites across Pennsylvania, Massachusetts, Rhode Island, New Jersey, and Maryland. A small sample of the Witnesses' photographs is shown here, and more can be found at www.witnessestohunger.org.

Food Insecurity among Children and Adolescents   Maternal depressive symptoms are associated with food insecurity and with poor child development and behavior, though the direction of causality is still in question (Casey et al., 2004; Whitaker, Phillips, & Orzol, 2006; Zaslow, Bronte-Tinkew, Capps, Horowitz, Moore, & Weinstein, 2009). Investigations indicate that caregivers in food-insecure households with children are more likely than those in food-secure households to report potentially harmful parenting practices (Bronte-Tinkew, Zaslow, Capps, Horowitz, & McNamara, 2007). Infants and toddlers are likely to suffer a host of negative consequences as a result of living in food-insecure households. Studies find that young children in food-insecure homes have an increased developmental risk relative to their counterparts living in food-secure households (Bronte-Tinkew et al., 2007; Rose-Jacobs et al., 2008). This has strong implications for a child's school readiness, which is so critical for well-being and success later in life (Heckman, 2006). Among adolescents and children, poor mental health and food insecurity are also strongly linked (Alaimo, Olson, & Frongillo, 2001a; Bhattacharya et al., 2004b, Gundersen & Kreider, 2009; Kleinman et al., 1998; Murphy, Wehler, Pagano, Little, Kleinman, & Jellinek, 1998). Compared to low-income school-age children living in food-secure households, their counterparts in food-insecure households were more likely to have lower math and reading scores, to have repeated a grade, and to report strained social relationships (Alaimo et al., 2001b, Howard, 2011; Jyoti, Frongillo, & Jones, 2005). Alaimo and colleagues found that family food insufficiency was positively associated with depression and suicidal ideation among adolescents (Alaimo, Olson, & Frongillo, 2002).

FIGURE 5.7   Hungry Child Asking Caseworker for Something to Eat

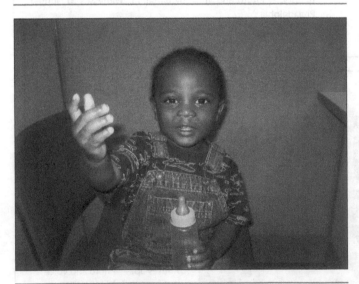

"I was thinking, 'I'm not going to lie to you miss, he's hungry.'" — Photo and voice by Imani S., Witnesses to Hunger Philadelphia.

Most of the research on child food insecurity is based on parental report, and the prevailing interpretation of the self-reports of caregivers is that children, especially young children, are shielded by their parents from experiencing food insecurity (Hamelin, Habicht, & Beaudry, 1999; Radimer, Olson, Green, Campbell, & Habicht, 1992; Rose & Oliveira, 1997). Recent research, however, has shown that children ages nine to sixteen are often emotionally, physically, and cognitively aware of food insecurity, despite their parents' attempts to shield them (Fram et al., 2011). A child-centered conceptualization by Fram and coauthors (2011) reveals that children have distinct experiences of food insecurity, characterized by managing immediate food resources for themselves and their parents, worrying about their parents' levels of stress, and feeling angry and helpless when not enough food is available. Figure 5.7 depicts a young child asking a caseworker for food.

NUTRITION ASSISTANCE PROGRAMS

The nutrition assistance programs administered by the USDA's Food and Nutrition Service (FNS) (see table 5.2) are considered the first line of defense in addressing household food insecurity.

TABLE 5.2   Nutrition Assistance Programs Administered by the USDA FNS

Program	Description	Eligibility	Participation
Supplemental Nutrition Assistance Program (SNAP)	Formerly called the Food Stamp Program, SNAP provides eligible families with funds to purchase food via electronic benefits transfer.	Households with income less than 130 percent of the federal poverty level (FPL); other income, asset, and cost-of-living criteria used	45 million people participated in 2011 (1)
Women, Infants, and Children (WIC)	WIC provides supplemental foods, health care referrals, and nutrition education for low-income pregnant, breastfeeding, and nonbreastfeeding postpartum women, and to infants and children up to age five who are found to be at nutritional risk. In most states participants also receive vouchers through WIC's Farmers Market Nutrition Program.	Household income at or below 185 percent of FPL with a child age zero to five and a pregnant or postpartum woman	8.96 million women, infants, and children participated in 2011 (2)
School Meals	This umbrella term includes the National School Lunch Program (NSLP), the School Breakfast Program, the Fresh Fruit and Vegetable Program providing fresh produce to selected low-income elementary schools, and the Special Milk Program for children without access to other meal programs.	Through the NLSP, children eighteen and younger in households with income less than 130 percent of FPL receive free lunch; those with incomes between 130 percent and 185 percent of FPL receive reduced price lunch up to $0.40.	More than 31 million children participated in 2012 (3)
Summer Food Service Program (SFSP)	SFSP provides free, nutritious meals and snacks to help children in low-income areas get the nutrition they need throughout the summer months when they are out of school. Works in tandem with the National School Lunch Program. (2)	No income requirements; children eighteen and younger and adults who are in a school programs because of a mental or physical disability	2.79 million children served through a combination of SFSP and NSLP in July 2011 (4)
Child and Adult Care Food Program (CACFP)	CACFP provides meals and snacks to children in day care, emergency shelters, and after-school care programs, and to adults in nonresidential adult day care centers.	Based on population served by facility; varies by type of facility	3.2 million children and 112,000 adults served daily (5)

(Continued)

TABLE 5.2   Nutrition Assistance Programs Administered by the USDA FNS (Continued)

Program	Description	Eligibility	Participation
Food Assistance for Disaster Relief	In the case of disaster emergency, this program provides food for shelters and other mass feeding sites, distributes food packages to households in need, and issues emergency SNAP benefits.	Based on FEMA disaster and emergency declarations	Varies based on disasters faced (6)
Food Distribution	Direct food distribution goes through the Schools/Child Nutrition Commodity Programs, the Food Distribution Program on Indian Reservations, Commodity Supplemental Food Program, and the Emergency Food Assistance Program. Food is distributed to food banks, schools, or directly to households, depending on the program.	Criteria vary based on program	N/A (7)

Sources: (1) US Department of Agriculture, Food and Nutrition Service, 2014a; (2) US Department of Agriculture, Food and Nutrition Service, 2013a, 2014b; (3) US Department of Agriculture, Food and Nutrition Service, 2013b; (4) Cooper, Anderson, and FitzSimons, 2012; (5) US Department of Agriculture, Food and Nutrition Service, 2013b; (6) US Department of Agriculture, Farm Service Agency, 2014; (7) US Department of Agriculture, Food and Nutrition Service, 2014c.

SNAP

Supplemental Nutrition Assistance Program (SNAP)
Federal food assistance for qualifying low-income households; formerly known as the Food Stamp Program and also referred to as EBT (electronic benefits transfer)

entitlement program
Program that guarantees access to certain benefits for all who qualify (e.g., Social Security benefits)

The **Supplemental Nutrition Assistance Program (SNAP),** formerly called the Food Stamp Program and also referred to as EBT (electronic benefits transfer), is the largest food and nutrition program in the country. Its primary goal is to prevent and treat food insecurity. Currently one in seven Americans participates in SNAP and approximately half of SNAP participants are children. SNAP is an **entitlement program**, meaning anyone who is eligible to participate in the program is entitled to participate (by contrast, other programs restrict participation after cost thresholds are reached). This ensures the program can respond to economic trends, ebbing and flowing with the needs of the US population. It also ensures that SNAP benefits can be provided to people in crisis after hurricanes and other disasters.

Overall, research has shown that SNAP reduces the severity of food insecurity and promotes health for children and families. SNAP has a dramatic, positive impact on young children's health and well-being, beginning at birth. Newborns whose mothers received SNAP for at least three months before birth had healthier birth weights (Almond, Hoynes, & Whitmore Schanzenbach, 2011). Young children receiving SNAP were less likely to be food insecure than children who were likely eligible but did not receive it (Frank et al., 2010). In addition to direct physical and mental health benefits, children who received SNAP between first and third grade, compared to eligible low-income children who did not receive SNAP benefits, had improved reading and math scores (Frongillo, Jyoti, & Jones, 2006). Clearly, SNAP's benefits go beyond improving nutrient intake to improving learning and reducing family stress.

Although SNAP helps to provide more available income to be spent on food, its benefits are insufficient to cover the cost of a healthy, nutritious diet (Breen, Cahill, Ettinger de Cuba, Cook, & Chilton, 2011), as depicted in figure 5.8. The **Thrifty Food Plan (TFP)**, on which SNAP allotments are based, does not account for regional variability in food prices or cost of living (Alaska and Hawaii are exceptions), nor for the lack of access to healthy food options in many communities. It comes as no surprise, then, that families report running low on SNAP benefits and thus low on nutritious foods toward the end of the month (US Department of Agriculture, Food and Nutrition Service, Office of Research and Analysis, 2013). The Institute of Medicine has also reported empirical evidence that SNAP benefits, as they are currently calculated, do not cover the cost of a healthy diet (Institute of Medicine, National Research Council, 2013). In addition, the time necessary to prepare the TFP foods is far greater than average food preparation time spent by the general population. The allotment amount does not take into consideration the added time costs that are now considered an important aspect of poverty (Rose, 2007).

FIGURE 5.8   Oodles of Noodles

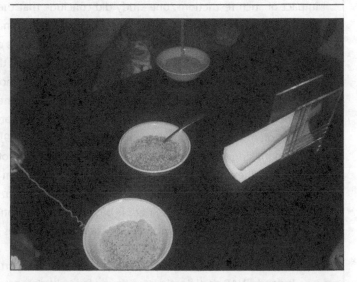

"Come leave your world just for one week and live in my world. Tell me how you're going to make it and survive; how emotionally, you're going to keep yourself together. To day-by-day look at your kids and tell them, 'I don't have any money to take you to the store.' Or, 'We're eating Oodles of Noodles today because the food stamps didn't last.'"—Photo and voice by Erica S., Witnesses to Hunger Philadelphia.

Thrifty Food Plan (TFP) Low-cost food plan providing adequate nutrition, used as the basis for USDA calculations of SNAP allotments

Although the evidence suggests that participation in SNAP improves nutritional intake and health, participants are permitted to use SNAP dollars to purchase any foods other than hot prepared foods.

Restricting Food Choices in SNAP   Much discussion has centered on whether SNAP can play a bigger role in fighting obesity without harming its other positive outcomes. For instance, some have suggested that restricting SNAP consumers' choice might combat obesity among low-income people. Perspectives 5.2 and 5.3 present two perspectives on this topic. What do you think?

Perspective 5.2. The Wrong Path Forward: Restricting Food Choices in SNAP

Heather Hartline-Grafton

Restricting food choices is a narrow strategy that distracts from the real issue—the inadequacy of SNAP benefits. There are many problems with the rationale, practicality, and potential effectiveness of restricting the use of SNAP benefits for certain food purchases in order to address obesity (Hartline-Grafton, Vollinger, & Weill, 2013; US Department of Agriculture [USDA], 2007). Although limited research currently exists exploring the potential impact of such restrictions, one study did conclude that the possible consequences made it an impractical, ineffective strategy to change behavior (Alston, Mullally, Sumner, Townsend, & Vosti, 2009).

Furthermore, according to the USDA, "as the problems of poor food choices, unhealthy diets, and excessive weight characterize all segments of American society, the basis for singling out low-income food stamp recipients and imposing unique restrictions on their food choices is not clear" (USDA, 2007a, p. 7). SNAP participants use a variety of savvy shopping practices to stretch their limited food dollars, and USDA research shows that foods commonly proposed for restriction (e.g., sweets and sugar-sweetened beverages) represent a small proportion of total SNAP food purchases (Cohen et al., 1999). Keeping poor people from the usual streams of decision making and commerce may emanate from a stereotypical belief that the culture or behavior among the poor is different and dysfunctional. In reality, people from the wealthiest to the poorest choose to distribute their grocery store food dollars in a strikingly similar manner.

Avoiding singling out poor people based on misconceptions or exaggerations is just one reason restricting food choices in SNAP is the wrong path. There are numerous others:

- SNAP does not cause poor diets or contribute to the current obesity problem, as described in this chapter. Indeed, SNAP participation can have a favorable impact on dietary quality and obesity risk.

- There are no agreed-on and easily applicable standards—in science or policy—that can be used to determine the foods to target for restriction. Consider the following example: some candy bars have fewer calories from fat than a serving of cheddar cheese. If the focus for restrictions was foods high in fat, would candy bars be eligible but cheddar cheese ineligible (USDA, 2007a)? Similar practical problems in how ineligible foods were defined surfaced when New York City and the state of Minnesota requested waivers from USDA to restrict certain foods in SNAP. Additionally, the effort to identify foods for disallowance would inevitably lead to endless political "food fights" over lists of "good" and "bad" foods.

- Implementing food restrictions would increase the program's complexity and costs for participants, retailers, and administrators. USDA would need to inventory and track the hundreds of thousands of foods and beverages on the market and continuous stream of new and reformulated products, creating a logistical nightmare that would increase administrative costs for the program (USDA, 2007a). Costs would also increase for campaigns to communicate ineligible items to participants and retailers.

- Limiting food purchases will be particularly ineffective in changing behavior if SNAP consumers do not have reasonable access to eligible foods at affordable prices. Many low-income communities have limited access to healthy, affordable foods. Further, many low-income consumers stretch food dollars by purchasing energy-dense, relatively inexpensive foods.

- There is no evidence that restricting food choices will improve diets or reduce obesity. Most SNAP households receive only partial benefits and are expected to use some of their own money to purchase food;

they could thus still purchase ineligible foods with other payment methods. In addition, food choices are affected by a number of factors, including cost, taste, convenience, personal preference, and availability. Restricting food choice would not substantially change most of these factors.

- Purchasing restrictions likely would increase confusion and stigma at grocery checkout, potentially causing a decline in SNAP participation that could worsen food insecurity and increase obesity risk among this vulnerable group (Alston et al., 2009; Metallinos-Katsaras, Sherry, & Kallio, 2009). Program administrators and advocates have worked for decades to reduce the stigma associated with SNAP participation and to reduce program complexities that lead to confusion and frustration on the part of participants. Even pilot program changes that risk decreasing or discouraging SNAP participation are ill-advised, especially at a time when SNAP participation and food insecurity rates are so high, yet approximately one in five Americans eligible for the program are not enrolled (Eslami & Cunnyngham, 2014).

SNAP reaches millions of vulnerable Americans and plays a critical role in alleviating food insecurity and improving health. There are promising strategies that can strengthen SNAP's role in improving health outcomes without creating unnecessary challenges for program beneficiaries. These include increasing program participation, improving benefit levels, and increasing access to healthy, affordable foods. Such thoughtful, comprehensive strategies need to be the priority in discussions about SNAP's impacts on diet, obesity, and health.

Perspective 5.3. A Defense of Excluding Foods of Minimal Nutritional Value from SNAP

Anne Barnhill

Americans' use of food stamps has reached an all-time high. Now more than ever, SNAP funds need to be deployed as efficiently as possible to achieve SNAP's aims of alleviating hunger and improving the nutrition and health of low-income people. One way to work toward this goal is to modify SNAP to exclude foods that have minimal nutritional value, such as sweetened beverages.

For example, in late 2010, New York State petitioned the USDA for permission to conduct a demonstration project, in which sweetened beverages would be excluded from the food items able to be purchased with SNAP benefits in New York City (New York State Office of Temporary and Disability Assistance, 2010). Eight other states have also sought stricter standards for the use of SNAP benefits (Brownell & Ludwig, 2011).

The Case for Excluding Foods of Minimal Nutritional Value from SNAP

SNAP's aims are to alleviate hunger and improve the nutrition and health of low-income people (Food and Nutrition Act of 2008). Funding SNAP participants' purchase and consumption of foods of minimal nutritional value does not further these aims. Such foods do not improve nutrition, because they have minimal nutritional value. Certain foods of minimal nutritional value, such as sweetened beverages, do not even alleviate hunger because they do not satiate (DiMeglio & Mattes, 2000). The addition of foods of minimal nutritional value simply makes the diets of SNAP participants worse by adding excess calories and sugar, which contribute to overweight, obesity, diabetes, and other chronic diseases.

(Continued)

(Continued)

Multiple Objections Have Been Raised to SNAP Exclusions

Nutrition education and financial incentives to purchase fruits and vegetables will be more effective at improving the diets of SNAP participants. Response: education, incentives, and exclusions are not mutually exclusive policies. Exclusions could be paired with incentives and education. Even if it's true that education and incentives would be more effective than exclusions in improving SNAP participants' diets, that does not show that exclusions will be ineffective.

New exclusions could increase confusion and embarrassment at the checkout, thereby stigmatizing SNAP participants and deterring use of SNAP. Response: in 2010, only 75 percent of eligible people received SNAP assistance (Eslami, Leftin, & Strayer, 2012). There is a need to increase eligible people's use of SNAP assistance, and reducing the stigma associated with use of SNAP is crucial to achieving that end. It is important to determine whether new exclusions are likely to cause embarrassment and stigma for a significant number of SNAP participants and whether any such effect would persist long enough to significantly deter SNAP use. But these are empirical issues that should not be prejudged, but rather examined as part of a pilot program of SNAP exclusions.

SNAP participation does not make people's diets worse, and SNAP participants' purchasing habits are as good as, or better than, the purchasing habits of nonparticipants. Response: the justification of SNAP exclusions is not that SNAP causes people to make bad choices or that SNAP participants have worse eating habits than nonparticipants and therefore SNAP should be changed. Rather, the justification is that the SNAP program could be modified to be more efficient and to more effectively promote good nutrition and health. Whether or not SNAP participants currently have worse nutrition and health than nonparticipants isn't relevant; what's relevant is whether SNAP participants' nutrition and health could be improved by modifying the program.

SNAP exclusions single out low-income SNAP participants and restrict only their choice, even though unhealthy diet is a problem for Americans of all income levels. Response: policies that disproportionately burden low-income people do raise ethical concerns and must be ethically justified. But it is important to recognize what kind of burden is and isn't at stake here. Suppose that sweetened beverages were excluded from SNAP. SNAP participants would not experience a reduction in their level of assistance (i.e., the dollar amount). They would not experience a reduction in their ability to feed their families a nutritionally adequate diet. They would just experience a reduction in the kinds of beverages they can choose among when choosing how to feed themselves and their families. They would have fewer beverages to choose among than higher-income people have.

It is ethically justifiable to modestly limit the consumer choice afforded by SNAP in order to improve the nutrition and health of SNAP participants, just as it is ethically justifiable to limit choice of unhealthy products in other settings such as schools, day care centers, hospitals, and places of employment. Such limitations are, in fact, already built into SNAP. SNAP is not cash assistance that participants use to maximize their consumer choice; rather, it is assistance to buy food and food only.

Significant limitations on SNAP participants' consumer choice or the exclusion of necessary food items from SNAP would be unjustifiable. However, the exclusion of sweetened beverages does not rise to this level because sweetened beverages are food products with little nutritional value that add nothing but excess calories to the diet. Though some consumers, both SNAP participants and nonparticipants, consider sweetened beverages to be a necessary part of their families' diet, this is precisely the mind-set that the exclusion of sweetened beverages is meant to challenge.

School Breakfast and Lunch

The USDA has found that the **School Breakfast Program** improves the quality of children's diets. For instance, children in the school breakfast program doubled their intake of fruits and vegetables, reduced overall fat intake, and had improved consumption of micronutrients compared to those not participating (Basiotis, Lino, & Anand, 1999; Bhattacharya et al., 2004a) (see figure 5.9). In addition, the program reduces the number of children's complaints of stomachaches and headaches (Wahlstrom & Begalle, 1999). Although the School Breakfast Program has been shown to improve the health of children, the data on health impacts of the **National School Lunch Program (NSLP)** are less conclusive. Some studies have pointed to the NSLP as a contributor to childhood obesity (Millimet, Tchernis, & Husain, 2010; Schanzenbach, 2009); others find the program to be protective (Magryta, 2009); and other studies find no correlation (Hofferth & Curtin, 2005). Experts agree, however, that improving the nutritional quality of the meals served through the NSLP will help to improve the health of children in the United States. Perspective 5.4 argues that making all school meals free would have numerous benefits for children and society.

FIGURE 5.9 Child Enjoys a Crisp Apple at Lunch

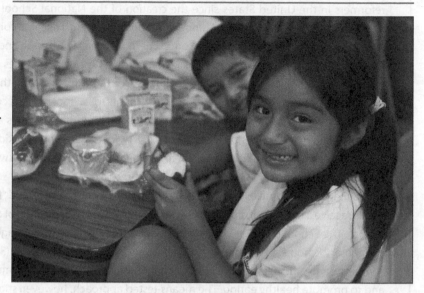

Source: USDA (2011).

School Breakfast Program
Federal program providing cash assistance to states to operate nonprofit breakfast programs in schools and residential child-care institutions

National School Lunch Program (NSLP)
Federally assisted meal program operating in public and nonprofit private schools and residential care institutions to provide nutritious meals to children at low or no cost

Perspective 5.4. The Public Health Case for Universal Free School Meals

Janet E. Poppendieck

For the health of our children, we need to change the way we pay for school food in the United States. In lieu of selling food to students, and then providing subsidies for those deemed too poor to purchase it, we need to integrate school meals with the curriculum and offer them without charge as a regular part of the school day. There may indeed be "no such thing as a free lunch," but the way we pay for it is a social choice we have made. A policy of universal free school meals, without regard to parental income, is a key to ensuring child health now and building healthy food habits for the future.

(Continued)

(Continued)

"Universal," as this approach is known within the school food community, has been a goal of school food reformers in the United States since the creation of the National School Lunch Program in 1946. In years of research for my book, *Free for All: Fixing School Food in America*, I became convinced that no other reform will fully succeed without this change. In the context of today's fiscal tightrope and the dominance of market ideology, however, an effort to shift responsibility from parents to taxpayers faces daunting obstacles. It seems worthwhile, therefore, to lay out the public health case for shifting away from the current means-tested approach.

The three-tier system for federal reimbursements for school meals is complicated, cumbersome, and costly to administer. Children are eligible for free meals if their family incomes are below 130 percent of the federal poverty level (FPL)—currently a cut-off of $24,817 for a mom and two kids. They qualify for a sharply reduced price (not to exceed $.40 or $.30 for breakfast) if family incomes are between 130 percent and 185 percent of the FPL, currently up to $35,317 for a family of three.

Children from families above this threshold pay a locally determined "full price," a misnomer because these meals receive a federal subsidy of $0.27 per meal as well as an allocation of donated federal commodities (USDA, 2013b). The School Nutrition Association reports that the national average price for a school lunch is $1.93 for elementary schools, $2.14 for middle schools, and $2.20 for high school (School Nutrition Association, 2011).

From a health perspective, the fundamental goals of the federal meal programs are to prevent hunger and to promote healthy eating. The means-tested approach, however, stigmatizes children who eat free or at a reduced price, thereby deterring some from participating in the program. By creating eligibility based on family income, it creates the conditions under which some students can look down on others. The stigma quickly attaches to the food itself. In some schools, the meals are seen as "welfare food," and some students who are eligible for free and reduced price meals may forego them to avoid the poverty label (Poppendieck, 2010).

The eligibility process creates an enormous administrative burden, absorbing resources that could be better spent on healthier food. Further, it is notoriously error-prone. In a USDA study, a third of applicants who had been denied benefits were found to have been eligible for them (USDA, 2007b). Even when the process is accurate, children in real need may be denied free and reduced-priced meals. One-fifth of the households with the most severe form of food insecurity in a recent Household Food Security Survey had incomes too high to qualify for reduced price meals. Further, the eligibility criteria penalize families with incomes near the threshold (Harper, Wood, & Mitchell, 2008).

Apart from the flawed three-tier system, the whole notion of selling food to school children undermines the health potential of these vital programs. At the most basic level, the relationship established between students and school food operators is a business relationship; we are selling food to children, and menu planners must keep a steady eye on children's tastes and preferences. The children who have been prematurely placed in this customer role, however, are not blank slates; their preferences are shaped by thousands of hours and billions of dollars of advertising for the nation's least healthy foods.

Further, in many schools, students are permitted to leave at lunchtime to procure their meals at fast food restaurants or convenience stores. With this sort of competition, it is not surprising that many school cafeterias offer an array of "carnival food," such as pizza, chicken nuggets, and fries. In many schools, the situation is made worse by the presence of á la carte lines and vending machines from which students can select their favorite foods in addition to or instead of the nutritionally regulated, federally subsidized meal. Why should a student try an unfamiliar vegetable when a favorite snack is on sale beside the cashier?

Conversion to universal free meals can remove this competition and free schools to incorporate healthier items. It will not happen overnight, but eating the school meal will become the norm—especially in schools that work actively to integrate the school menu with food education. Experiences in Sweden, Finland, and Brazil, all of which have universal school meals, suggest that healthy school food can indeed become a regular part of the school day. A trip through the cafeteria need not contradict what is being taught in the classroom, but rather reflect and reinforce health messages.

WIC

Fostering the health and nutrition of very young children is particularly important in establishing a solid foundation for future growth and development. The **Special Supplemental Nutrition Program for Women, Infants, and Children (WIC)** is a federal program for eligible pregnant, breastfeeding, postpartum women, and young children who are living at or below 185 percent of the federal poverty line. It provides access to nutrient-rich food, information about healthy eating, seasonal vouchers to farmers markets, and referrals to health care. Currently, 50 percent of children born in the United States participate in the WIC program. On the one hand, such high participation rates demonstrate the breadth and reach of a successful public health nutrition intervention. On the other hand, this indicates that over one-half of American children are born into households at or near poverty.

Special Supplemental Nutrition Program for Women, Infants, and Children (WIC) Federal program for eligible pregnant, breastfeeding, postpartum women, and young children who are living at or below 185 percent of the federal poverty line

WIC participation is associated with a reduction in nutrition-related child health problems, including anemia, nutrition deficiency, and failure to thrive (Black et al., 2004; Lee, Mackey-Bilaver, & Chin, 2006). As expected, WIC participants are less likely to be food insecure compared to eligible households that do not participate (Casey et al., 2004). WIC is also associated with positive growth and health, and improved social, cognitive, and emotional development among children under age three (Black et al., 2012). WIC also has a positive effect on mothers. Female caregivers receiving WIC were less likely to report depressive symptoms compared to women who did not receive WIC (Black et al., 2012).

Policy makers and researchers alike laud the WIC program for saving health care costs. As an example, for every dollar spent on WIC during pregnancy, between $1.77 and $3.13 is saved in Medicaid costs within the first sixty days after a child's birth (Devaney, Bilheimer, & Schore, 1992).

Emergency Food Provisions: Federal and Nonfederal Programs

The emergency food system in the United States is composed of local and national responses. Food pantries, which provide free grocery items, and soup kitchens, which provide prepared meals, many of them linked to faith communities, often participate in the national food bank network called Feeding America. This network currently provides emergency food assistance to thirty-seven million people, or one in eight people living in the United States. Often, these programs are inadequate to bridge the gap clients face, and many resort to hazardous practices in order to obtain adequate food (see focus 5.1).

The emergency food programs receive food from a variety of sources: food donations from corporate manufacturers and retailers, foundations and individual donors, and federal food distribution programs, including **The Emergency Food Assistance Program (TEFAP)**. These donations go to regional and local food banks, which then distribute the food to soup kitchens, food pantries, and homeless shelters.

The Emergency Food Assistance Program (TEFAP) Program that provides US Department of Agriculture commodities to states, which distribute the food through local emergency food providers

As the United States dealt simultaneously with a recession and cutbacks of social programs in the 1980s and 1990s, a large number of emergency food programs sprouted up to address an increased demand for food assistance. The emergency food assistance programs have continued to address that need in the decades since, with donations from individuals, business, and government (Poppendieck, 1998). The emergency food system provides immediate short-term support to individuals and families in need. However, there is no research evidence that such programs can effectively address or prevent food insecurity (Tarasuk, 2001a). An unintended consequence may be that, as Poppendieck describes, the neighborly kindness and goodwill demonstrated through emergency food services enables inaction on a systemic level. Broader action would help address the root causes of the hunger faced by families forced to rely on these charitable services (Poppendieck, 1998).

FOCUS 5.1. WHAT DO PEOPLE DO WHEN THEY ARE WORRIED ABOUT FEEDING THEIR FAMILIES?

Andrea S. Anater

Hunger is not readily seen in the United States. Unlike the televised commercials soliciting aid for starving individuals in developing countries, we see neither newscasts showing US children with distended bellies nor legions of thin, frail people lined up at soup kitchens. In large part this can be attributed to a combination of public and private financial and feeding assistance programs. Considering the suite of assistance programs, in theory, and as a matter of policy, food insecurity should not then be a widespread problem. Yet, in addition to or in place of participation in these programs, many households still struggle to acquire sufficient food directly or to obtain the resources to purchase it, and thus rely on using informal food acquisition coping strategies. For example, food pantry clients often report receiving SNAP and borrowing money or working odd jobs to buy food (Anater, McWilliams, & Latkin, 2011). This makes sense considering that about 59 percent of US households who reported difficulties in securing enough food received assistance from one or more of the three largest federal food and nutrition assistance programs (Coleman-Jensen, Nord, & Singh, 2013).

To better understand the coping strategies employed by food-insecure households and whether they constitute a public health concern, I conducted a first quantitative study on the topic (Anater, 2010; Anater et al., 2011). I sought to verify the use of previously identified coping strategies, determine their frequency, and begin to examine the relationship between employment of these strategies and sociodemographic, psychosocial, household, and environmental-level influences.

I interviewed 492 clients at fifty randomly selected emergency food providers. Participants confirmed use of seventy-eight coping strategies, with 50 percent reporting using at least nineteen. (See table 5.3 for select coping strategies reported.) Of the 9,638 total coping strategies (nonunique) reported used in the year before the survey, 52 percent posed potential risk to users. Specifically, 19 percent (1,853 strategies) potentially posed nutritional risk, 16 percent (1,590) food safety risk, 10 percent (955) financial risk, 6 percent (544) illegal or regulatory risk, and 1 percent (71) physical risk to the user. Ninety-nine percent of participants used more than one nutritionally risky strategy (e.g., diluting baby formula); 92 percent used more than one strategy that posed a food safety risk (e.g., consuming food from dumpsters); 83 percent used more than one financially risky strategy (e.g., avoiding paying bills); 80 percent used more than one potentially illegal strategy (e.g., shoplifting food); and 41 percent used more than one physically risky strategy (e.g., prostituting for food).

TABLE 5.3 Percentage of People Using Select Coping Strategies When Concerned about Food Sufficiency

Strategy	(%)
Skipped paying bills to have more money for food	58
Went to a soup kitchen	47
Been paid under the table for odd jobs to have money for food	41
Ate as much as possible when food was available	40
Avoided inviting guests to home, if expected to serve food	37
Pawned or sold items to get money for food	28
Begged for money for food	13
Lived in abandoned buildings to have more money for food	12
Shoplifted food	12
Switched price tags on food to purchase it at a lower cost	10
Ate food that was thrown away	10
Removed slime from lunch meat before eating	10
Left a restaurant without paying for food	6
Committed a crime to be sent to jail in order to get meals	3

Further, as might be expected, when concerned about maintaining an adequate food supply, those who were less food secure used more coping strategies and more potentially risky strategies than those with greater food security (see figure 5.10). Significantly, participants with very low food security (VLFS) used at least six times more coping strategies than individuals at all other levels of food security, including those with low food security. VLFS predicted increased engagement in risky strategies.

FIGURE 5.10 Comparison of Select Coping Strategies by Food Security Level

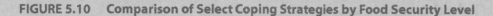

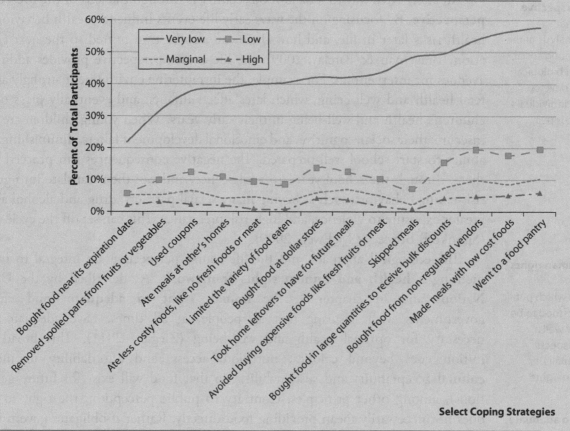

Source: Anater.

Understanding the coping strategies and the attributes associated with them and recognizing those individuals who are most likely to use certain strategies can provide researchers, advocates, and policy makers actionable information to better address the needs of the most vulnerable.

BROADER PERSPECTIVES

Though public assistance programs may buffer families from health effects of severe deprivation, these programs, in and of themselves, cannot help families to break the cycle of hunger and poverty. The United States must take broader, more systematic approaches to understanding and addressing food insecurity. In the following, we share three complementary frameworks that can help us identify opportunities for intervention to treat the underlying causes of food insecurity, not only the symptoms.

ecological approach
Framework rooted in the notion that multiple factors such as economic, social, cultural, political, and institutional structures shape outcomes such as food insecurity or public health

life-course perspective
A framework that incorporates analysis of the relationship among social, behavioral, and biological factors as they develop throughout an individual's life and social context

health and human rights framework
A lens through which public health is understood to be shaped by how well a government respects, protects, and fulfills its people's human rights

human right to adequate food
Realized when every man, woman, and child, alone or in community with others, has physical and economic access at all times to adequate food or means for its procurement, according to the United Nations (United Nations Economic and Social Council, 1999)

Food insecurity is not solely an individual or household-level phenomenon. It is related to political, economic, and social contexts most often beyond control of the household. An **ecological approach** to food insecurity emphasizes the importance of the structural conditions that affect food insecurity. These can be educational attainment, employment opportunities, corporate pay scales, labor laws, and socioeconomic factors. This approach enables us to see how policies and programs and corporate structures can shape the contours of the agriculture and food systems, and thus individual experiences.

An alternative way to look at food security is through the lens of the **life-course perspective.** By focusing on the ways early life events influence health behavior and health risks later in life, and how these can also be transmitted to the next generation (Braveman & Barclay, 2009), the life-course perspective provides additional avenues for intervention. For example, the intrauterine environment strongly affects fetal health and well-being, which later affects infants, and eventually plays out in children's health and well-being in their early years. When young children are food insecure, their social, cognitive, and emotional development falters, diminishing their ability to start school well-prepared. The negative consequences can proceed from there, through the school years, to adolescence, and can then translate into greater risk-taking behaviors, such as having many sexual partners, drug and alcohol abuse, greater exposure to violence, and high-risk pregnancy. This can set off the cycle again (Shonkoff, Boyce, & McEwen, 2009).

The ecological approach and the life-course perspective are integral to implementing a **health and human rights framework**. As described by the United Nations and in chapter 1, the **human right to adequate food** charges governments with ensuring that all people, at all times, have adequate food necessary for optimal health and well-being (Ziegler, 2011). This broad definition goes beyond calories, nutrition, access, and affordability to include cultural acceptability and sustainability (so that food will exist for future generations), among other principles. Contrary to public perception, the right to food does not necessarily mean providing food directly. Rather it obligates governments to respect (not get in the way of), protect (make sure others do not get in the way of), and fulfill (do what is needed to enable people to nourish themselves) the right to food (Riches, 2002). Viewing food security as a human rights issue means good nutrition should not be ensured through simple benevolence or charity, but is instead a duty and obligation of a country to its people. The United States has not yet ratified the international covenant that covers the right to food and has not agreed with the rest of the international community that food is a basic human right. Still, there is much value in using a rights framework to encourage the United States to take a more comprehensive approach; further, the concept that food is a basic right can be transformative in mobilizing advocacy (Chilton & Rose, 2009).

Solutions

Taking into account the described broad frameworks, in the following we describe several strategies for treating and preventing food insecurity and its negative health effects.

Strengthen the Safety Net As demonstrated, there is strong evidence that nutrition-assistance programs work. Thus, the first and most immediate solution available is to strengthen the federal programs providing nutrition and income assistance and ensure more seamless coordination between programs—including between those that assist with food, housing, and utilities—so as to prevent trade-offs.

Improve the Minimum Wage and Reassess Labor Laws Eighty-five percent of SNAP participants work; 70 percent work full time. Their low incomes are below "living-wage" standards and are thus subsidized by SNAP. Improving incomes would have an enormous impact on working households' ability to pay for food and other basic needs. Many low-income working parents struggle to find jobs that can help them care for their families. For example, many have work schedules that are not conducive to accessing regular child-care settings, making it difficult to find safe, adequate child care. Such jobs are also more likely to have variable and inconsistent hours, leading to major fluctuations in income month by month, and are associated with increases in food insecurity (Coleman-Jensen, 2011). In addition, many low wage jobs offer workers neither health insurance nor paid sick days to care for themselves or a sick child (Chavkin & Wise, 2002). Improvements to the minimum wage and more family-friendly labor laws requiring coverage for sick days will take government intervention and incentives to encourage businesses to improve their wage and family-leave structures.

Develop State or Regional Plans Regional and state interventions may also show some promise. Approximately half of the variation in food insecurity rates by state was accounted for by state-to-state differences in average wages, rental costs, housing policies and programs, and participation in nutrition assistance programs such as SNAP and school breakfast and lunch programs. State initiatives to improve wages and lower household costs and tax burdens can have a positive impact on lowering food security (Bartfield, Dunifon, Nord, & Carlson, 2006). Current statewide efforts on food insecurity, specifically, are targeted to improving school breakfast and lunch participation.

Develop a National Plan to End Food Insecurity The United States needs a national strategy on food security, with a strong implementation and accountability mechanism that ensures the participation of multiple government agencies. Based on the number of issues involved, an interagency national plan would need to include the US Department of Agriculture, the Department of Health and Human Services, the Department of Housing and Urban Development, the Department of Education, the Department of Labor, and the Department of Energy. Having a national plan is also the first step toward implementing the right to food (Chilton & Rose, 2008).

In 1999, the United States did present such a plan. The USDA and other agencies developed a report called the *US Action Plan on Food Security: Solutions to Hunger* (US Department of Agriculture Food and Nutrition Service [USDA-FAS], 1999). This report includes language asserting the US responsibility for ensuring the right to food. The first recommendation to redress food security is to promote policies that help to improve economic security, such as encouraging individuals to move into well-paid work and to focus on the most vulnerable groups—American Indian nations, immigrants, and other groups that have been disenfranchised or oppressed, children, people with disabilities or suffering with substance abuse, and others. Since a progress report in 2000 (USDA-FAS, 2000), there is no further evidence of deliberate national focus on food insecurity. Accordingly, it must be emphasized that a plan must include mechanisms to ensure action proceeds.

Encourage Adoption of the Right to Food More than twenty countries have some constitutional provision ensuring the right to food. Some may think that integrating the right to food into the US constitution would have little real-world effect. Evidence from these forward-thinking countries, however, shows that putting this right into the constitution enables the government to harness its law-making, programmatic, and surveillance abilities to document and track progress toward the goals of respecting, protecting, and fulfilling the right to food.

SUMMARY

Food insecurity remains a major yet underrecognized public health problem in the United States. Although food insecurity affects at least one in five children in this country, and more than fifty million people across the United States, the US public often fails to recognize its immediate and long-term health implications. These include increased rates of diet-related diseases and depression in adults, and poor school performance and poor physical and mental health among children. The social and emotional effects of food insecurity are also alarming and have consequences that go far beyond immediate nutrition-related issues. There are major gender, racial, ethnic, and age disparities in rates of food insecurity. Female-headed households, households with children, and African American and Latino households have a higher prevalence of food insecurity than white and two-parent families and households with no children. Food insecurity is a complex phenomenon that stretches beyond simply providing food to the hungry. Nutrition assistance and other public assistance programs can help keep food insecurity at bay, but evidence shows that without attention to ensuring economic security among low-income families, food insecurity rates will stay alarmingly high. Food insecurity should be viewed as not just an individual or household problem but also related to the political, economic, and social contexts beyond the control of the household. Strengthening the federal safety net, improving the minimum wage and reassessing labor laws, developing state or regional plans and a national plan to end hunger, and encouraging the adoption of the right to food are all important steps to creating solutions to the food insecurity problem in the United States.

KEY TERMS

Ecological approach

Entitlement program

Food insecurity

Food security

Health and human rights framework

Household Food Security Survey Module (HFSSM)

Human right to adequate food

Life-course perspective

National School Lunch Program (NSLP)

School breakfast program

Special Supplemental Nutrition Program for Women, Infants, and Children (WIC)

Supplemental Nutrition Assistance Program (SNAP)

The Emergency Food Assistance Program (TEFAP)

Thrifty Food Plan (TFP)

DISCUSSION QUESTIONS

1. Why did food insecurity rates drastically increase during the recession beginning in 2008?

2. American Indians and Latino immigrants have especially high rates of food insecurity and are among the communities most difficult to reach. Knowing the complexity of food insecurity, what structural

factors do you think affect these communities, which may increase their food insecurity rates? How might they be reached more effectively?

3. As explained in this chapter, the United States has not ratified the international covenant on the human right to adequate food. Why do you think this has not happened? What could be done to encourage adoption of this document?

4. Perspectives 5.2 and 5.3 present two views about whether SNAP benefits should be permitted for use in purchasing items such as sugar-sweetened beverages. Which arguments did you find most persuasive on each side? More broadly, what is your opinion? There are some stakeholders on both sides of the issue who may be motivated by concerns other than those they state. What might these concerns be?

5. In perspective 5.4, Janet Poppendieck argues for universal school meals. What are the main counterarguments to her perspective? What is your opinion?

REFERENCES

Alaimo, K., Olson, C. M., & Frongillo Jr., E. A. (2002). Family food insufficiency is associated with dysthymia and suicidal symptoms in adolescents: Results from NHANES III. *Journal of Nutrition, 132,* 719–725.

Alaimo, K., Olson, C. M., & Frongillo Jr., E. A. (2001a). Food insufficiency and American school-aged children's cognitive, academic, and psychosocial development. *Pediatrics, 108*(1), 44–53.

Alaimo, K., Olson, C. M., Frongillo Jr., E. A., & Briefel, R. R. (2001b). Food insufficiency, family income, and health in U.S. preschool and school-age children. *American Journal of Public Health, 91,* 781–786.

Almond, D., Hoynes, H. W., & Whitmore Schanzenbach, D. (2011). Inside the war on poverty: The impact of food stamps on birth outcomes. *The Review of Economics and Statistics, 93*(2), 387–403.

Alston, J. M., Mullally, C. C., Sumner, D. A., Townsend, M., & Vosti, S. A. (2009). Likely effects on obesity from proposed changes to the US food stamp program. *Food Policy, 34*(2), 176–184.

Anater, A. S. (2010). *Exploring food acquisition practices of food insecure individuals in New Jersey.* PhD dissertation. Baltimore: Johns Hopkins University.

Anater, A. S., McWilliams, R., & Latkin, C. A. (2011). Food acquisition practices used by food-insecure individuals when they are concerned about having sufficient food for themselves and their households. *Journal of Hunger and Environmental Nutrition, 6*(1), 27–44.

Barbosa-da-Silva, S., Fraulob-Aquino, J. C., Lopes, J. R., Mandarim-de-Lacerda, C. A., & Aguila, M. B. (2012). Weight cycling enhances adipose tissue inflammatory responses in male mice. *PLOS One, 7*(7), e39837.

Bartfeld, J., Dunifon, R., Nord, M., & Carlson, S. (2006). *What factors account for state-to-state differences in food security?* Washington, DC: US Department of Agriculture.

Basiotis, P., Lino, M., & Anand, R. (1999). *Eating breakfast greatly improves schoolchildren's diet quality* (Report No. Nutrition Insight 15). Washington, DC: US Department of Agriculture.

Bauer, K. W., Widome, R., Himes, J. H., Smyth, M., Rock, B. H., Hannan, P. J., et al. (2012). High food insecurity and its correlates among families living on a rural American Indian reservation. *American Journal of Public Health, 102*(7), 1346–1352.

Bhattacharya, J., Currie, J., & Haider, S. (2004a.). *Breakfast of champions? The school breakfast program and nutrition of children and families.* Washington, DC: US Department of Agriculture.

Bhattacharya, J., Currie, J., & Haider, S. (2004b). Poverty, food insecurity, and nutritional outcomes in children and adults. *Journal of Health Economics, 23*(4), 839–862.

Black, M. M., Cutts, D. B., Frank, D. A., Geppert, J., Skalicky, A., Levenson, S., et al. (2004). Special supplemental nutrition program for women, infants, and children participation and infants' growth and health: A multisite surveillance study. *Pediatrics, 114*(1), 169–176.

Black, M. M., Quigg, A. M., Cook, J., Casey, P. H., Cutts, D. B., Chilton, M., et al. (2012). WIC participation and attenuation of stress-related child health risks of household food insecurity and caregiver depressive symptoms. *Archives of Pediatrics & Adolescent Medicine, 166*(5), 444.

Braveman, P., & Barclay, C. (2009). Health disparities beginning in childhood: A life-course perspective. *Pediatrics, 124*(Suppl. 3), S212–S213.

Breen, A. B., Cahill, R., Ettinger de Cuba, S., Cook, J., & Chilton, M. (2011). *The real cost of a healthy diet*. Philadelphia: Children's HealthWatch.

Bronte-Tinkew, J., Zaslow, M., Capps, R., Horowitz, A., & McNamara, M. (2007). Food insecurity works through depression, parenting, and infant feeding to influence overweight and health in toddlers. *The Journal of Nutrition, 137*(9), 2160–2165.

Brownell, K., & Ludwig, D. (2011). The supplemental nutrition assistance program, soda, and USDA policy: Who benefits? *JAMA, 306*(12), 1370–1371.

Casey, P., Goolsby, S., Berkowitz, C., Frank, D., Cook, J., Cutts, D., et al. (2004). Maternal depression, changing public assistance, food security, and child health status. *Pediatrics, 113*(2), 298–304.

Chavkin, W., & Wise, P. H. (2002). The data are in: Health matters in welfare policy. *American Journal of Public Health, 92*(9), 1392–1395.

Chilton, M., Black, M. M., Berkowitz, C., Casey, P. H., Cook, J., Cutts, D., et al. (2009). Food insecurity and risk of poor health among US-born children of immigrants. *American Journal of Public Health, 99*(3), 556–562.

Chilton, M., & Booth, S. (2007). Hunger of the body and hunger of the mind: African American women's perceptions of food insecurity, health and violence. *Journal of Nutrition Education and Behavior, 39*(3), 116–125.

Chilton, M., & Rose, D. (2009). A rights-based approach to food insecurity in the United States. *American Journal of Public Health, 99*(7), 1203–1211.

Chung, W. T., Gallo, W. T., Giunta, N., Canavan, M. E., Parikh, N. S., & Fahs, M. C. (2011). Linking neighborhood characteristics to food insecurity in older adults: The role of perceived safety, social cohesion, and walkability. *Journal of Urban Health, 89*, 1–12.

Cohen, B., Ohls, J., Andrews, M., Ponza, M., Moreno, L., Zambrowski, A., & Cohen, R. (1999). *Food stamp participants' food security and nutrient availability*. Alexandria, VA: US Department of Agriculture Food and Nutrition Service, Office of Analysis and Evaluation.

Coleman-Jensen, A. (2011). Working for peanuts: Nonstandard work and food insecurity across household structure. *Journal of Family and Economic Issues, 32*, 84–97.

Coleman-Jensen, A., Nord, M., Andrews, M., & Carlson, S. (2012). *Household food security in the United States in 2011*. Washington, DC: US Department of Agriculture.

Coleman-Jensen, A., Nord, M., & Singh, A. (2013, September). *Household food security in the United States in 2012* (ERR-155). Washington, DC: US Department of Agriculture Economic Research Service.

Cooper, R., Anderson, S., & FitzSimons, C. (2012). *Hunger doesn't take a vacation: Summer nutrition status report 2012*. Food Research and Action Center. Retrieved from http://frac.org/pdf/2012_summer_nutrition_report.pdf

Cutts, D. B., Meyers, A. F., Black, M. M., Casey, P. H., Chilton, M., Cook, J. T., et al. (2011). US housing insecurity and the health of very young children. *American Journal of Public Health, 101*(8), 1508.

Devaney, B., Bilheimer, L., & Schore, J. (1992). Medicaid costs and birth outcomes: The effects of prenatal WIC participation and the use of prenatal care. *Journal of Policy Analysis and Management, 11*, 573–592.

Dietz, W. (1995). Does hunger cause obesity. *Pediatrics, 95*(5), 766–767.

DiMeglio, D., & Mattes, R. (2000). Liquid versus solid carbohydrate: Effects on food intake and body weight. *International Journal of Obesity and Related Metabolic Disorders, 24*(6), 794–800.

Drewnowski, A., & Darmon, N. (2005). The economics of obesity: Dietary energy density and energy cost. *American Journal of Clinical Nutrition, 82*(1 Suppl.), 265S–273S.

Eslami, E., Leftin, J., & Strayer, M. (2012). *Supplemental nutrition assistance program participation rates: Fiscal year 2010*. Alexandria, VA: US Department of Agriculture Food and Nutrition Service.

Eslami, E., & Cunnyngham, K. (2014). *Supplemental Nutrition Assistance Program Participation Rates: Fiscal Years 2010 and 2011*. USDA Food and Nutrition Service: Washington, DC.

Food and Nutrition Act of 2008. (2008). Retrieved from www.fns.usda.gov/snap/rules/legislation/pdfs/pl_110–246.pdf

Fram, M. S., Frongillo, E. A., Jones, S. J., Williams, R. C., Burke, M. P., DeLoach, K. P., et al. (2011). Children are aware of food insecurity and take responsibility for managing food resources. *The Journal of Nutrition, 141*(6), 1114–1119.

Frank, D. A., Casey, P. H., Black, M. M., Rose-Jacobs, R., Chilton, M., Cutts, D., et al. (2010). Cumulative hardship and wellness of low-income, young children: Multisite surveillance study. *Pediatrics, 125*(5), e1115.

Frank, D. A., Chilton, M., Casey, P. H., Black, M. M., Cook, J. T., Cutts, D. B., et al. (2010). Nutritional-assistance programs play a critical role in reducing food insecurity. *Pediatrics, 125*(5), e1267; author reply e1267–e1268.

Frongillo, E. A., Jyoti, D. F., & Jones, S. J. (2006). Food stamp program participation is associated with better academic learning among school children. *Journal of Nutrition, 136*(4), 1077–1080.

Gundersen, C. (2008). Measuring the extent, depth, and severity of food insecurity: An application to American Indians in the USA. *Journal of Population Economics, 21*(1), 191–215.

Gundersen, C., & Kreider, B. (2009). Bounding the effects of food insecurity on children's health outcomes. *Journal of Health Economics, 28*(5), 971–983.

Hamelin, A. M., Beaudry, M., & Habicht, J. P. (2002). Characterization of household food insecurity in Québec: Food and feelings. *Social Science and Medicine, 54*(1), 119–132.

Hamelin, A. M., Habicht, J. P., & Beaudry, M. (1999). Food insecurity: Consequences for the household and broader social implications. *Journal of Nutrition, 129*(2 Suppl.), 525S–528S.

Harper, C., Wood, L., & Mitchell, C. (2008). *The provision of school food in 18 countries*. School Food Trust, UK. Retrieved from www.childrensfoodtrust.org.uk/assets/research-reports/school_food_in18countries.pdf

Hartline-Grafton, H., Vollinger, E., & Weill, J. (2013). *A review of strategies to bolster SNAP's role in improving nutrition as well as food security*. Washington, DC: Food Research and Action Center.

Heckman. J. J. (2006). Skill formation and the economics of investing in disadvantaged children. *Science, 312*(5782), 1900–1902.

Hofferth, S. L., & Curtin, S. (2005). Poverty, food programs, and childhood obesity. *Journal of Policy Analysis and Management, 24*(4), 703–726.

Howard, L. L. (2011). Does food insecurity at home affect non-cognitive performance at school? A longitudinal analysis of elementary student classroom behavior. *Economics of Education Review, 30*(1), 157–176.

Institute of Medicine. (2001). *Promoting health: Intervention strategies from social and behavioral research*. Washington, DC: National Academies Press.

Institute of Medicine and National Research Council. (2013). *Supplemental nutrition assistance program: Examining the evidence to define benefit adequacy*. Washington, DC: The National Academies Press.

Jeng, K., Ettinger de Cuba, S., Coleman, S., Meyers, A., Rose-Jacobs, R., Frank, D., et al. (2010). *Healthcare cost "trade-offs" with basic needs: Impact on maternal and child health in five cities*. American Public Health Association annual meeting, November 8, Denver, CO.

Jones, S. J., & Frongillo, E. A. (2007). Food insecurity and subsequent weight gain in women. *Public Health Nutrition, 10*(2), 145–151.

Jyoti, D. F., Frongillo, E. A., & Jones, S. J. (2005). Food insecurity affects school children's academic performance, weight gain, and social skills. *Journal of Nutrition, 135*(12), 2831–2839.

Kleinman, R. E., Murphy, J. M., Little, M., Pagano, M., Wehler, C. A., Regal, K., et al. (1998). Hunger in children in the United States: Potential behavioral and emotional correlates. *Pediatrics, 101*(1), E3.

Lee, B., Mackey-Bilaver, L., & Chin, M. (2006). *Effects of WIC and Food Stamp program participation on child outcomes* (Contractor and Cooperator Report No. 27). Washington, DC: US Department of Agriculture.

Magryta, C. J. (2009). School lunches: A strategy to combat childhood obesity. *Explore, 5*(6), 352–353.

Melchior, M., Caspi, A., Howard, L. M., Ambler, A. P., Bolton, H., Mountain, N., et al. (2009). Mental health context of food insecurity: A representative cohort of families with young children. *Pediatrics, 124*(4), e564–e572.

Metallinos-Katsaras, E., Sherry, B., & Kallio, J. (2009). Food insecurity is associated with overweight in children younger than 5 years of age. *Journal of the American Dietetic Association, 109*(10), 1790–1794.

Millimet, D. L., Tchernis, R., & Husain, M. (2010). School nutrition programs and the incidence of childhood obesity. *Journal of Human Resources, 45*(3), 640–654.

Mullany B., Neault, N., Tsingine, D., Powers, J., Lovato, V., Clitso, L., et al. (2012). Food insecurity and household eating patterns among vulnerable American-Indian families: Associations with caregiver and food consumption characteristics. *Public Health Nutrition, 16*, 1–9.

Murphy, J. M., Wehler, C. A., Pagano, M. E., Little, M., Kleinman, R. E., & Jellinek, M. S. (1998). Relationship between hunger and psychosocial functioning in low-income American children. *Journal of the American Academy of Child & Adolescent Psychiatry, 37*(2), 163–170.

National Research Council. (2006). Food Security and Hunger in the United States: An Assessment of the Measure. Washington, DC: National Academies Press.

New York State Office of Temporary and Disability Assistance. (2010). *Request for waiver to modify allowable purchases under the supplemental nutrition assistance program.* Retrieved from www.idfa.org/files/Healthy_NY_SNAP_Demo_Project_Proposal_Final_092910.pdf

Nord, M., Andrews, M., & Carlson, S. (2002). *Household food security in the United States* (Report No. 29). Washington, DC: US Department of Agriculture Economic Research Service.

Nord, M., Andrews, M., & Carlson, S. (2007). *Household food security in the United States, 2006.* Washington, DC: US Department of Agriculture, Economic Research Service.

Olson, C. M., Bove, C. F., & Miller, E. O. (2007). Growing up poor: Long-term implications for eating patterns and body weight. *Appetite, 49*(1), 198–207.

Olson, C. M., & Strawderman, M. S. (2008). The relationship between food insecurity and obesity in rural childbearing women. *Journal of Rural Health, 24*(1), 60–66.

Poppendieck, J. (1998). *Sweet charity? Emergency food and the end of entitlement.* New York: Viking Press.

Poppendieck, J. (2010). *Free for all: Fixing school food in America.* Berkeley: University of California Press (especially chapter 7).

Quandt, S. A., Shoaf, J. I., Tapia, J., Hernandez-Pelletier, M., Clark, H. M., & Arcury, T. A. (2006). Experiences of Latino immigrant families in North Carolina help explain elevated levels of food insecurity and hunger. *Journal of Nutrition, 136*(10), 2638–2644.

Radimer, K., Olson, C., Green, J., Campbell, C. C., & Habicht, J. P. (1992). Understanding hunger and developing indicators to assess it in women and children. *Journal of Nutrition Education, 24*, 36S–44S.

Riches, G. (2002). Food banks and food security: Welfare reform, human rights and social policy. *Social Policy & Administration, 36*(6), 648–663.

Rose, D. (1999). Economic determinants and dietary consequences of food insecurity in the United States. *Journal of Nutrition, 129*(2 Suppl.), 517S–520S.

Rose, D. (2007). Food stamps, the thrifty food plan, and meal preparation: The importance of the time dimension for us nutrition policy. *Journal of Nutrition Education and Behavior*, *39*(4), 226–232.

Rose, D., & Oliveira, V. (1997). Nutrient intakes of individuals from food-insufficient households in the United States. *American Journal of Public Health*, *87*(12),1956–1961.

Rose-Jacobs, R., Black, M. M., Casey, P. H., Cook, J. T., Cutts, D. B., Chilton, M., et al. (2008). Household food insecurity: Associations with at-risk infant and toddler development. *Pediatrics*, *121*(1), 65–72.

Scarpellini, E., & Tack, J. (2012). Obesity and metabolic syndrome: An inflammatory condition. *Digestive Diseases*, *30*(2), 148–153.

Schanzenbach, D. W. (2009). Do school lunches contribute to childhood obesity? *Journal of Human Resources*, *44*(3), 684–709.

School Nutrition Association. (2011). *School nutrition operations report, 2011* (p. 42). National Harbor, MD: School Nutrition Association.

Seligman, H. K., Davis, T. C., Schillinger, D., & Wolf, M. S. (2010). Food insecurity is associated with hypoglycemia and poor diabetes self-management in a low-income sample with diabetes. *Journal for Health Care for the Poor and Underserved*, *21*(4), 1227–1233.

Sharkey, J. R., Dean, W. R., & Johnson, C. M. (2011). Association of household and community characteristics with adult and child food insecurity among Mexican-origin households in Colonias along the Texas-Mexico border. *International Journal for Equity in Health*, *10*(1), 19.

Shepard, D., Setren, E., & Cooper, D. (2011). *Hunger in America: Suffering we all pay for*. Washington, DC: Center for American Progress.

Shonkoff, J. P., Boyce, W. T., & McEwen, B. S. (2009). Neuroscience, molecular biology, and the childhood roots of health disparities: Building a new framework for health promotion and disease prevention. *Journal of the American Medical Association*, *301*(21), 2252–2259.

Tarasuk, V. (2001a). A critical examination of community-based responses to household food insecurity in Canada. *Health Education & Behavior*, *28*(4), 487–499.

Tarasuk, V. (2001b). Household food insecurity with hunger is associated with women's food intakes, health and household circumstances. *Journal of Nutrition*, *131*, 2670–2676.

US Department of Agriculture Farm Service Agency. (2014). *Disaster assistance programs*. Retrieved from www.fsa.usda.gov/FSA/webapp?area=home&subject=diap&topic=landing

US Department of Agriculture, Food and Nutrition Service. (2007a). *Implications of restricting the use of food stamp benefits—Summary*. Retrieved from www.fns.usda.gov/ora/MENU/Published/snap/FILES/ProgramOperations/FSPFoodRestrictions.pdf

US Department of Agriculture, Food and Nutrition Service. (2007b). *Erroneous payments in the national school lunch program and school breakfast program: Summary of findings*. Retrieved from www.fns.usda.gov/sites/default/files/APECSummaryofFind.pdf

US Department of Agriculture, Food and Nutrition Service. (2013a). *Summer food service program*. Retrieved from www.fns.usda.gov/cnd/summer/FAQs.htm

US Department of Agriculture, Food and Nutrition Service. (2013b). *Child and adult care food program*. Retrieved from www.fns.usda.gov/cnd/care/CACFP/aboutcacfp.htm

US Department of Agriculture, Food and Nutrition Service. (2013c). *National school lunch program*. Retrieved from www.fns.usda.gov/sites/default/files/NSLPFactSheet.pdf

US Department of Agriculture, Food and Nutrition Service. (2014a). *Supplemental nutrition assistance program*. Retrieved from www.fns.usda.gov/snap

US Department of Agriculture, Food and Nutrition Service. (2014b). *WIC program*. Retrieved from www.fns.usda.gov/pd/wisummary.htm

US Department of Agriculture, Food and Nutrition Service. (2014c). *Food distribution programs*. Retrieved from www.fns.usda.gov/fdd/food-distribution-programs

US Department of Agriculture, Food and Nutrition Service, Office of Research and Analysis (2013). *SNAP food security in-depth interview study*, by Kathryn Edin, Melody Boyd, James Mabli, Jim Ohls, Julie Worthington, Sara Greene, Nicholas Redel, Swetha Sridharan. Project Officer Sarah Zapolsky. Alexandria, VA: Author.

US Department of Agriculture, Foreign Agricultural Service. (1999). *U.S. action plan on food security: Solutions to hunger*. Washington, DC: Interagency Working Group on Food Security and Food Security Advisory Committee.

US Department of Agriculture, Foreign Agricultural Service. (2000). *A millennium free from hunger: U.S. national progress report on implementation of the U.S. action plan on food security and World Food Summit commitments*. Washington, DC: Author.

UN Committee on Economic, Social and Cultural Rights, (1999). *General Comment No. 12. The Right to Adequate Food (Art. 11 of the Covenant)*.

Wahlstrom, K. L., & Begalle, M. S. (1999). More than test scores: Results of the universal school breakfast pilot in Minnesota. *Topics in Clinical Nutrition*, *15*(1), 17–29.

Wehler, C., Weinreb, L. F., Huntington, N., Scott, R., Hosmer, D., Fletcher, K., et al. (2004). Risk and protective factors for adult and child hunger among low-income housed and homeless female-headed families. *American Journal of Public Health*, *94*(1), 109–115.

Whitaker, R. C., Phillips, S. M., & Orzol, S. M. (2006). Food insecurity and the risks of depression and anxiety in mothers and behavior problems in their preschool-aged children. *Pediatrics*, *118*(3), e859–e868.

Zaslow, M., Bronte-Tinkew, J., Capps, R., Horowitz, A., Moore, K. A., & Weinstein, D. (2009). Food security during infancy: Implications for attachment and mental proficiency in toddlerhood. *Maternal and Child Health Journal*, *13*(1), 66–80.

Ziegler, J. (2011). *The fight for the right to food: Lessons learned*. Basingstoke, UK: Palgrave Macmillan.

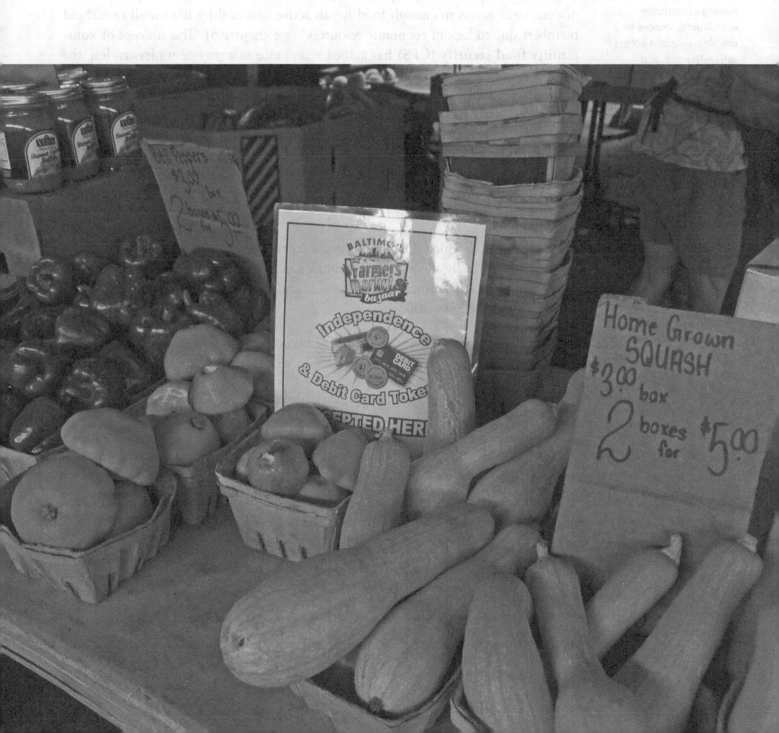

Chapter 6

Community Food Security

Anne M. Palmer, Wei-Ting Chen, and Mark Winne

food insecurity
Having inadequate economic resources to enable consistent access to safe, adequate, and nutritious food to support an active and healthy life for all household members (low food security: reduced quality, variety, desirability of diet; very low food security: multiple indications of disrupted eating patterns and reduced food intake)

community food security (CFS)
A condition in which all community residents obtain a safe, culturally acceptable, nutritionally adequate diet through a sustainable system that maximizes community self-reliance, social justice, and democratic decision making

The US Department of Agriculture (USDA) defines **food insecurity** as "the lack of consistent access to enough food for an active and healthy life for all household members due to lack of economic resources" (see chapter 5). The concept of **community food security (CFS)** has gained acceptance as a way of understanding the broader context of household food security by examining it in relation to factors such as food environment and poverty. By looking at the context, CFS activists seek to understand the strengths and weaknesses of the food system serving a jurisdiction (i.e., state, county, city, neighborhood), with a focus on low-income citizens.

Advocates have described CFS as an *analytic tool* for understanding the issue of food security, as a *method* for developing food-secure communities, and as a *goal* in and of itself (Winne, Joseph, & Fisher, 1997). The most widely cited definition of community food security is as follows:

> A condition in which all community residents obtain a safe, culturally acceptable, nutritionally adequate diet through a sustainable system that maximizes community self-reliance, social justice, and democratic decision-making. (Hamm & Bellows, 2003)

This definition provides a vision of the ideal community food system and highlights the multidimensional nature of CFS, of which concern about hunger is a key component.

Community food security projects include a wide range of activities that reflect most components of the food system. Following are examples:

- *Production:* Sustainable agriculture groups conduct beginner farmer training to increase younger generations' capacity to farm.

- *Processing:* Entrepreneurs build incubator kitchens that provide small businesses an opportunity to turn raw ingredients into value-added food products such as jam.

- *Distribution and selling:* Urban farmers take mobile produce trucks to neighborhoods that have few fresh food options and sell produce at a reasonable price (see figure 6.1).

- *Consumption:* Food educators teach students the importance of good nutrition and cooking skills to influence their food choices.

- *Waste:* Local compost operations accept food waste and create rich soil for community gardens and others.

Organizations and individuals working on CFS also bridge these domains. They build direct links between producers and consumers by starting farmers markets, helping low-income consumers access fresh local produce, expanding the customer base for local farmers, and contributing to overall local economic development.

The CFS movement grew out of the efforts of three distinct but overlapping groups: community nutritionists and educators, progressive sustainable agricultural researchers and activists, and antihunger and community development researchers and activists (Anderson & Cook, 1999). In 1994, representatives of these groups formed the Community Food Security Coalition

FIGURE 6.1   Mobile Produce Truck

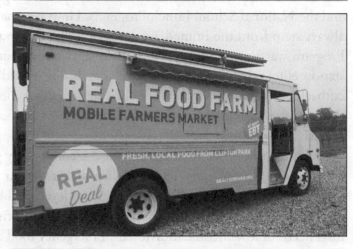

Source: Ruth Burrows, CLF.

(CFSC), the North American organization responsible for much of the policy and programming progress on CFS. The CFSC founders identified six principles with which to structure ongoing consensus in their efforts:

- Focus on the food needs of low-income populations.

- Define food security as a product of wide social issues and policies.

- Encourage consumption of locally grown food.

- Emphasize community self-reliance and empowerment, rather than emergency and charity food relief.

- Promote a democratic, community-responsive food system.

- Include the talents and participation of diverse peoples in the community (Community Food Security Coalition [CFSC], 2011).

For some participants, joining with the other groups helped them recognize that an environmentally unsustainable food production system is a significant risk to long-term food security for all (Gottlieb & Fisher, 1996). For others, working together was an opportunity to overcome the political and practical struggles of incorporating social justice components into the definition and promotion of sustainable agriculture. The framework of CFS provides an opportunity for these different groups to work through the practical issues of environmental sustainability and hunger alleviation.

HISTORY AND EVOLUTION OF CFS

The evolutionary paths leading toward CFS—its development from antihunger, community development, and sustainable agriculture activism to community food security—are nonlinear trajectories marked by slow growth and sudden halts in different areas. Political and financial support for projects in each of these areas has waxed and waned depending on the political climate of the time and place.

As described in chapter 8, between 1936 and the late 1970s, the US government had incrementally increased its support for nutritional social safety net programs such as Food Stamps (now SNAP), WIC, and the National School Lunch Programs. However, the impetus for food assistance programs did not always stem from the immediate needs of individual food security. For example, the first Food Stamp Program was started in 1939 to balance agricultural surpluses and hunger. When economic circumstances eliminated farm surpluses, such as during World War II, food assistance programs experienced cutbacks. The pattern of serving the dual needs of the agricultural sectors and the poor continued through the 1960s, during which citizen groups advocated for social programs designed to directly combat hunger (Allen, 1999).

Efforts to improve food security at the community level arose out of an eroding social safety net for the poor. In the early 1980s, policy makers began cutting back social safety net programs. The US Congress reduced food stamp benefits to levels well below those considered necessary for adequate diets (Allen, 1999). The reductions forced state and private charities to increase their support for the food needs of low-income individuals. Emergency food assistance programs, such as food pantries and soup kitchens, multiplied to bridge the gaps. To avoid hunger, people have had to supplement their federal food assistance by navigating the system of private food assistance programs, which often have limited stock, hours, and uncertain operational longevity. The need for emergency food assistance has increased over time. In 1991, there was a national network of 180 food banks, 23,000 food pantries, and 3,300 soup kitchens (Clancy, 1993). As of 2014, there is a national network of 203 food banks that stock more than 61,000 emergency food assistance sites including food pantries, soup kitchens, and shelters; together, these services provide food to an estimated 37 million low-income people, including 14 million children (Feeding America, 2014). The problem of urban hunger also worsened during the 1980s when supermarkets left city centers and moved into the suburbs (Clancy, 1993). All of these changes and events further marginalized urban residents, particularly the poor and politically weak, from many institutions within the food system (Clancy, 1993). The political and economic changes in the food security safety net contributed to the consensus that a more unified, community-driven approach was needed to "reweave the food security safety net" (Allen, 1999, p. 117).

Similar to antihunger and other food system social justice advocates in the 1980s, supporters of sustainable agriculture also saw the need to establish new forms of community empowerment that would provide greater support and create new economic opportunities for farmers practicing sustainable methods. By the early 1990s, a coalition of CFS supporters began working together to move their agenda into the 1995 US Farm Bill. The lobbying effort drove the institutionalization of existing but unconnected efforts nationwide to address simultaneously, at the local level, household food security and sustainable agriculture concerns (Hamm & Bellows, 2003).

Officially founded in 1994, the CFSC successfully lobbied for the passage of the Community Food Security Act in the 1996 Farm Bill, which provided initial funding for the Community Food Project Competitive Grant Program (CFP). The USDA CFP program supports projects that meet the food needs of low-income people, increase community self-reliance in meeting food needs, or promote comprehensive responses to local food, farm, and nutrition issues. Funded CFPs have included community gardens with market stands, farmers markets, farm to school projects, faith-based community food assessments, and food hubs (see focus 6.1), all of which involved low-income participants. Since 1996, about four hundred projects have been funded, and the program is widely cited as a key funding source for local food system activities. Together, these projects have elevated the importance of CFS on the political and public agenda (Anderson & Cook, 1999).

FOCUS 6.1. FOOD HUBS: SUPPORTING HEALTHY FARMS, HEALTHY PEOPLE, HEALTHY ECONOMY

John Fisk

The demand for local and regionally produced food is growing; however, in many parts of the country channeling locally produced food into wholesale markets is difficult. Due to consolidation trends over recent decades, farms and the infrastructure needed to handle farm products are no longer available to meet the demand for locally produced food. For example, when the Kansas City branch of Sysco, a national food distributor, wanted to offer more local food to its customers they found that their usual suppliers could not provide these products. However, by connecting with Good Natured Family Farms, a nearby cooperative of more than one hundred small family farms, they could begin to source the desired products (Cantrell, 2010).

USDA identified key barriers to building a region's capacity to supply more local foods, including the lack of small- and mid-sized packing houses, processors, and distributors; lack of mechanisms for **product traceability** (the ability to track a food product back to the farm from which it came); and the need to build farmer capacity for meeting the volume and quality demands of wholesale markets, such as retail stores and food service companies (Barham, Tropp, Enterline, Farbman, Fisk, & Kiraly, 2012). Additionally, farm-to-school advocates have identified "insufficiencies in local supply chains (e.g., production volume and quality, processing, storage, etc.) as a major barrier to continued growth" (US Department of Agriculture, 2011, p. i).

product traceability
The ability to track a food product back through the distribution system to the farm from which it came

At the heart of any supply chain is an efficient and effective means of aggregating products for quantity, quality, packing, storing, and distributing them to buyers. A working definition of a food hub offered by the USDA is "a business or organization that carries out or actively coordinates the aggregation, distribution and marketing of primarily source-identified local and regional food products from small- and mid-sized producers to wholesalers, retailers and/or institutional buyers" (Barham et al., 2012, p. 4). By offering these and a number of producer and community services, the more than two hundred food hubs currently in operation are poised to bridge the gap in infrastructure necessary to increase the flow of healthy local foods into areas with limited access. Hubs are providing wider access to institutional and retail markets for small- and mid-sized producers, creating new jobs along the supply chain, and—crucially—increasing access to fresh healthy food for consumers through more mainstream food system outlets, such as retail stores, corner stores, schools, and hospitals. Regional food hubs can also encourage the retention of agricultural jobs by helping to keep farming a profitable and viable business.

In order for aggregation and distribution businesses to be considered food hubs they need to express values-based characteristics, such as the following:

- Commitment to buying from small- to mid-sized local producers at a fair price

- Differentiate products from commodities through identity preservation, group branding, sustainable production practices, and other approaches

- Build the capacity of producers to help them meet market requirements

- Operate as triple bottom line businesses that seek to be financially viable and have positive economic, social, and environmental impacts

The 2013 National Food Hub Survey (Fischer, Hamm, Pirog, Fisk, Farbman, & Kiraly, 2013) found a surge in food hub development in recent years with 62 percent in operation for five years or less. Forty-seven

(Continued)

(Continued)

percent of surveyed hubs were started by entrepreneurs, another 13 percent by cooperatives, and 34 percent were nonprofit organizations. On average, food hubs sold more than $3.25 million in products annually (with a wide range reported) from a median of thirty-six producers. On average, hubs had eleven full-time employees, and a number of them also had part-time and seasonal staff and used volunteers. Food hubs play an important role in addressing food access. Many food hubs were working to increase healthy food access in communities underserved by full-service food retail outlets; and 35 percent reported selling to public schools, many with significant free and reduced-price food programs. Seventy five percent of hubs reported making donations of fresh products to food banks. Additionally, food hubs work with producers to increase their capacity to meet standards and specifications required by schools and hospitals.

FIGURE 6.2   Local Food Hub Warehouse

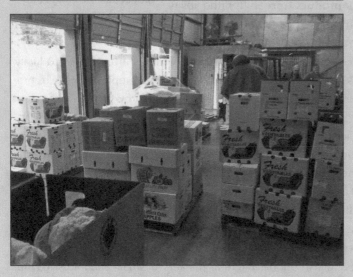

Source: Local Food Hub. "Farm to School Week Madness at the Warehouse." Used with permission.

Local Food Hub (LFH) in Charlottesville, Virginia, exemplifies the breadth of food hub activities and the potential impact. Founded in 2009, LFH works with farmers to coordinate their production and product packing with market demand, bringing together products from more than seventy-five small- and mid-sized family farms within one hundred miles from Charlottesville. At LFH's warehouse, products are checked for quality, labeled, kept in cold storage at the appropriate temperatures, and eventually delivered in refrigerated trucks (see figure 6.2). LFH offers fresh produce, meat, eggs, and value-added products to more than 150 customers including schools, college dining halls, restaurants and caterers, retail stores, senior centers, hospitals, and several larger distributors and processors. As a result, LFH has reinvested more than $1.3 million in the local farming community, created fifteen paid jobs at their distribution and farm operations, and their services have helped to retain and support more than two hundred agriculture-related jobs. The hub's educational farm offers apprenticeships and high school internships to budding farmers. Local Food Hub considers it part of their mission to contribute to the public health of the community. They supply hospitals with local food for cafeteria and patient meals and a weekly food market. They also work with forty-five schools to put food on children's plates and have donated over 130,000 pounds to hunger groups.

By working with small farmers and larger buyers, food hubs are providing the essential glue needed to increase the role of local food in the more conventional food system and thus its impact on the lives of farmers, families, and communities.

Though there remain tensions between CFS stakeholders (for example, the cost of sustainably grown foods is often beyond the reach of low-income consumers), there are instances of successful CFS projects that integrate goals and stakeholders from multiple sectors. The effort to increase SNAP redemption in farmers markets is an example (see figure 6.3). Although the number of farmers markets has been growing around the nation, and a rising number of markets accept food assistance benefits, farmers market SNAP redemption rates remain low, accounting for only 0.016 percent of total SNAP redemption in FY2010–2011 (USDA Food and Nutrition Services, via Farmers Market Coalition). Antihunger groups and community nutrition educators already lead efforts to increase SNAP use, but the coalition of supporters behind farmers market SNAP acceptance brings in local agriculture advocates.

FIGURE 6.3   Mayor Stephanie Rawlings Blake Announcing SNAP EBT Program at Baltimore Farmers Market

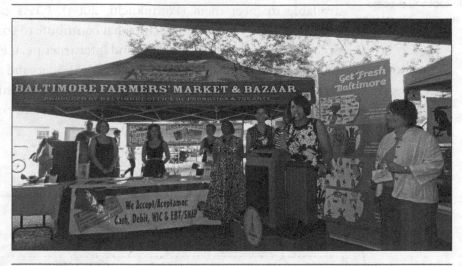

Source: USDA. "20120708-OSEC-LSC-0074." http://www.flickr.com/photos/usdagov/75318 63328

MEASURING COMMUNITY FOOD SECURITY

Measurement of CFS can identify areas for improvement, track progress, and evaluate program impact. To date, few studies have attempted to measure a particular CFS program's effect on a community. Measurement is challenging for many reasons. For one, whereas food security related to hunger is typically measured at the *household* and *individual* levels (see chapter 5), CFS considers *communities* of households and individuals to be the unit of analysis, that is, whether the community in question, as a whole, is able to access adequate nutrition at all times. Yet, even the term **community** evokes highly differentiated interpretations that vary according to geographic characteristics (sizes, locations), local **political economy** (how local political activities shape food-related economic activities), demographic characteristics of those who define local food security, and purpose (Hamm & Bellows, 2003). For example, in a 2004 publication that summarized the methods and results of nine community food assessments, the communities in question ranged from a single neighborhood, select zip codes within a city, entire cities, a collection of counties, and a state. The population sizes in these communities ranged from 24,000 to 4.7 million (Pothukuchi, 2004). Without a clear definition of community, it is difficult to determine whether a CFS project has improved food security. Whether or not there is a standard definition among practitioners and academics, each CFS project needs to specify what unit or measurement it intends to use. Differing definitions can inform one another with comparisons at the appropriate scale. CFS as a goal may also be relative rather than absolute. Accordingly, the CFS status of a community may be best described on a relative severity scale similar to the USDA household food security scale (described in chapter 5) rather than in binary terms such as whether or not CFS is achieved.

community
The unit of analysis in community food security; as defined by stakeholders, may refer to a neighborhood, town, county, or even a region

political economy
Generally refers to study of social relations, particularly the power relations that mutually constitute the production, distribution, and consumption of resources; in the context of CFS, refers to how political and policy processes shape the way food is produced, distributed, and consumed

community food assessment (CFA)
The main tool and process used to measure a local food system

A **community food assessment (CFA)** is the main tool used to measure a local food system. CFAs profile a given community's food needs and the local resources available to meet them (Pothukuchi, 2004). CFAs can also evaluate the performance of other food system sectors that contribute to community food security—for example, transportation, land use, and infrastructure. CFAs provide baseline measures of the food security status of a community so that community leaders and agencies can devise appropriate strategies to improve status and can measure progress. The process behind CFAs can also encourage collaborations across sectors and connect CFS stakeholders in different parts of the local food system. Figure 6.4 shows how CFAs contribute to change efforts.

FIGURE 6.4   The Role of CFAs in the Design of Strategies for Change

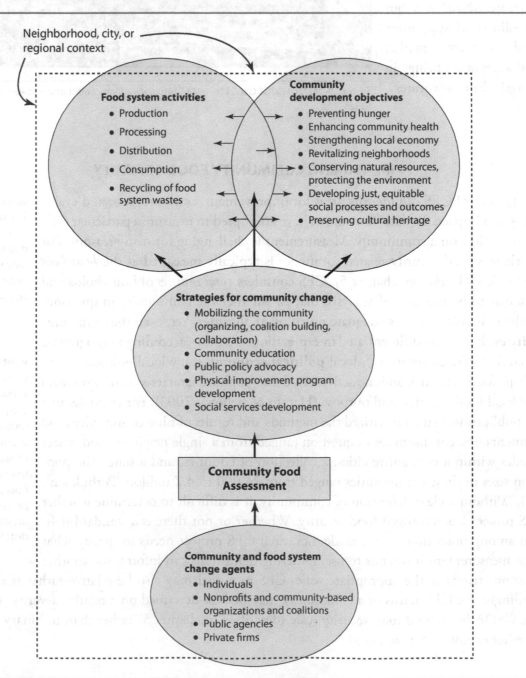

Source: Pothukuchi (2004).

There are two general approaches to conducting CFAs. Stakeholders can collect and analyze original data on the community food system or they can aggregate and analyze secondary data collected for other purposes (Cohen, Andrews, & Kantor, 2002). It is common to combine both approaches. A wide array of indicators may be included, ranging from local community demographic and socioeconomic indicators to the number and types of community food resources. The USDA *Food Environment Atlas* includes more than 130 county-level indicators relevant to a community's food security status (USDA Environmental Research Service, 2010).

Beyond basic CFAs, comprehensive CFAs may also be performed, requiring collection of community-specific original data. These are resource-intensive endeavors requiring strong quantitative and sometimes qualitative research expertise. The secondary (preexisting) data approach is more cost-effective, but there may be inadequate available data to reflect community realities. For example, the USDA annually publishes survey data about food security, but the information is available at only the national and state levels. Reflecting the challenges, to date, only two teams of researchers have published purely quantitative CFAs in peer-reviewed journals (Bletzacker, Holbem, & Holcomb, 2009; Lopez, Drake, Martin, & Tchumtchoua, 2008). These studies used relative measures to describe CFS, ranking communities' food security statuses in each element of CFS.

Another type of comprehensive CFA assessment is practice-based and builds on existing community knowledge. For example, in 2007, the Food Security Partners of Middle Tennessee (FSP) initiated a new, comprehensive community food assessment process that would be cost-effective and engage a wide spectrum of stakeholders. The stakeholders felt strongly that the challenge in Tennessee was not a shortage of knowledge about the food system. Instead, they realized that the researchers, agency staff, advocates, and residents lacked a mechanism and process to communicate and share their knowledge. The staff and collaborators of FSP created a figure (see figure 6.5) to illustrate the dynamic CFA model they developed. This model recognized the expertise of the community, made public the research that had already been conducted on the local food system, and could help meet FSP's other strategic goals (Johnson et al., 2011). Further, the model creators understood that local social, political, and economic contexts greatly influence CFS work.

FIGURE 6.5   Dynamic Community Food Assessment Process

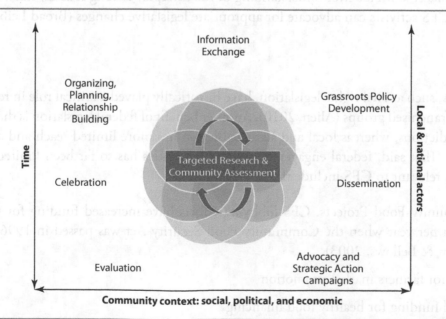

Source: Johnson, Freedman, Joosten, and Duke (2011).

In 2008, the group held a food security summit for the greater Nashville community. The event provided an opportunity for exchanging information and developing a grassroots policy and program platform. FSP staff also used the event to gather data from the more than three hundred participants; the data were then synthesized into an actionable agenda to guide change. The information gathered before and during the event resulted in thirty-three local policy and program recommendations.[1] The group convened another summit three years later to celebrate the accomplishments (ranging from engaging public health officials in policy efforts to planting school gardens) and reassess ongoing food security assessment needs in the community. The sequence of the two summits highlights CFA as a process that needs time to unfold. To the creators of this particular CFA model, the summits and the CFA process serve as means to mobilize action and reflection by advocates and residents.

In addition to, and building on, measurement of a community's food security, there is a need to evaluate specific CFS activities. The CFSC has examined the collective effects of the previously described federally funded CFP program. Evaluations of these projects use simple outcome and indicator measurements of food security, such as number of jobs created and pounds of food handled. They also use a participant survey to report changes in knowledge, attitudes, and behaviors of program participants. The combined measures are intended to indicate changes toward a more food-secure community. Outside of the CFP, unfortunately to date, the great majority of CFS activities have been executed with little or no evaluation, sometimes because of a lack of resources and sometimes because of a lack of expertise or interest. This represents a substantial missed opportunity for programs to learn about how to improve their work and contribute to generalizable knowledge.

CFS POLICIES AT MULTIPLE LEVELS

According to Anderson and Cook (1999, p. 145), beliefs "held by CFS advocates are based largely in a progressive political philosophy stressing egalitarianism and democratic governance." This philosophy drives the values within the movement toward greater inclusion, particularly of citizens who are not typically included in the political process. It also drives the types of policies that are proposed. Policy is important because it can help or hinder the social, political, and financial environment in which CFS activities take place. With a better understanding of the interplay among federal, state, and municipal governments, CFS activists can advocate for appropriate legislative changes (Broad Leib, 2012).

Federal

Federal policies, such as civil rights legislation, have historically played a critical role in representing the rights of disenfranchised groups (Allen, 2010). Another benefit of federal legislation is that it potentially affects all jurisdictions, whereas local and state legislation has more limited reach and scope (Born & Purcell, 2006). That said, federal engagement in CFS priorities has so far been limited. Examples of federal policies relevant to CFS include the following:

- Community Food Projects. CFS lobbying efforts have increased funding for CFPs from $1 million per year when the Community Food Security Act was passed in 1996 to $5 million (Hamm & Bellows, 2003).

- Funds for farmers market promotion

- Federal funding for healthy food financing

- Support for a USDA research project on food deserts
- USDA's "Know Your Farmer, Know Your Food" initiative

Total funds for these programs represent a small portion of overall federal funds for food and agriculture.

State and Local Food Policy

Knowing a state's laws is helpful in understanding municipal laws. Technically, municipalities only have powers given to them by the state, and state laws preempt most municipal laws (focus 8.3) (Broad Leib, 2012). But in practice, the situation is much more nuanced. For example, local jurisdictions regularly challenge preemption; even when unsuccessful, these challenges draw desired attention to issues important to them.

Following are examples of state policies relevant to community food security:

- Pennsylvania enacted the Fresh Food Financing initiative that provided financing to supermarkets to locate in underserved areas. The program resulted in eighty-eight fresh food retail projects in thirty-four Pennsylvania counties, more than five thousand jobs, and improved access to healthy food for an estimated five hundred thousand people (Broad Leib, 2012).

- Mississippi passed the Healthy Student Act that creates strict guidelines for vending, school stores, snack bars, and fund-raisers.

- New York passed laws encouraging all government agencies to give procurement preference to New York products (Broad Leib, 2012).

Local food policy typically includes regulatory changes, land use, and zoning changes; removing barriers for local food producers; and comprehensive planning efforts that incorporate sustainability metrics. Relationships developed at the local level provide a human-scale interaction that can encourage accountability and enhance opportunities for transformational change (Allen, 2010).

Following are examples of local food policies:

- Seattle's comprehensive plan requires at least one community garden for every 2,500 households in an urban village or neighborhood.

- The San Luis Local Food Coalition successfully advocated for the Colorado Cottage Foods Act, which allows locally produced home goods to be sold to consumers.

- The Baltimore Food Policy Initiative updated the zoning code to support urban agriculture by removing the permit requirement for hoop houses and for community gardens (see figure 6.6), permitting farm

FIGURE 6.6   Rose Street Garden, Baltimore

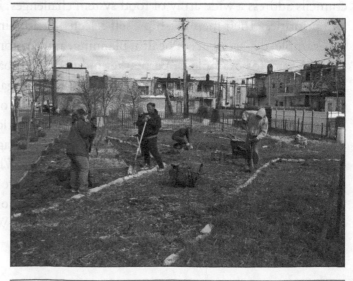

Source: Brent Kim, CLF

stands in community-managed open space, and allowing urban agriculture with a conditional-use permit (use is allowed with certain conditions applied by the zoning authorities) and management plan.

HOW DOES CFS CHANGE HAPPEN?

Changes in a community's food security tend to occur when a critical mass of community food system stakeholders appreciate the concept of a food system and begin to recognize their roles in that system. CFS programs and policies and partnerships among food system stakeholders are all indicators of change (Winne, 2008). Participation is a key attribute of CFS activities. Ideally, community members are brought together to create physical and social spaces where they can actually engage with the food system and their fellow residents, and test out different possibilities for change (Feenstra, 2002). Parents and school administrators can work together to improve school food, city planning departments can zone areas for urban agriculture, and neighborhoods can transform vacant lots into gardens. Additional indicators of improved community food security are thoughtfully managing community-based emergency food programs by providing nutritious food, focusing on empowerment approaches such as job training, and organizing action to improve food access. Community participation grounds CFS efforts in a practical context that enables place-based programs and policy solutions and provides residents an opportunity to give input (McCullum, Desjardins, Kraak, Ladipo, & Costello, 2005). Participation can, however, present its own equity challenges, because stakeholder groups tend to attract people with time, money, and access to resources; low-income citizens may have less capacity to get involved.

Stakeholder groups such as food policy councils are often indicators that change is afoot at the local level, and they are also often the most important bodies that bring about changes (Feenstra, 1997; McCullum et al., 2005; Winne, 2008). Food policy councils, which often go by other names such as food system councils, food councils, or food and agriculture networks, are designed to accomplish two basic goals: coordinate the work of food system stakeholders within a specific jurisdiction or region and influence the food and farm-related policies of one or more specific units of government (Burgan & Winne, 2012). Additionally, they contribute to a shared vision of a food-secure community and form the foundation to engage with local and state public policy makers in city councils, county commissions, and state legislatures. As an extension of the community food security concept, food policy councils address a wide array of food system challenges, issues, and opportunities based on local needs and priorities. Their memberships, self-selected or appointed, are usually drawn from the public sector, for example, departments of health, planning, and economic development; and the profit and nonprofit food sectors, for example, supermarket industry, food bank, and community gardening organizations (Scherb, Palmer, Frattaroli, & Pollack, 2012). The organizations can be formally created by government as in a local ordinance or resolution, state statute, or executive order, or they can be independent. Although there are pros and cons of different organizational models (Schiff, 2008), a key indicator of a food policy council's effectiveness is its ability to engage closely with government officials, administratively and legislatively (Burgan & Winne, 2012). When food and farming and their relationships to health, economic development, and quality of life are placed firmly on the public agenda, improvements in community food security should be evident; or, at the very least, the community builds the capacity to work productively for food system change (Winne, 2003).

Local and state-level food advocates had been seeking support for their work from their respective governments since at least the 1970s; however, these early efforts tended to be piecemeal, short-term, and narrowly focused. The first US city food policy council formed in Knoxville, Tennessee, in 1981, and it became the model for all future endeavors. The idea, however, grew from there in fits and starts. Several new councils were formed throughout the 1980s, but many ceased operation after a few years because of lack of adequate funding and, to a lesser degree, lack of acceptance by private and public food system stakeholders. Starting with the formation of the City of Toronto Food Policy Council in 1992 and City of Hartford (Connecticut) Advisory Commission on Food Policy in 1993, a second wave of food policy councils emerged, a wave that now sustains 270 food policy councils across North America (Center for a Livable Future, 2014) (See focus 6.2 for a brief case study of one in Iowa.)

FOCUS 6.2. CASE STUDY: IOWA FOOD SYSTEMS COUNCIL, A SECOND-GENERATION FOOD POLICY COUNCIL

Angie Tagtow

The Iowa Food Policy Council (IFPC) was established in March 2000 by Iowa governor Vilsack through Executive Order 16 and was administered by Drake University Agricultural Law Center. The IFPC consisted of twenty-one citizen members, appointed by the governor and representing diverse food-related sectors. When the governor changed, the executive order was not reissued and the IFPC dissolved.

Former IFPC members and interested stakeholders acknowledged the need to reestablish a state-level food policy council. From 2008 to 2010, more than 165 stakeholders across Iowa engaged in strategic planning and assessment activities in an effort to reestablish a state food policy council. Initiatives included identifying a governance structure and conducting a comprehensive assessment of Iowa's food, farming, and health landscape.

On a thorough evaluation of state food policy council governance structures, stakeholders decided that a member-based 501(c)(3) nonprofit organization would provide the greatest opportunities for supporting the mission and vision. This next generation state food policy council in Iowa became the Iowa Food Systems Council (IFSC).

The IFSC is governed by an eighteen-member board of directors who represent diverse food system sectors and domains. State government agency representatives serve in an ex officio, nonvoting capacity. The IFSC has work groups that include Food Access & Health, Environment, Economic, Fair Food and Farming, and Education/Outreach. Workgroups are guided by the recommendations in the report, *Cultivating Resilience: A Food System Framework that Advances the Health of Iowans, Farms and Communities* (Tagtow & Roberts, 2011).

Food policy councils have become a popular way to put the partnership and policy aspects of community food security into practice. As the number of community-based food system players grew through the 1990s and 2000s at the local and state levels, so did the need for coordination and more intentional forms of food system planning. At the same time, individual food security activists and organizations recognized the need for more direct engagement with local and state governments in order to press their expanding agendas. Up until this point, most broad food policy work in the United States had been directed at the national government and was almost exclusively focused on federal programs, for example, SNAP, WIC, and farm production and conservation programs.

CFS AND PUBLIC HEALTH

There are many reasons for public health professionals to be concerned about CFS. In the following, we describe these and provide examples of public health professionals' contributions to CFS work. Food insecurity and the resultant unhealthy diets are highly correlated with chronic diseases such as type 2 diabetes and obesity, two major public health concerns. The examples provided throughout this chapter show that CFS work has the potential to mitigate the rise of noncommunicable chronic diseases.

Public health professionals have long recognized that community-level food security and nutritional status have important implications for their work, and CFS projects often include public health goals. As far back as 1973, in a special supplement to the *American Journal of Public Health,* George Christakis, then president of the American Public Health Association, urged public health professionals to assess nutritional status at the community level. Such assessments, he said, "paint a picture of the health of the community, its ecology and the factors influencing the way its people live" (Christakis, 1973, p. 1).

Public health professionals are concerned with population-based health and quality-of-life measures that often occur as the result of disparities. Disparities in the food system, including food production and access, have been described as reflections of systemic social disparities, which are correlated with numerous public health challenges (see chapter 4). The cycle of systemic social and health disparities perpetuates itself: research has established negative associations between food insecurity and health in social, psychological, physical, and behavioral outcomes (see chapter 5). CFS projects, such as those that focus on community and economic development, go beyond addressing food access disparities; many of these initiatives aim to reduce the degree of social inequality, thus holding the potential to improve public health outcomes at a more fundamental level. For instance, focus 17.3 describes how urban gardens in Denver not only provide access to healthy food but also motivate participants to eat healthfully and involve them in the process of food security and food system transformation. Meanwhile, some public health departments in North America include food security, hunger, and food systems planning in their work. The Toronto Department of Public Health has recognized food insecurity and hunger as public health challenges since the 1980s by creating programs that focus on health promotion and hunger alleviation, as described in perspective 4.5. The San Francisco Department of Public Health's (SFDPH) work on improving access illustrates ways in which public health agencies can leverage their positions to improve coordination between federal policies and local actions. Since 2002, SFDPH has led the city's urban food policy and planning initiatives, including providing structural interventions to advance and integrate health, equity, and resource conservation priorities (Jones & Bhatia, 2011).

CHALLENGES FOR THE CFS FIELD

As this chapter shows, the CFS field has been successful at changing the conversation in many locales, at bringing together diverse stakeholders, and at implementing policies to improve community food security. There are also well-recognized challenges. The CFS field has tried to encompass multiple orientations to food system change, including sustainable agriculture, food system planning, community development, antipoverty, antihunger, economic development, and others. Each of these movements has distinct beliefs about what would improve, reform, or transform the food system, which has created additional challenges in building a comprehensive and coordinated approach to CFS. Grappling with these various beliefs and challenges will help advance the movement.

Community food systems, similar to local food systems (Anderson & Cook, 1999; Delind, 2011), are often assumed to have desirable attributes (i.e., healthy, sustainable, just) simply because they are not perceived to be part of the industrial food system. It is important to understand, however, that there is nothing inherently just or sustainable or healthy about scale. In fact, the concept of "scale," whether local or national, is socially constructed: the boundaries are not objectively defined but delineated by those in charge (Allen, 2010; Born & Purcell, 2006). In this way, as described in perspective 4.2, any scale of food system activities can replicate the same social problems found in global industrial food systems. Local food politics and programs can exacerbate the racial and economic inequities within a community; under such tensions, even thoughtful programs do not necessarily translate to greater community food security.

Another challenge is that communities can be global, national, statewide, or local, and each connotes a different set of assumptions, so CFS projects are not consistent in scale (Born & Purcell, 2006). A related challenge is the lack of a shared theoretical framework (Anderson & Cook, 1999). Theory is rarely considered when groups are working together on specific projects, but it assumes great importance when making the connection between CFS and related concepts understandable, and in deciding how to measure progress toward community food security goals. In addition to helping build new CFS interventions, good theory may also improve evaluations of the effectiveness of existing community food security efforts.

There is a need for solid evidence regarding the impact of CFS approaches. And, as mentioned previously, most CFS projects lack rigorous evaluation and evidence of long-term impact because of a lack of human and financial resources. As a possible remedy, Born and Purcell (2006) suggest an analysis of the desired outcome before determining what strategy and at what scale will enable one to achieve that outcome. Certain indicators and outcomes may be better suited to measuring CFS, which would help practitioners select the right tools to assess progress (Anderson & Cook, 1999). An evaluative feedback loop also offers CFS leaders and participants' data and information to decide how to prioritize their efforts.

Two final challenges are more fundamental to the mission of CFS. First, some critics maintain that many CFS programs have failed to adequately address issues germane to changing the CFS landscape at a deeper level, such as living wage legislation, racial inequities, a lack of diversity in leadership positions, class differences, and farmworker rights (Guthman, 2008; Holt-Gimenez & Wang, 2011; Slocum, 2007). In response, some organizations have turned to a **food justice** framework, which focuses less on reforming the current food system and more on understanding and transforming the dominant structures that have shaped the aforementioned inequities (Holt-Gimenez & Wang, 2011). These organizations believe that a food justice approach represents an opportunity to acknowledge differences between food system reformers and those seeking radical transformation, while also building alliances for change (Holt-Gimenez & Wang, 2011).

food justice
Movement seeking to address ways in which racial and economic inequalities pervade food system practices and processes from production to consumption

Food justice can be understood in several different ways. First, and perhaps the broadest expression of food justice, is that it is synonymous with food security—that everyone, regardless of income, location, or race has access to healthy and affordable food. In other words, without good food there is no social or economic justice, and it is unjust for one class of society to have access to the best and healthiest food while another class sources its food from food banks, federal food assistance programs, and food deserts (Winne, 2008).

More recently, food justice has been considered in terms of who is leading the movement, an organization, or project. The language of "white privilege" and "dismantling racism" have been used to sensitize leadership, participants, and funders as well as to ensure that people of color have a "seat at the table," and more explicitly, actually lead the organizations engaged in local food system work. Two organizations that have come to embody this understanding of food justice are Growing Power based in Milwaukee, Wisconsin, and The People's Grocery based in West Oakland, California. Increasingly, funders that have supported community food security work have developed special funding categories and language that states that they give preference to applicants who are people of color or who can concretely demonstrate that people of color and other vulnerable populations actively participate in the organization.

A third and even more recent dimension of food justice revolves around food chain workers, namely, those engaged in the lower paid aspects of farming, processing, preparing, and serving food. Although poor working conditions, unfair labor practices, and low wages have been the concern of union organizers and other economic justice activists for some time, it is only in the last few years that they have been joined more explicitly to the interests of community food security advocates. Fair trade is one manifestation of the food chain worker struggle—to ensure that producers of food in developing nations receive fair compensation for their products. Living wages for restaurant workers and workers in big box retail stores such as Walmart have also become the focus of the food justice and CFS movements. At root is the growing recognition that household and community food security are highly dependent on earning sufficient income to purchase healthy food, and that just as the food system's environmental harms are problematic, so too are its harms to other humans.

Future Directions

Community food security programs have experienced significant growth since the 1990s and have attracted interest from a wide variety of disciplines. Given the uncertainty of the US economy, CFS programs are likely to see a decrease in available resources at the federal level and from private foundations. At the same time, the growth in food policy councils and other food system programs indicate that interest in the food movement continues to gain traction. Food seems to have unlimited drawing power, although shrinking resources may trigger a corresponding decline in activity.

Some advocates believe CFS can best be advanced through incremental reforms (McCullum et al., 2005) and others call for a revolution that builds a community-based food system with cooperative ownership structures (Holt-Gimenez & Wang 2011). Most recognize that there is value in each approach and that sustained change will happen only through partnerships and collective action (Valdivia, 2009). Perspective 6.1 provides an inspiring example of one city that took broad food system reform action.

Perspective 6.1. The City That Ended Hunger
Frances Moore Lappé

In writing *Diet for a Small Planet*, I learned one simple truth: hunger is not caused by a scarcity of food but a scarcity of democracy. But that realization was only the beginning, for then I had to ask, What does a democracy look like that enables citizens to have a real voice in securing life's essentials? Does it exist anywhere? Is it possible or a pipe dream? With hunger on the rise here in the United States—one in seven of us is now turning to food stamps—these questions take on new urgency.

To begin to conceive of the possibility of a culture of empowered citizens making democracy work for them, real-life stories help—not models to adopt wholesale, but examples that capture key lessons. For me, the story of Brazil's fourth largest city, Belo Horizonte, is a rich trove of such lessons. Belo, a city of 2.5 million people, once had 11 percent of its population living in absolute poverty and almost 20 percent of its children going hungry. Then in 1993, a newly elected administration declared food a right of citizenship. The officials said, in effect, If you are too poor to buy food in the market—you are no less a citizen. I am still accountable to you.

The city agency developed dozens of innovations to ensure everyone the right to food, especially by weaving together the interests of farmers and consumers. It offered local family farmers dozens of choice spots of public space on which to sell to urban consumers, essentially redistributing retailer mark-ups on produce—which often reached 100 percent—to consumers and the farmers. Farmers' profits grew, because there was no wholesaler taking a cut. And poor people got access to fresh, healthy food.

In addition to the farmer-run stands, the city makes good food available by offering entrepreneurs the opportunity to bid on the right to use well-trafficked plots of city land for "ABC" markets, from the Portuguese acronym for "food at low prices." Today there are thirty-four such markets, where the city determines a set price—about two-thirds of the market price—of about twenty healthy items, mostly from in-state farmers and chosen by store owners (see figure 6.7). Everything else they can sell at the market price.

"For ABC sellers with the best spots, there's another obligation attached to being able to use the city land," a former manager within this city agency, Adriana Aranha, explained. "Every weekend they have to drive produce-laden trucks to the poor neighborhoods outside of the city center, so everyone can get good produce."

Another product of food-as-a-right thinking is three large, airy "People's Restaurants" (*Restaurante Popular*) (see figure 6.8), plus a few smaller venues, that daily serve twelve thousand or more people using mostly locally grown food

FIGURE 6.7   ABC Bulk Produce Market
These markets stock the items that the city determines will be sold at a fixed price, about 13 cents a pound.

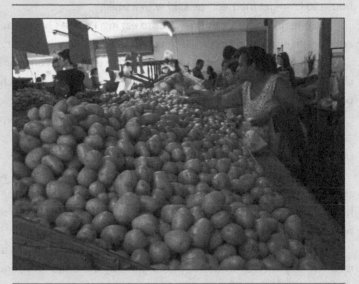

Source: Leah Rimkus.

FIGURE 6.8   The Line for One of Three "People's Restaurants" a Half Hour before Opening Time
Meals at these restaurants cost about 50 cents, and diners come from all socioeconomic groups.

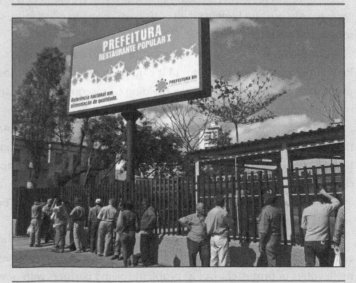

Source: Leah Rimkus.

(Continued)

(Continued)

for the equivalent of less than 50 cents a meal. When my daughter Anna and I ate in one, we saw hundreds of diners—grandparents and newborns, young couples, clusters of men, mothers with toddlers. Some were in well-worn street clothes, others in uniform, still others in business suits.

"I've been coming here every day for five years and have gained six kilos," beamed one elderly, energetic man in faded khakis.

"It's silly to pay more somewhere else for lower-quality food," an athletic-looking young man in a military police uniform told us. "I've been eating here every day for two years. It's a good way to save money to buy a house so I can get married," he said with a smile.

No one has to prove they're poor to eat in a People's Restaurant, although about 85 percent of the diners are. The mixed clientele erases stigma and allows "food with dignity," say those involved.

Belo's food security initiatives also include extensive community and school gardens as well as nutrition classes. Plus, money the federal government contributes toward school lunches, once spent on processed, corporate food, now buys whole food mostly from local growers.

"We're fighting the concept that the state is a terrible, incompetent administrator," Adriana explained. "We're showing that the state doesn't have to provide everything; it can facilitate. It can create channels for people to find solutions themselves."

For instance, the city, in partnership with a local university, is working to "keep the market honest in part simply by providing information," Adriana told us. They survey the price of forty-five basic foods and household items at dozens of supermarkets, then post the results at bus stops, online, on television and radio, and in newspapers so people know where the cheapest prices are.

The result of these and other related innovations? In just a decade Belo Horizonte cut its infant death rate—widely used as evidence of hunger—by more than half, and today these initiatives benefit almost 40 percent of the city's 2.5 million population. One six-month period in 1999 saw infant malnutrition in a sample group reduced by 50 percent. And between 1993 and 2002 Belo Horizonte was the only locality in which consumption of fruits and vegetables went up.

The cost of these efforts? Around $10 million annually, or less than 2 percent of the city budget. That's about a penny a day per Belo resident.

Behind this dramatic, life-saving change is what Adriana calls a "new social mentality"—the realization that "everyone in our city benefits if all of us have access to good food, so—like health care or education—quality food for all is a public good."

The Belo experience shows that a right to food does not necessarily mean more public handouts (although in emergencies, of course, it does.) It can mean redefining the "free" in "free market" as the freedom of all to participate. It can mean, as in Belo, building citizen-government partnerships driven by values of inclusion and mutual respect.

Before leaving Belo, Anna and I had time to reflect a bit with Adriana. We wondered whether she realized that her city may be one of the few in the world taking this approach—food as a right of membership in the human family. So I asked, "When you began, did you realize how important what you are doing was? How much difference it might make? How rare it is in the entire world?"

"I knew we had so much hunger in the world," Adriana said. "But what is so upsetting, what I didn't know when I started this, is it's so easy. It's so easy to end it."

Adriana's words have stayed with me. They will forever. They hold perhaps Belo's greatest lesson: that it is easy to end hunger if we are willing to break free of limiting frames and to see with new eyes—no longer as mere voters or protesters, but as problem-solving partners with government accountable to us.

Source: Excerpted and updated from Lappé (2009). See also Small Planet Institute, www.smallplanet.org.

In 2012 the CFS movement's flagship organization, the CFSC, closed its doors because of funding challenges. This change could signify that CFS work is under threat. Yet, the movement remains thriving albeit disjointed (Fisher, 2013). Since CFSC's founding in 1994, dozens of new organizations have formed. Many of them have distinguished themselves as leaders in their own right and many are deliberately tackling more entrenched problems such as race and class through meaningful programs and policies. Discussions about regional organizing recognize the value in the embedded levels of community and embedded levels of food systems.

There will always be a need to build coalitions of organizations that advocate for CFS in federal legislation (i.e., the Farm Bill), and it is likely that these networks will play an increasingly valuable role in keeping the work going. The CFS model, as it exists now, may prove to have inadequate convening power given the diversity of issues that have arisen over the past twenty years. Other models and paradigms may gain relevance and speak to those issues that have struggled under the CFS mantle. Two recent articles—one on the state of the movement and one addressing "wicked" problems in food policy—provide valuable insights on the state of organizing efforts to affect community food security (Fisher, 2013; Winne, 2013). Ultimately, how these different stakeholders work together for change will prove to be the biggest accomplishment of remaking and rethinking the current food system.

SUMMARY

Community Food Security (CFS) is concerned with providing a long-term guarantee of food security within a community. A diverse group of stakeholders from fields including sustainable agriculture, antihunger, public health, and community development initially gathered with the idea that the context in which people live affects their ability to meet their households' food needs. Public health advocates have championed its potential contribution to improving rates of diet-related disease. CFS practitioners vary in approach, from those working incrementally to reform current food production and distribution practices; to others, such as food justice advocates, who aim to radically transform the food system from a social justice angle. The field's historical strength has been in convening divergent organizations and types of food system stakeholders to work on shared goals. Practitioners and academics have struggled to develop standard measures of community food security. More rigorous research and evaluation of CFS efforts is needed. The findings can help direct resources to the most effective programs and enable sharing across communities.

KEY TERMS

Community	Food justice
Community food assessment (CFA)	Political economy
Community food security (CFS)	Product traceability
Food insecurity	

DISCUSSION QUESTIONS

1. How do you define community? What factors determine whether the entire community has been fully represented in working toward community food security (CFS)? What are some important characteristics of a community that could help build CFS?

2. The authors state that the "delineation between traditional antihunger and community food security work is blurry." Do you agree with this statement? If so, what causes the overlap between these two ideas to be "blurry"? What implications does this blurriness have for local governments from a policy perspective?

3. What are some difficulties that researchers might face in accurately measuring community food security? How might they overcome them?

4. What are some ways in which the difficulty of achieving CFS in a sparsely populated rural area can be addressed and overcome? How can policy makers and community members balance the present needs of the local population with their low density?

5. Who do you think has more influence over CFS policies—the national government that holds the funding or the small, nonprofit programs whose workers include citizens who are experiencing food insecurity themselves and are actively voicing their opinions? Is the synergistic effect of these programs enough to have more influence than the money holders in this equation? How should the balance of power be distributed and how can it be changed for the better?

6. Imagine your community has achieved a high level of CFS. What will have changed? What did it take to get there?

7. If you were in charge of an organization working on CFS in your community, what are some ideas you would implement to address the current CFS challenges?

NOTES

1. Conversation with former executive director of FSP, Cassi Johnson, on February 20, 2012.

REFERENCES

Allen, P. (1999). Reweaving the food security safety net: Mediating entitlement and entrepreneurship. *Agriculture and Human Values*, *16*(2), 117–129.

Allen, P. (2010). Realizing justice in local food systems. *Cambridge Journal of Regions, Economy and Society*, *3*(2), 295–308.

Anderson, M. D., & Cook, J. T. (1999). Community food security: Practice in need of theory? *Agriculture and Human Values*, *16*(2), 141–150.

Barham, J., Tropp, D., Enterline, K., Farbman, J., Fisk, J., & Kiraly, S. (2012). *Regional Food Hub resource guide*. Washington, DC: US Department of Agriculture, Agricultural Marketing Service.

Bletzacker, K. M., Holben, D. H., & Holcomb, J. P. (2009). Poverty and proximity to food assistance programs are inversely related to community food security in an Appalachian Ohio region. *Journal of Hunger & Environmental Nutrition*, *4*(2), 172–184.

Born, B., & Purcell, M. (2006). Avoiding the local trap: scale and food systems in planning research. *Journal of Planning Education and Research*, *26*(195), 195–201.

Broad Leib, E. (2012). *Good laws, good food: Putting local food policy to work for our communities*. Harvard Law School Food Law and Policy Clinic. Retrieved from www.law.harvard.edu/academics/clinical/lsc/documents/FINAL_LOCAL_TOOLKIT2.pdf

Burgan, M., & Winne, M. (2012) *Doing food policy councils right: A guide to development and action*. Retrieved from www.markwinne.com/wp-content/uploads/2012/09/FPC-manual.pdf

Cantrell, P. (2010). *Sysco's journey from supply chain to value chain: 2008–2009 final report*. Arlington, VA: Wallace Center at Winrock International.

Center for a Livable Future. (2014). *Food policy council directory*. Retrieved from www.jhsph.edu/research/centers-and-institutes/johns-hopkins-center-for-a-livable-future/projects/FPN/directory/index.html

Christakis, G. (1973). *Nutritional assessment in health programs*. Washington, DC: American Public Health Association.

Clancy, K. L. (1993). Sustainable agriculture and domestic hunger: Rethinking a link between production and consumption. In P. Allen (Ed.), *Food for the future: Conditions and contradictions of sustainability* (pp. 251–318). New Jersey: John Wiley & Sons.

Cohen, B., Andrews, M., & Kantor, L. (2002). *Community food security assessment toolkit*. Retrieved from www.ers.usda.gov/publications/efan02013/efan02013.pdf

Community Food Security Coalition. (nd). *What is community food security?* Retrieved from www.foodsecurity.org/views_cfs_faq.html

Community Food Security Coalition. (2011). *About Community Food Security Coalition*. Retrieved from http://foodsecurity.org/aboutcfsc.html

DeLind, L. B. (2011). Are local food and the local food movement taking us where we want to go? Or are we hitching our wagons to the wrong stars? *Agriculture and Human Values*, *28*(2), 273–283.

Feeding America. (2014). *Overview of our mission and impact*. Retrieved from http://feedingamerica.org/how-we-fight-hunger/about-us/mission-and-values.aspx

Feenstra, G. W. (1997). Local food systems and sustainable communities. *American Journal of Alternative Agriculture*, *12*(1), 28–36.

Feenstra, G. W. (2002). Creating space for sustainable food systems: Lessons from the field. *Agriculture and Human Values*, *19*, 99–106.

Fischer, M., Hamm, M., Pirog, R., Fisk, J., Farbman, J., & Kiraly, S. (2013, September). *Findings of the 2013 National Food Hub Survey*. Michigan State University Center for Regional Food Systems & The Wallace Center at Winrock International. Retrieved from http://ngfn.org/resources/ngfn-cluster-calls/state-of-the-food-hub-national-survey-results

Fisher, A. (2013). *Who is minding the movement?* Civil Eats. Retrieved from http://civileats.com/2013/03/14/whos-minding-the-movement

Gottlieb, R., & Fisher, A. (1996). Community food security and environmental justice: Searching for a common discourse. *Agriculture and Human Values*, *13*(3), 23–32.

Guthman, J. (2008). Bringing good food to others: Investigating the subjects of alternative food practice. *Cultural Geographies*, *4*, 431–447.

Hamm, M. W., & Bellows, A. C. (2003). Community food security and nutrition educators. *Journal of Nutrition Education and Behavior*, *35*(1), 37–43.

Holt-Giménez, E., & Wang, Y. (2011). Reform or transformation? The pivotal role of food justice in the US food movement. *Race/Ethnicity: Multidisciplinary Global Contexts*, *5*(1), 83–102. Retrieved from www.jstor.org/stable/10.2979/racethmulglocon.5.1.83

Johnson, C., Freedman, D., Joosten, Y., & Duke, M. (2011). Cultivating an agenda for change: A dynamic model for community food assessments. *Journal of the College of Social Work: The University of South Carolina*, *32*(2).

Jones, P., & Bhatia, R. (2011). Supporting equitable food systems through food assistance at farmers' markets. *American Journal of Public Health*, *101*(5), 781–783.

Lappé, F. M. (2009, February 13). The city that ended hunger: A city in Brazil recruited local farmers to help do something U.S. cities have yet to do: End hunger. *Yes!* Retrieved from www.yesmagazine.org/issues/food-for-everyone/the-city-that-ended-hunger

Lopez, R. A., Drake, L. T., Martin, J., & Tchumtchoua, S. (2008). Assessing community food security across Connecticut towns. *Journal of Hunger & Environmental Nutrition*, *3*(1).

McCullum, C., Desjardins, E., Kraak, V. I., Ladipo, P., & Costello, H. (2005). Evidence-based strategies to build community food security. *Journal of the American Dietetic Association, 105*(2), 278–283.

Pothukuchi, K. (2004). Community food assessment: A first step in planning for community food security. *Journal of Planning Education and Research, 23*(4), 356–377.

Scherb, A., Palmer, A., Frattaroli, S., & Pollack, K. (2012). Exploring food system policy: A survey of food policy councils in the United States. *Journal of Agriculture, Food Systems, and Community Development, 2*(4), 3–14.

Schiff, R. (2008). The role of food policy councils in developing sustainable food systems. *Journal of Hunger & Environmental Nutrition, 3*(2–3), 206–228.

Slocum, R. (2007). Whiteness, space and alternative food practice. *Geoforum, 38*(3), 520–533.

Tagtow, A., & Roberts, S. (2011). *Cultivating resilience: A food system framework that advances the health of Iowans, farms and communities.* Retrieved from http://iowafoodsystemscouncil.org/cultivating-resilience

US Department of Agriculture. (2011). *Farm to school team, 2010 summary report.* Retrieved from www.fns.usda.gov/sites/default/files/2010_summary-report.pdf

US Department of Agriculture Environmental Research Service. (2013). *Food environment atlas.* Retrieved from www.ers.usda.gov/data-products/food-environment-atlas.aspx#.Ubnmt_k8BBk

Valdivia, Y. (2009). *Broadening discourse and centering social justice: Struggles for a more just food system in Seattle, WA.* University of Washington at Seattle. Retrieved from www.seattleglobaljustice.org/wp-content/uploads/foodjusticethesis.pdf

Winne, M. (2003). *Community food security: Promoting food security and building healthy food systems.* Retrieved from www.foodsecurity.org/PerspectivesOnCFS.pdf

Winne, M. (2008). *Closing the food gap: Resetting the table in the land of plenty.* Boston: Beacon Press.

Winne, M. (2013). *Warriors, workers, and weavers: Choreographing the food policy dance.* Mark's food policy blog. Retrieved from www.markwinne.com/warriors-workers-and-weavers-choreographing-the-food-policy-dance

Winne, M., Joseph, H., & Fisher, A. (1997). *Community food security: A guide to concept, design and implementation.* Community Food Security Coalition. Retrieved from www.foodsecurity.org/CFSguidebook1997.PDF

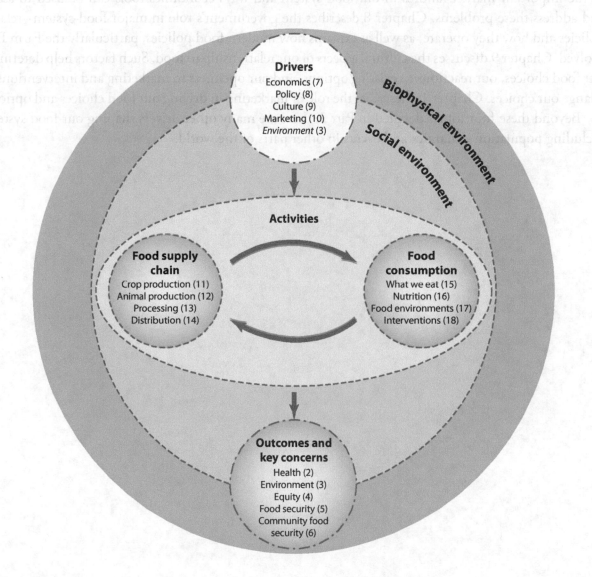

Part 2

Drivers of the Food System

Part 2 Chapters

Part 2 focuses on four of the major driving forces that shape our modern food system and its potential alternatives (economics, policy, culture, and marketing). Many of the chapters also use these concepts to discuss ways to shape change. Although the food system's biophysical environment is also a driver, given its dual role, the relevant chapter on environment is in part 1, "Outcomes," as shown in the figure.

Chapter 7 uses case study examples to illustrate key economics concepts and to describe some of the important market failures in our food system and ways economics tools can be used to assess and address these problems. Chapter 8 describes the government's role in major food-system–related policies and how they operate, as well as explains how modern food policies, particularly the Farm Bill, evolved. Chapter 9 discusses the cultural aspects of our relationship to food. Such factors help determine our food choices, our reactions to existing options, and our openness to marketing and interventions to change our choices. Chapter 10 describes the role of marketing in driving our food choices and options.

Beyond these four topics detailed in Part 2, there are many other drivers shaping our food system, including population dynamics and events in other parts of the world.

Chapter 7

Food System Economics

Rebecca Boehm, Sean B. Cash, and Larissa S. Drescher

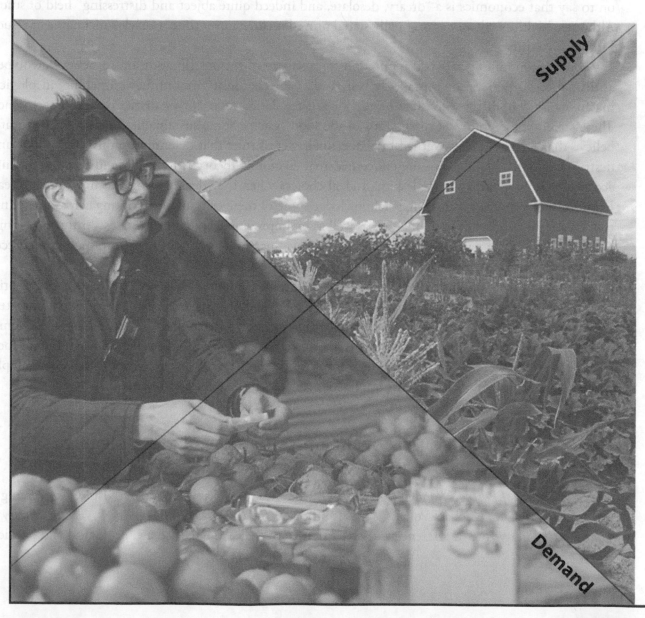

Price

Supply

Demand

Quantity

Learning Objectives

- Differentiate between the colloquial use of *economics* to refer to the financial aspects of a system or problem and the disciplinary toolbox of economics.

- Define basic concepts of microeconomic analysis, particularly the concepts of optimizing under constraints and market failures.

- Apply these concepts to important topics in food systems and public health.

- Discuss some strengths and limitations of traditional economic analysis of food systems.

In 1849 historian Thomas Carlyle gave the academic discipline of economics an unfortunate nickname: "the dismal science." He did so in evaluating Thomas Malthus's theory that the world's population would ultimately reach an upper limit because of constraints on food production. Carlyle went on to say that economics is a "dreary, desolate, and indeed quite abject and distressing" field of study. Although Malthus's theory as originally stated proved incorrect over time, Carlyle's nickname has stuck for over a century.

Today, economics gets a bad reputation for a variety of reasons (in addition to being stereotyped as dismal or boring). Some mistakenly believe that all economists are number-crunching, ideological machines for whom the "invisible hand," or self-regulating behavior of marketplaces, is sacrosanct. These stereotypes abound in discussions of the food system. Some sustainable food system advocates believe that economics is governed by a doctrinaire set of rules that defend an unjust, unhealthy, and destructive food system. Some are concerned that economic theory is too rigid and fails to take into account that people may make less-than-ideal choices when they decide what and how much to eat. Economists themselves increasingly acknowledge some of these critiques by working across disciplines to increase the validity of their analyses as well as by improving research techniques. At the same time, researchers from the natural and health sciences have increasingly sought to incorporate explicit economic components into their models of food systems.

In this chapter, we illustrate the usefulness of specific economic tools and concepts through brief examples of pressing food system challenges. Although we do not have the space to discuss completely how economics applies to food systems issues, we instead seek to introduce the concept of an economic model and then discuss instances of how economic concepts can improve our understanding of food systems and how economic tools can help improve the health and sustainability of our food supply. More detail on how these models are applied is available in the online supplement.

ECONOMICS BOILED DOWN: MODELS, OPTIMIZATION, EQUILIBRIUM, AND SOCIAL OPTIMALITY

In *The Pleasures of Eating*, Wendell Berry (1990), American novelist and food activist, wrote, "eating is an agricultural act." Michael Pollan (2009), author of *The Omnivore's Dilemma: A Natural History of Four Meals*, later wrote in reference to Berry's statement that eating is also an "ecological and political act." You can probably guess the punch line: ask any economist, and she or he will tell you that eating is also an economic act. Deciding whether to purchase food in a supermarket or at your local farmers market involves financial and time costs. How many more buttermilk biscuits to prepare from scratch in your kitchen involves decision making on the margin (i.e., consideration of the benefits and costs of one more unit of production or consumption)? How much food you can purchase in a given month is based on your preferences. But you can't spend all of your money on food (or else how would you pay your rent!) and so your monthly food spending is constrained by your income, also known as your budget constraint. Whatever the food

FIGURE 7.1 Some shoppers are willing to pay higher prices for healthy or organic food.

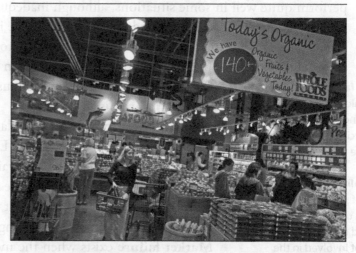

Source: A Healthier Michigan. Flickr Commons.

decision might be, people are, in economics lingo, engaging in **optimization** under constraints. The basic underlying assumption of economic thought, indeed, is that people, firms, organizations, families, and farms are all optimizing, or doing the best they can with what they have. The many optimizing individuals in the world tend to interact and reach an **equilibrium** with one another in market transactions. The moment you hand your money to the grocery store clerk is the moment at which you've reached what an economist would call an equilibrium. For this transaction to occur your willingness to pay for that food item must be at least as great as the direct cost to someone of having provided it. Optimization and equilibrium are two of the most basic principles underlying economic theory.

optimization
Doing the best one can with available resources

equilibrium
The balance achieved when many optimizing individuals interact with one another in markets

Many people mistakenly believe that economics is only about math and numbers or about shifting curves on complicated graphs. But at its core the discipline is interested in studying how optimizing individuals or firms make decisions while interacting with others and the factors that influence how they respond to changes in the environment in which they make these decisions. One can rightly object that this assumption of optimizing behavior is a fairly limited picture of human endeavor. And, indeed, most economists recognize that and intend it to be a model of human behavior rather than a complete description. Models, by design, are simplified stories of how complex systems work. If a model is too complex, the data needed to analyze it and make predictions become intractable, whereas if a model is too simple, it will fail to provide us with useful predictions. Consider a paper map, which is simply a model of spatial relationships of natural and built environments. A map with too little detail will be useless in helping you get from the train station to your cousin's house in Chicago. A map with a scale of one meter equals one meter will be extremely detailed but equally useless for navigation purposes: such a map of Chicago would fill the entire city itself when unfolded!

Economics models often use graphs or equations to provide simplified representations of behavior in the same way that a map uses red and blue lines to represent roads and rivers. As the statistician George Box noted, "All models are wrong, but some are useful" (Box & Draper, 1987, p. 74). The proper assessment of a model's quality is therefore not its accuracy at a detailed level, but rather the usefulness of its predictions for a given application or problem. And it is often the case that a simple model can perform quite well in some situations, although inadequate for other purposes. The fact that the basic economic models of consumer and human behavior are incomplete and therefore "wrong" should not, in itself, be a reason to disregard the insights they can provide. Moreover, economists have worked hard to develop more complex models that can be useful in those situations when the basic models have not been yielding accurate predictions (for example, see the behavioral economics discussion later in this chapter).

One primary implication of standard economic models is that under ideal conditions, market outcomes are efficient. Efficiency requires that no more social benefits can be achieved given the resources available for a given task. Although this may seem to be an overly broad conclusion to be able to draw from aggregate models of human behavior, it is a powerful one in that it also provides insights into the factors that prevent efficient outcomes from taking place.

Market failure exists when the most efficient market outcome is not achieved. Market failures originate from a variety of sources. One type occurs when there is an **externality** in a market, meaning that all the costs or benefits of production or consumption of a good or service are not internalized in its market price, so buyers are not paying the optimal amount from a social perspective. Another type of market failure occurs when a market is imperfectly competitive (i.e., there are not many buyers and sellers), leading to disproportionate power, which affects prices. A special case of this failure is when there is only one seller in the market for a particular good or service. This is called a *monopoly*. Market failures can also occur when there are **information asymmetries** between buyers and sellers about a particular product. For example, in some cases sellers have more information about a product than buyers do, prohibiting the buyers from making correct decisions about what the value of the product is to them. Another type of market failure is when there are behavioral constraints on individual optimization. These four sources of market failure are common in the food system and will be detailed in this chapter.

Identifying market failures in food consumption and production is an important step in identifying interventions or remedies that can improve our health, environmental quality, and overall well-being. The large and growing field of food economics is therefore largely focused on applying economic frameworks to understanding these failures and finding ways to improve on current outcomes. Some of the tools and frameworks that economists use to understand consumer behavior, food production, and market failures are discussed in the following sections using the following examples from across the food system:

- Water pollution stemming from agricultural production, which illustrates the market failure of externality, and which may be remedied through **taxes** and **subsidies** or **cap-and-trade systems**

market failure
Economic concept describing the occurrence of an inefficient market outcome

externality
A cost of providing a product or service that is imposed on people who were not involved in the transaction, including future generations; also called *external cost*; can be negative (costs imposed on others) or positive

information asymmetry
When buyers in a market have less information about goods or services than the sellers or the reverse

tax
Government policy charging a per-unit fee on the consumption or production of a good or service

subsidy
Government policy providing consumers or producers with a per-unit discount on consumption or production of a good or service

cap-and-trade systems
Systems by which a government entity sets an upper limit on total pollution in a particular industry or economy sector, and each firm in that sector is allotted pollution credits

- Market structure in the food system and whether bigger is good because it enables us to take advantage of **economies of scale** in food production or is harmful because it leads to **market concentration** and the market failure of imperfect competition across the food supply chain

- Income and price interventions designed to increase access of low-income consumers to food, steer consumers away from unhealthy foods, or encourage them to make more healthy choices

- The market failure of information asymmetry and how it can hamper good food consumption decisions

- **Behavioral economic** models of food choice that incorporate psychological factors to account for the fact that sometimes we unwittingly make decisions we later regret and how some argue that these insights may also provide new policy tools for improving health and well-being

economies of scale
The advantages occurring when quantity of production becomes large and a firm has lower total costs than at lower levels of output; can level off or be reduced after a certain size

market concentration
The extent to which market shares in an industry are owned by a small number of companies

behavioral economics
Subfield of economics that assumes consumers do not make perfectly rational decisions; incorporates theories and models from psychology and other adjacent fields

AGRICULTURE AND FOOD PRODUCTION

Economics tools and frameworks can be used to understand how and why the agricultural and food production sectors operate as they do and to pinpoint inefficiencies that negatively affect the environment and public health. In this chapter we provide examples of how economic principles play out in the agricultural and food production system. We also show how the discipline of economics can shed light on solutions to even the most challenging problems in this part of the food system.

Dealing with the Dead Zone in the Gulf of Mexico

One stubborn environmental problem associated with today's agriculture production is runoff and leaching of fertilizers into waterways; economics tools may provide some answers. As described in chapter 3, fertilizers are often applied in excess of agronomic needs. Fertilizer runoff contributes to hypoxic (dead) zones in water systems, where animals and plants die off for lack of sunlight and oxygen. In the Gulf of Mexico, hypoxia not only affects marine ecosystem health as such but also it threatens the economic viability of fisheries and marine-based recreational activities.

Sixty-five percent of the nitrogen loadings carried by the Mississippi River come from agricultural production across the midwestern and central United States (Gulf of Mexico Hypoxia Task Force, 2011). In an economic framework, we recognize this added and unaccounted for cost as a negative externality of agricultural production. In general, a negative externality is an additional cost associated with the consumption or production of goods and services, which has not been fully accounted for in the market price of the product. These additional costs are borne by third parties not directly involved in the consumption or production decisions. Ideally, producers of all types of goods, food or otherwise, internalize (i.e., pay for) most costs of production. But in many cases, not all costs of production are internalized by the producer, which results in negative externalities. As in the case of the Gulf dead zone, the cost of agricultural production to the marine environment and fisheries is not easily internalized by farmers or agribusinesses without regulation. If negative externalities are not addressed, the market outcome generally involves too much production and consumption associated with the harmful activity, in that the excess damage outweighs the social benefits of some of this consumption and production.

FIGURE 7.2 Underwood Farm Feedlot Runoff, North Dakota

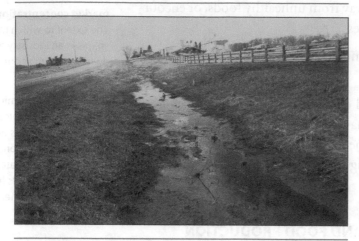

Source: Kathleen M. Rownland, 2011, USGS. Public domain. Cropped. http://gallery.usgs.gov/photos/07_14_2011_m52Tkw7JJe_07_14_2011_3# .U3JXuSgWl0o

Reducing nitrogen runoff from agricultural land is complicated. Pinpointing the location from which nitrogen contamination originated is nearly impossible because water runoff cannot be easily monitored on each farm. As a result, policy experts and researchers have struggled for decades to determine how effectively to reduce nitrogen loading in the Mississippi River Basin while ensuring high crop yields. Figure 7.2 shows how animal production contributes to the problem of nutrient runoff. Although the Environmental Protection Agency has established some laws to regulate waste produced from livestock production, runoff is still a major issue in this sector.

Economic tools provide some promising solutions. For example, the US Department of Agriculture (USDA)-led Mississippi River Basin Healthy Watershed Initiative provides subsidies to producers to implement on-farm conservation practices that reduce nitrogen runoff and leaching (USDA Natural Resources Conservation Service, 2013). In general, a subsidy is a financial incentive that redirects production or consumption of goods and services to better meet specific environmental, social, or economic goals. In this example, reducing nitrogen fertilizer runoff may increase costs for agricultural producers, so the subsidy is used to offset these added costs. One downside is that, even when they improve the social good, subsidies cost governments money, which may either be politically unpopular or difficult to sustain financially over the long term.

Other economic mechanisms have been proposed to reduce nitrogen runoff and leaching from farm fields. A tax is one possible method. When a tax is designed to achieve specific environmental, social, or economic goals that are hampered by externalities (rather than simply to raise revenue), it is sometimes referred to as a *Pigovian tax*. According to economic theory, taxes can be directed toward the level of a negative externality during goods production in order to reduce the quantity of the externality.

deadweight loss
Loss when some external force causes a market to move away from its free market equilibrium; takes form of decreased revenues, increased prices, and reduced quantity produced versus what would happen in a free market

A tax levied on nitrogen fertilizer used by agricultural producers could help reduce total nitrogen use or promote more careful application. The revenue raised from taxation could also be used to support programs that help farmers better manage nitrogen fertilizer on their farms. The primary downside to a tax is that in addition to reducing the level of harm caused by the externality, it also reduces the quantity produced of the agricultural good itself. This creates **deadweight loss** in the economy. Deadweight loss takes the form of decreased revenues for firms, increased prices for consumers, and reduced quantity of a good or service produced as compared to levels produced and consumed in a market free of taxes.

Another potential method for reducing the negative externalities associated with agricultural nonpoint source pollution is by using market-oriented trading schemes. The rationale for this mechanism was inspired by the Coase Theorem developed in 1960 by Nobel prize–winning economist, Ronald Coase. Coase theorized that if those affected by an externality could bargain with polluters over the cost incurred by the pollution, then the externality could be eliminated or reduced. If fishers had a right to a clean environment, then farmers (or agribusinesses) would have to pay the fisher, recreational businesses, and Gulf Coast residents for damages caused by hypoxia. Given that there are many farmers who may be contributing to the pollution, many anglers who may be affected, and difficulty in determining whose pollution is affecting whose catch, it might seem unlikely that such an arrangement could be achieved simply through private negotiation alone. A more widely workable alternative based on similar reasoning is a cap-and-trade system. In a cap-and-trade system, a government entity sets an upper limit on total pollution in a particular industry or economy sector, and each firm in that sector is allotted pollution credits, which may be bought and sold. Although this system does not eliminate pollution entirely and relies on government defining the interests of anglers and other affected parties, it can be effective at reducing environmental damage significantly. It also provides flexibility for producers, some of whom may have difficulty controlling nitrogen runoff whereas others may be better adapted to do so. The Environmental Protection Agency (EPA) recently introduced a Water Quality Trading program in select US watersheds; its effectiveness, and the appropriate scale for such trading schemes, remain open questions (US EPA, 2012).

Just as pollution can be modeled as a negative externality to agriculture, there can also be positive externalities in food systems. A positive externality is when parties that are not part of a transaction receive benefits not accounted for in the marketplace. The ecosystem services delivered by agriculture (discussed in chapter 3) are an example of positive externalities. Whereas negative externalities are associated with overproduction and damage, positive externalities are also a market failure in that the market outcome is inefficient—some benefits accruing to parties other than the buyers or sellers are not being taken into account, so we are not producing enough of them and thus failing to "do the best with what we've got." The subsidy approach discussed previously is one way to try to increase production of ecosystem services if unaddressed positive externalities exist.

Why Are So Many Farms So Big?

There is much discussion about the size of farms in the United States and how they are becoming larger and fewer in number. From an economic point of view, this raises the question of whether this represents a market failure or not. What does this actually mean, why is this true, and are big farms always bad farms? We use a *New York Times* article about tomato production in California to address these questions and to explain some of the structural changes seen in agriculture both in the United States and more broadly over the last several decades.

New York Times food writer Mark Bittman wrote a column in August 2013 entitled "Not All Industrial Food Is Evil." He traveled to California's Sacramento Valley to learn about large-scale tomato production (Bittman, 2013). The Sacramento Valley is one of the most productive agricultural regions in the United States. It has a **comparative advantage** in producing some crops because of ample sunshine and warm temperatures throughout the year. Comparative advantage implies that a firm has lower costs compared to other firms producing the same good or service. Although California's climate helps give tomato producers a comparative advantage, the region depends almost exclusively on irrigation as its water source. Water is becoming scarcer in California as population grows, and as a result, agricultural water usage is hotly debated. Bittman toured a large-scale tomato farm (see figure 7.3) and

comparative advantage
The climatic, labor, or geographic advantage of one area to produce a product more efficiently and at cheaper cost than another

FIGURE 7.3   Rominger Brothers Farm

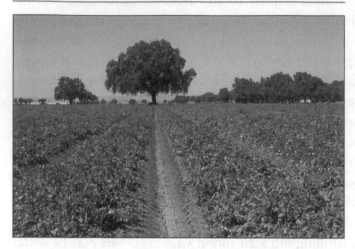

Source: Pacific Coast Producers.

fixed costs
Costs of production that do not vary depending on the number of units produced

variable costs
Costs of production that vary with number of units produced

total costs
Sum of fixed and variable costs

total average cost
Total cost divided by the number of units produced

an equally large tomato packinghouse during his visit. Bruce Rominger, the tomato farmer he met with, relied on an efficient subsurface drip irrigation system to water the plants and a thirty-five-foot-long machine for harvesting. Other inputs used in tomato production include fertilizer, seeds, fuel, and human labor; each carries a cost.

Some costs are the same no matter how many tomato units are produced. These are called **fixed costs** because they do not change with the amount of output; they are often one-time upfront costs. For Rominger, one fixed cost is the tomato-harvesting machine, which "cuts the vine underground and lifts it into its belly, where belts and sensors return dirt, vine, root and green tomatoes to the soil" on which sheep will later graze. Rominger incurred a one-time upfront cost to buy the harvester. **Variable costs**, by contrast, vary with the amount of output produced. Fertilizer is a variable cost in tomato production because the amount of fertilizer increases as the number of tomatoes produced increases. Summing the fixed and variable costs gives **total costs** that the producer must incur to produce tomatoes. As the number of units produced increases, total costs increase because variable costs increase.

Dividing total costs by the number of units produced gives the **total average cost** of production. We can also examine average fixed costs and average variable costs separately. Average fixed costs decrease as the number of units produced increases. The average fixed cost of the tomato harvester declines as the number of tomatoes harvested increases, all else being equal. However, average variable costs typically decrease at first and then increase as more and more of a good is produced. For example, when little or no fertilizer is being applied to a plot of land, a small amount may increase yields considerably, but this yield effect may decline quickly, greatly raising the cost of using fertilization as an approach to increase quantities. At some point, no additional amount of fertilizer will help production, and could well lower it. So above certain levels of production, but below an upper threshold, the total cost per unit of output can be minimized. In cases when the fixed costs are very high, or when variable costs continue to decline as production levels rise, this level of minimal cost is reached only at fairly sizable production levels, creating economies of scale. For example, only at higher levels of production will a tomato farmer be able to have employees specialize in particular aspects of production, such as when some employees harvest crops and others focus on sorting and packing. This technological innovation of sorts creates economies of scale in tomato production by reducing the cost of labor per tomato produced. Innovations at higher levels of production, such as labor specialization, have led to economies of scale across many portions of the agricultural sector.

Most commercial farms and producers of goods and services generally seek to minimize the cost of production in order to increase profits or leave resources available to pursue other goals of their operations. They may do this by achieving economies of scale or other production advantages. Purchasing a mechanical harvester, for example, may enable a farmer to beat competitors on production costs by lowering labor costs. More profit can be earned with lower labor costs, which may drive nearby farms out of business. When this happens farmers can use excess profits to purchase nearby competitors' land and use it to grow even more tomatoes. This situation illustrates one way in which farms in the United States have grown in size. (There are other factors, including a minor yet important role for government policies, such as direct payment subsidies and crop insurance, which reduce costs or risks of agricultural production. These have also favored larger producers and have made financial resources available to farms, which have been used to buy out other operations) (MacDonald, Korb, & Hoppe, 2013).

As will be discussed in chapters 11 and 14 and perspective 11.2, many farms in the United States are getting very large or small, whereas the "agriculture of the middle" is declining. As Bittman (2013) notes in his article, mechanization and the related increase in size of some farms is not necessarily a bad thing. He writes, "fifty years ago, tomatoes were picked by hand, backbreaking piecework that involved filling and lugging fifty-pound boxes. Workers had few rights and suffered much abuse, as did the land: irrigation and fertilizer were more wasteful." At Rominger's farm, according to Bittman, "workers aren't paid by the piece, they get shade, water and breaks, and the fields are managed conscientiously." This example demonstrates the benefits of large-scale production. Some consumers, however, all things being equal, might prefer supporting the livelihoods of smaller farms, even if some the benefits of this type of agriculture extend to consumers in the form of lower prices and some social and environmental benefits. In the face of such competing preferences, it is perhaps not paradoxical that we see a vibrant number of smaller farms alongside increasing concentration of farmland.

Food as Fuel for Cars: The Renewable Fuel Standard

Ethanol from corn starch is an important market for corn farmers in the United States and for other stakeholders in the US biofuel industry. Nearly 40 percent of US corn is used to produce ethanol, which is mixed into regular gasoline to fuel cars and other vehicles (USDA, 2013). The Renewable Fuel Standard (RFS), a federal law passed in 2007, requires fuels sold in the United States to contain a minimum amount of fuel from renewable sources, including ethanol and biodiesel (Schnepf & Yacobucci, 2013). RFS mandates that thirty-six billion gallons of biofuels be brought to market by 2022. In economics terms, the RFS production target is called a **quota**. A quota is used to increase production of a particular good or service to either address a market failure or pursue other social goals. The quota established in RFS (along with historical subsidies to ethanol processors and distributors) is partly responsible for the ethanol industry's growth in the United States (see figure 7.4).

quota Government policy mandating level of production for a good or service, typically above what would be produced in a free market

FIGURE 7.4 Corn Production

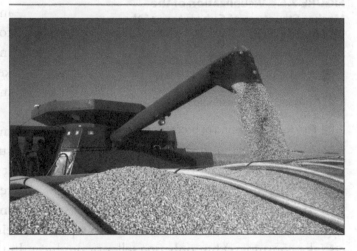

Source: South Dakota Corn.

demand expansion
A government policy that increases demand for a particular good or service

This growth has led to higher corn prices, which have been a boon to corn farmers both in the United States and globally (Ajanovic, 2011). In other words, the mandate has led to what economists call **demand expansion** for corn. Prior to development of the US ethanol industry, corn was primarily a raw ingredient in livestock feed and human foods, and these two industries primarily determined corn demand. Overall the RFS policy, aimed at demand expansion, has raised corn prices because ethanol processors can pay more than had previously been charged when corn was used other purposes.

Although ethanol reduces dependence on foreign and domestic oil and has helped corn farmers with the growth of a new agricultural subsector, its production is not without downsides. First, higher corn prices resulting from policies that promote biofuel production from food crops, such as RFS, have negatively affected populations in developing countries, many of whom are highly sensitive to changes in food prices (Rosengrant, 2008). These populations spend a larger fraction of their income on food than those in more developed countries, and so price changes have a bigger effect on their food spending and overall welfare. Additionally, in poorer countries corn is more commonly consumed directly by people, meaning that price changes for corn have a greater effect on food costs. By contrast, people in developed countries commonly consume corn and soybeans indirectly, in the form of animal products or processed foods, so changes in the price of raw commodities have a relatively smaller effect on food prices than in poor countries.

FOOD MANUFACTURING AND THE FOOD SUPPLY CHAIN

Once food leaves the farm gate it enters the hands of distributors, processors, in some cases more processors, retailers, and finally the consumer. For economic and other reasons the number of sellers at each stage along the supply chain varies dramatically. In this next section we discuss why certain sectors are highly concentrated and why the number of sellers matters to the efficiency of market outcomes.

The Shape of Things: Market Structure in the US Food System

As mentioned in the chapter introduction, a market is not efficient if it is imperfectly competitive. Across the subsectors of the US food economy there exist some markets in which there are a limited number of sellers and buyers. This is illustrated in figure 7.5. The many farms sell their goods to a small handful of marketing and processing firms, including retailers such as supermarkets. And these retailers finally sell their goods to many consumers.

Table 7.1 summarizes common types of market structure in the US food system. Market structure is important to understand because it helps to determine how governments can regulate a particular market for a good. A **monopoly** market structure, for example, can negatively affect consumer welfare, for example, well-being. A monopoly is characterized by many buyers (aka consumers) but only one seller or producer. In the food system, monopolies may exist because

FIGURE 7.5 Visualization of the Market Structure of Subsectors of the US Food System

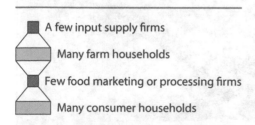

A few input supply firms

Many farm households

Few food marketing or processing firms

Many consumer households

Source: Adapted with permission of William A. Masters, Tufts University.

TABLE 7.1   Types of Market Structure in the US Food System

Market Type	Number of Sellers	Number of Buyers
Monopoly	One	Many
Duopoly	Two	Many
Oligopoly	A few	Many
Monopsony	Many	One
Duopsony	Many	Two
Oligopsony	Many	A few
Perfect competition	Many	Many

of economies of scale and technological innovations that enable one firm or a few firms to dominate a particular market. When markets approach a monopoly structure, government intervention is often needed because firms that operate like monopolies can increase their profits by lowering production to raise a good's price, which makes consumers worse off in that (1) their access to the good is lowered and (2) those who do still obtain it are paying a higher price, often much higher than would otherwise be the case.

The degree of monopoly or market concentration can be characterized by a **four-firm concentration ratio (CR4)**. A CR4 ratio can range from zero to 100. A score of 65 means that four firms control 65 percent of the market for a good. Table 7.2 illustrates CR4 scores for various manufacturing sectors in the food system. The cane sugar–refining sector is particularly concentrated compared to other sectors. Four firms control 95 percent of market shares. Meanwhile, the fruit, vegetable, and frozen food processing sector is more competitive (i.e., less concentrated). Four firms control only 22 percent of market shares in this sector.

Monopoly or oligopoly power provides an incentive for firms to lobby the government, compared to if they operated in more competitive market structures. This is because regulations have a greater

monopoly
Market characterized by one seller and many buyers

four-firm concentration ratio (CR4)
Represents level of concentration (i.e., the number of sellers) in a market for a good or service (e.g., if the CR4 score = 65 that means 65 percent of the market is controlled by only four firms)

TABLE 7.2   CR4 Scores for Food Manufacturing Industries

Manufacturing Industry	CR4
Cane sugar refining	95
Breakfast cereals	80
Butter	79
Bottled water	72
Cookies/crackers	69
Grains and oilseeds	52
Soft drinks/water	52
Poultry	46
Frozen fruits, vegetables, juice	41
Meat	38
Sugar and sweets	38
Dairy	24
Bakery	22
Fruits and vegetables and frozen foods	22

Source: Wilde (2013).

impact on their operations when there is only one firm or a few firms in the market for a particular good or service. The cane sugar industry presents an interesting example of how market concentration can lead to government lobbying, which leads to policy changes that can affect consumers. In March 2013 National Public Radio's *Planet Money* aired a story about how US sugar growers have lobbied Congress for price subsidies, import quotas, and other protections. Import quotas limit the amount of a good or service that can enter a country and are used to protect domestic producers. The policies lobbied for by sugar producers keep sugar prices twice as high as the world price, which benefits US sugar growers but hurts food manufacturers who use sugar as an input (Chace, 2013). What is interesting about this example is that one could make a case that higher sugar prices are actually better for consumers' health than lower ones because they reduce the quantity of sugar demanded. This could affect the amount of sugar and thus the total calories that people consume. High sugar prices, however, have led some food manufacturers to substitute high fructose corn syrup (HFCS) for other types of sweeteners, such as cane sugar, and encouraged technological developments that have lowered the production costs of these alternatives. In actuality, it is unlikely that higher sugar prices would have led consumers to consume less sugar anyway, because the price of sugar as a raw ingredient in food or beverage products constitutes a relatively small share of the overall price of food.

Overall, market structure has changed in the food marketing system, as described in detail in chapter 14. For consumers this shift comes with the advantage of lower food prices. This isn't because firms are exerting monopoly power, however. Instead firms exhibit monopsonistic market power in purchasing food from producers. When a firm acts as a monopsonist it can lower the price it pays to a producer and demand less than if more than one buyer existed in the market. A firm can become a monopsonist in the same way that some firms exert monopoly market power—through innovation or economies of scale in purchasing. In practice, pure monopsonies or monopolies rarely exist. In most cases, markets that are imperfectly competitive have few buyers or sellers, meaning they are oligopsonies or oligopolies, respectively.

It should be noted that although market power can play an important role in shaping prices, there are also many examples in which industries are powerful, but yet prices are in fact shaped by other, often complex, forces. Focus 7.1 describes reasons why grocery store prices may not reflect what you hear on the news about farm prices.

FOCUS 7.1. PRICE TRANSMISSION IN THE DISTRIBUTION SYSTEM: RETAIL RESPONSES TO SUPPLY PRICE CHANGES

Edward W. McLaughlin

After noting the modest and often highly volatile prices at the production stages of the distribution channel, some observers have been critical of retail level prices that do not appear to move in concert with changes in supply prices. For example, although the farm gate prices for most vegetables vary considerably during the calendar year because of seasonality, the retail prices generally exhibit modest, infrequent variation. Although the observation is correct, the reasons are complex. There exist at least six explanations for the phenomenon, each of which provides partial illumination.

First, retailers do not set their prices based on production price; they rely more on local competition, the prices of other retailers. Second, as reported annually by the USDA, about three-quarters of all consumer food spending goes to cover marketing costs—packaging, transportation, risk taking, storage, handling, promotion, and profit—and only about one-quarter returns to the farmer (USDA, 2013). For some foods, such as fresh fruits and vegetables, the percent returning to the grower is even less. Thus, supply price can change considerably but has little impact at the retail shelf because production costs are such a small fraction of the total system costs. Third, nearly all foodstuffs are characterized by an "inelastic price elasticity of demand," that is, sales are not very sensitive to price changes. Specifically, if prices of individual food items are lowered (or raised), consumers are not likely to radically change their purchase behavior. This theory is well substantiated in empirical research. Thus, attempting, say, to legislate lower prices for food or to establish certain limited ranges for retail price movement as is done in many states for products such as milk (e.g., Massachusetts and New York) (Bolotova & Novakovic, 2011), to induce consumers to buy more may not have the intended effect, at least not at the magnitude that would otherwise be expected. Fourth, sometimes retailers do not change prices consistent with supply price changes, because a conventional retail assumption is that consumers do not like price changes, except for retail price promotions (sales). This may or may not be strictly true, but nevertheless, it drives some retail price decisions.

Fifth, in order for price changes—particularly price reductions—to be effective, consumers must perceive them and respond. As supermarkets have grown in size, this has become much more difficult. In the 1960s, the average supermarket carried fewer than five thousand different products. By 2012, the average supermarket carried more than forty-two thousand products (Food Marketing Institute, 2014); it is challenging for one simple price change to break through the advertising clutter to get noticed by shoppers. What's more, even if the new, lower price is perceived, will the consumer respond? That is, will the price change be of sufficient magnitude to induce a behavior change?

Finally, the retailer's objective is not necessarily to maximize sales and profits of each department separately, but of the entire store. Because there are many opportunities for shopping substitution between departments (e.g., processed deli meat for fresh meat or frozen vegetables for fresh vegetables), the retailer attempts to establish pricing and merchandising policies that will make the entire store profitable, not each individual product or even department. Moreover, the dilemma faced by all multiproduct firms, such as supermarkets, is that there is no specific economic theory that guides the spreading of overhead costs that are shared by all departments. This economic reality makes it difficult to follow individual product prices and their markups through the distribution system.

Source: Based on McLaughlin (2004).

FOOD CONSUMPTION

Our health is greatly affected by the quality and amount of food we eat, which in turn is influenced by the prices of various foods on offer. Understanding the economics of food purchase decisions enables us to consider whether and how economic tools might be able to help address concerns such as obesity and malnutrition.

Taxing the Junk out of Junk Foods

Earlier in this chapter we illustrated how taxes can be used to address environmental externalities caused by agricultural production. Taxes could similarly be used to eliminate or reduce negative externalities associated with consuming unhealthy food products, such as the health care costs associated with

law of demand
Refers to the marketing concept that when the price of a (normal) good rises, the quantity demanded will decline

treating diet-related diseases. To reduce consumption of unhealthy foods we rely on the **law of demand** which states that as the price of a good rises the quantity consumed falls, all else being equal. This means that as a tax on a food product would increase its price, it would reduce demand.

A growing body of research examines the effectiveness of taxes to curb consumption of energy-dense and high-sugar food items to reduce rates of obesity and overweight. One food category in the crosshairs of this research is sugar-sweetened beverages (SSBs). SSBs include sodas and other beverages that contain added sugars. It is hypothesized that SSB consumption has played a major role in the obesity epidemic in the United States (Fletcher, Frisvold, & Tefft 2010). Perspectives 5.2 and 5.3 presented views on the desirability of restricting food choices in the SNAP program, essentially making some foods more costly to participants. Another frequently discussed strategy for changing the relative prices of less healthy foods is cutting farm subsidies. Focus 7.2, at the end of this section, shares evidence suggesting this change may not be effective. Here we look at taxation—another way to make selected foods more costly—with an economist's lens.

Economic analysis can provide some evidence for or against the effectiveness of a tax by examining the price elasticity of demand of foods and beverages. The price elasticity of demand measures how the quantity demanded of a particular good, expressed as a percent, changes with respect to a 1 percent change in the price of a good. The **own-price elasticity of demand** of a product is a measure of how a price change for a good affects the quantity demanded of that good itself, whereas the cross-price elasticity of demand provides an estimate of how consumer demand for a good will change when the price of *another* good changes. For example, the cross-price elasticity of milk with respect to coffee would provide information about the change in milk demanded if the price of coffee changed, all else being equal. Positive cross-price elasticities of demand are associated with **substitute goods** (e.g., margarine and butter), whereas negative cross-price elasticities indicate that the two goods in question are **complementary goods** (e.g., bread and butter). The following equation can be used to calculate the own-price elasticity of demand for a good (η):

own-price elasticity of demand
A measure of consumer responsiveness to price changes for a particular good

substitute goods
Goods whose demand increases when the price of another good increases, all else being equal

complementary goods
A good, *a*, whose demand decreases when the price of a good, *b*, decreases, all else being equal

$$\eta = \frac{\% \ change \ in \ quantity \ demanded}{\% \ change \ in \ price} = \frac{\Delta Q / Q}{\Delta p / p}$$

where ΔQ *and* Δp represent the observed change in quantity demanded and price, respectively, and Q and p represent the original quantity and price. In table 7.3, own-price elasticity estimates are presented for a number of food and beverage categories, including SSBs (see figure 7.6). For simplicity, own-price elasticities are often reported in absolute value (i.e., a 1 percent drop in the quantity demanded is reported as 1, rather than −1). The reported own-price elasticity of demand for SSBs is 0.79. This implies that when the price of soft drinks increases by 1 percent the quantity demanded falls by 0.79 percent.

The magnitude of a product's own-price elasticity has important implications for determining whether or not a tax will alter consumer demand. Economists classify products into categories based on the value of their own-price elasticity of demand, which helps determine the relative effectiveness of a tax. If a good's elasticity is between zero and one in absolute value, demand for that good is said to be **inelastic**, which means that price changes have a relatively small effect on the quantity consumed. If the elasticity is equal to one

inelastic
Consumers being relatively unresponsive to price changes

TABLE 7.3 Estimates of Price Elasticities for Major Food and Beverage Categories

Food and Beverage Category*	Absolute Value of Mean Price Elasticity Estimate (95% CI)	Range	No. of Estimates
Food away from home	0.81 (0.56, 1.07)	0.23-1.76	13
Soft drinks	0.79 (0.33, 1.24)	0.13-3.18	14
Juice	0.76 (0.55, 0.98)	0.33-1.77	14
Beef	0.75 (0.67, 0.83)	0.29-1.42	51
Pork	0.72 (0.66, 0.78)	0.17-1.23	49
Fruit	0.70 (0.41, 0.98)	0.16-3.02	20
Poultry	0.68 (0.44, 0.92)	0.16-2.72	23
Dairy	0.65 (0.46, 0.84)	0.19-1.16	13
Cereals	0.60 (0.43, 0.77)	0.07-1.67	24
Milk	0.59 (0.40, 0.79)	0.02-1.68	26
Vegetables	0.58 (0.44, 0.71)	0.21-1.11	20
Fish	0.50 (0.30, 0.69)	0.05-1.41	18
Fats/oils	0.48 (0.29, 0.66)	0.14-1.00	13
Cheese	0.44 (0.25, 0.63)	0.01-1.95	20
Sweets and sugars	0.34 (0.14, 0.53)	0.05-1.00	13
Eggs	0.27 (0.08, 0.45)	0.06-1.28	14

Note: Values were calculated based on the 160 studies reviewed. Absolute values of elasticity estimates are reported. The price elasticity of demand measures the percentage change in purchased quantity or demand with a 1% change in price.
*Including restaurant meals and fast food.
Source: Andreyeva, Long, and Brownell (2010).

in absolute value, then the good is **unit elastic**, meaning that the quantity demanded responds proportionally to a price change. If the price elasticity is greater than one in absolute value, the good is said to exhibit **elastic** demand. When the price of an elastic good changes there is a relatively large effect on the quantity consumed. The reported elasticity of SSBs, 0.79, means they are an inelastic good. To reduce the quantity demanded of SSBs would require a relatively large tax because consumers are not very sensitive to price changes. If policy makers want to reduce consumption by a specific amount the elasticity estimate can be used to determine what price increase would be required to lower demand by a target amount.

The debate over whether a tax on SSBs will lead to health improvements is a hot topic in the fields of nutrition and applied economics. Economists believe that a tax may reduce consumption of SSBs; however, consumers may consume substitute goods that are just as dense in calories (Johnson, 2011). Others estimate that a 1 cent per ounce national tax on SSBs would cut calorie consumption by 8 to 10 percent and

FIGURE 7.6 Sugar-Sweetened Beverages

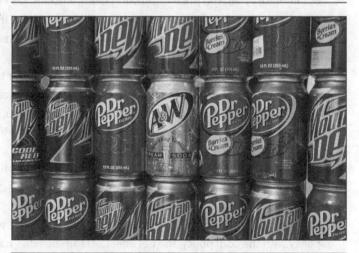

unit elastic
Consumer demand responds proportionally to price changes

elasticity
Consumers being relatively responsive to price changes

raise $15 billion per year in government revenue (Runge, Johnson, & Runge, 2011). Recent research estimates that a tax on SSBs would reduce the body mass index for a broad range of Americans, but that the magnitude of the effect would be quite small (Fletcher et al., 2010). Such taxes are also regressive in that lower-income households are disproportionately affected by them. In the case of SSBs, there is evidence that they pay more not just in a relative sense (i.e., as a percent of income) but also in an absolute sense (i.e., that lower-income households will continue to purchase more SSBs even after a tax is imposed, and would therefore pay more in dollars on average) (Lin, Smith, Lee, & Hall, 2011). Continued research—and economic analysis of policy experimentation—will help determine whether or not taxing SSBs is a good policy for reducing obesity rates in the United States.

FOCUS 7.2. US FARM SUBSIDIES DO NOT MAKE AMERICANS FAT

Julian M. Alston and Bradley J. Rickard

America's rising obesity rates are exacting a high cost on society. In looking for solutions, many people blame federal farm subsidies for the current obesity problems. It may seem obvious that subsidies make certain foods cheaper, therefore contributing to overconsumption, but every serious analysis of the relationship by economists has found the notion untrue. In fact, US farm policies have had generally modest and mixed effects on prices and quantities of farm commodities. The overall effect on the prices paid by US consumers for food has been negligible; consequently, eliminating farm policies would have a negligible influence on dietary patterns and obesity.

Farm subsidies have at times resulted in lower US prices of some farm commodities, such as certain food grains or feed grains, and consequently lower costs of producing breakfast cereal, bread, or livestock products. But in these cases, the price-depressing (and consumption-enhancing) effect of subsidies has been contained (or even reversed) by the imposition of additional policies that restricted acreage or production. In addition, for more than a decade, about half of the total subsidy payments have provided limited incentives to increase production because the amounts paid to producers were based on past acreage and yields rather than current production. Moreover, for the commodities that are subject to US import barriers, the effect of the policy is to increase farm and food prices domestically, providing a disincentive to consume foods that use these commodities as ingredients. Trade barriers that apply to imported sugar, dairy, orange juice, and beef cause the prices of these agricultural commodities to increase, and thereby increase the cost and discourage consumption of foods that use these commodities.

What about corn? Farm subsidies are responsible for the growth in the use of corn to produce HFCS as a caloric sweetener, but not in the way it is often suggested. The culprit here is not corn subsidies; rather, it is sugar policy that has restricted imports, driven up the US price of sugar, and encouraged consumers and food manufacturers to replace sugar with alternative caloric sweeteners, especially HFCS. Combining the sugar policy with the corn policy, the net effect of farm subsidies has been to increase the price of caloric sweeteners generally and to discourage total consumption while causing a shift in sweetener use between sugar and HFCS. This discouragement has been enhanced recently by US biofuels policy. The current US ethanol policy benefits US corn growers by driving up the demand for corn as feedstock. This effective subsidy to corn growers much more than offsets any impact of other farm policies that might increase the availability of corn for use in food and livestock feed. So the overall effect of the full set of policies is to make all of the corn-based food products more expensive, not less expensive to consumers.

Even if the effects of policy on the prices of farm commodities were large and in a direction that would contribute to obesity, the ultimate impacts on food prices would be comparatively small. Farm commodities used as ingredients represent a small share of the total cost of retail food products, and this share has been shrinking for all farm commodities since the 1970s. On average the farm commodity cost share is approximately 20 percent, but it varies widely: for grains, sugar, and oilseeds, it is less than 10 percent; for soda, a food product that is often associated with obesity, the share is approximately 2 percent.

US farm policies might well be seen as unfair and inefficient, but whether we like these policies or not for other reasons, their effects on obesity are negligible. The 2014 Farm Bill eliminated direct payment subsidies and increased crop insurance subsidies. The other reasons for the effects being negligible, however, have not changed and the general effects of farm policy on consumption will remain modest. Farm subsidies are a red herring in the obesity context just as obesity is a red herring in the context of farm subsidy policy. Our careful quantitative analysis of these issues indicates that US farm subsidy policies, for the most part, have not made food commodities significantly cheaper and have not had a significant effect on caloric consumption. In fact, eliminating all farm subsidies, including those provided indirectly by trade barriers, may, if anything, lead to an *increase* in annual per capita consumption of calories and an increase in body weight. Farm policies have more likely slowed the rise in obesity in the United States—but any such effects must be small. Compared with other factors, the policy-induced differences in relative prices of farm commodities have played only a tiny role in determining excess food consumption and obesity in the United States.

For further information, look at the following resources.

Alston, J. M., Rickard, B. J., & Okrent, A. M. (2010). Farm policy and obesity in the United States. Choices. Retrieved from www.choicesmagazine.org/magazine/article.php?article=138

Alston, J. M., Sumner, D. A., & Vosti, S. A. (2008). Farm subsidies and obesity in the United States: National evidence and international comparisons. *Food Policy, 33*(6), 470–479.

Can the Price Make It Right? Using Subsidies to Make Healthy Food Cheaper

Getting Americans to eat healthier foods such as fruits and vegetables has been a decades-long challenge. Americans on average consume 1.03 cups of fruits and 1.58 cups of vegetables per day, about half the amounts recommended by USDA's MyPlate, which is based on the 2010 Dietary Guidelines for Americans (Dietary Guidelines Advisory Committee, 2010). Likewise, only 14.0 percent of adults and 9.5 percent of adolescents consume the recommended servings of fruits and vegetables per day (Centers for Disease Control and Prevention, 2013). To tackle this problem, the USDA developed the Healthy Incentives Pilot (HIP) program, a randomized controlled trial to evaluate the effect of subsidies for fruits, vegetables, and other healthy foods on purchases of these products among SNAP recipients. A subsidy can be used to increase demand for goods or services. Similar to when governments use a tax to address a negative externality, subsidies can be used to address positive externalities in a market.

The price of healthier food items in the United States is a barrier to purchases for some households, and food prices for healthier items, such as fruits, vegetables, and whole grains, have risen over time faster than for unhealthier foods such as red meat and refined grain products (Kuchler & Stewart 2008). To address this issue HIP made healthier foods such as fruits and vegetables less expensive. In the HIP trial, SNAP recipients in Massachusetts were randomly assigned to receive immediate $0.30 credits to their EBT cards for every dollar they spent on targeted fruits and vegetables (Abt Associates, 2011; USDA Food and Nutrition Service, 2013) or no credits. Preliminary results indicate that those receiving the subsidy consumed 25 percent more of the targeted fruits and vegetables per day than those who did not receive the subsidy (Bartlett et al., 2013). In addition, both groups reported that they bought more and a greater variety of fruits and vegetables because of the HIP incentive (Bartlett et al., 2013). Another randomized controlled trial in the Netherlands found that a 50 percent discount on fruits and vegetables increased purchases of these items by 8.59 pounds per household biweekly (Waterlander, de Boer, Schuit, Seidell, & Steenhuis, 2013). Other studies, based on simulation approaches using price elasticity estimates such as those shown in table 7.3, have suggested that such subsidies can translate into reduced rates of conditions such as heart attack and stroke (Cash, Sunding, & Zilberman, 2005). Although these results seem promising, more controlled trials are needed to determine the degree to which subsidies increase consumption of fruits and vegetables and, more important, how they can translate into long-term improvements in consumers' health.

On-Package Nutrition Labeling

credence attributes
Food attributes, such as nutritional quality, that cannot readily be ascertained by the consumer even after consuming a product

In addition to taxes on unhealthy food and subsidies for healthy foods, food labels are another strategy to promote healthy diets. Food attributes, such as nutritional quality, that cannot readily be ascertained by the consumer even after consuming a product are called **credence attributes**. When only the manufacturer or producer knows about the existence of a credence attribute such as nutritional quality, there exists an information asymmetry in the market. Labels are used to correct information asymmetries in food and beverage products.

US readers have probably seen the Nutrition Facts Panel on the back of packaged foods and beverage products (similar labeling requirements exist in many other countries as well). This label contains information about the quantity of calories, fat, sugar, and micronutrients contained in the product as a percentage of recommended daily intake. In early 2014 the USDA Center for Nutrition Policy and Promotion proposed changes to the design of the Nutrition Facts Panel, intended to make it easier to use. As described in focus 10.2, research has suggested that consumers find back-of pack nutrition labels confusing, especially the numerical information and terminology used (Feunekes et al., 2008). As a result, nutritionists and public health experts have proposed "front-of-pack" labeling schemes, and a variety of voluntary front-of-pack labeling schemes exist in the United States and in other countries. Ongoing research is examining which front-of-pack label is most effective at communicating nutrition information to consumers and in promoting healthful eating.

There is evidence that overcoming information asymmetry can have significant economic benefits (Cash, 2011). In the United States, the inclusion of trans fatty acid content on the nutrition facts panel became mandatory on January 1, 2006. The rule requiring this addition had originally been proposed years before, but implementation had been stalled within the Food and Drug Administration (FDA). The Office of Management and Budget (OMB) issued a letter to the FDA prompting along the process on the basis of a preliminary weighing of likely benefits of the label. OMB is charged with conducting regulatory impact analyses of proposed major changes to federal rules. These analyses are a form of **benefit-cost analysis**, in which the total social benefits and costs of a project are estimated and used to provide insight into whether an initiative will be a net winner or loser to society (Cash, 2011). Some critics feel that regulatory impact analyses are often used to block or delay environmental and health protection measures, but in this case the economic evidence strongly pointed

benefit-cost analysis
Method of analysis that estimates total social benefits and costs of a project; used to provide insight into whether an initiative will be a net winner or loser to society

to great net benefits from completing the rule-making process (Graham, 2007). The OMB's analysis and "prompt letter" led not only to the eventual labeling of trans fat levels in packaged foods but also indirectly to a considerable reduction of trans fats in the US food supply, because many food manufacturers responded to the new labeling requirement by reformulating their products to reduce or remove the trans fat content.

This example demonstrates the power of regulation to shift industry practices by motivating additional voluntary action. Focus 7.3 provides a broader description of food industry voluntary actions to promote health and the factors that motivate them, from an author who has worked for change from within the food industry.

FOCUS 7.3. RECENT PROGRESS IN PRIVATE SECTOR VOLUNTARY INITIATIVES TO PROMOTE HEALTHY EATING

Derek Yach

Over the past century, the food industry has laid the basis for intergenerational improvements in health and economic development (Floud, Fogel, Harris, & Hong, 2011). Now it is addressing obesity.

The underlying causes of obesity are complex. Sir David King stressed in a major UK report that "no one policy will fix the problem of obesity" and that solutions will take time and need to be designed and implemented through "structured comprehensive collaboration" involving industry and government (Foresight, 2007). Industry actions include increased investments in research and development linked to product formulation aimed at calorie reduction (natural sweeteners, smaller portions sizes, lower fat contents being a few), shifts in marketing of the highest calorie products to children, and introduction of labeling efforts aimed at better informing consumers and supporting innovative community-based programs (Epode, 2012; Tufts University Friedman School of Nutrition Science and Policy, 2012).

Until recently multinational food and beverage companies relied on a business model that favored product quantity over quality. Similar to the energy sector, the food industry increasingly recognizes that to change, it has to change its business model. Better nutrition, not more calories, will become the future business and social goal.

Industry Progress

The food and beverage industry has undertaken several important voluntary initiatives to address obesity. In the United States, more than 210 organizations joined together in the Healthy Weight Commitment Foundation [HWCF], a CEO-led partnership to reduce childhood obesity by 2015. HWCF food companies have pledged to reduce 1.5 trillion calories from the marketplace by 2015 (HWCF, 2010). These commitments are independently evaluated by the Robert Wood Johnson Foundation. Beverage companies partnered with the Alliance for a Healthier Generation to remove full-sugar soda from US schools starting in 2006, resulting in an 88 percent calorie reduction from beverages shipped to schools (ABA, 2010).

It is likely that the combined impact of public and industry-led initiatives to reduce childhood obesity is responsible for recent reports of the slowdown and decline in rates across parts of the United States (Robbins, Mallya, Polansky, & Schwarz, 2012). Globally, a partnership of ten multinational companies made commitments to support WHO's Global Strategy on Diet, Physical Activity, and Health that included product development and reformulation, nutrition information, responsible advertising, and awareness on healthy diets and activity (Accenture, 2012; IFBA, 2008).

(Continued)

(Continued)

There have also been more individual company activities. Competition is emerging regarding doing more for health. In 2009 PepsiCo pledged to eliminate the direct sale of full-calorie sodas from all schools worldwide and has made progress in more than one hundred countries. In the United States, the total volume of PepsiCo beverages sold in the mid- and low-calorie range has sharply increased from 24 percent in 1997 to nearly 50 percent today (PepsiCo, 2012). That represents millions of calories removed from beverages. This is matched by a range of related efforts by other food companies. These changes occurred during a recession, suggesting that future progress will accelerate.

Progress by companies has been motivated by many factors: leading CEOs know that change is the right thing to do, investors increasingly reward companies who address health as part of broader sustainability efforts, consumer demand for healthy foods is increasing, and the regulatory and litigation environment remains of concern to many companies (Dow Jones Sustainability Indexes, 2012; Global Reporting Initiative, 2012; Ketchum, 2012). Bank of America Merrill Lynch's (BoA's) recent influential report entitled "Globesity: The Global Fight Against Obesity" identified investment opportunities in fifty companies most likely to play important roles in reducing obesity over the next two decades (BoA, 2012). Within the food sector, Danone, Dole, General Mills, PepsiCo, and Darden Restaurants are among those mentioned. BoA analysts focused on trends underway that will contribute to reversing obesity and not just on today's portfolios.

The Way Forward

Benjamin Franklin said that "a man convinced against his will is of the same opinion still." That is particularly true with respect to food choices. Researchers such as Cass Sunstein, Kevin Volpp, and Brian Wansink have suggested using a range of simple interventions that nudge people into healthy choices and present them with healthier default options. The use of broad-based incentives to encourage healthy eating (and reduce consumption of unhealthy foods) has been shown to be effective in shifting diets in a large population and is evidence of the type of innovation possible through voluntary corporate actions (An, Patel, Segal, & Strum, 2013).

Overall, the food system needs an approach that draws on the power of markets. Smarter incentives for food companies to change, subsidies for healthy food, shifts in defaults to reverse supersizing, more activity built into our daily lives, better use of social networks, and rewards for health professionals and teachers who promote healthy eating and more activity, when combined with public policies will make healthy choices the economically easy and readily available choices (Yach, Stuckler, & Brownell, 2006).

Improving Behavior Models of Food Consumption

As noted, the basic economic model of optimizing behavior in the face of constraints is a powerful one, but may fall short in explaining some behavior—particularly around individual aspects of food consumption. Behavioral economics is a growing field that formally models how emotional and psychological factors influence consumer choice. This subfield of economics presumes that consumers are not perfectly rational, in part because automatic psychological systems play a role in our decision-making processes (Kahneman, 2011). These automatic systems may force us to make decisions using **heuristics** (i.e., rules of thumb) or emotions instead of rationality (i.e., when we engage in a cognitive process of weighing the costs and benefits of each choice). Such heuristics are important time-savers as we navigate through our daily lives, but they can also lead us astray in that they were often adapted for situations very different from our modern food environments. For example, researchers conducted a blinded experiment in which participants were asked to sit at a table and consume bowls of soup. Participants in the

heuristics
Rules of thumb consumers use to make choices

treatment group had soup bowls that were automatically refilled from beneath the table as they consumed the soup, unbeknownst to them! Individuals eating from the auto-refill bowls ate 73 percent more soup than participants with normal bowls (Wansink, 2006). There are a variety of other clever examples that highlight ways in which we make less-than-rational food choices on a regular basis (Wansink, 2006).

When traditional economic theory fails, behavioral economics may be successful and illuminating. Some of the theories that behavioral economists have developed are intuitive but can yield valuable ideas for nutrition policy and promotion. Here is a sampling (excerpted from Just, Mancino & Wansink, 2007, p. 1):

- **People often prefer "default options."** Experimental studies have shown that people tend to overvalue the potential of loss. As a result, we often prefer the status quo, as it both requires less mental effort and provides protection from losses that may result from change. This suggests that making the default option a healthier one can provide healthier outcomes. For example, many restaurants advertise that a sandwich comes with French fries, but allow consumers to substitute a salad. If instead the default was the salad and people could substitute fries, they are likely to make the healthier choice while still having the same options (i.e., fries or a salad) available.

- **Food decisions are often based more on emotion than rational thought**. The presentation of a food item can influence impulsive behavior. By drawing attention to healthier food items, such as by placing them under better lighting or in more attractive containers, school cafeteria managers have increased children's selection of fruits and vegetables.

- **People have problems with self-control when choosing food**. This means that consumers seek immediate satisfaction and often choose things in the "heat of the moment" that they might not choose if selecting foods for later consumption. One way to address this challenge is to provide opportunities to preselect healthier choices, such as workers choosing their cafeteria lunches ahead of time.

- **External cues can have a major effect on the food selected, the amount consumed, and an eater's perception of how much was consumed**. If the designers of a workplace food court wished to encourage more "mindful eating" so that people were more aware of how much they were consuming, they could reduce the amount of noise and distraction. In another example, as people often perceive taller beverage containers as being larger and providing a better bargain than shorter containers holding the same volume, serving healthier beverages in bottles and less preferred ones in cans might encourage people to make the healthier choice.

Although interesting in their own right, the insights behavioral economics provide into food consumption may have important implications for formulating better food policies. Some have suggested that behavioral economics can improve food choices through simple interventions in school lunchrooms, fast food restaurants, and within households, including small environmental manipulations meant to make healthier options the default option. This approach has been termed *libertarian paternalism* by its proponents, who argue that the seemingly objectionable phrase is apt in that it is "libertarian in that it can shift individual behavior without limiting freedom of choice, but it is paternalistic in that it inevitably involves some judgments about what those best outcomes should be" (Cash & Schroeter, 2010, p. 2).

CONCLUSION

As we noted in our introduction, many observers (mistakenly, in our opinion) feel that economics relies on assumptions that undervalue environmental and health concerns or promote the interests of industry over those of neighborhoods and families. This may be based in part in confusing economic forces in the marketplace with economics as an analytical discipline. In truth, economic frameworks can and do readily encompass health and environmental concerns and are in fact particularly well suited for balancing competing social interests, such as access to nutritious food, corporate profits, environmental protection, and ethical preferences for some forms of production over others. When markets have failed to provide and balance these benefits appropriately, it is often a failure of society to measure the benefits, rather than of economics as a discipline to account for them. In our view, those looking to improve the performance of food systems should embrace economic models and analyses as a vehicle for quantifying environmental and health benefits and ensuring they make it onto the social balance sheet.

SUMMARY

This chapter provides an overview of the discipline of economics and how it can be used to diagnose and remedy inefficiencies in the food system. It illustrates key economic concepts as they play out in a series of real-world examples: the external costs of water contamination from agricultural production, large-size farms, income and price interventions to improve food access among low-income consumers and encourage healthier food choices, and consumer access to information about what is in foods. These examples and the chapter's discussion show that economics is not solely about finances. The real bottom lines of economics are efficiency and individual optimization. When a market does not operate efficiently there exists a market failure, which in many instances can be remedied only with governmental intervention. Likewise, certain behavioral constraints limit an individual's ability to optimize. Market failures occur in the food system for a variety of reasons, including presence of positive or negative externalities, lack of competition in markets, information asymmetries, behavioral constraints on optimization, and others. Behavioral constraints are rooted in human psychology and behavior. When market failures occur or when human behavior overrides optimal decision making, a remedy must be sought. The discipline of economics can help to provide sustainable solutions for improved food systems and public health.

KEY TERMS

Behavioral economics	Elastic
Benefit-cost analysis	Equilibrium
Cap-and-trade systems	Externality
Comparative advantage	Fixed costs
Complementary goods	Four-firm concentration ratio (CR4)
Credence attributes	Heuristics
Deadweight loss	Inelastic
Demand expansion	Information asymmetry
Economies of scale	Law of demand

Market concentration

Market failure

Monopoly

Optimization

Own-price elasticity of demand

Quota

Subsidy

Substitute goods

Tax

Total average cost

Total cost

Unit elastic

Variable costs

DISCUSSION QUESTIONS

1. Obesity has been framed as a major US public health challenge since the 1990s. What are some economic theories and principles that might help public health practitioners better understand the epidemic's causes and potential policy solutions?

2. How does market structure influence consumers' available food choices and the decisions they make in retail settings?

3. What are some shortcomings of economics as a discipline to dissect and resolve long-standing challenges facing the food system? How can economists and practitioners in disciplines such as public health work together to better address these issues?

4. What are some sources of market failure in the food system? Why is market failure or inefficiency a problem?

5. What types of intervention might be useful to address these?

6. The word *paternalism* is sometimes used in describing behavioral economics approaches; in fact, it might be used to describe many interventions using economic tools. Why is paternalism typically criticized? What (if anything) makes some kinds of paternalism acceptable and others objectionable?

REFERENCES

Abt Associates. (2011). *Updated study plan: Healthy incentives pilot evaluation*. US Department of Agriculture Food and Nutrition Service. Retrieved from www.fns.usda.gov/sites/default/files/study_plan.pdf

Accenture. (2012). *2011 Compliance monitoring report for the international food & beverage alliance*. Retrieved from https://www.ifballiance.org/sites/default/files/IFBA%20Accenture%20Monitoring%20Report%202011%20FINAL%20010312.pdf

Ajanovic, A. (2011). Biofuels versus food production: Does biofuels production increase food prices? *Energy, 36*(4), 2070–2076.

Alston, J. M., Rickard, B. J., & Okrent, A. M. (2010). Farm policy and obesity in the United States. Choices. Retrieved from www.choicesmagazine.org/magazine/article.php?article=138

Alston, J. M., Sumner, D. A., & Vosti, S. A. (2008). Farm subsidies and obesity in the United States: National evidence and international comparisons. *Food Policy, 33*(6), 470–479.

American Beverage Association (ABA). (2010). *Alliance school beverage guidelines progress report*. Retrieved from www.healthiergeneration.org/uploadedFiles/About_The_Alliance/SBG%20FINAL%20PROGRESS%20REPORT%20(March%202010).pdf

An, R., Patel, D., Segal, D., & Strum, R. (2013). Program for healthy food purchases in South Africa. *American Journal of Health Behaviors, 37*(1), 56–61.

Andreyeva, T., Long, M. W., & Brownell, K. D. (2010). The impact of food prices on consumption: A systematic review of research on the price elasticity of demand for food. *American Journal of Public Health, 100*(2), 216–222.

Bank of America Merrill Lynch. (2012). *Efforts to tackle global obesity shaping a new investment megatrend, says new BoA Merrill Lynch report.* Retrieved from http://newsroom.bankofamerica.com/press-release/economic-and-industry-outlooks/efforts-tackle-global-obesity-shaping-new-investment-me

Bartlett, S., Klerman, J., Wilde, P., Olsho, L., Blocklin, M., Logan, C., & Enver, A. (2013). *Healthy incentives pilot interim report.* US Department of Agriculture Food and Nutrition Service. Retrieved from www.fns.usda.gov/sites/default/files/HIP_Interim.pdf

Berry, W. (1990). *The pleasures of eating. What are people for?* New York: North Point Press.

Bittman, M. (2013). Not all industrial food is evil. *New York Times,* August 17, online edition, sec. Opinionator. Retrieved from http://opinionator.blogs.nytimes.com/2013/08/17/not-all-industrial-food-is-evil

Bolotova, Y. V., & Novakovic, A. M. (2011). *The effect of the New York State milk price gouging law on the performance of fluid whole milk market: An empirical analysis.* Retrieved from http://ssrn.com/abstract=1865302

Box, G.E.P., & Draper, N. R. (1987). *Empirical model-building and response surfaces* (p. 424). New York: Wiley.

Cash, S. B. (2011). Policy evaluation and benefit-cost analysis. In J. L. Lusk, J. Roosen, & J. F. Shogren (Eds.), *The Oxford Handbook of the Economics of Food Consumption and Policy* (ch. 22). Oxford: Oxford University Press.

Cash, S. B., & Schroeter, C. (2010). Behavioral economics: A new heavyweight in Washington? *Choices, 25*(3). Retrieved from www.choicesmagazine.org/magazine/article.php?article=142

Cash, S. B., Sunding, D. L., & Zilberman, D. (2005). Fat taxes and thin subsidies: Prices, diet and health outcomes. *Acta Agriculturae Scandinavica Section C, 2*(3–4), 167–174.

Centers for Disease Control and Prevention. (2013). *State indicator report on fruits and vegetables.* Atlanta, GA: US Department of Health and Human Services. Retrieved from www.cdc.gov/nutrition/downloads/State-Indicator-Report-Fruits-Vegetables-2013.pdf

Chace, Z. (2013). *The lollipop wars.* Retrieved from www.npr.org/blogs/money/2013/04/26/179087542/the-lollipop-war

Dietary Guidelines Advisory Committee. (2010). *Report of the Dietary Guidelines Advisory Committee on the Dietary Guidelines for Americans, 2010.* US Department of Agriculture Center of Nutrition and Policy Promotion. Retrieved from www.cnpp.usda.gov/Publications/DietaryGuidelines/2010/DGAC/Report/2010DGACReport-camera-ready-Jan11–11.pdf

Dow Jones Sustainability Indexes. (2012). Retrieved from www.sustainability-index.com

Epode. (2012). Retrieved from www.epode-european-network.com

Feunekes, G.I.J., Gortemaker, I. A., Willems, A. A., Lion, R., & van den Kommer, M. (2008). Front-of-pack nutrition labelling: Testing effectiveness of different nutrition labelling formats front-of-pack in four European countries. *Appetite, 50*(1), 57–70.

Fletcher, J. M., Frisvold, D., & Tefft, N. (2010). Can soft drink taxes reduce population weight? *Contemporary Economic Policy, 28*(1), 23–35.

Floud, R., Fogel, R. W., Harris, B., & Hong, S. C. (2011). *The changing body: Health, nutrition and human development in the western world since 1700.* Cambridge, UK: Cambridge University Press.

Food Marketing Institute (2014). *Supermarket Facts.* Retrieved from www.fmi.org/research-resources/supermarket-facts.

Foresight. (2007). Tackling obesity: Future choices. Retrieved from www.bis.gov.uk/assets/foresight/docs/obesity/17.pdf

Global Reporting Initiative. (2012). *About GRI.* Retrieved from www.globalreporting.org/Pages/default.aspx

Graham, J. D. (2007). The evolving regulatory role of the U.S. Office of Management and Budget. *Review of Environmental Economics and Policy, 1*(2), 171–191.

Gulf of Mexico Hypoxia Task Force. (2011). *Moving forward on Gulf hypoxia annual report 2011*. US Environmental Protection Agency. Retrieved from http://water.epa.gov/type/watersheds/named/msbasin/progress.cfm

Healthy Weight Commitment Foundation. (2010). *Food and beverage manufacturers pledging to reduce annual calories by 1.5 trillion by 2015*. Retrieved from www.healthyweightcommit.org/news/Reduce_Annual_Calories

International Food and Beverage Alliance (IFBA). (2008). *Our commitments*. Retrieved from www.ifballiance.org/our-commitments.html

Johnson, R. S. (2011). Caloric sweetened beverage taxes: The good food/bad food trap. *Choices Magazine*, *26*(3), 3.

Just, D. R., Mancino, L., & Wansink, B. (2007). *Could behavioral economics help improve diet quality for nutrition assistance program participants?* SSRN Scholarly Paper ID 1084548. Rochester, NY: Social Science Research Network. Retrieved from http://papers.ssrn.com/abstract=1084548

Kahneman, D. (2011). *Thinking, fast and slow*. New York: Macmillan.

Ketchum. (2012). *Food 2020*. Retrieved from www.ketchum.com/sites/default/files/food_2020_infographic_07_12_v12.pdf

Kuchler, F., & Stewart, H. (2008). Price trends are similar for fruits, vegetables and snack foods (No. ERR-55). US Department of Agriculture Economic Research Service. Retrieved from www.ers.usda.gov/publications/err-economic-research-report/err55.aspx#.UqKL72RDtyw

Lin, B.-H., Smith, T. A., Lee, J.-Y., & Hall, K. D. (2011). Measuring weight outcomes for obesity intervention strategies: The case of a sugar-sweetened beverage tax. *Economics and Human Biology*, *9*(4), 329–341.

MacDonald, J. M., Korb, P., & Hoppe, R. A. (2013). *Farm size and the organization of U.S. crop farming* (No. ERR-152). US Department of Agriculture Economic Research Service. Retrieved from www.ers.usda.gov/publications/err-economic-research-report/err152.aspx#.UqCdlGRDtyw

McLaughlin, E. W. (2004). The dynamics of fresh fruit and vegetable pricing in the supermarket channel. *Preventive Medicine*, *39S2*, 81–87.

PepsiCo. (2012). *PepsiCo beverages: Facts to know and share*. Retrieved from www.pepsico.com/Download/PepsiCo_Beverages_Balanced_Choices.pdf

Pollan, M. (2009). *The omnivore's dilemma: A natural history of four meals*. New York: Penguin.

Robbins, J. M., Mallya, G., Polansky, M., & Schwarz, D. F. (2012) Prevalence, disparities, and trends in obesity and severe obesity among students in the Philadelphia, Pennsylvania, School District, 2006–2010. *Prevention of Chronic Disease*, *9*, 120118.

Rosengrant, M. W. (2008). *Biofuel and grain prices: Impacts and policy responses*. Testimony for the US Senate Committee on Homeland Security and Governmental Affairs, May 7. Washington, DC. Retrieved from www.ifpri.org/publication/biofuels-and-grain-prices

Runge, C. F., Johnson, J., & Runge, C. P. (2011). Better milk than cola: Soft drink taxes and substitution effects. *Choices*, *26*(3), 3.

Schnepf, R., & Yacobucci, B. D. (2013). *Renewable fuel standard (RFS): Overview and issues*. R40155. Congressional Research Service. Retrieved from www.fas.org/sgp/crs/misc/R40155.pdf

Tufts University Friedman School of Nutrition Science and Policy. (2012). *Shape up Somerville*. Retrieved from www.nutrition.tufts.edu/index.php?q=research/shapeup-somerville

US Department of Agriculture. (2013). *Corn backgrounder*. Retrieved from www.ers.usda.gov/topics/crops/corn/background.aspx#.Uqi7UWRDtyw.

US Department of Agriculture Food and Nutrition Service. (2013). *Supplemental nutrition assistance program (SNAP)*. Retrieved from www.fns.usda.gov/snap/supplemental-nutrition-assistance-program-snap

US Department of Agriculture Natural Resources Conservation Service. (2013). *Mississippi River Basin healthy watershed initiative*. Retrieved from www.nrcs.usda.gov/wps/portal/nrcs/detail/wi/programs/?cid=nrcs142p2_020764

US Department of Agriculture Food and Nutrition Service. (2013). *Healthy incentives pilot basic facts*. Healthy Incentives Pilot Program. Retrieved from www.fns.usda.gov/hip/healthy-incentives-pilot-hip-basic-facts

US Environmental Protection Agency. (2012). *Water quality trading*. Retrieved from water.epa.gov/type/watersheds/trading .cfm

Wansink, B. (2006). *Mindless eating: Why we eat more than we think*. New York: Random House.

Waterlander, W. E., de Boer, M. R., Schuit, A. J., Seidell, J. C., & Steenhuis, I.H.M. (2013). Price discounts significantly enhance fruit and vegetable purchases when combined with nutrition education: A randomized controlled supermarket trial. *The American Journal of Clinical Nutrition, 97*(4), 886–895.

Wilde, P. (2013). *Food policy in the United States: An introduction*. New York: Earthscan.

Yach, D., Stuckler, D., & Brownell, K. (2006). Epidemiologic and economic consequences of the global epidemics of obesity and diabetes. *National Medicine, 12*(1) 62–66.

Chapter 8

Policies That Shape the US Food System

Mark Muller and David Wallinga

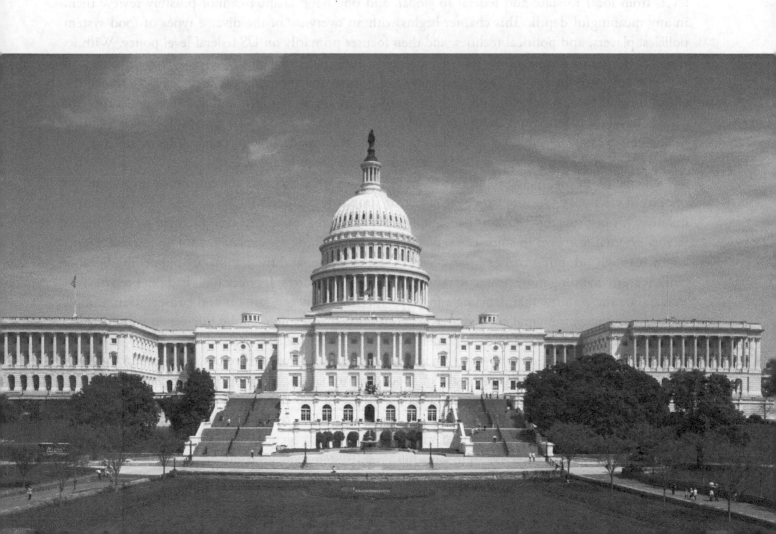

Learning Objectives

- Understand food systems policies as critical drivers of public health and health disparities.

- Describe the process for policy proposals to become legislation and then receive federal funding.

- Appreciate the role of alliances, stakeholders, and other political factors in policy change.

- Become familiar with a brief history of food and agriculture policy in the United States.

- Identify ways food system policies can affect price and thus shape the food system.

- Recognize strengths and limitations of working in state and local versus federal policy arenas.

Policy refers to institutional rules: for example, governmental programs to perform functions including regulating, taxing, providing incentives, creating mandates, and building infrastructure. For decades, elected officials have been crafting laws on food and agriculture; government agencies also devise policy to implement these laws. Until recently, those creating food and agriculture policy have rarely considered the compatibility of programs affecting food production and food demand. Instead, policies were traditionally siloed into sectors such as agriculture, health, food safety, transportation, environment, and business.

Government policy and food systems interact extensively and with great complexity at multiple levels from local to state and federal to global, and one book chapter cannot possibly review them in any meaningful depth. This chapter begins with an overview of the diverse types of food system policies, players, and political realities, and then focuses primarily on US federal level policy. With its size and enormous ramifications for food and agriculture, we place particular emphasis on the Farm Bill. Focusing still further on four important food policy topics we discuss fair prices for farmers, the elimination of food-borne illnesses, greater food security for all families, and access to and supply of nutritious foods. Information about state and local policy can be found throughout this book, including in chapters 6 and 18. Table 8.1 provides examples of the broad range of policy interventions at the federal, state, and local levels that can be used to advance the public's health.

Policy is often considered to be a driver of behavior, with consumers and businesses responding to the incentives policy creates. That is a somewhat simplistic perspective. The process is actually more iterative, history suggests. Rather than simply driving change, policy makers often are responding to factors external to them. In some cases, policy becomes a vehicle for expressing public interest. Farms are increasingly adopting conservation practices, for example, and these shifts are happening because citizens are demanding more protections for soil and water resources. If policy tools had not been devised to facilitate these shifts, then labeling efforts, partnerships between farmers and conservation groups, and other nongovernmental tools may have been created to express public interest in conservation. Other policies are promoted by stakeholders with more narrow self-interests.

In US food and agriculture policy, most major initiatives have been responses to crises: the Dust Bowl, the Great Depression, outbreaks of food contamination, to name a few. It is unsurprising, therefore, that legislation is often assembled hastily, and the potential for collateral food system effects other than those intended is rarely considered. The compartmentalizing of food policy development and implementation into various departments, agencies, and committees contributes to the consideration of these issues in isolation. Food system policies come before Congress through

TABLE 8.1   Examples of Food System Policies That Could Potentially Advance Public Health

Food Sector	Federal	State	Local
Production Farming, gardening, aquaculture, wild foods	• Incentives to increase production of health-promoting foods • Moratorium on livestock producers using nontherapeutic antibiotics and synthetic growth hormones in healthy animals • Requirement that foods served to children through USDA programs be produced without antibiotics, synthetic hormones, pesticides, or chemical fertilizers • Requirement that USDA food programs procure at least 10 percent of foods from local producers	• Fruit and vegetable production included in economic development plans • Land-use policies that halt excessive encroachment of urban development on agricultural land • Procurement priorities for local food in state-funded programs and institutions • Requirement to integrate gardening and food preparation into school curriculum • Tax incentives for roof gardens • Partnership with tribal governments to establish productive lands supporting native food systems	• City ordinances allowing residents to keep chickens, ducks, rabbits, and beehives • Enforcement of land-use protections for urban agriculture, community gardens, and farmers markets • Resolution recognizing importance of local, healthy, sustainably produced foods • Compost and water made available to community gardens • Allowances for organizations to lease nondevelopable city-owned property for community gardens • Chemical-free pest management and lawn care for city- and county-owned property • Business development assistance for small-scale, women-, and minority-owned farms • Edible landscaping on city- and county-owned property
Transformation Processing, packaging, labeling, marketing	• Labeling laws identifying foods containing genetically engineered ingredients • Prohibition on marketing foods of low nutritional value to children • Prohibition on misleading health claims in advertising and food package labels • Requirement that franchise restaurants provide nutritional information on menu items • Mandate contributions to a national nutrition campaign based on dollars spent marketing foods of low-nutritional value	• Tax incentives for small- to mid-sized industries that process, store, and distribute perishable foods grown in state	• Standards, secondary labels, and logos for foods produced within specific geographic region • Establishment of community kitchens and mobile processing units

(Continued)

TABLE 8.1   *(Continued)*

Food Sector	Federal	State	Local
Distribution Transportation, wholesaling, warehousing	• USDA grant programs leveraged to build local foods infrastructure	• Establishment of cooperative transportation and warehousing opportunities for local producers • Tax incentives for regional transportation, warehousing, and wholesaling of locally produced foods	• Permitting, regulatory, and other taxes eased for food business incubation • Zoning requirements creating transit routes (sidewalks, pedestrian malls, bicycle paths) from all neighborhoods to grocery stores and food assistance providers
Access Retail, food safety, food and nutrition security	• Coordinated food safety regulations • WIC and **Senior Farmers' Market Nutrition Program** fully supported in all states	• Zoning restrictions limiting fast food outlets within specified distance of schools and youth-centered facilities • Food access strategies incorporated into emergency preparedness plans to build local reserves and ensure maintaining food supplies in times of crisis	• Licensing requirements eased for new farm stands • Feeding program access expanded to all children and youth throughout the year • City ordinance allowing mobile fruit and vegetable vendors in low-income neighborhoods • Fast-food–free zones in and near schools and hospitals
Consumption Purchasing, preparing, preserving, eating	• Requirement that food in food and nutrition programs (SNAP, SLP, WIC) meet US dietary guidelines • Prioritize local and sustainably produced foods in purchasing requirements • Farm-to-school efforts expanded through Child Nutrition Act • Sustainability and other criteria incorporated into US dietary guidelines	• Minimum percentage established for locally produced food purchasing by public entities • Establish and expand education and training programs for culinary arts and sciences	• Preservation of native and ethnic food cultures • Requirement that city agencies purchase above minimum percentage of food from local farmers • New food enterprise zones providing zoning and tax incentives to attract food retailers to underserved areas and restrict number of fast food restaurants • Tax abatement for retail outlets selling healthy food; elimination of tax subsidies for fast food restaurants • All schools providing (locally grown) fruit and vegetable snacks to all children • Soft drink and snack industries' access to schools limited

TABLE 8.1 *(Continued)*

Food Sector	Federal	State	Local
			• Incentives for community kitchens that prepare and preserve locally produced food for schools and other institutions
			• Provisions expanding access to public land for community gardeners
			• Food preparation courses as part of city parks and recreation activities
Resource and Waste Management Disposal, recycling	• Tax credits for food production, processing, transportation, and retail entities using alternative energy • Standards for food industry water use and water recycling	• Tax incentives for using food waste for biofuel production • Award program recognizing communities that reduce food waste in landfills	• Community composting initiative providing composting bins to residents and businesses; compost provided to area farms

Source: Modified from Muller, Tagtow, Roberts, and MacDougall (2009).

different bills with different **renewal cycles** and are administered by different governmental agencies and departments. Some federal agencies, such as the US Food and Drug Administration and Department of Agriculture, have substantial focus on policies pertaining to food and agriculture (though they rarely present these policies within the food systems paradigm). Other agencies and policies significantly affect food systems but are rarely viewed as food or agriculture policy, such as US Environmental Protection Agency regulations affecting land and water use by farmers, federal tax policies that affect food businesses, and US Immigration and Customs Enforcement policy that profoundly affects the availability and treatment of labor in the food system. These separate—and sometimes competing—**jurisdictions** do not lend themselves to consideration of how individual policies or programs affect the food system as a whole.

FEDERAL FOOD SYSTEM LEGISLATION: THE PROCESS

The long and often confusing course of policy, as it moves from an idea to enactment to implementation, generally begins with Congress and makes its way to the president for a signature or a veto, as explained further in focus 8.1.

Congressional legislation is grouped into three categories. **Authorizing legislation** refers to bills creating new programs or extending or repealing old ones. **Appropriations bills** passed annually allocate federal funds for specific programs.

Senior Farmers' Market Nutrition Program
Provides grants to states, territories, and tribes to provide coupons to seniors for food at farmers markets, roadside stands, and from community-supported agriculture

renewal cycles
Length of time before a piece of legislation expires and requires new authorization; the Farm Bill is expected to be renewed every five years

jurisdictions
The subjects and functions assigned to a committee of Congress

authorizing legislation
Bill that creates a new federal program, extends the life of an existing program, or repeals existing law, though it does not provide program funding

appropriations bills
Legislation that sets money aside for specific spending

entitlement program
Program that guarantees access to certain benefits for all who qualify (e.g., Social Security benefits)

And **entitlement programs** provide certain benefits, such as SNAP or Medicare, to all persons who meet eligibility requirements. Entitlement legislation does not require a corresponding appropriations bill, just initial authorizing legislation.

FOCUS 8.1. TURNING POLICY IDEAS INTO LEGISLATIVE REALITIES
Mark Muller

Any House or Senate member can introduce legislation onto the floor of their respective body, but their ability to move that legislation is far from equal. Pieces of legislation fall within jurisdiction of different committees. Both the House and Senate, for example, have committees dedicated to agricultural matters. Chairs of these committees generally have the most say in crafting such legislation, followed by other committee members. The majority political party selects the chairperson, and the minority party selects the ranking member (next in leadership order) of each committee.

chairman's mark
Draft bill that the chairperson of a committee or subcommittee uses as the starting point for developing legislation

reporting out
Act of finalizing a committee's drafting of legislation and bringing it to the attention of the broader Congressional body

Most committees delegate specific issues to subcommittees. Policy options can be considered in detail at that level, with recommendations made back to the full committee. Subcommittees, similar to full committees, will often solicit public input, hold public hearings, and invite written comments. Committee and subcommittee chairs often provide a **chairman's mark** that serves as the draft version of the legislation, and then facilitates discussion about the merits of its different aspects. At some point the chair calls for a vote among committee members; if a majority give their approval, the bill is subject to **reporting out** to the House or Senate. Committee staff provide a written report explaining the purpose and scope of the bill, as well as any dissenting comments from committee members.

A bill is then brought up to the floor of the House or Senate based on the rules of each body. The House and Senate leadership have oversight of their respective legislative calendars, and at times the leadership may attempt to effectively kill a piece of legislation by not providing time on the calendar. Individual members may add amendments to the bill, which generally have to be deemed germane to the bill (although riders are sometimes added, which are amendments that pertain to less-related or sometimes unrelated topics). Both supporters and opponents of the legislation are provided the chance to speak, and a majority vote is taken to approve or defeat the bill.

After a bill passes the House and Senate, and to reconcile any differences between the two versions, it must go to a conference committee consisting of Congressional members from both bodies and both parties. If compromise is achieved, a conference report is submitted to both chambers for a final vote to approve the legislation and then it goes to the president for a signature or veto.

HOW ALLIANCES SHAPE POLICY

Major policy initiatives rarely succeed without aggregating the support of an array of separate interests. Some constituencies favor a policy change because they see profit potential, others are driven by perceived moral or public benefits, and still others may get involved simply because they are trading their political support in order to call in a favor in a completely different policy realm.

Alliances between divergent political interests are sometimes referred to as coalitions of "bootleggers and Baptists" (Buck & Yandle, 2001). In the nineteenth century, several states passed "blue laws" banning alcohol sales on Sundays. Many Baptists publicly supported these laws on moral and religious grounds, whereas bootleggers discreetly provided their support because of the profit potential they would enjoy with Sunday sales of illicit alcohol. Despite the fact that these two constituencies probably had little that they would agree on, the messy reality of politics brought them together to pass the legislation. Food systems policy is full of these alliances of divergent interests, from the Homestead Act of 1862 that merged opportunities for new immigrants to obtain land with railroad profit motives—to today's SNAP program that is supported by both antihunger advocates and food and agriculture industries seeking to expand markets. Such alliances are often effective because they combine political interests across traditional lines of division, such as political party, rural versus urban communities, and geographic regions of the country.

Other political alliances between diverse interests form regularly. Former New York City mayor Michael Bloomberg's proposal to cap the size of sugary drinks created an array of interesting alliances for and against the policy, including a partnership between the NAACP and the American Beverage Association (Grynbaum, 2013). The rapid adoption of genetically modified crops in the United States has created a diverse coalition of corporations, organic farmers, public health organizations, and consumer rights organizations that are demanding the labeling of foods made with these crops. And alliances with farm organizations are regularly touted by a variety of **special interests** that seek to benefit from the overall positive public opinion of farmers.

special interests
A group of people acting together to influence the legislative process

One hard-earned lesson from past fights over food system policy is that significant legislation rarely passes solely because it provides a public benefit. Benefits to society are often too diffuse or unclear, and potential economic losses to business interests invested in the current policy paradigm are too concentrated and tangible (Stone, 2001).

The public health interest in reducing the overuse of antibiotics in animal agriculture provides a clear example. As will be described in chapter 12, the widespread use of antibiotics in animal production already has contributed to the decreased effectiveness of certain antibiotics for human medicinal use, adding to the public health threat. Yet the beneficiaries of legislation that would limit antibiotic use are "diffuse and unclear" (for instance, most of us don't spend much time worrying about getting antibiotic-resistant infections, and even if we do, we are usually not focused on animal agriculture as a cause), whereas the opponents are concentrated (such legislation would directly threaten the business models of animal feedlot operators and certainly reduce pharmaceutical company sales). Accordingly, policy progress on this issue has been limited. It is possible that substantial legislative progress will be delayed until more groups stand to gain directly from increased antibiotic regulation. For example, regulation could provide financial gains for livestock farmers with antibiotic-free production practices, veterinarians with treatment alternatives, water treatment operators and other entities with concerns about water contamination, or patient advocacy groups. When will the time be right? Focus 8.2 describes theories regarding how issues make it onto the policy agenda.

FOCUS 8.2. A BRIEF LOOK AT AGENDA-SETTING, POLICY ANALYSIS, AND FOOD SYSTEMS

Linnea Laestadius

agenda-setting
Process by which problems and alternative solutions to address them rise to the attention of the public and policy makers

window of opportunity
Time-limited opportunity for taking action, when chances of success are relatively high

At any given time in the food system there are myriad issues to be addressed and even more potential solutions. What determines which of these are brought forward for political debate? **Agenda-setting** is the name for the process by which problems and the alternative solutions to address them rise to the attention of the public and policy makers (Birkland, 2005). One of the most straightforward and commonly used theories of agenda-setting is John Kingdon's "multiple-streams framework" (Kingdon, 2002).

Although we might like to think that agenda-setting is rational—a problem is identified and a series of solutions are compared to find the best one to act on—in truth, the process can be anything but linear. Oftentimes policy makers or advocacy groups already have a solution in mind and are simply looking for a problem to couple it with (Kingdon, 2002). In place of a rational decision-making model, Kingdon proposes that there are three separate streams at work in the agenda-setting process: problems, politics, and policies. When something causes these streams to intersect, a **window of opportunity** opens and the probability of successful action on an issue rises.

The problem stream considers how much information is available on a problem, the problem's characteristics, and how it has come to be defined by the public and policy makers. Although many problems are identified thanks to the collection of routine statistics, for example, a spike in a reportable disease such as *Salmonella,* other problems become known through *focusing events,* such as natural disasters or other crises. The 2010 heat wave, which dramatically affected Russian grain production, serves as an example of a focusing event that brought attention to food prices and food security. There is also a large body of literature documenting the importance of the media in bringing recognition to problems and serving as an agenda-setting tool in its own right (McCombs, 2005). To help bring an item onto the agenda, it is valuable to raise public and policymaker awareness, and to frame the issue so as to stress urgency and importance.

The political stream considers the national mood, political administration and party distribution in Congress, and activities of interest groups. Changes in the political stream can dramatically affect the feasibility of an item rising onto the agenda of policy makers. The political stream can be influenced not only by supporting political candidates who favor food systems reform but also through lobbying and grassroots advocacy campaigns undertaken by interest groups.

The policy stream consists of all the possible alternative solutions to problems at hand. Policies might be developed by researchers, Congressional staff, interest groups, or policy analysts, but all of their ideas commingle in what Kingdon (2002) terms the *policy primeval soup.* Ideas grow and are shaped by one another through discourse within communities of policy specialists. Only the ideas that meet specific criteria make it out of this process to become viable alternatives to solving a problem. Kingdon (2002) also stresses the importance of *policy entrepreneurs,* who champion a particular solution or idea. These individuals, for example, an advocate who seeks to promote incentives for organic farming, work to bring the three streams together and look to promote their desired policy when a window of opportunity finally does open.

Examining potential policies through the lens of policy analysts can provide useful insights. Although there are a number of potential policy analysis criteria to consider, the following are those most commonly used: effectiveness, efficiency, equity, liberty (i.e., does the policy affect people's rights or choices), political feasibility, social acceptability, administrative feasibility, and technical feasibility (Kraft & Furlong, 2007). Additional criteria are valuable for some food system policies, such as health or ecosystem impacts. A policy that compares well against alternative solutions based on these criteria is more likely to make it onto the agenda and be acted on favorably.

Although the agenda-setting process can be complicated and irrational, it is important to become familiar with it in order to be strategic in promoting desired change.

THE POLICY-MAKING PROCESS AND THE ROLE OF STAKEHOLDERS: THE FARM BILL AS AN EXAMPLE

The most substantial piece of legislation affecting the food system is the Farm Bill, a roughly $100 billion per year piece of legislation that funds most USDA programs, from SNAP to crop insurance to wastewater treatment. Farm Bill programs generally are authorized for five years, which means Congress needs to bring the legislation up for **reauthorization** within that time frame. The legislation affects all US citizens, yet the Senate and House agriculture committees are dominated by **farm state** Congressional members, providing overrepresentation to the Midwest, Great Plains, and South (see figure 8.1). This makes sense given the history of the policy and because farms and rural communities in those states are among those most affected by the legislation—though it also creates inertia for maintaining the status quo. By several measures it can be argued that "specialty crops," which include fruits and vegetables and are often grown outside of traditional farm states, are shortchanged in Farm Bill legislation in favor of farm state **commodity** crops, such as corn, soybeans, wheat, rice, and cotton. Commodity crops tend to be grown in larger quantities and sold more in bulk than specialty crops, whereas specialty crops tend to have a much higher value per acre.

reauthorization
The legislative process by which Congress renews, amends, or terminates existing programs

farm state
States that have commodity agriculture as an important part of their rural economy, usually referring to states in the Midwest and southeast United States

commodity
Agricultural crop produced at a large scale; commonly refers to corn, soybeans, wheat, rice, cotton, and animal products

Agriculture committee and subcommittee leaders in Congress often call hearings and hold listening sessions to gain exposure to multiple perspectives on the merits of proposed legislation. Within this context, the success of advocates for a particular Farm Bill often hinges on their ability to patch together a "bootleggers and Baptists" coalition of Congressional members and senators with concern for diverse issue areas within the Farm Bill including farming, conservation, food aid, and public health. Nutritional support programs in the Farm Bill, for example, have benefited from the agribusiness corporate lobbying interests that have converged to support lobbying efforts of the antihunger community (Simon, 2012).

The story isn't over after the president signs legislation. The Farm Bill provides the authorization for funds to be used on certain programs, but as described previously, funding for these programs needs to be appropriated annually with separate legislation. Multiple appropriations bills need to be passed each year, including one that is specifically focused on "Agriculture, Rural Development and Food." In the appropriations process, it is not uncommon for already-authorized programs to receive far less funding than is being requested, or even no funding.

The final component is policy implementation. Congress enacts legislation, but governmental departments and agencies need to create the infrastructure for laws to be implemented. For the Farm Bill, naturally, this takes place primarily within the USDA. For example, Congress may enact legislation that provides payments to farmers for implementing practices that improve wildlife habitat, but then

FIGURE 8.1   Geographic Distribution of Districts of House (above) and Senate (below) Agriculture Committee Members in the 113th Congress (2013–2014)

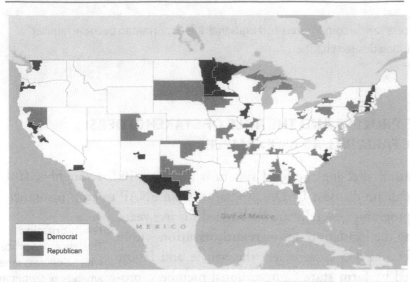

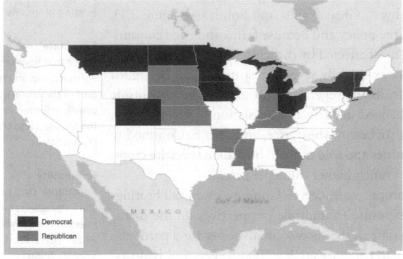

Note: The concentration of members in Great Plains, Midwest, and Southeastern states generally results in agricultural policies that more closely reflect the priorities of those regions.
Source: Roswell and Bowman (2013).

it is up to the USDA to develop requirements for who is eligible for the payments and a structure for disbursing them. Agencies develop these parameters, called *rules*, often with the assistance of Congressional committees. Rules are generally subject to comment periods allowing for public input.

After going through rule making and implementation, the reality of legislation can look far different from what Congress intended. Entities that opposed legislation passed by Congress can sometimes use the administrative process to water down the impact of that legislation. It is not surprising that policy advocates sometimes fail to pay adequate attention to rule making; it takes significant time to sit in on committee meetings, provide formal comments, and make use of other avenues for input. Typically, industry or trade groups who may financially benefit from administrative decisions have greater capacity for these tasks than do groups working on behalf of the public's interest.

THE HISTORY OF US FOOD AND AGRICULTURE POLICY: AN OVERVIEW

From the start, agricultural production has been integral to the growth of the US economy and the prosperity of its citizens. Historically, the primary concern of policymakers has been the economic conditions of farming and the safety of the food supply. The agricultural economy is erratic, however. Production can vary dramatically based on weather, drought, and pests; demand for agricultural products also can vary based on the health of regional and global economies.

A government has many interests in ensuring that the agricultural economy thrives, but foremost is the fact that its primary product, food, is essential. A host of other concerns, beyond simply producing adequate calories, invite government involvement in food and agriculture policy, from food safety to healthy eating to conservation. History suggests a long trend of rising government involvement, sometimes marked by success and sometimes by a large and somewhat ineffective bureaucracy.

The Economic Viability of Farming, 1840s to 1990s

A nation cannot have economic and social stability without a stable food supply. From the Great Famine in Ireland in the late 1840s to high food prices contributing to the Arab Spring, history is full of reminders that political unrest, mass migrations, and even wars have ensued from food insecurity. Providing an economic climate that supported agricultural production and a stable food supply was clearly the original driver of US farm policy, but over time, perhaps in part because of the successful growth in agricultural production, concerns about the stability of the US food supply have waned in favor of policies that support farmer income, increase food availability for families in poverty, and conserve natural resources.

The birth of US agricultural policy can in many ways be pinpointed to the Lincoln administration. In just a three-month span in 1862, President Lincoln established the US Department of Agriculture, signed the Homestead Act (which provided applicants with farm land at little or no cost), and signed the Morrill Land Grant College Act. The Homestead Act still affects us today, because the promise of free land drove new migrants to the Midwest and Great Plains, well beyond existing population centers. Those farmers focused production on storable, durable commodities such as corn and wheat, which could be transported via rail back to population centers on the East Coast. The Morrill Land Grant College Act initiated the creation of colleges and universities that conducted agricultural research and outreach, which contributed to the rapid development and adoption of new technologies and overall increases in production.

Throughout the late nineteenth century and much of the twentieth, farmers faced dramatic fluctuations in commodity prices. This is largely because of the fact that farmers are challenged with incorporating crop production—a biological process with significant variability—into a market system. The volume of agricultural production varies tremendously with weather and pests, making it difficult to forecast future supply and price.

A second challenge for farmers is that unlike in most industries, they do not have the ability to adjust production; for example, a television factory can idle part of its production if television sales slow. Farmers can make production decisions only once a year, and then, over the next several months until harvest, they are unable to respond to market fluctuations.

Third, given the structure of agricultural commodity markets that have thousands of individual farmers primarily selling to a few large food corporations, farmers producing commodity crops are in a weak bargaining position, with extremely limited ability to set prices. Farmers must largely accept whatever prices commodity markets provide. Most commodities are not sold directly to the consumer, but instead are sold to animal feeding operations, food processing corporations, or biofuel facilities. These entities make purchasing decisions driven not by crop quality, but rather by the need for large quantities of a certain minimum quality. The vast majority of corn and soybeans grown in the United States are different crops than sweet corn and edamame!

Given these market constraints, one of the only ways an individual farmer can improve his or her farm income is to increase overall levels of production on the farm. And although that decision may make sense for that individual farmer, the impact cumulated over thousands of farmers often is to create a crop glut so that supply exceeds demand and prices drop for those raw crops.

Willard Cochrane popularized the term *technology treadmill* to describe how farmers continually adopt new technologies to increase production in the hopes of increasing income. Expanded production instead contributes to lower prices and reduced income, thereby creating the visual of farmers running hard and yet not moving, as if on a treadmill (Levins, 2003). This model of expanding production and falling prices has worked to the advantage of grain buyers and the food processing industry, seeking inexpensive inputs, and to the detriment of farmers.

FIGURE 8.2   Eroded Land During the Dust Bowl

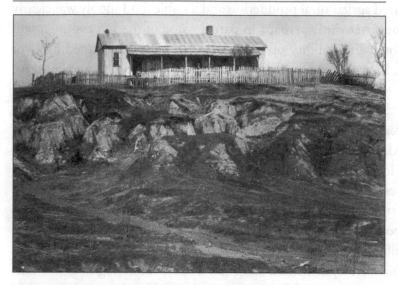

Source: USDA Natural Resources Conservation Service. NRCSDC01001. Public domain.

The economic challenges for farmers came to a head in the 1930s during the Great Depression. The stock market crash in October 1929 caused a rapid decline in income and overall economic activity, resulting in a severe reduction in demand for agricultural products and subsequently causing commodity prices to plummet. On top of these economic challenges was the Dust Bowl, caused by dry weather and inappropriate farming practices that devastated Great Plains farmers (see figure 8.2). A growing sentiment among many workers and farmers was that capitalism had failed them. Policy makers felt increasingly obliged to act in order to quiet a restless population.

Henry Wallace was President Franklin D. Roosevelt's Secretary of Agriculture from 1933 to 1940 and a visionary. He understood that these forces were beyond the control of each individual farmer, were caused by excessive market volatility, and could be mitigated with federal intervention. He realized that to address the low prices that left farmers reeling in the Great Depression, excess supply required management attention (**supply management policies**). Because grains and oilseeds (such as soybeans) store well, part of the harvest could be taken off the market and put into reserve when prices were too low. Then, when prices recovered, the crops could be sold for a profit. By using this simple concept of buying low and selling high, government-operated storage facilities could actually make money for taxpayers while smoothing out price spikes that could be devastating for farmers, food processors, and consumers. This program, advertised in figure 8.3, meant better food affordability for all Americans.

supply management policies
Policies that use incentives, taxes, and regulation to affect the available supply of an agricultural commodity; most often used as a mechanism for reducing large fluctuations in commodity prices; less common than in the past

In addition to reserves, a program was instituted that supported soil conservation, thereby maintaining the land's ability to produce future harvests. Although farmers and consumers may at first benefit from maximizing production, the short-term benefits are offset if future production is harmed by the loss of healthy soils. An industry that operates at maximum production for too long becomes less resilient and sets itself up for disaster. Electric utilities, for example, are usually planned to operate at just a portion of their total capacity so they have sufficient reserve capacity to meet periods of peak demand. Food is the perfect example of a commodity in which we always need to have a buffer of reserve production capacity, and maintaining the health of soil and other resources is crucial for creating that buffer.

Thus the 1930s, the era of a financial and an ecological disaster—the Great Depression and the Dust Bowl—led to the framework for a modern agricultural policy that is still used today. The most significant change since then has been a shift away from programs that support farmer livelihoods by managing the supply and price of commodities (supply management) to programs that instead support farmers directly by providing them with government payments and federally subsidized crop insurance. This transition was strongly supported by grain buyers and other businesses that purchase commodities from farmers and thereby benefit from lower prices. This shift has increased government spending on agriculture considerably and has also affected the structure of US agriculture. These government payments are based on bushels of crop produced and the historic cropping history of the land, providing farmers with an even greater incentive to maximize production and take more risk. These policies, in conjunction with other factors such as unequal access to capital and the availability of labor-saving technologies such as tractors, have likely contributed to greater financial returns to larger farms and subsequently an increasingly large scale of farms in the United States.

It is important to point out that not all farmers

FIGURE 8.3 A Poster Advertising "Plenty of Food for Everyone"

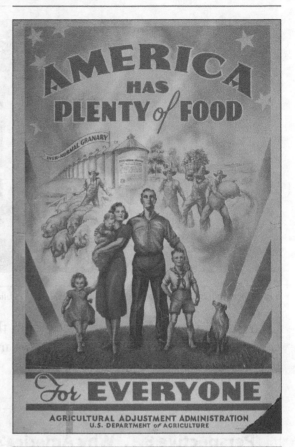

The agricultural program under Franklin Roosevelt meant savings for taxpayers and steady incomes for farmers.
Source: USDA Agricultural Research Service. Special Collections, Permission received.

or potential farmers had similar experiences with agricultural policy. The Homestead Acts and other nonagricultural policies largely benefited people of European descent, whereas the experience of African Americans, whose involvement in US agriculture at that time was largely in the shackles of slavery, was far different. Unfortunately, the USDA has a long, documented history of discriminatory practices in its farmer programs. In a landmark 1997 case, the USDA settled with African American farmers over the denial or untimely processing of loans (the Pigford Settlement). The USDA subsequently settled a discrimination case with Native American farmers for denying them equal access to credit (the 2010 Keepseagle settlement) and also started a claims process for Hispanic and women farmers (Ackerman, Bustos, & Muller, 2012).

Food Safety Policy, 1900 to 1970s

A second set of food system policy concerns, driven by consumer concerns, emerged in the first half of the twentieth century. Upton Sinclair's 1906 novel, *The Jungle*, famously exposed the abhorrent worker conditions and health concerns associated with meatpacking. The resultant public outcry gave Congress no choice but to react. Congress passed the Meat Inspection Act and the Pure Food and Drug Act of 1906, legislation that eventually resulted in the creation of the Food and Drug

FIGURE 8.4   Government Inspectors at a Nebraska Meatpacking Plant in 1910

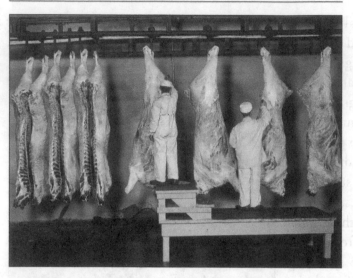

Source: National Archives. "Inspection of Carcasses, 1910." Public domain.

Administration in 1930. Interestingly, Sinclair was not a supporter of the 1906 legislation because the cost of food inspections was paid for by taxpayers rather than by the food industry (see figure 8.4). It has been over a century since that early legislation, and inspection costs are still largely borne by the government rather than the food industry.

One of the most dramatic changes to food safety regulation occurred with the passage of the Food Safety Modernization Act (FSMA) of 2010. This legislation increased the FDA's ability to prevent outbreaks of food-borne illness and provided FDA with more oversight of foods grown in the United States and imported from other countries. Despite widespread support for food safety, the legislation's implementation has been delayed and contentious, partly because of the cost and tracking burden that food safety legislation can impose on farmers and food processors and handlers. Perspective 8.1 describes ongoing challenges in governmental oversight of food safety.

Perspective 8.1. Why America's Food Is Still Not Safe
Adam Sheingate

Each year, forty-eight million Americans suffer from illnesses caused by dangerous microbial pathogens lurking in the food they eat. For most people, food poisoning just leads to temporary stomachaches or diarrhea. But the effects can be much more serious. According to the Centers for Disease Control and Prevention, more than 125,000 Americans are hospitalized and 3,000 die each year from pathogens in our food. Estimates of the cost of food-borne illness exceed $75 billion a year—taking into account the cost of health care and lost time on the job for people who get sick. The actual suffering and economic cost could be much greater, because many incidents of mild illness caused by tainted food go unreported.

That eating dinner can result in disability or death comes as a shock to most Americans. Most of us believe that the United States fixed these problems more than a century ago, after Upton Sinclair's famous book, *The Jungle*, revealed the ghastly facts about unsafe methods of commercial food processing for a mass market economy. But in fact, the rules and regulations we assume will protect us are inadequate. Duplication and gaps in government responsibilities leave Americans highly vulnerable to a variety of risks from industrial food production.

Government must have more effective tools to prevent food-borne illness. Problems of administrative overlap must be remedied so that we can manage the risks of our modern food system. Successful reform also requires that we reframe the food safety issue so that industry and government accept greater responsibility for illness outbreaks when they occur—rather than place much of the responsibility for food safety on consumers themselves.

Why Food Safety Administration Often Falls Short

In 1906, Congress took important steps toward protecting consumers by passing both the Pure Food and Drug Act and the Meat Inspection Act. The two laws divided authority for food safety between the US Department of Agriculture and the Food and Drug Administration. Since then, authority and oversight have fractured even further (see figure 8.5).

Today, responsibility for ensuring US food safety is scattered across at least twelve federal departments and agencies. Responsibilities are divided in ways that make little sense, and resources often do not match responsibilities. Here are some telling examples.

Five different agencies share authority over frozen pizza, with responsibilities divided according to the type of food top-

FIGURE 8.5   A Sampling of Governmental Agencies with Partial Oversight of US Food Safety

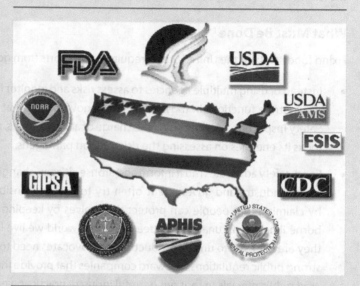

Source: Food Safety Council. Used with permission.

ping. Cheese pizza facilities are inspected by the Food and Drug Administration, and companies that make pepperoni pizza are assigned to the Food Safety Inspection Service in the Department of Agriculture.

Federal rules require on-site inspectors to be stationed at all meat-processing plants, and the Food Safety Inspection Service employs more than seven thousand inspectors to carry out this task. Meanwhile, other food-processing facilities do not require on-site inspections, so fewer than three thousand inspectors monitor sixty-five thousand domestic plants and oversee food imports. More than half of all the facilities in the United States have gone five or more years without a single inspection.

In 2010, Congress passed the Food Safety Modernization Act to begin to address longstanding problems. The Food and Drug Administration now has the authority to order mandatory recalls of tainted food (previously the recalls were voluntary). It can also conduct more frequent inspections and exercise greater control over imported foods.

But serious risks remain. For example, 80 percent of all antimicrobials sold in the United States are delivered to food animals, mostly as low-dose feed additives, for the purpose of speeding growth, increasing feed efficiency, or offsetting infection risk. For decades, farmers have been able to use these drug products without prescriptions, buying them from feed stores, even online. Since 1977, the Food and Drug Administration acknowledged that its prior approval of human antibiotics for use in animal feed constitute a threat to public health. Rather than use its authority to restrict antibiotic use in animal agriculture, however, the agency instead proposed "voluntary" guidelines. In effect, the FDA is asking the pharmaceutical industry to regulate itself, by voluntarily reducing sales of its own products for use in animal feeds.

(Continued)

(Continued)

Dubious political practices create obstacles to ensuring food safety. The food industry enjoys tremendous influence over the way government regulates safety. A revolving door enables food industry officials to move back and forth between companies and government bureaus and congressional offices throughout their careers. Presidential appointees come and go, and administrations often bring in individuals with industry experience to oversee rules and regulations that affect their former employers. Campaign contributions keep the machine well oiled, guaranteeing industry access to Congress and the executive branch.

What Must Be Done

Fixing food safety in the United States requires new efforts from government and citizen advocates alike.

- Instead of using multiple agencies to assess risks and monitor food production, a smarter alternative would concentrate functions in those parts of the government that can do the job best. For instance, the Food Safety Inspection Service could take charge of all inspections, freeing the Food and Drug Administration to focus its energies on assessing the risks of food pathogens.

- Food-safety advocates must inform and arouse citizens, changing the way we talk and think about the issue. Today, industry and government often try to shift responsibility to everyday consumers—for example, by claiming that people can protect themselves by keeping clean kitchens or by suggesting that food-borne illness is an unavoidable feature of the world we live in. But increasingly, people get sick because they are exposed to unsafe products. Food advocates need to get this message out and make the case for strong public regulations to reward companies that provide the safest food and enable adequately empowered public officials to root out harmful industry practices well before people get sick or die.

America knows enough to make our food safe. We just need to remove political obstacles and overcome governmental inefficiencies to get the job done.

Source: Excerpted from Sheingate (2012).

Our food system is global, and accordingly, our food safety policy must be global, too. Perspective 8.2 describes the magnitude of our produce imports and discusses some of the policy changes needed to ensure that our fruits and vegetables are safe.

Perspective 8.2. Produce Imports
Food & Water Watch

Americans are consuming more imported fresh fruits and vegetables, frozen and canned produce, and fruit juice than ever before (see figure 8.6). An examination of US consumption of produce that is commonly eaten as well as grown in America found that Americans' consumption of imported fresh fruits and vegetables doubled from 1993 to 2007, but border inspection has not kept pace with rising imports, and less than 1 percent of the imported produce is inspected by the federal government.

Food & Water Watch studied fifty common fruit and vegetable products, such as fresh apples, frozen broccoli, fresh tomatoes, orange juice, and frozen potatoes. Food & Water Watch found the following:

- Imports made up one out of ten fresh fruits and one out of nine fresh vegetables Americans ate in 1993 but by 2007 the import consumption share doubled to more than one out of five fresh fruits and fresh vegetables.

- The share of imported processed (canned or frozen) produce tripled, from 5.2 percent of frozen packages or cans in 1993 to 15.9 percent in 2007.

- The share of imported fruit juice (orange, apple, and grape) grew by 61 percent, from about a third of US consumption in 1993 to about half of consumption in 2007.

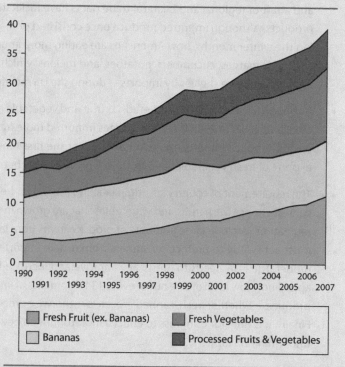

FIGURE 8.6   Total US Fresh and Processed Produce Imports (in Billions of Pounds)

Fresh Fruit (ex. Bananas)   Fresh Vegetables
Bananas   Processed Fruits & Vegetables

Source: Food & Water Watch, 2008.

- On average, each American consumed twenty pounds of imported fresh fruit, thirty-one pounds of imported fresh vegetables, and twenty-four pounds of imported processed produce, and drank three gallons of imported juice in 2007.

- Imports of fresh fruits (except bananas), fresh vegetables, and processed produce essentially tripled, rising from ten billion pounds in 1990 to thirty billion pounds in 2007.

- Imported produce was more than three times more likely to contain the illness-causing bacteria *Salmonella* and *Shigella* than domestic produce, according to an FDA survey of imported and domestic produce (Beru & Salsbury, 2002). Imported fruit was four times more likely to have illegal levels of pesticides and imported vegetables were twice as likely to have illegal levels of pesticide residues as domestic fruits and vegetables (FDA, 2008).

The hidden dangers on imported fruits and vegetables can enter US supermarkets because the FDA inspects only the tiniest fraction of imported produce. Less than 1 percent of imported fresh produce shipments were inspected at the border in recent years (US GAO, 2008).

In 2007, the FDA performed only eleven thousand border inspections on thirty-three billion pounds of imported fresh produce (US GAO, 2008). Only 3 percent of FDA's food safety funding and only 4 percent of its food safety manpower were used to monitor domestic and imported fresh produce (US GAO, 2008). Other findings include the following:

(Continued)

(Continued)

- International trade deals such as the North American Free Trade Agreement, the World Trade Organization, and a raft of regional and bilateral trade pacts have facilitated the surging imports of fruit and vegetable products. Although imported produce once consisted primarily of tropical fruits and fresh vegetables during the winter months, now Americans are eating more imported fruits and vegetables year-round. Crops such as tomatoes, cucumbers, potatoes, and melons, which can be grown in the United States, are being replaced on store shelves by imports—during the US growing season.

- Although imports have skyrocketed, US fruit and vegetable product exports had minimal growth between 1993 and 2007. In 2007 the United States imported more fresh fruit than it exported for the first time, processed produce imports exceeded exports for the first time in 2002, and the gap between imports and exports of fresh vegetables and fruit juice grew steadily between 1993 and 2007.

- The requirement of country-of-origin labeling (COOL) for fresh and frozen fruits and vegetables helps consumers choose fresh fruits and vegetables that are grown in the United States. But exemptions in the COOL regulations exclude large amounts of produce items from labeling requirements. The federal government must act swiftly to protect consumers from unsafe imported produce and stop expanding a failed trade model. The FDA needs to drastically improve and increase its inspection of imported produce above the appallingly low level of one out of every 134 shipments of imported produce. Consumers need all imported produce—whether fresh, canned, frozen, or otherwise processed—to be labeled with its country of origin. Finally, it is time for Congress to enact a moratorium on new free trade pacts that threaten consumers and undermine US farmers.

Source: Excerpted from Food & Water Watch (2008).

Food Insecurity and Nutrition Policy, 1930s to Present

The Great Depression reminded citizens that they not only needed to think about what was in their sausages but also that so many of their fellow citizens did not have enough food on the table. The fact that children were hungry in the United States—and subsequently had difficulty learning and succeeding in school—was of particular concern. Providing school lunches to students at a free or reduced cost was a direct way of supporting those students, and several cities instituted local programs. Local school boards, however, had difficulty financially subsidizing school lunches, and various New Deal programs provided federal aid for this purpose. Then in 1936 Congress passed legislation that encouraged school lunch programs to use surplus agricultural commodities, complementing previously described programs to reduce the oversupply of commodities in government reserves. The program increased profits for farmers and provided food to children in need (Poppendieck, 1985). Legislation was introduced in 1946, largely because of malnutrition-related health issues found in many World War II military recruits, to permanently authorize the school lunch program and to prescribe minimum calorie requirements (see figure 8.7).

The Food Stamp program, now known as the Supplemental Nutrition Assistance Program (SNAP), was similarly initiated in the late 1930s; it lasted at first for four years. The legislation finally became permanent when President Lyndon Johnson signed the Food Stamp Act of 1964. Whereas originally participants received paper coupons, today benefits are electronic. Participation, based on income, waxes and wanes due to economic conditions and legislative tweaks to the program. SNAP allows participants to buy any food or food product excepting hot food, whether considered healthy or otherwise, from a certified retailer.

The final major federal food system program to mention is the Special Supplemental Food Program for Women, Infants, and Children (WIC), which was introduced as a temporary program in 1972 and became permanent in 1975. Congress had determined that pregnant women, infants, and young children were at special risk for physical and mental health problems because of poor or inadequate nutrition and health care. In contrast to the SNAP program, WIC specifically promotes healthy diets and has always had strong nutritional guidelines for allowable foods. Food-security–related policies are described in more detail in chapter 5.

Interwoven with addressing food security have been the USDA's efforts to provide consumers with guidance on how to maintain healthy diets through regularly issued dietary guidelines. The controversy generated over any federal nutrition advice provided by the USDA, with independent public health professionals often at odds with representatives of industry, demonstrates the magnitude of food industry power and the impact that nutrition guidance can have on an industry's bottom line (Nestle, 2007).

FIGURE 8.7 "Every Child Needs a Good School Lunch," 1941–1945

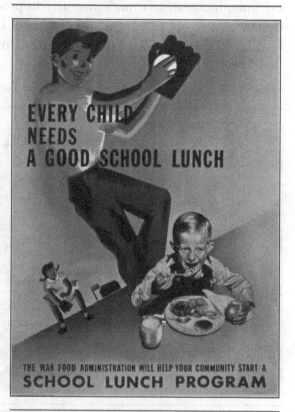

Source: National Archives. Every Child Needs a Good School Lunch, 1941–1945. Public domain.

THE POLITICS OF FOOD SYSTEM POLICY: THE FARM BILL AS AN EXAMPLE

It can be challenging to parse out what drives changes in policy. Federal funding for food security, for example, could increase because the need has become greater, because society has placed a greater priority on feeding hungry people, or because state governments, churches, and nonprofit organizations are not playing as large a role in feeding people as in previous years. In this section, we turn to a discussion of the politics of food system policy, using the Farm Bill as an example.

The majority of groups active in Farm Bill outreach and lobbying are involved in order to achieve specific policy priorities, such as increasing the financial safety net for farmers, increasing food assistance to people in poverty, or increasing wildlife habitat on agricultural lands. These divisions are further exacerbated by the structure of the Farm Bill. Similar to that of most other **omnibus bills,** it has separate **titles** (sections) for different topics. Thus farm groups focus their energy on getting funding for programs in the commodity title and crop insurance title, conservation groups focus on the conservation title, and antihunger groups focus on the nutrition title. This narrow focus contributes to

omnibus bills
Legislation covering multiple diverse or unrelated topics

titles
Similar to book chapters, but for legislation: breaking a bill into topics

advocacy success but limits the opportunity to promote policies that take the entire food system into consideration, which sometimes leads to conflicting policies. Federally subsidized crop insurance, for example, increases a farmer's incentive to produce more crops, whereas programs in the conservation title often attempt to mitigate the impact of that production. Some coalitions have formed to address broader food system issues in the Farm Bill; it will be valuable to observe their progress.

FIGURE 8.8   Pesticide Applied to Lettuce in Yuma, Arizona

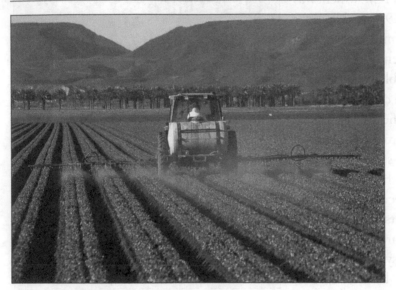

Source: USDA, Natural Resource Conservation Service. NRCSAZ02083. 2011.

An important player in the changes to food system policy that is not represented by these interest groups is *agribusiness,* a term used to generally describe the businesses engaged in producing the input supplies (including seed companies, pesticide, and fertilizer manufacturers) used on farms, and in the processing, storage, trade, and distribution of farm commodities (e.g., grain traders and processors that convert crops into food products and bioenergy). After World War II the United States experienced a proliferation of chemical inputs and explosive growth in the use of energy-intensive farm equipment (see figure 8.8) as well as dramatic growth in the size of agribusiness corporations. As these corporations increased in economic clout, they gained more influence over federal policy making as well. Further, they often promote a political agenda different from that of farmers or consumers. Many farmer groups, for example, have traditionally favored policies to stabilize commodity prices, including some form of supply management, and at a level determined to provide farmers with adequate income. As discussed previously, the programs most effective at maintaining this price stability tend to use some form of supply management.

Grain buyers, however, have financial interests in grains costing less. They have also learned how to profit from price volatility. Although the policy interests of the wide array of agribusiness companies are diverse, the overall impact of the expanded influence of this special interest group on food system policy has been profound. Commodity policy has shifted from supply management to an emphasis on opening up new markets for farm products, including international exports and new opportunities in bioenergy such as ethanol. US farmers now produce, for example, about eleven billion bushels of corn, far more than can be consumed by its traditional use as a livestock feed, and research-driven expansion into other uses for corn, such as ethanol and high fructose corn syrup, have taken up some of the excess supply. Despite these changes, the Farm Bill continues to focus its programs on influencing farmer behavior and consumer behavior, and rarely recognizes the impact that agribusiness has on the food system.

HOW POLICY DRIVES THE FUTURE FOOD SYSTEM: THE ROLE OF PRICE

Perhaps the most important—and least understood—aspect of food system policy is how policy drives the future decisions of farmers, agribusiness, food retailers, and consumers. Some decisions have a short time horizon—the decisions that a grocery shopper makes today may affect what his or her family has for dinner later in the week. Other decisions have an impact for years—a farmer that buys a new corn combine harvester has likely committed to growing corn for many years into the future. And still other decisions have a huge impact potentially for decades—a corporation that decides to site a large corn wet milling facility (a plant to separate corn kernels into parts for different uses) in a town will likely affect the local economy, the nearby air quality, and the cropping decisions of local farmers far into the future.

A central factor in nearly all of these decisions is price. In these examples, low corn prices might make the farmer less likely to invest in the new combine, make the corporation more likely to invest in a new wet mill, and make the grocery shopper more likely to purchase products such as corn tortillas and meat from corn-fed livestock. Even if policy contributes to slight deviations in price, the impacts could snowball to create major changes in the food system. A credible argument can be made that policy drivers contributed to corn prices averaging well below the farmers' cost of production in recent decades (USDA, 2013c), which incentivized the use of corn rather than grass as an animal feed, high fructose corn syrup rather than cane sugar as a sweetener, and corn-based ethanol as a fuel additive. These policy-driven shifts in the agricultural economy distort future investment, research, and infrastructure and lessen the industry's responsiveness to future price changes. The 2008 food crisis and the sharp rise in corn prices provide such an example. The skyrocketing corn prices created challenges for large-confinement livestock farmers, yet most of these farmers could not even consider a shift to feeding their animals grass, because they had invested heavily in buildings and equipment dedicated to feeding animals corn.

There are five primary mechanisms by which food system policies affect prices and subsequently affect investment and procurement decisions made by farmers, food businesses, and consumers.

Supply Management Programs

As described, these programs, which were an initial goal of Farm Bill policy, explicitly attempt to keep commodity prices above **price floors** or below **price ceilings**. Many commodities formerly had federal supply management programs; now sugar is the only major commodity crop for which this mechanism is used. Dairy policy also includes some supply management provisions, but those mechanisms have been diluted over several Farm Bills.

Subsidy Payments and Subsidized Crop Insurance

This may be the most widely known and controversial part of the Farm Bill. Subsidies have received criticism for deadening the price signals that farmers would receive from market forces. These government payments to farmers are based on a complicated array of policies, but the overall impact is to pay farmers largely based on the bushels of commodity produced or acreage historically planted in certain crops, and for subsidized crop insurance to (some would say inordinately) reduce farmers' risk in commodity crop production. It logically follows that if farmers receive payments for commodity crops such as corn, soybeans, wheat, and cotton—and do not receive payments for specialty crops such as fruits and vegetables—then farmers will grow more of the commodity crops than they would in a market without this interference. Studies have countered, however, that the impact of these payments is negligible or much smaller than often assumed (Ray & Schaffer, 2007; Wise, 2004), as is described in focus 7.2. Subsidies for **conservation practices** and other **public goods** can also

price floors
Price levels used in supply management policies that designate the price which an agricultural commodity should not go below

price ceilings
Price levels used in supply management policies that designate the price which an agricultural commodity should not go above

conservation practices
Farming practices that reduce loss of soil and water and often improve their quality

public goods
Benefits, such as clean air and public libraries, for which it is not possible to exclude only some people and for which one person's usage does not reduce availability for others

affect price, because land that is taken out of production for conservation may reduce overall crop production and subsequently increase commodity prices.

Creating New Demand for Agricultural and Food Products

As supply management grew out of favor since the 1980s, the federal government has shifted its focus toward maintaining adequate commodity prices by expanding demand for commodities. Some of the most well-known market expansion efforts came from **checkoff** programs, which are essentially government-facilitated taxes on commodities that raise funds for outreach and promotion of the commodity. "Got Milk" and "Beef. It's What's for Dinner" are two checkoff-funded advertising slogans heavily promoted by industry that became part of popular culture. The Farm Bill also contains other marketing programs to support fruits and vegetables and farmers markets. As described in chapter 10, marketing interventions more broadly can affect food demand and thus price. Although these policies support marketing, there is also a small body of policy outside the Farm Bill seeking to limit marketing of unhealthy foods.

Even with marketing, there is only so much food a person can eat, and so the two largest opportunities for greater commodity use have been in international exports and expanding the market for energy produced from organic matter (bio-based energy). Efforts to expand export opportunities for US agriculture have been mixed; the volume of US agricultural exports has not expanded dramatically since the 1980s (USDA, 2013b). By contrast, consumption of commodities for bio-based energy—primarily corn used for ethanol production—has exploded. A combination of **tax incentives**, **tariffs**, and **mandates** promoted by federal legislation has largely facilitated that growth.

Regulation

The USDA is not largely a **regulatory body**. Environmental regulation is managed by the Environmental Protection Agency and state agencies; food safety is predominantly managed by the Food and Drug Administration, state and local health agencies, and the USDA; and workplace safety is handled by the Occupational Safety and Health Administration and agencies in some states. Regulation can make certain management practices more expensive and make alternative options more attractive to industry. The regulation of water and air quality, for example, can limit a farmer's ability to use certain chemical applications that benefit production, thereby potentially affecting a farmer's cost of production. The effectiveness of regulation depends on factors including, in the language of deterrence theory, the "certainty, severity, and swiftness" of enforcement, as well as end-user understanding and how well the regulation is applied. Often national implementation is far from uniform.

Public Research

Public research has played a key role in the dramatic increases in agricultural productivity in recent decades. Public agricultural research takes place in universities, especially land grant universities, the

checkoff
Commodity checkoff programs are funds collected through small fees placed on farmers producing commodities such as corn, milk, or beef; checkoff programs fund research and promotion for their specific commodities

tax incentives
Policies that aim to incentivize behavior change by reducing the amount of taxes paid (or providing exemptions) for those who make change

tariffs
Taxes levied on goods as they enter a country

mandates
Policies that use incentives or penalties to encourage certain actions across an industry, such as the renewable fuels standard, which requires a certain level of renewable fuel use in the United States

regulatory body
An agency or other government entity mandated under the terms of a legislative act to ensure compliance with its provisions

USDA, and also on farms and in communities, through partnerships. Research is conducted in nearly every area of the food system.

Much research has concentrated on ways to improve productivity and reduce costs in industrial agriculture. Such research is considered a key contributor to US agriculture's remarkable gains in total productivity—a 170 percent increase between 1948 and 2008 (USDA, 2013a). Indeed, agricultural economists have consistently estimated a 40 to 60 percent return for every dollar invested in public agricultural research (Muller & Pursell, 2012). These gains, although helpful at times to farmers, have provided substantial benefit to the companies that could take advantage of the expanding supply by purchasing commodities more cheaply. Accordingly, much food and agricultural research, including at public institutions, is supported by corporate funds (Food & Water Watch, 2012).

Public research also affects business investment decisions. The majority of crop research is conducted on commodity crops. For example, specialty crops comprise about half of total agricultural sales but receive only 14 percent of public research expenditures. To the extent this disparity makes it more profitable to produce commodity crops and more affordable to purchase them, it incentivizes farmers to grow more commodity crops, and contributes to agribusinesses' motivations to find ever more ways of using these crops. Public research emphasis on commodity crops has also likely contributed to the use of certain farm management practices, such as raising animals in confinement facilities (which use corn and soybeans as the primary feedstock) at the expense of practices considered more sustainable, such as intensive grazing (as described in chapter 12).

• • •

There is inadequate attention to these five policy opportunities for affecting prices and thus shaping the future food system. Take the example of antibiotics administered to farm animals. Straightforward approaches, such as Congress legislating the regulation of agricultural antibiotic use or the FDA taking its own regulatory action, have faced barriers because of industry opposition. Even if regulations emerge, they may be watered down to a point that public health advocates would find unacceptable.

An alternative legislative approach could emphasize increasing funds for public research on grass-fed livestock and other practices that tend to use fewer antibiotics. Such an approach could eventually reduce the price premium for antibiotic-free meat, though it would take some years to bear fruit. Another approach would be to support policies leading to higher prices for corn and soybeans, which would raise the input costs for raising animals in confinement. The most straightforward approach is not always the most politically expedient approach.

STATE AND LOCAL POLICY

Although this chapter focuses primarily on federal policy, it is important to recognize the role of local and state policy in shaping food systems, as outlined in table 8.1. Advocates have increasingly looked to policy opportunities in state and local governments for multiple reasons:

- State and local governments can serve as laboratories for piloting policies that might later be scaled up.

- Sentiment in some geographic areas may be more supportive of particular policy options than at a national scale.

- State and local policies can more effectively respond to specific conditions and needs of an area.

- Some policy tools are available at state and local levels and not at the federal level.

- Federal legislative gridlock has made state and local policy work more attractive to advocates.

- The more than two hundred multistakeholder food policy councils in North America have expanded opportunities at the local level (see chapter 6).

An example of an issue that has received significant local level attention is discouraging sugar-sweetened beverage (SSB) consumption through taxes or restrictions (see also: chapter 7). Although federal legislation to tax SSBs has been challenged by the strong lobbying effort of the food industry, moving the debate to the state and local levels means the sugary beverage industry must prepare numerous counter-campaigns rather than only one. The Healthy Food Financing Initiative is one policy that originated at the state level (Pennsylvania) and is now scaled up to federal policy. This initiative provides financing to supermarkets to incentivize them to locate in underserved areas.

Another type of policy addresses agricultural land. Several states have anticorporate farming laws that limit the ability of corporations to own farmland, as well as incentives for organic agriculture and farmland conservation. Tax policy is likely one of the most important state policy drivers of the food system, because property taxes often inadvertently disincentivize agricultural land ownership and incentivize urban sprawl on former farmland. Additionally, many localities have been active in zoning policy to open opportunities for urban agriculture.

Regarding food safety, state and local health agencies serve at the front lines for prevention and response. Local health departments are responsible for food inspections in restaurants, grocery stores, day-care facilities, hospitals, schools, and some manufacturing plants. Food safety efforts can only be as successful as the implementation, outreach, and education provided by their respective state and local governments.

A final component at the state level is the implementation of many federal policies. Though nutrition programs such as SNAP and WIC are federally funded, they are implemented by state (both) and local (WIC) governments, and state rules can affect participant eligibility and level of support. State-level innovations, such as allowing participants to spend their funds in farmers markets, have proliferated.

Although state and local policy making has emerged as a primary area for food system efforts, there are also limitations compared to trying to enact changes at the national level, including the fact that these policies may be preempted by federal policies (see focus 8.3), the risk that inequalities across states may be exacerbated, and the need to stretch advocacy resources to multiple legislative arenas (although, it is not a zero-sum game, and these efforts may also tap new pools of supporters).

FOCUS 8.3. PREEMPTION AND LOCAL FOOD AND AGRICULTURE POLICIES

Lainie Rutkow and Jennifer L. Pomeranz

Law influences the food system in countless ways at the federal, state, and local levels. The US legal system determines where food growers and producers are located, the sanitation standards under which foods are manufactured, and the parameters for advertising food. Because states and localities tend to have differing concerns, their laws may vary in areas such as zoning and land-use regulation.

States and localities may, however, find that their efforts to regulate the food system are limited by a legal doctrine called **preemption**. Preemption occurs when a higher level of government limits actions that can be taken by a lower level (Rutkow, Vernick, Hodge, & Teret, 2008). Preemption derives from the US Constitution's Supremacy Clause, which states that federal law is the country's

preemption
Limitation by a higher level of government on what actions can be taken by a lower level of government

highest law. Thus, the federal government can preempt, or prevent, states and localities from regulating in particular areas. State governments can similarly prevent localities from acting. When a preemptive law is enacted, states or localities may be unable to respond to their communities' specific health or safety concerns (Pomeranz, Teret, Sugarman, Rutkow, & Brownell, 2009).

Preemption has advantages and disadvantages. Through preemption, the federal government can ensure consistent national laws versus a patchwork of state and local laws. This is desirable when a single standard is beneficial (e.g., federal safety standards that require disclosure of common food allergens on packaging [42 USC. §§ 343 et seq.]), or when states or localities might enact weak regulations not adequate to protect the public. But preemption may frustrate states and localities, particularly if it prevents them from addressing issues faced by their constituents (O'Reilly, 2006). Sometimes localities may want stricter regulations than those established by a state or federal government, but preemption prohibits this. Additionally, preemption can curtail localities' innovative approaches, including those relevant to the food system (e.g., menu labeling and regulation of confined animal feeding operations [CAFOs]).

A useful lens to examine preemption is through the challenges preemption has posed for localities seeking to regulate CAFOs. As described in chapter 12, the EPA noted public health harms associated with CAFOs, including water, soil, and air pollution attributable to "mismanagement of wastes" such as manure (US Environmental Protection Agency, 2012). When individuals learn of a CAFO planned for their community, they may seek local regulation. However, state preemption of local law sometimes nullifies these efforts. For example, in 2001 the board of supervisors in Worth County, Iowa, passed the Rural Health and Family Farm Protection Ordinance (*Worth County Friends of Agric. v. Worth County [Worth County]*, 2004). The ordinance regulated air emissions, indoor air quality, and water monitoring for the county's CAFOs. Agricultural organizations challenged the ordinance, arguing that Iowa law preempted it.

In 2004 the Iowa Supreme Court concluded that Worth County's ordinance was preempted by state law, noting that "our legislature intended livestock production in Iowa to be governed by statewide regulation, not local regulation" (*Worth County*, 2004). Courts have similarly determined that local efforts to regulate CAFOs were preempted in Kansas, North Carolina, and Minnesota (*Board of Sup'rs of Crooks Tp., Renville County v. ValAdCo*, 1993; *Craig v. County of Chatham*, 2002; *David v. Board of Com'rs of Norton County*, 2004). State laws, however, vary in the extent to which they preempt local efforts to regulate CAFOs. Because not all state laws on a particular subject will preempt local governments' ability to regulate in that area, it is important for localities to understand what, if any, latitude they have when drafting ordinances. For example, a Missouri appellate court ruled that local ordinances that regulate CAFOs to protect the public's health are not preempted by state law (*Borron v. Farrenkopf*, 1999).

Advocates should work with lawyers who understand the nuances of relevant state laws. Attorneys can provide advice about whether an ordinance is likely to be preempted and guidance about language that may withstand a preemption-based legal challenge. Pertschuk and colleagues published a framework that details the questions grassroots advocates should consider when facing preemption, which may serve as a useful resource for localities (Pertschuk, Pomeranz, Aoki, Larkin, & Paloma, 2013). Although preemption of food and agriculture ordinances may limit communities' regulatory options in some states, opportunities exist in other states for local legal action in a wide variety of areas, including agricultural zoning, pesticide usage, and food safety and sanitation. By working with lawyers to understand a state's preemption of local regulation, localities may be better able to enact legally permissible ordinances that address the public health challenges that modern food systems raise for their communities.

CONCLUSION

Look at the juggernaut of food systems policy and it would be easy to conclude there are too many forces maintaining inertia in the system to truly change it. This chapter's example of so-far unsuccessful efforts to legislate the use of antibiotics in livestock production demonstrates that progress can be slow.

Yet there are also plenty of examples of rapid policy change, often in response to perceived crises in the food system. *The Jungle* instigated food safety legislation in 1906, and the Great Depression and Dust Bowl instigated Farm Bill legislation in the 1930s.

Individuals, too, can make a difference. High school students frustrated with the quality of school lunches have been instrumental in making policy change at all levels, from the school district to federal policy, and college students have worked for changes in campus food (see focus 18.3). Most often, policy change happens through the concerted and strategic efforts of multiple individuals and organizations. Successful policy advocacy often requires developing proposals attractive to people with many different perspectives, rather than only the already converted. It also helps to prepare well, marshaling resources, scientific evidence, and effective arguments, enabling rapid response on that future day when a crisis does arise.

Change is possible, in other words, but patience is necessary. After all, crisis is virtually certain. Issues already affecting food systems and thus the public's health—and likely to drive future policy change—include climate change, the obesity epidemic, high fossil fuel prices, and the continued economic concentration of the agribusiness industry.

SUMMARY

Federal legislation currently does not lend itself to thinking of the food system as a whole. An array of policies has been developed instead to support the abundant production of food and address impacts of food production, processing, transportation, and consumption. The intersections between government policy and food systems are extensive and complex and occur at multiple levels from local to state to federal to global. This chapter focuses primarily on US federal-level policy, with a particular emphasis on the Farm Bill, and also provides more in-depth discussion on topics such as farmer income, food safety, food security, and public health. Although federal policy draws the most advocacy activity, other jurisdictions may be more appropriate for some food systems efforts. Policy change is often slow, yet it also develops—albeit in fits and starts—when Congress perceives that a crisis needs to be addressed. Many other factors affect policy change, including advocacy and lobbying from stakeholders, the economic climate, public perceptions about the role of government, and other issues that compete for the attention of policy makers.

KEY TERMS

Agenda setting

Appropriations bills

Authorizing legislation

Chairman's mark

Checkoff

Commodity

Conservation practices

Entitlement program

Farm state

Jurisdiction

Mandates

Omnibus bills

Preemption

Price ceilings

Price floors

Public goods

Reauthorization

Regulatory body

Renewal cycles

Reporting out

Senior Farmers' Market Nutrition Program

Special interests

Supply management policies

Tariffs

Tax incentives

Titles

Window of opportunity

DISCUSSION QUESTIONS

1. Consider a potential piece of food system legislation, such as increasing access to healthy foods or reducing agriculture's impact on natural resources. What constituencies would support your initiative? What messages or strategies would help draw support from atypical allies?

2. The USDA administers antihunger programs including SNAP, WIC, and the National School Lunch Program. These were created at different points in time and address different target populations. Consider the challenges and benefits of having multiple antihunger programs. What policy reforms could make these programs more efficient?

3. Farm programs have changed significantly since the New Deal, most notably when most commodity programs shifted from policies maintaining prices at a level that supported farmers, to policies that subsidized farmers when prices were too low. How do these changes in policy affect farm size and the types of crops grown? What would happen if all government intervention in commodities was eliminated?

REFERENCES

Ackerman, L., Bustos, D., & Muller, M. (2012). *Disadvantaged farmers: Addressing inequalities in federal programs for farmers of color*. Retrieved from www.iatp.org/files/04_DisadvantagedFarmers_f.pdf%20

Beru, N., & Peter, A., & Salsbury, P. A. (2002,). FDA's produce safety activities. *Food Safety Magazine* (February–March).

Birkland, T. (2005). *An introduction to the policy process: Theories, concepts, and models of public policy making* (2nd. ed.). New York: M. E. Sharp.

Board of Sup'rs of Crooks Tp., Renville County v. ValAdCo (Minn. App. 1993).

Borron v. Farrenkopf, 5 S.W.3d 618 (Mo. App. 1999).

Buck, S., & Yandle, B. (2001). *Bootleggers, Baptists, and the global warming battle*. Retrieved from http://ssrn.com/abstract= 279914

Craig v. County of Chatham, 565 S.E.2d 172 (N.C. 2002).

David v. Board of Com'rs of Norton County, 89 P.3d 893 (Kan. 2004).

Food & Water Watch. (2009). *The poisoned fruit of American trade policy*. Retrieved from www.foodandwaterwatch.org/tools-and-resources/the-poisoned-fruit-of-american-trade-policy

Food & Water Watch. (2012). *Public research, private gain: Corporate influence over university agricultural research.* Retrieved from www.foodandwaterwatch.org/tools-and-resources/public-research-private-gain-corporate-influence-over-university-agriculture

Grynbaum, M. (2013). In N.A.A.C.P., industry gets ally against soda ban. *New York Times,* January 23. Retrieved from www.nytimes.com/2013/01/24/nyregion/fight-over-bloombergs-soda-ban-reaches-courtroom.html?_r=0

Kingdon, J. (2002). *Agendas, alternatives, and public policies* (2nd. ed.). New York: Longman.

Kraft, M., & Furlong, S. (2007). *Public policy: Politics, analysis, and alternatives* (2nd. ed.). Washington, DC: CQ Press.

Levins, R. A. (2003). *Willard Cochrane and the American family farm.* Lincoln: University of Nebraska Press.

McCombs, M. (2005). The agenda setting function of the press. In G. Overholser & K. H. Jamieson (Eds.), *The institutions of American democracy: The press* (pp. 156–168). New York: Oxford University Press.

Muller, M., & Pursell, M. (2012). *Making public agriculture work for the public: Research and the Farm Bill.* Retrieved from www.iatp.org/documents/making-public-agricultural-research-work-for-the-public-research-and-the-farm-bill

Muller, M., Tagtow, A., Roberts, S., & MacDougall, E. (2009). Aligning food system policies to advance public health. *Journal of Hunger and Environmental Nutrition, 4,* 225–240.

Nestle, M. (2007). *Food politics: How the food industry influences nutrition and health.* Berkeley: University of California Press.

O'Reilly, J. T. (2006). *Federal preemption of state and local law.* Chicago: American Bar Association.

Pertschuk, M., Pomeranz, J. L., Aoki, J. R., Larkin, M. A., & Paloma, M. (2013). Assessing the impact of federal and state preemption in public health: A framework for decision makers. *Journal of Public Health Management and Practice, 19*(3), 213–219.

Pomeranz, J. L., Teret, S. P., Sugarman, S. D., Rutkow, L., & Brownell, K. D. (2009). Innovative legal approaches to address obesity. *Milbank Quarterly, 87*(1), 185–213.

Poppendeick, J. (1985). *Breadlines knee-deep in wheat: Food assistance in the Great Depression.* Rutgers, NJ: Rutgers University Press.

Ray, D. E., & Schaffer, H. D. (2007). How U.S. farm policies in the mid-1990s affected international crop prices: A harbinger of what to expect with further world-wide implementation of WTO-compliant policy modifications. In K. Niek & P. Pinstrup-Andersen (Eds.), *Agricultural trade liberalization and the least developed countries.* Wageningen UR Frontis Series, Vol. 19. Dordrecht, The Netherlands: Springer.

Roswell, M., & Bowman, D. (2013). *The Farm Bill primer.* Retrieved from www.farmbillprimer.org

Rutkow, L., Vernick, J. S., Hodge, J. G., & Teret, S. P. (2008). Preemption and the obesity epidemic: State and local menu labeling laws and the Nutrition Labeling and Education Act. *Journal of Law, Medicine, and Ethics, 36*(4), 772–789.

Simon, M. (2012). *Are corporations profiting from hungry Americans?* Retrieved from www.eatdrinkpolitics.com/wp-content/uploads/FoodStampsFollowtheMoneySimon.pdf

Stone, D. (2001). *Policy paradox: The art of political decision making.* New York: W. W. Norton.

Sheingate, A. (2012). Still a jungle. *Democracy: A Journal of Ideas, 25*(9), 48–59.

US Environmental Protection Agency. (2012). *How do CAFOs impact the environment?* Retrieved from www.epa.gov/region7/water/cafo/cafo_impact_environment.htm

US Department of Agriculture, Economic Research Service. (2013a.) *Overview of agricultural productivity in the United States.* Retrieved from www.ers.usda.gov/data-products/agricultural-productivity-in-the-us.aspx

US Department of Agriculture, Economic Research Service. (2013b). *Summary of exports shares of the volume of U.S. agricultural production* (Table 2). Retrieved from www.ers.usda.gov/topics/international-markets-trade/us-agricultural-trade/export-share-of-production.aspx#.UURj1UqeCcx

US Department of Agriculture, Economic Research Service. (2013c). *Commodity costs and returns: Overview.* Retrieved from www.ers.usda.gov/data-products/commodity-costs-and-returns.aspx

US Food and Drug Administration, Center for Food Safety and Applied Nutrition. (2008). *Pesticide monitoring program 2004–2006: Results and Discussion FY 2006*. Retrieved from www.fda.gov/Food/FoodborneIllnessContaminants /Pesticides/ucm125183.htm

US General Accountability Office. (2008). *Food safety: Improvements needed in FDA oversight of fresh produce. GAO-08–1047*. Retrieved from www.gao.gov/products/GAO-08–1047

Wise, T. (2004). *The paradox of agricultural subsidies: Measurement issues, agricultural dumping, and policy reform* (GDAE Working Paper 04–02). Somerville, MA. Retrieved from www.ase.tufts.edu/gdae/pubs/wp/04–02agsubsidies.pdf

Worth County Friends of Agric. v. Worth County, 688 N.W.2d 257 (Iowa 2004).

Chapter 9

Food, Culture, and Society

Sarah Chard and Erin G. Roth

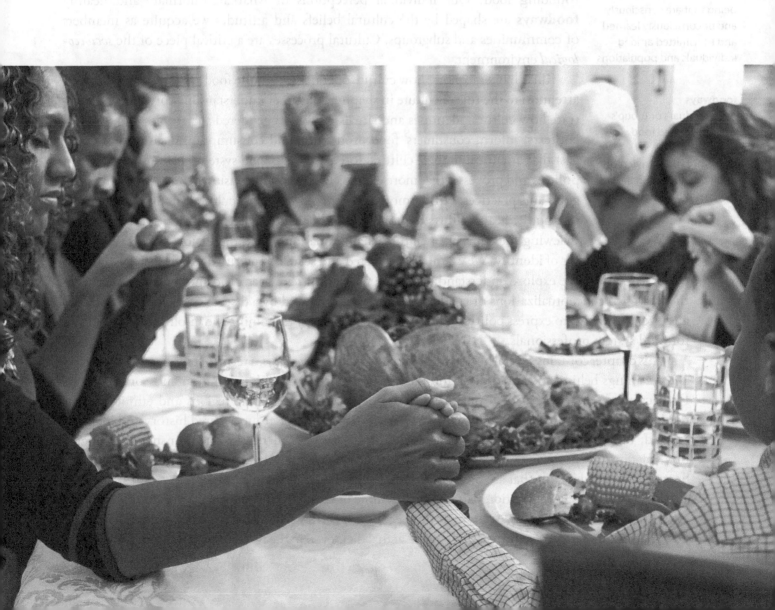

Learning Objectives

- Understand culture as a powerful but contested and modifiable influence on individuals' foodways, their beliefs about the relationship between food and health, and their assumptions regarding gender and food.

- Identify how food serves as a vehicle for establishing identity and group belonging and is a tool for reinforcing a group's values and expectations.

- Recognize how cultural beliefs about gender and gender roles influence food preferences and practices.

- Understand foodways as expressions of political ideology and their role in social movements.

culture
Beliefs, behaviors, traditions, customs, and other ways of being that are consciously and unconsciously learned and transmitted among individuals and populations

foodways
An individual's or group's culturally based food preparation and consumption behaviors and traditions, including the material production of food

Culture is a powerful though often invisible force within food systems. Human groups develop complex meanings, behaviors, customs, traditions, and rituals surrounding food. Our individual perceptions of what are "normal" and healthy **foodways** are shaped by the cultural beliefs and attitudes we acquire as members of communities and subgroups. Cultural processes are a critical piece of the *socioecological* environment.

This chapter explores how culture operates within the food system, with particular attention to the role of culture in shaping consumer understandings of food. We illustrate how cultural identities and rituals, as well as gendered social roles and political contexts, inform consumers' food production and consumption decisions. We suggest that attention to these cultural forces can help food system professionals develop policies and processes that more effectively respond to consumers' ever-changing food goals and practices. Furthermore, deeper recognition of cultural foodways can facilitate public health efforts to modify individual and societal consumption patterns.

We begin by reviewing the concept of culture, the foundation of this discussion. Next, we explore how food is a marker of identity. We examine how sacred and secular food rituals teach social values and preserve identity. We explore understandings of the relationship between food and health. The chapter then turns to conceptualizations of gender and foodways, followed by a discussion of food movements and the use of food to express political ideology. We conclude by examining the implications of culture for food system professionals.

This chapter contains several key themes regarding cultural *foodways,* a term that refers to the decisions and meanings behind food traditions and the material culture of food preparation and consumption. First, cultural variations in food practices are common across geographic regions and ethnic groups; these food practices often become prominent markers of a region or group's shared history and identity. Second, humans continually adapt their learned food practices in response to transnational migration, media, and popular trends. Third, many persons hold strong beliefs regarding the relationship between food and health that are based on cultural principles and personal experience. Cultural norms also label foods and consumption patterns as masculine or feminine and inform understandings of food responsibilities across genders. At the same time, economic and environmental contexts—especially work demands—can critically influence individuals' actual diets even in the presence of strong cultural beliefs.

CULTURE AND FOOD

Culture commonly refers to "traditions and customs transmitted through learning that guide the beliefs and behaviors of the people exposed to them" (Kottak, 2006, p. 4). Although our palates are highly individual, social interactions impart expectations regarding appropriate tastes. Food norms and preferences are taught within the home starting in infancy and are further informed by peers, schools, and media. These learned beliefs about what is or is not food and "correct" taste experiences often remain throughout adulthood. In addition, because beliefs, values, and behaviors are often internalized, they may seem wholly instinctual or "natural" and biologically predetermined (Bourdieu, 1990). Entomophagy (eating insects), for example, is uncommon and perhaps even repulsive to many in North America, but related arthropods such as crabs and lobster are considered a delicacy (see figure 9.1). That one person's visceral "yuck" is another person's equally visceral "yum" demonstrates how food preferences are strongly influenced by the experiences of early life.

Although cultural forces serve to maintain food practices over time, cultures change within and across generations. The increasing popularity of sushi throughout the United States is one example of changing food norms (Mintz, 2002). Cultural practices also are contested—that is, individuals may violate norms for personal, social, or political reasons. Thus, culture is a powerful but flexible influence on foodways. Perspective 9.1 presents the example of white bread, showing how our attitudes toward this product have evolved over time and how we can read into these attitudes to derive insights about the broader culture.

FIGURE 9.1   Bugs and Scorpions in Market, China

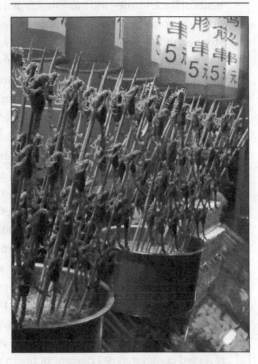

Source: istolethetv. "Mostly scorpions." 2006. https://www.flickr.com/photos/istolethetv/3189658885.

Perspective 9.1. Beyond White Bread, a Better Society?

Aaron Bobrow-Strain

Most foodie discourse assumes that once people have knowledge about the difference between "good" and "bad" food, along with improved access to the former, they will automatically change their diets. But what about those who know and could change, but don't? I wrote a book about ultrasoft, mass-produced, sliced white bread because I wanted to understand America's fraught relationship to industrial eating in all its contradictory ferment. We no longer get 25 to 30 percent of our daily calories from bread. But anyone paying attention to the rising cries for slow, local, organic, and healthful food will find America's battles over bread surprisingly fresh.

Over the last one hundred years, few foods have been as revered and reviled as industrial white bread. When Americans connect the decline of mom's home-baked bread with a loss of moral virtue, as they have periodically since the 1840s, they are also making claims about the proper place of women in society. When

(Continued)

(Continued)

industrial tycoons of the late 1800s lauded inexpensive white bread churned out by factories as a foundation for social harmony, they were also arguing against labor organizing and government regulation. When proponents of back-to-the-land movements of the 1850s and 1960s rejected dreams of industrial abundance, praising hearty, whole wheat bread baked on independent family farms as a bedrock of American democracy, they rarely stopped to ask who got left out of this invariably white, propertied vision.

As with today's calls for food justice (focused primarily on consumers' unequal access to safe, healthy food), bygone battles over what bread Americans should eat contained uplifting visions of the connection between good food and strong communities, insightful critiques of unsustainable status quos, and earnest desires to make the world a better place. Efforts to reform American bread habits have also been replete with smug paternalism, misdirected anxieties, sometimes neurotic obsessions with health, narrow visions of what counts as "good food," and open discrimination against people who choose "bad food."

For foodies in America today, yesteryear refers to a time when everyone grew up instinctively knowing the difference between "real" and "fake" food—wisdom we seem to have lost. This attitude has crystallized in a popular axiom: if your great-grandmother wouldn't recognize it as food, don't eat it. It's a simple, homey rule with immediate nostalgic appeal. But what if great-grandmother was just as conflicted about food as we are? As a young mother in the 1910s and 1920s, my great-grandmother Farrell baked twelve to sixteen loaves of bread a week for seven children. She enjoyed the sense of community when neighbors crowded into her kitchen on baking day. Her husband insisted on homemade bread. Store-bought loaves were just "sacks of hot air," he proclaimed—and expensive, too. Yet, by the early 1930s, the family bought its bread.

No one remembers why the Farrells switched, but they were not alone. In 1890, 90 percent of the country's bread was baked in homes. The rest was purchased from tiny neighborhood bakeries. By 1930, this trend had reversed completely: 90 percent of bread was purchased, and purchased from increasingly large, increasingly distant factories. Despite their success, industrial bakers lived in constant fear that bread would lose its place on the nation's tables. Compared with newfangled fruit arriving by refrigerated train or the novelty of modern wonders such as Jell-O, bread was just basic. But something remarkable happened during the first three decades of the twentieth century. Not only did Americans switch to store-bought bread but also per-capita bread consumption increased.

Food politics in the 1920s and 1930s in the United States were distinguished by heated debates over what bread the country should eat. Legions of food reformers, social workers, public health officials, advertising executives, and an astonishing number of diet gurus worked frantically to convince Americans that choosing the wrong bread would lead to serious problems. Some pinpointed newfangled loaves as the source of cancer, diabetes, criminal delinquency, tuberculosis, kidney failure, overstimulated nervous systems, and even "white race suicide." Others heralded modern bread as a savior, delivering the nation from drudgery, hunger, and dangerous contagions carried by unscientific bread.

But they could all agree on one thing: incorrect food choices were the root cause of nearly all of the nation's moral, physical, and social problems. So, in a fashion reminiscent of many community-garden and antiobesity campaigns today, well-meaning reformers poured into the country's urban tenements to spread "the gospel of good eating." What happened next entangled choice of bread with high-stakes questions of race, responsibility, and citizenship. Small immigrant-run bakeries came under intense scrutiny, with sanitary inspectors and women's groups painting pictures of dank, vermin-infested cellar workrooms where sewage dripped into dough-mixing troughs.

Even that sentimental icon of all that is good—"mother's bread"—was denounced under the banner of a safe and efficient diet. *Scientific American,* women's magazines, and home economics textbooks portrayed careless home baking as a threat to family health, while other observers wondered whether even the most careful housewife should bake at all.

Whether or not bread from small bakeries and home ovens was actually unsanitary—it probably wasn't—anxiety over unclean bread was a gift for industrial bakers (see figure 9.2). "I want to know where my bread comes from!" an affluent woman demanded in a national advertising campaign. Strange as it might seem, especially to contemporary foodies, the language of "knowing where your food comes from" was a publicity coup for industrial food.

The question of what to eat can't be contained in easy rules or glossed through the assumption that "if you only knew how evil your processed foods were, you would change." What remains to be seen is whether foodies can effectively counter these affective attachments to industrial eating—create new dreams of good food—without reinforcing the stark social inequalities of elite consumerism. When making the food system better is understood largely in terms of an enlightened "us" helping an uneducated "them" access "good food" (i.e., not white bread), we miss the real root causes of our dietary crises—not consumer ignorance, but soaring inequality, declining prospects for large segments of the population, and concentration of power in the food industry.

Source: Excerpted from Bobrow-Strain (2012).

FIGURE 9.2   "In Homes Where Children Are Well-Cared-For, You Will Usually Find Bond Bread," 1928 advertisement

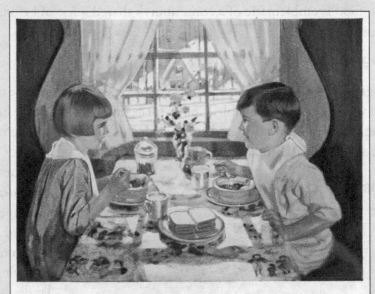

In homes where children are well-cared-for,
you will usually find Bond Bread

A FRIENDLY loaf, brown-crusted, firm, deliciously home-like. How their appetites quicken at the thought of its goodness! In what an agreeable form it brings to them the food elements necessary to healthy growth!

And mothers enjoy the happy knowledge that the bread their children like best nourishes sturdy frames and vigorous muscles. The richness of its flavor, its inviting aroma when toasting, tell of pure

and wholesome ingredients. Of such only is Bond Bread made. In the uniform excellence of each loaf is the assurance of thorough, perfect baking. That's why the children in more than a million homes find Bond Bread a daily temptation to be cheerful and healthy.

Bond
The *home-like* bread

© 1928 G. B. C.

November 1928 Good Housekeeping

Source: Public domain.

The following section explores how group identity is expressed and revealed through foodways. We focus on two of the more prominent influences on foodways—region and ethnicity. Through examples, we demonstrate how food traditions and preferences become imbued with individual and collective meaning. We then explore how sacred and secular food rituals teach and reinforce these meanings and identity.

FOODWAYS AND IDENTITY

The phrase "we are what we eat" describes the power of food as a marker of one's identity. Communities that share an identity based on geographical region or ethnicity frequently use foodways to establish lines of inclusion and exclusion (Kalcik, 1992). For example, for those who grew up in the historically German town of Evansville, Indiana, batter-fried brain sandwiches are a powerful marker of place and community. Still served in taverns locally, ordering foods such as specially prepared offal (organ meat) indicates an individual is an insider in part *because* offal is reviled by many outsiders. Beyond sustenance, then, food is emblematic of a community's shared sense of belonging.

Geographic Regional Identity

Geography heavily influences foodways; the types of food people traditionally prepare often derive from what was historically available. Chiles, for example, thrive in the hot climate of the southwestern United States. Human innovation and creativity led to the development of the Southwest's unique red or green chile sauce and accompanying cuisine.

FIGURE 9.3　Crabs

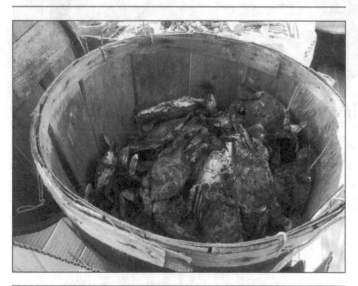

Source: Rashida S. Mar B. Flickr Commons.

The blue crab is an important symbol of coastal Maryland, a region defined by the Chesapeake Bay. People gather around paper-covered tables, piled with steaming, Old Bay seasoning–encrusted crabs (see figure 9.3). Knowing how to eat a crab connects Marylanders with each other. Picking crabs is tedious and time consuming, yet many Marylanders relish crab feasts as a time to socialize with friends and family, usually accompanied by several pitchers of "Natty Boh" (National Bohemian, a local beer). Although much of the blue crab meat eaten in Maryland today is imported from Southeast Asia due to pollution and overfishing in the Chesapeake Bay, the symbolism of the blue crab remains strong. Indeed, Marylanders' identification with the crab and crab feasts has galvanized support for antipollution campaigns (Paolisso, 2007).

Ethnic Identity

An ethnic group is a group of people who perceive a shared ancestry or a common cultural, religious, linguistic, political, or geographic heritage. Persons who share an ethnic identity may have common foodways traditions. It is important, however, not to presuppose an individual's beliefs and practices based on ethnicity.

Ethnic foods serve as a material tie to the past, real or idealized. For immigrants, maintaining food traditions is a way to preserve memories of home (D'Sylva & Beagan, 2011; Mankekar, 2005) and to resist assimilation (Beagan, Chapman, D'Sylva, & Bassett, 2008). Food traditions thus take on an added significance by symbolizing the preservation of culture (see, for example, figure 9.4). This is especially true for immigrant parents seeking to ensure children continue cultural traditions.

For other immigrants, however, the desire for assimilation competes with the pull of tradition. Ethnic foods may be rejected when children seek to "fit in" by consuming foods that are encouraged by media and are popular among school peers. Resolving this tension can involve a conscious or unconscious blending of customs and food preferences. For example, Arab Americans in Detroit report serving "American" Thanksgiving dishes, such as turkey, pumpkin pie, and bread stuffing with *hashwa*, a traditional Arab dish of rice, meat, and nuts (Lockwood & Lockwood, 2002).

As ethnic food traditions change through processes of assimilation, these modifications can significantly alter the nutritional content of immigrants' diets. Indeed, although sub-

FIGURE 9.4   Halal Food Store, Minneapolis

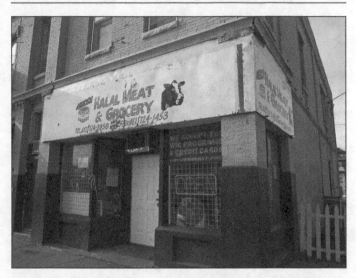

Source: Ed Kohler, 2009. https://www.flickr.com/photos/edkohler/4169867343/in/set-72157613846391752/.

group differences exist, immigrants to the United States who show higher levels of assimilation tend to have poorer diets than those who maintain more traditional lifestyles. For example, among Hispanic immigrants, assimilation is associated with lower fruit, rice, and bean consumption and higher sugar consumption (Ayala, Baquero, & Klinger, 2008). The correlation among assimilation, diet, and health, however, is complex, and multiple factors, including the availability of ingredients, work demands, and socioeconomic factors, also likely influence immigrant foodways (Creighton, Goldman, Pebley, & Chung, 2012; Fitzgerald, 2010).

The frequency with which foodways are adapted and shared indicates the flexibility of food traditions. Over the centuries food ideas have continually dispersed across ethnic groups and regions, which often results in the creation of new foodways and food meanings (Mintz, 1998). Cajun cuisine, for example, developed as French speakers from Nova Scotia moved to south Louisiana in the mid-eighteenth century, blending French traditions with Native American, African, and Latin foodways. Over many years, what was a strictly ethnic food type has taken on regional importance. Louisiana tourism offices are aware of the symbolic power of all things Cajun and that the unique style of food draws many tourists to the state (Gutierrez, 1992). Cable cooking shows and the Internet are now accelerating the diffusion and blending of food practices.

Whatever its origins, food expresses group identity and may serve to demarcate the borders between "us" and "them." At the same time, the borders between groups are constantly flexing and bending as individuals come to embrace multiple identities.

FOOD AS RITUAL

Rituals, sacred and secular, often reinforce identification with a community's social values and beliefs. Sacred or religious rituals impart a standard of morality, social values, and religious teachings. Many sacred rituals involve food as symbols. The Protestant Christian Eucharist, for example, culminates with

FIGURE 9.5   Seder Plate

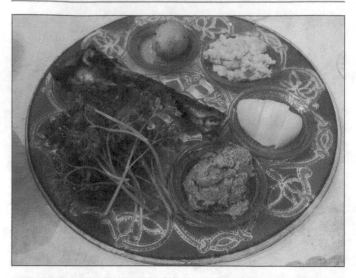

Source: Edsel Little, 2011. Passover Seder Plate http://www.flickr.com/photos/edsel_/5638974836/

the consumption of wine and bread or wafer, symbolizing Christ's blood or body. Consumption is a means for renewing one's commitment to Christ's teachings. Similarly, the food included on the Jewish seder plate serves as a reminder of Jews' enslavement in Egypt (bitter herbs), their tears (salt water), and the lamb's blood markings that spared Jewish families from the spirit of death (lamb shankbone). In the seder ritual, the message of overcoming hardship through faith is remembered and passed across generations (see figure 9.5). This link between food and faith is seen throughout history from religion to religion, as further exemplified in focus 9.1.

FOCUS 9.1. FOOD AND FAITH
Angela Smith

Numerous faith traditions speak of the theological implications of food production and consumption (see table 9.1). Sacred texts talk about eating, producing, and giving thanks for food as a spiritual act; and religious rituals and holidays celebrate and include certain foods as a central element. Laws in many religions mandate care for other people, the environment, and farm animals. For thousands of years, food cultivation and harvesting offered a spiritual experience; in many traditions, connecting with the land was/is connecting with one's creator.

As societies moved from being largely agrarian to primarily urban, the spiritual significance of agriculture diminished. That a growing number of faith communities are now rediscovering how eating relates to spiritual beliefs is merely a return to these traditions. Of course, their actions have a distinctly modern twist.

community-supported agriculture (CSA) Program in which consumers and farmers share the risks and benefits of agriculture; there are many models, but most commonly consumers pay a farmer at the beginning of a season and receive weekly produce distributions

The Baltimore Food and Faith Project of the Johns Hopkins Center for a Livable Future has been partnering with local faith communities, religious schools, and other faith-based organizations since 2007. Participating groups engage their communities in numerous ways. Some study how food and agriculture relate to religious teachings; some change institutional practices by, for example, switching to fair-trade coffee or purchasing locally grown food for events. Many have started food gardens, hosted **community-supported agriculture (CSA)** drop-off sites, and weighed in on key food-related policies. The Franciscan Center and Congregation Netivot Shalom, both in Baltimore, Maryland, provide two examples of the ways that faith communities are mobilizing to improve the food system.

TABLE 9.1   Faith Traditions and Selected Food-Related Texts

Faith Tradition	Selected Text
Buddhism	**Grace of the Bodhisattva Buddhists** This food comes from the Earth and the Sky, It is a gift from the entire universe and the fruit of much hard work; I vow to live a life which is worthy to receive it.
Christianity	**Psalms 104:10–15** You make springs gush forth in the valleys; they flow between the hills Giving drink to every wild animal … You cause the grass to grow for the cattle, and plants for people to use, to bring forth food from the earth, and wine to gladden the human heart, oil to make the face shine, and bread to strengthen the human heart.
Hinduism	**Chāndogya Upanishad 7.25.2** When one's food is pure, one's being becomes pure.
Islam	**Qu'ran 6:141** It is He who produceth gardens with trellises and without and dates and tilth with produce of all kinds and olives and pomegranates similar [in kind] and different [in variety]: eat of their fruit in their season but render the dues that are proper on the day that the harvest is gathered. But waste not by excess: for Allah loveth not the wasters.
Judaism	**Kohelet Rabbah 7:13** When the Holy One created the first man, He took him around all the trees in the Garden of Eden and said to him: See how beautiful and wonderful my works are. Everything I have created, I have created for you. Be mindful that you do not ruin or devastate my world, for if you ruin it, there is no one to repair it after you.

The Franciscan Center, founded by the Franciscan sisters of Baltimore, serves a hot lunch meal to as many as 650 people each weekday. The center's clients are often at increased risk of diet-related diseases, such as diabetes or high blood pressure. Despite this, historically the center had to serve food high in sodium, fat, and sugar, reflecting the donations it received. Realizing that people could not live up to their full potential if they weren't eating properly, the center began revamping its food service program in 2010. First, a meatless option was put on the menu each Monday. Second, the food pantry began asking donors for healthier foods. Third, the center began providing several clients with CSA shares—fresh produce to feed a family of four during the growing season (see figure 9.6). The center's late executive director,

(Continued)

(Continued)

FIGURE 9.6 Picking up a CSA Share at the Franciscan Center

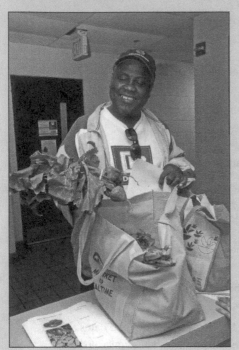

Source: Franciscan Center.

Ed McNally, liked to say that "you can't serve an unhealthy meal with a smile ... There is nothing more dignified than a nutritious meal."

Another example is the Orthodox Jewish congregation Netivot Shalom, which made environmental stewardship a priority from its establishment in 2004. One way the congregation tangibly represents its care for the earth is through a "Kiddush Garden." The garden is used to teach adults and children to nurture soil organically through the use of compost made on-site, and prepare healthy dishes for the communal gatherings that follow weekly services. The opportunity to share food grown by congregants lends a deeper spiritual meaning to the meal because participants understand the work that goes into tending a garden and are that much more grateful for its gifts. The synagogue's sense of shared purpose is also heightened in this way. Netivot Shalom further extends the connections being made to others in the greater community by inviting them to participate in the garden and by giving fresh garden produce to area food banks. The Franciscan Center and Netivot Shalom are part of a growing movement not only in Baltimore but also throughout the United States as faith communities of every size, tradition, and background work to bring about a healthier, more sustainable, and just food system.

The everyday rituals of where and with whom to eat also carry important meanings and preserve identity (Marshall, 2005). Often predictable and routinized, people frequently eat in the same places each day, for example, in front of the TV or computer, in the dining room, or even over the kitchen sink. No matter how ordinary, these routines help us to establish who we are. When sharing meals with children, for example, parents impress cultural beliefs and expectations regarding emotions and behavior (Barlow, 2010). A prayer before a meal confirms and imparts religious values, an admonition to eat one's vegetables teaches health values, and "clean your plate" becomes a lesson in social or environmental consciousness.

Patronizing specific food stores and restaurants, from the local Starbucks to a particular ethnic restaurant, also can become a regular ritual integrated into the everyday structure of an individual's life, further confirming one's identity (Warde & Martens, 2000). Buying and consuming junk food is part of the ritual of "hanging" among teenagers (Chapman & Maclean, 1993), and some urban school children's before-school ritual of visiting a corner store for a sweet or salty breakfast also has been documented (Cannuscio, Weiss, & Asch, 2010). Finally, many immigrants make ritualized weekly shopping expeditions to ethnic food markets in order to experience aromas and sounds reminiscent of their country of origin and to catch up on community news (Mankekar, 2005). These rituals serve to reduce stress and provide a sense of order and belonging. At the same time, rituals that involve foods high in fat or sugar, whether a daily stop for a Starbuck's Frappuccino or a bag of chips at the corner store, can contribute to the establishment of lifelong food habits that have unintended negative health consequences.

FOOD, HEALING, AND HEALTH BELIEFS

What we choose to eat to prevent or cure illness at times reflects deeply held beliefs. Individual beliefs regarding the connection between food and health often combine **folk traditions** and popular ideas obtained from family, friends, media, and social media, and may or may not reflect current nutritional evidence. In addition, such health beliefs frequently are unconscious and conscious, dynamic, and contradictory (Kleinman, 1980).

folk traditions
Informal beliefs or customs that are usually handed down orally from one generation to the next

Many beliefs regarding the relationship between food and health have an underlying logic or rationale that is distinct from biomedicine's conceptualization of nutrition and immunology. For instance, traditional Chinese medicine (TCM), a formalized, professional healing system, is based on Chinese cosmology, particularly ideas regarding flows of energy. Traditional Chinese medicine categorizes foods by their heating, cooling, and strengthening properties (Anderson, 1997). Persons may add hot, cold, wet, or dry foods to their diets to address illness or restore the body's yin and yang balance. As Simpson (2003, p. 835) explains, "medicine is used for diseases, and food is used for longevity. Food can be used as medicine, but medicine cannot be used as food."

Even in regions where biomedicine is the dominant healing system, food-health beliefs may still be grounded in folk medicine, that is, informal, tradition-based healing methods. Food-health beliefs also develop from idiosyncratic personal and familial experiences and lay food discourses on popular topics—the latter accelerated with the rise of the Internet and social media.

Social media and marketing often work together to shape health beliefs regarding foods. As one example, **superfoods** are often popularized through informal social media, which link onto formal marketing efforts for discussions of phytochemicals and antioxidants that rationalize consumption and costs. Superfoods include a range of products, from bean sprouts and oat bran, to goji berries and chia seeds (Grotto, 2008), and often become fetishized, that is, promoted as the dietary key to health, energy, or long life and contrasted with processed foods.

superfoods
Foods promoted as having unusually high nutritional or health values

Individuals also may develop their own interpretations of nutritional advice in order to accommodate local beliefs. Research in the rural southern United States, for example, has found that many older adults in this setting distinguish "raw" salt that is added to food at the table from salt that is added during food preparation. Participants in this study reported they had eliminated using raw salt in order to adhere to their doctor's recommendation to restrict salt consumption. At the same time, they continued to add salt during cooking because this use of salt was seen as essential for the correct preparation of foods (Smith, Quandt, Arcury, Wetmore, Bell, & Vitolins, 2006).

Although many professions historically have tended to dismiss cultural beliefs and practices as "quackery," food system professionals must recognize that food beliefs may be based on internal logics and experiences that legitimize those beliefs to the individual. Failing to acknowledge and appreciate the multiple beliefs that orient individuals' views of food, health, and illness can create distance between professionals and the communities within which they work (Brady, 2001), limiting the acceptance of food system policies and interventions.

Public health efforts to reduce the diabetes burden of Native Americans, the leading cause of morbidity and mortality in that population (Buxton, 2012), for example, often focus on diet and weight loss; but nutritional advice at times runs contrary to local beliefs regarding body size, disease processes, and food (Joos, 1992). Among the Seminole in Florida, being overweight is traditionally a sign of good health, whereas diabetes is conceptualized as largely related to eating sweets. Nutritionists discourage consumption of *sofki,* a thin gruel-like drink made from corn; yet *sofki* is a crucial marker of Seminole identity and a cultural superfood that is perceived as a source of health and vitality. Recommendations to reduce sugar intake correspond with Seminole understanding of the disease process; however, *sofki* presents an added cultural challenge for public health efforts.

FOOD AND GENDER

In many societies foodways are heavily gendered, with specific tasks and foods viewed as the purview of men or women (see figure 9.7). Although persons may contest such norms, that is, preferring the foods and behaviors designated for the opposite gender, local beliefs and values regarding gender and food remain strong. This section examines the gender norms and expectations influencing the roles that men and women play in food production in the United States. We then explore the relationships among gender, food consumption, and idealized body size.

Gender and Food Production

FIGURE 9.7 "Danger—Men Cooking"

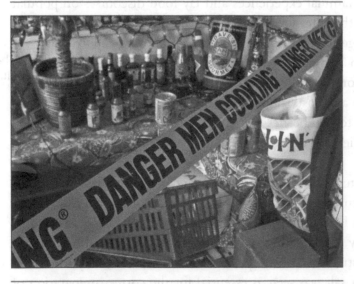

Source: Justin Marty. Danger Men Cooking, 2007. https://www.flickr.com/photos/jmarty/418854968

Throughout the United States, food production is gendered, that is, specific jobs are viewed as the domain of men or women. Women are often the preferred employees for preparing chickens and picking crabs, in part based on idealized assumptions about the nimbleness of women's fingers (Allen & Sachs, 2012; Warren, 2007). These stereotypes also fuel women's participation in the industrial production of precooked and packaged meals, wherein women typically have limited access to management positions (Allen & Sachs, 2012).

Within the home, women tend to have greater responsibility for household food shopping and cooking, although the amount of household work contributed by men has increased over past decades (Jabs & Devine, 2006). Women also may be judged by others based on how their partners and children are fed (Beagan et al., 2008; Blake, Devine, Wethington, Jastran, Farrell, & Bisogni, 2009). Within many immigrant communities or groups experiencing social change, women are further responsible for "preserving the culture," which is symbolized by the maintenance of food traditions (D'Sylva & Beagan, 2011).

Qualitative studies suggest that both men and women may rationalize women's larger role in household food production by suggesting that women are "just better at it" (Lake, Hyland, & Mathers, 2006), it is "just easier" and avoids conflict, or that women are more concerned about nutrition (Beagan et al., 2008). Ironically, the pressure to be "good" and responsive mothers can lead women to prioritize the food desires of spouses and children, at times sacrificing nutrition in the process (Inglis, Ball, & Crawford, 2005).

Same-gender couples may challenge traditional gender roles, but they are not immune to the influence of stereotypical gender expectations. One study found lesbian couples played up their partner's contribution to food production, and gay male couples played it down, reinforcing traditional gender role expectations (Carrington, 1999).

Considerable debate exists regarding how to view women's ongoing role in food production. Although the expectation that women will be the primary food preparers can be seen as a sign of gender discrimination that overburdens women, others argue that control over household food production provides women with a source of power. Indeed, D'Sylva and Beagan's (2011) reworking of the concept of "culinary capital" argues that being in charge of a household's foodways gives women tremendous social control.

Food, Work Life, and Gender

Increasing cultural shifts in gender roles, changes in family structure, and the overall decline in financial well-being have had a significant impact on how the work of feeding the family is managed. When parents are formally employed outside the home the consistent production of nutritious meals can be difficult. Work and household roles often must be negotiated among household members. Both the structure of the workplace, including the regularity of work schedules, the timing and number of work hours, job stability, and the resources available at work (microwaves, refrigerators, and nearby food sources), as well as family characteristics, including having a significant other within the household, children's ages and activities, other caretaking responsibilities, and household income, influence how a household resolves food and work demands (Devine, Farrell, Blake, Jastran, Wethington, & Bisogni, 2009; Devine, Jastran, Jabs, Wethington, Farrell, & Bisogni, 2006).

Work spillover, the disruption of family life because of work, is a common outcome of employment today, particularly for low- and middle-income workers (Blake et al., 2009). In the face of work-related fatigue and time pressures, eating becomes something that is checked off a list rather than an enjoyable process. Parents frequently employ short-term coping mechanisms to address work spillover or "role overload" (Devine et al., 2006). Conventional means for coping include the use of fast food and prepared quick foods for family meals (Devine et al., 2009; Jabs & Devine, 2006). These foods, however, are often high in calories, fat, salt, and sugar, carrying nutritional deficits that add up over time. Furthermore, parents express disappointment and guilt over resorting to fast food and prepared foods, which can exacerbate work-family tension (Devine, Connors, Sobal, & Bisogni, 2003).

Efforts to alter family foodways in the context of working households thus require considering the characteristics of individual workplaces and family life and their interrelationships. Changing foodways involves difficult negotiations regarding the types, quantities, and timing of food preparation, as well as food tasks, including shopping and cleanup.

Gender, Food Consumption, and Body Size

Similar to food production, many gender norms and values exist regarding food consumption. Across many societies, certain foods are considered to be more appropriate for a specific gender. Within the

United States, for example, beef historically was viewed as a "male" food, whereas "lighter" foods, such as chicken, yogurt, and salads, were seen as "female" (Counihan, 1999). Such categorizations were based on cultural assumptions of taste preference and nutritional needs. Although men today enjoy both chicken and salads and women relish a good steak without their respective gender identities being questioned, gendered consumption behaviors still exist in the United States. Women, particularly non-Hispanic white and college-educated women, are more likely than men to moderate the amount they eat and refrain from eating in social settings where others are not eating in order to avoid appearing unfeminine (Counihan, 1999).

Across ethnic groups, consumption, health, and body size also are commonly linked, particularly for women. Among non-Hispanic white women, thinness often is associated with health and self-control, but among non-Hispanic white men, weight is a sign of power and masculinity (Counihan, 1999). By contrast, among many Puerto Ricans, weight gain after marriage symbolizes that newlyweds are doing well (Massara, 1989). Many African Americans similarly view a curvy body as more sexually desirable; thinness signals poor health (Hughes, 1997; Randall, 2012). As Randall (2012, p. SR5) writes of growing up in the 1960s, "I asked God to give me big thighs like my dancing teacher, Diane. There was no way I wanted to look like Twiggy, the white model whose boy-like build was the dream of white girls."

Thus, many interpretations of body size exist. Professionals must recognize how cultural constructions of body size underlie individuals' assessments of their own and their children's dietary needs and health. In addition, young persons, particularly non-Hispanic white and ethnic minority females, are vulnerable to conflicting messages regarding body size, which can contribute to their body dissatisfaction and the development of eating disorders (Cheney, 2011; Counihan, 1999).

FOOD, POWER, AND POLITICS: FOOD MOVEMENTS

In addition to serving as an essential expression of gender and cultural identity, foodways also hold broader social and political significance for governments and are a means for groups and individuals to contest political, economic, and social ideologies. This section examines how governments have used food policies as mechanisms for social control. It then explores how foodways have served as the cornerstone of many recent social movements, symbolizing a movement's social and political values and beliefs.

First, foodways policies, such as sales restrictions and taxes on food and beverages, at times are enacted by governments to regulate or encourage desired social behavior. For instance, in 2012 New York City's Board of Health voted to ban the sale of high-sugar drinks in containers larger than sixteen ounces in order to reduce the city's obesity and diabetes burden (the ban was contested legally and at the time of publication is not enacted). Many states tax alcohol at a higher level than other foodstuffs and limit consumption locations. At the federal level, the US government regulates the content of school meals. Although health, economic, and civics arguments are used to justify restrictions on sales of alcohol, sugar, and other products, such measures at times are rooted in moral judgments and are perceived by some as an infringement on the rights of the individual.

Second, groups and individuals worldwide have used foodways to express dissatisfaction with national and global events and trends. As Michael Pollan (2010, p. 32) describes, food movements are in part "about carving out a new social and economic space removed from the influence of big corporations on the one side and government on the other." To many in these groups, food is not merely something that fuels the body—food represents political and economic ideology. The counterculture movement of the 1960s and 1970s, for example, saw highly processed foods as symbolic of the problematic political and cultural mainstream. The counterculture's "natural food movement" helped pave the way for much of the current interest in whole foods, organic farming, and food cooperatives. Similarly, the **slow food** movement, which began in Italy in the 1980s, developed in opposition to the rise of fast food restaurants. Now a formal organization with more than 150 chapters worldwide (see www.slowfood.com), slow food supporters advocate that "food must be 'good, clean, and fair.' The 'good' refers to taste; the 'clean,' to local, organic, sustainable means of production; and 'fair,' to a system committed to social justice" (Schlosser, 2008, p. 4).

slow food
An international food movement in which supporters promote local production and preparation of food for individual health, creating community, and enjoyment

Supporters of the related "local food" movement further argue that diets should be structured around locally produced food in order to sustain regional economies and to minimize the use of petroleum in food distribution. The demand for local produce and direct farm-consumer connections has contributed to a rise in farmers markets across the United States and have subsequently become mechanisms for economic development (Bubinas, 2011).

Perspective 9.2 argues that some of the central food movement writers so problematize the industrial food system that their discourse becomes apocalyptic, and actually resembles that of recent zombie movies.

Perspective 9.2. Zombies, Food Writing, and Agribusiness Apocalypse
Michael Newbury

In *Zombieland* (Fleischer, 2009), a zombie outbreak originates in tainted hamburger served at a gas station mini-mart. A small group of survivors travels through the wreckage of civilization, avoiding the infected monsters that would eat them, in search of the world's last Twinkie. *28 Days Later* (Boyle, 2003), another contemporary zombie movie, begins with its protagonist awakening from a coma and wandering through the food wrapper– and cup-strewn streets of a chaotically abandoned London. He searches for signs of human life and something to eat, finding only chips, soda, and other kinds of junk food.

Similar to these and other recent zombie movies, an almost staggering number of best sellers, trade books, periodicals, and acclaimed film documentaries find themselves preoccupied with dystopian imaginings of industrial food. But, unlike the zombie films, these journalistic works routinely offer a compensatory dream of and hope for social reintegration, an order in which food becomes the basis for an intimate connection to the natural and the local. Through the unapologetic indulgence of exploitative violence and gore, the zombie films work instead to crush this dream, offering a critique far more radical than—even beyond the imagination of— the public intellectuals and journalists more commonly associated with warnings of food-related catastrophes.

Although not all journalistic critiques of industrial food are equally apocalyptic, such books and documentaries have developed a shared language and common metaphors of crisis. Michael Pollan's *The Omnivore's Dilemma* and, even more intensely, Eric Schlosser's *Fast Food Nation* have at their heart a bleak mixture of animal abuse, corporate malfeasance, and government corruption. Indeed, the slaughtering of livestock and systematically manipulative marketing techniques have provided the most ready flow of shared, predictable, even routinized dystopian imagery. Schlosser emphasizes that the stench and filth produced by feedlots and slaughterhouses have made the areas around them all but unlivable for long-time, small-town residents (Schlosser, 2005, p. 150). Pollan follows a calf from newborn to hamburger, only to be mortified by the inhumanity of the system, its obliteration of the good, the humane, and the natural (Pollan, 2009, p. 66). Taking a different tack, Marion Nestle emphasizes not the brutality of the blood-soaked slaughterhouse, but the antiseptic environs

(Continued)

(Continued)

of the food science laboratory, the cynically manipulative world of corporate advertising that places logos on baby bottles and recruits cheerleaders at local high schools to drink particular soft drink brands (Nestle, 2007, p. 185). The promotional trailer for Robert Kenner's *Food, Inc.* may be the most striking synthesis of all of these familiar images because it cuts frenetically in a kind of horror-movie pastiche from frenziedly spinning bottles of Heinz ketchup to trembling cameras gliding through supermarket aisles to imprisoned cattle ankle-deep in their own feces.

But for all of their visions of collapse and disaster that rely on atrocity, nightmarish bureaucracies, and mad food scientists, popular documentarians of the industrial food apocalypse also routinely turn to the dream of a pastoral antidote. Pollan and Kenner (2008), for example, both feature the self-proclaimed "beyond organic" yeoman farmer, Joel Salatin. Salatin, in his broad-brimmed straw hat, white t-shirt, and suspenders, emerges as the embodiment of folksy, Thoreauvian common sense, self-reliance, and authenticity. He lives and eats with his extended family at a long outdoor table covered with a gingham cloth and rides an almost antique tractor through fields pulling a cart piled high with old-fashioned square bales, the blue sky lit brilliantly behind him. Salatin stands in for the redemptive power of pastoral landscapes, farmers' markets, individual agency, and "beyond organic" alternatives that promise to save civilization from the looming food system collapse sponsored by industrial agribusiness.

FIGURE 9.8   Zombie

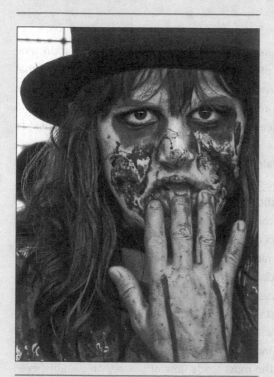

Source: Bob Jagendorf. Zombie girl having a snack, Zombiewalk, Asbury Park NJ. 2007. https://www.flickr.com/photos/bobjagendorf/3978897574/.

Contemporary zombie movies, by contrast, extinguish with brutal enthusiasm all aspiration to retrieving alternatives to the industrial food chain. When the zombie movie does narrate temporary returns to the pastoral, it does so only to undermine the plausibility of the "natural" or the "local" as effective responses to the crisis at hand. In Zack Snyder's (2004) remake of *Dawn of the Dead*, for example, survivors attempt to convert a coffee franchise modeled on Starbucks into an intimate haven for candlelit dinners and personal friendships only to find this fantasy unsustainable in the face of the zombie threat. Indeed, when survivors in these films seek out alternatives to or the reshaping of the wreckage of the industrial food system, predatory zombies, haunting figures of indiscriminate appetite, seek them out and attack. Accordingly, the postapocalyptic landscape of the recent zombie film is not only littered with junk food but also displaces humans from the top of the food chain, offering them no escape from the institutional and corporate power feared by food documentarians. The survivors themselves become fast food for the mindless but ravenous zombies, the ideal embodiments of the indiscriminate food consumers of our age.

Zombie movies, then, lie at some temperamental distance from the sources usually invoked by those thinking about food systems and ecology. But the films are, if anything, routinely overburdened by the apocalyptic imagining of a food crisis. Scholars and activists ought to pay attention to how the imagining of food crisis circulates beyond the realm of its most obvious intellectual and political sympathizers. Zombie movies, with their lavish interest in gore and lowbrow aesthetic, challenge the sometimes sentimental attachment to the pastoral visions present in much writing on industrial food. Whereas the recent zombie films are less given to systematic, linear, and coherent exposition on the catastrophic potential of agribusiness than many documentarians, they offer a visually spectacular, shockingly impressionistic but total critique of producers and consumers of industrial food.

Source: Adapted from Newbury (2012).

Vegetarianism and **veganism** are two additional food movements that often are motivated by similar political and social agendas. To the political issues raised within the counterculture, slow, and local food movements, many vegetarians and vegans add concern for the ethics and environmental toll of **animal husbandry**. Vegetarianism and veganism also are fueled by increasing numbers of nutritional studies that associate meat and dairy consumption with a higher risk of metabolic disease and certain types of cancer (Ferrucci et al., 2010; Pan et al., 2012; Wu et al., 2012). Although individuals vary considerably in the extent to which they share these concerns, being vegetarian or vegan often becomes a defining part of an individual's identity and provides a sense of group belonging. Social media, particularly blogs, have helped to further popularize vegetarianism and veganism, offering instruction on the use of unfamiliar products and recipe exchanges.

These contemporary food movements, particularly the emphasis on slow and local food, however, have been heavily critiqued for the significant time and financial costs they can carry (Simonetti, 2012). As discussed elsewhere in this textbook, on the macro level implementing these social and political beliefs across the food system would require large-scale rethinking of food production. On the local level, the time costs of slow and local food participation can be gendered in households where women are the primary cooks or in regions where women are responsible for harvesting produce for market sale (Allen & Sachs, 2012; Simonetti, 2012). In addition, food discourses and spaces such as farmers markets are seen by some as expressing a middle-class non-Hispanic white orientation that subtly excludes persons of color (Guthman, 2012; Harper, 2012). Others note, however, that farmers markets and related local produce ventures can represent important, low-cost sources of fresh produce in urban and minority neighborhoods (see figure 9.9).

vegetarianism
Diet that includes no animal meat or fish, but may include eggs and dairy

veganism
Diet that includes no foodstuffs with animal origins, including animal meat, fish, dairy, eggs, and honey

animal husbandry
The branch of agriculture concerned with the care and breeding of domestic animals

FIGURE 9.9 Waverly Farmers Market

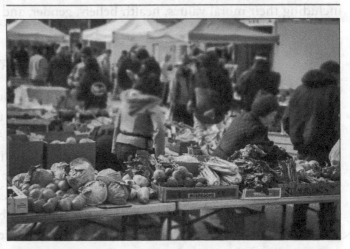

Source: Michael Milli, CLF.

IMPLICATIONS FOR FOOD SYSTEMS

Tremendous variation in foodways exists worldwide. Ritualized, symbolic meanings often are attached to foods, explaining correct food preparation and when and why foods are eaten. Foods also are endowed with properties of "wholesome," "healthy," or "wrong" regardless of actual nutritional value. Such beliefs and values are so firmly entrenched in understandings of food and food behavior that to violate those beliefs can seem not only unhealthy but also a threat to one's personal and group identity. These culturally grounded beliefs and practices often shape food systems from behind the scenes, that is, driving local or regional food demands and creating expectations regarding food production and distribution methods.

At the same time, humans clearly are capable of change, with friends, family, media, and structural factors, such as economic resources and work characteristics, all contributing to foodways transformations. Individual taste preferences, as well as social and political stances, likewise may lead individuals and groups to embrace foodways that are distinct from the dominant community or subgroup. Thus, culture should be viewed as a flexible rather than an immutable force within the food system.

Because cultural misunderstandings can hinder professional effectiveness, cultural competency training is now common in many fields. Such training is designed to increase workers' abilities to identify and respectfully respond to cultural beliefs and practices. In addition, food system professionals are encouraged to discuss the meaning and function of food with community members and other food system stakeholders. By increasing their understanding of the roles of culture in food decisions, from where to shop to what's for dinner, food system professionals at all levels can better serve the communities within which they work, developing food system plans, policies, and interventions that are culturally appropriate and feasible to implement.

Ultimately, this textbook argues that a socioecological perspective is critical for understanding and changing the food system. Cultural processes are a critical component of the socioecological environment. Meaningful change in the food system can be achieved only through thoughtful consideration of the ways in which food and food rituals express persons' understandings of themselves and society, including their moral values, health beliefs, gender, and group belonging.

SUMMARY

This chapter explores how cultural and social forces influence the foodways, or food rituals and behaviors, of individuals and social groups. Cultural beliefs regarding what is food, when to eat, and how food should taste are frequently learned in childhood. Although maintaining these customs can serve as a marker of one's geographic and ethnic identity, individual food practices change over time, particularly under the influence of peers and media. Cultural beliefs and individual experiences also guide understandings of the relationship between food and health. What we choose to eat to prevent or cure illness at times reflects deeply held beliefs. Individual beliefs regarding the connection between food and health often combine folk traditions and popular ideas obtained from family, friends, media, and social media, and may or may not reflect current nutritional evidence. Regardless of their source, such beliefs can powerfully influence our willingness to modify foodways in response to illness. Gender likewise can affect food behaviors, because many societies label specific foods and food consumption patterns as masculine or feminine. Both men and women, however, may contest or select not to enact gender-based norms. Broader societal changes, such as the increased presence of women in the workforce and increasing numbers of same gender households, also are leading to changes in food preparation patterns. Finally, food is not merely fuel for the body, but rather, food also connects to political, economic, and social systems and faith traditions. Changing foodways can be a means for changing these systems.

KEY TERMS

Animal husbandry

Community-supported agriculture (CSA)

Culture

Folk traditions

Foodways

Slow food

Superfoods

Veganism

Vegetarianism

DISCUSSION QUESTIONS

1. How has your geographic background or your ethnic heritage influenced your food preferences? Are there food norms from your home that you no longer share? What food norms or preferences would you find difficult to change or give up?

2. Are there specific foods that you believe should or should not be eaten when a person is sick? What foods are critical for maintaining health? What are the sources of your beliefs?

3. Who was in charge of food in your household when you were young? Why? Did other adults or children in the household affect food decisions? How?

4. What types of interventions could be developed to help households avoid processed convenience foods when faced with fatigue and time constraints? What variables might influence the success of such interventions?

5. Consider movies, TV shows, or advertisements that you have recently seen. How is the act of eating depicted, particularly among ethnic, regional, or socioeconomic groups? Similarly, how is being thin depicted? How is being overweight depicted? How could these depictions influence young persons' views of food?

6. Traditional and commonly consumed foods from some cultures are considered relatively unhealthy by nutritionists. As a health practitioner from outside the community, what is the most culturally sensitive way to approach this information? The most effective? Can you be effective without being culturally sensitive? How can those coming from outside a community best gain insight into its food-related beliefs, attitudes, and practices?

7. Did any of the messages from perspectives 9.1 (white bread) or 9.2 (zombies) cause you to question your own attitudes or assumptions?

REFERENCES

Allen, P., & Sachs, C. (2012). Women and food chains: The gendered politics of food. In P. Williams-Forson & C. Counihan (Eds.), *Taking food public: Redefining foodways in a changing world* (pp. 23–40). New York: Routledge.

Anderson, E. N. (1997). Traditional medical values of food. In C. Counihan & P. Van Esterik (Eds.), *Food and culture* (pp. 80–91). New York City: Routledge.

Ayala, G., Baquero, B., & Klinger, S. (2008). A systematic review of the relationship between acculturation and diet among Latinos in the United States: Implications for future research. *Journal of the American Dietetic Association*, 108(8), 1330–1344.

Barlow, K. (2010). Sharing food, sharing values: Mothering and empathy in Murik society. *Ethos*, 38(4), 339–353.

Beagan, B., Chapman, G. E., D'Sylva, A., & Bassett, B. R. (2008). "It's just easier for me to do it": Rationalizing the family division of foodwork. *Sociology: The Journal of the British Sociological Association*, 42(4), 653–671.

Blake, C. E., Devine, C. M., Wethington, E., Jastran, M., Farrell, T. J., & Bisogni, C. A. (2009). Employed parents' satisfaction with food-choice coping strategies. Influence of gender and structure. *Appetite*, 52(3), 711–719.

Bobrow-Strain, A. (2012). *White bread: A social history of the store-bought loaf.* Boston: Beacon Press.

Bourdieu, P. (1990). *The logic of practice* (R. Nice, Trans.). Stanford, CA: Stanford University Press.

Boyle, D. (Director), Macdonald A. (Producer). (2003). *28 Days Later* [DVD]. London: DNA Films and British Film Council.

Brady, E. (2001). Introduction. In E. Brady (Ed.), *Healing logics: Culture and medicine in modern belief systems* (pp. 3–12). Logan, UT: USU Press.

Bubinas, K. (2011). Farmers markets in the post-industrial city. *City & Society*, 23(2), 153–172.

Buxton, R. (2012). Diabetes no. 1 health problem among Native Americans. *Seminole Tribune*, February 21. Retrieved from http://seminoletribune.org/diabetes-no-1-health-problem-among-native-americans

Cannuscio, C. C., Weiss, E. E., & Asch, D. A. (2010). The contribution of urban foodways to health disparities. *Journal of Urban Health*, 87(3), 381–393.

Carrington, C. (1999). *No place like home: Relationships and family life among lesbians and gay men.* Chicago: University of Chicago Press.

Chapman, G., & Maclean, H. (1993). "Junk food" and "healthy food": Meanings of food in adolescent women's culture. *Journal of Nutrition Education*, 25(3), 108–113.

Cheney, A. (2011). "Most girls want to be skinny": Body (dis)satisfaction among ethnically diverse women. *Qualitative Health Research*, 21(10), 1347–1359.

Counihan, C. (1999). *The anthropology of food and body.* New York City: Routledge.

Creighton, M., Goldman, N., Pebley, A., & Chung, C. (2012). Durational and generational differences in Mexican immigrant obesity: Is acculturation the explanation. *Social Science and Medicine*, 75, 300–310.

Devine, C. M., Connors, M., Sobal, J., & Bisogni, C. (2003). Sandwiching it in: Spillover of work onto food choices and family roles in low- and moderate-income urban households. *Social Science and Medicine*, 56, 617–630.

Devine, C. M., Farrell, T. J., Blake, C. E., Jastran, M., Wethington, E., & Bisogni, C. A. (2009). Work conditions and the food choice coping strategies of employed parents. *Journal of Nutrition Education and Behavior*, 41(5), 365–370.

Devine, C. M., Jastran, M., Jabs, J., Wethington, E., Farrell, T. J., & Bisogni, C. A. (2006). "A lot of sacrifices": Work-family spillover and the food choice coping strategies of low wage employed parents. *Social Science and Medicine*, 63(10), 2591–2603.

D'Sylva, A., & Beagan, B. (2011). "Food is culture, but it's also power": The role of food in ethnic and gender identity construction among Goan Canadian women. *Journal of Gender Studies*, 20(3), 279–289.

Ferrucci, L., Sinha, R., Ward, M., Graubard, B., Hollenbeck, A., Kilfoy, B., et al. (2010). Meat and components of meat and the risk of bladder cancer in the NIH-AARP diet and health study. *Cancer*, 116(18), 4345–4353.

Fitzgerald, N. (2010). Acculturation, socioeconomic status, and health among Hispanics. *NAPA Bulletin*, 34, 28–46.

Fleischer, R. (Director). Kavanaugh, R., Reese, G., Swerdlow, E., Wernick, P. (Producers). (2009). *Zombieland* [DVD]. San Mateo, CA: Sony Entertainment.

Grotto, D. (2008). *101 foods that could save your life.* New York: Bantam Book.

Guthman, J. (2012). "If they only knew": Color blindness and universalism in California alternative food institutions. In P. Williams-Forson & C. Counihan (Eds.), *Taking food public: Redefining foodways in a changing world* (pp. 211–222). New York: Routledge.

Gutierrez, C. P. (1992). *Cajun foodways*. Jackson: University Press of Mississippi.

Harper, A. B. (2012). Going beyond the normative white "post-racial" vegan epistemology. In P. Williams-Forson & C. Counihan (Eds.), *Taking food public: Redefining foodways in a changing world* (pp. 155–174). New York: Routledge.

Hughes, M. (1997). Soul, black women, and food. In C. Counihan & P. Van Esterik (Eds.), *Food and culture* (pp. 272–279). New York: Routledge.

Inglis, V., Ball, K., & Crawford, D. (2005). Why do women of low socioeconomic status have poorer dietary behaviours than women of higher socioeconomic status? A qualitative exploration. *Appetite, 45*(3), 334–343.

Jabs, J., & Devine, C. M. (2006). Time scarcity and food choices: An overview. *Appetite, 47*(2), 196–204.

Joos, S. (1992). Economic, social and cultural factors in the analysis of disease: Dietary change and diabetes mellitus among the Florida Seminole Indians. In L. K. Brown & K. Mussell (Eds.), *Ethnic and regional foodways in the United States* (pp. 217–237). Knoxville: University of Tennessee Press.

Kalcik, S. (1992). Ethnic foodways in America: Symbol and the performance of identity. In L. K. Brown & K. Mussell (Eds.), *Ethnic and regional foodways in the United States* (pp. 37–65). Knoxville: University of Tennessee Press.

Kenner, R. (Director). (2008). Participant media. Theatrical trailer for *Food, Inc.* [Electronic Source]. Retrieved from www.youtube.com/watch?v=5eKYyD14d_0

Kleinman, A. (1980). *Patients and healers in the context of culture*. Berkeley: University of California Press.

Kottak, C. (2006). *Cultural anthropology*. New York: McGraw-Hill.

Lake, A., Hyland, R., & Mathers, J. (2006). Food shopping and preparation among the 30-somethings: Whose job is it? The ASH30 study. *British Food Journal, 108*(6), 475–486.

Lockwood, W. G., & Lockwood, Y. R. (2002). Being American: An Arab-American thanksgiving. In H. Walke (Ed.), *The meal: Proceedings of the Oxford Symposium on Food and Cookery 2001* (pp. 155–164). Devon, UK: Prospect Books.

Mankekar, P. (2005). "India shopping": Indian grocery stores and transnational configurations of belonging. In J. Watson & M. Caldwell (Eds.), *The cultural politics of food and eating* (pp. 197–214). Malden, MA: Blackwell.

Marshall, D. (2005). Food as ritual, routine or convention. *Consumption, Markets, and Culture, 8*(1), 69–85.

Massara, E. B. (1989). *Que gordita! A study of weight among women in a Puerto Rican community*. New York: AMS Press.

Mintz, S. (1998). The localization of anthropological practice: From area studies to transnationalism. *Critique of Anthropology, 18*, 117–133.

Mintz, S. (2002). Food and eating: Some persistent questions. In W. Belasco & P. Scranton (Eds.), *Food nations* (pp. 24–32). New York: Routledge.

Nestle, M. (2007). *Food politics: How the food industry influences nutrition and health*. Berkeley: University of California Press.

Newbury, M. (2012). Fast zombie/slow zombie: Food writing, horror movies, and agribusiness apocalypse. *American Literary History, 24*, 87–114.

Pan, A., Sun, Q., Bernstein, A., Schulze, M., Manson, J., Stampfer, M., et al. (2012). Red meat consumption and mortality. *Archives of Internal Medicine, 172*(7), 555–563.

Paolisso, M. (2007). Taste the traditions: Crabs, crab cakes, and the Chesapeake Bay blue crab. *American Anthropologist, 109*(4), 654–665.

Pollan, M. (2009). *The omnivore's dilemma: A natural history of four meals*. New York: Penguin.

Pollan, M. (2010). The food movement, rising. *New York Review of Books*. Retrieved from www.nybooks.com/articles/archives/2010/jun/10/food-movement-rising/?pagination=false

Randall, A. (2012, May 6). Black women and fat. *New York Times*, p. SR5,

Schlosser, E. (2005). *Fast food nation: The dark side of the all-American meal*. New York: Harper.

Schlosser, E. (2008, September 22). Slow food for thought. *The Nation*, 4–5.

Simonetti, L. (2012). The ideology of slow food. *Journal of European Studies, 42*(2), 168–189.

Simpson, P. B. (2003). Family beliefs about diet and traditional Chinese medicine for Hong Kong women with breast cancer. *Oncology Nursing Forum, 30*(5), 834–840.

Smith, S. L., Quandt, S. A., Arcury, T. A., Wetmore, L. K., Bell, R. A., & Vitolins, M. Z. (2006). Aging and eating in the rural, southern United States: Beliefs about salt and its effect on health. *Social Science & Medicine, 62*(1), 189–198.

Snyder, Z. (Director). Abraham, M, Bernstein, A., Bliss, T. et al. (Producers). (2004). *Dawn of the dead* [DVD]. Strike Entertainment.

Warde, A., & Martens, L. (2000). *Eating out: Social differentiation, consumption, and pleasure*. New York: Cambridge University Press.

Warren, W. (2007). *Tied to the great packing machine: The Midwest and meatpacking*. Iowa City: University of Iowa Press.

Wu, J., Cross, A., Baris, D., Ward, M., Karagas, M., Johnson, A., et al. (2012). Dietary intake of meat, fruits, vegetables, and selective micronutrients and risk of bladder cancer in the New England region of the United States. *British Journal of Cancer, 106*(11), 1891–1898.

Chapter 10

Promotional Marketing

A Driver of the Modern Food System

Corinna Hawkes

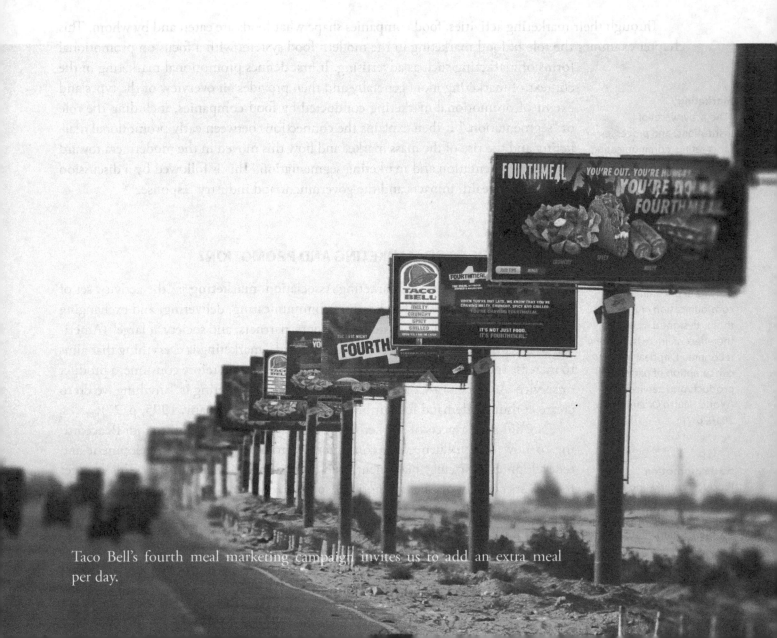

Taco Bell's fourth meal marketing campaign invites us to add an extra meal per day.

Learning Objectives

- Define food promotion in the context of food marketing more broadly.

- Describe the nature and extent of promotional food marketing and how it has changed over time.

- Understand that promotional marketing is not an isolated process but a fundamental part of the modern US food system.

- Explain in what ways promotional food marketing has been detrimental to public health and ways marketing techniques can be used to promote healthy foods.

- Discuss efforts to restrict food promotion to children and the ways such policies are perceived by different stakeholders.

Through their marketing activities, food companies shape what foods are eaten and by whom. This chapter examines the role of food marketing in the modern food system, with a focus on promotional forms of marketing such as advertising. It first defines promotional marketing in the context of marketing more generally and then provides an overview of the types and extent of promotional marketing conducted by food companies, including the role of "segmentation." It then explains the connections between early promotional marketing and the rise of the mass market and how this moved in the modern era toward product segmentation and marketing segmentation. This is followed by a discussion of its public health impacts and the government and industry response.

marketing
"The activity, set of institutions, and processes for creating, communicating, delivering, and exchanging offerings that have value for customers, clients, partners, and society at large" (AMA, 2007)

promotion
"Any form of commercial communication or message that is designed to, or has the effect of, increasing the recognition, appeal and/or consumption of particular products and services" (World Health Organization, 2010, p. 7)

trade promotion
Producers marketing to other actors in the food system, such as primary producers marketing their products to manufacturers or manufacturers promoting their products to retailers

WHAT ARE FOOD MARKETING AND PROMOTION?

According to the American Marketing Association, **marketing** is "the activity, set of institutions, and processes for creating, communicating, delivering, and exchanging offerings that have value for customers, clients, partners, and society at large" (American Marketing Association, 2007). In other words, marketing is everything that aims to increase the likelihood that customers will value, and therefore consume, a product or service. As the Coca-Cola Company once put it, marketing is "anything we do to create consumer demand for our brands" (Coca Cola Company, 1995, p. 27).

The different aspects of marketing are commonly categorized into four Ps according to how they influence the consumer environment: product development and redevelopment, pricing, placement, and promotion (Keegan, 2007). This chapter focuses specifically on the promotion aspect. **Promotion** is "any form of commercial communication or message that is designed to, or has the effect of, increasing the recognition, appeal and/or consumption of particular products and services. It comprises anything that acts to advertise or otherwise promote a product or service" (World Health Organization [WHO], 2010, p. 7). Though not dealt with here, promotion also includes **trade promotion**, in which producers market to other actors in the food system, such as primary producers marketing their products to manufacturers or manufacturers promoting their products to retailers.

All forms of promotion are designed to stimulate demand. The aim is to increase the *amount* purchased, the *frequency* of purchasing, and the *number of people* who purchase, including through brand switching (when a consumer decides to buy one brand rather than another). Demand can also be increased indirectly by building brand awareness and loyalty, thus increasing consumer preference for the product over the longer term.

TYPES OF FOOD PROMOTION

Food is promoted through many different types of communication channels using a wide range of techniques. Much of modern day promotion in the United States is by large food companies using a sophisticated array of **communications channels**, which are the media and venues through which marketing is conducted, such as television, the Internet, print, radio, video games, schools, stores, or restaurants (Hawkes & Harris, 2011). The marketing industry tends to categorize communications channels into two types: the **measured media** (or "above-the-line" or "traditional" media), such as television, cinema, radio, and print press, which are tracked by media research companies; and **nonmeasured media** (or "below the line" or "nontraditional"), such as the Internet, stores, or schools. Various marketing techniques—such as advertising, use of licensed characters, popular personalities or celebrities, packaging, product placements, sales promotions, interactive games, and text messaging—are used to promote foods through both of these channels (see figure 10.1).

A broad array of communications channels and marketing techniques are used in the United States to promote food to adults and children. In 2008, the Federal Trade Commission (FTC) identified the channels and techniques most commonly used by leading food and beverage companies to market to children (table 10.1). Although television advertising still dominates food promotion, a notable trend in the 1990s and 2000s has been the increasing use of nontraditional communications channels and techniques (McGinnis, Gootman, & Kraak, 2006). Marketing campaigns have also become increasingly **integrated**—that is, different channels and techniques are used together (e.g., product packaging, supermarket displays [see focus 10.1], advertising spots, and online contests) to increase impact.

communications channels Media and venues through which marketing is conducted, such as television, the Internet, print, radio, video games, schools, stores, or restaurants

measured media "Above-the-line" or "traditional" media, such as television, cinema, radio, and print press, which are tracked by media research companies

nonmeasured media "Below-the-line" or "nontraditional" media, such as the Internet, stores, or schools

integrated Different channels and techniques being used together

FIGURE 10.1   Mikaela Shiffrin Promotes Wheaties

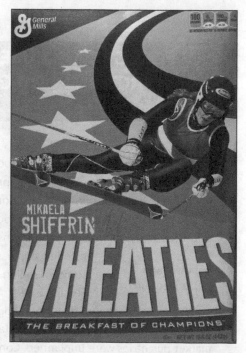

Source: Mike Mozart. "Mikaela Shiffrin Wheaties Cereal Box US Ski Team Olympics General Mills Breakfast Cereal Box." (2014). https://www.flickr.com/photos/jeepersmedia/14091279907/

TABLE 10.1   Communications Channels and Marketing Techniques Commonly Used by Leading US Food and Beverage Companies

Communications Channels	Examples of Marketing Techniques
TV	Sponsorship of TV programs
Radio	Advertising
Print	"Information" promotions in children's magazines
	Celebrity endorsements on billboards
Internet	Games, competitions, and so forth on company websites
	Social media marketing
Cinema	Product placement
Video games	Advertising
Cell phones	Digital messages (e-mail, text)
In-store	Displays
Packaging	In-pack premiums
	Box-top promotions
	Use of licensed characters and brand characters
Public entertainment events	Sponsorship
	Free samples
Consumers of the product	Viral
	Word-of-mouth
In-school	Sponsorship of sports teams and activities
	Educational programs
Philanthropic endeavors	Sponsoring charitable activities
	Holding charity auctions
	Organizing volunteer days

Source: Adapted from Federal Trade Commission [FTC] (2008).

FOCUS 10.1. "SUPERMARKETING" AND THE IMPACT ON FOOD CHOICE

Jared Simon

One of the most important influencers of food choice is the purchasing environment. Supermarkets are the predominant environment in which food purchasing decisions are made in the United States. In the supermarket setting, the four Ps of marketing (product choices, product placement, pricing, and promotions) all play important roles in the consumer decision-making process.

Supermarkets seek to maximize food sales and profits within their stores through store design, product selection, shelving, pricing, promotions, and other marketing efforts. These in-store stimuli help reinforce planned purchases and concurrently trigger unrecognized needs and desires of consumers, leading to additional unplanned purchases, or **impulse buys** (Inman, Winer, & Ferraro, 2009).

impulse buys
Unplanned purchases

Research has shown that most shoppers arrive at the supermarket undecided about what to buy across a variety of food categories and items. In fact, a study by Inman & Winer (1998) estimated that 59 percent of supermarket purchases were unplanned. Consumer decision making has been shown to be a modifiable behavior that can be influenced very late in the process. Even when consumers possess detailed knowledge of healthy foods and state strong preferences for healthy foods, these preferences may be overridden by factors in the supermarket or broader environment (Zachary, Palmer, Beckham, & Surkan, 2013).

Pricing

As discussed in previous chapters, pricing plays an important role in food choice, making supermarket price promotions an effective tool for influencing consumer behavior. Many supermarkets send weekly circulars highlighting their price discounts across hundreds of items and dedicate much signage to price promotions. Perhaps more than any other retail environment, supermarkets use price promotions with multiples (e.g., "Buy 2 for $1"), further encouraging greater purchase and consumption. Despite the prevalence of price promotions for less healthful foods, some retailers are choosing to focus more price promotions on healthful foods to attract consumers interested in healthful eating.

In-Store Design and Location

The in-store environment can have profound effects on a consumer's interest in and willingness to make healthy food choices. Key design elements in every store include the store configuration, shelving, lighting, and signage. Each of these elements is carefully chosen to communicate a message to consumers, which in turn influences the shopping experience and the types of products purchased by consumers.

The importance of location in the supermarket setting is well established. The most highly coveted spaces in any given store include those at the entrance, near the front registers, and at the end of each aisle. These are typically referred to as areas of "display." Items on display not only garner more attention from shoppers but also see a dramatic increase in sales compared to when these items are solely in their regular in-aisle locations. Beyond the display location, food manufacturers and retailers use materials at the **point of sale (POS)**, such as cardboard cutouts or banners, to draw further attention to the foods they are promoting.

point of sale (POS)
The place where purchases are made; can be specific to the register or refer more broadly to within a store

Shelf Placement

The shelf placement of a product within a supermarket can have a dramatic effect on consumer awareness, consideration, and ultimately purchase decisions. Using an eye-tracking experiment, one study demonstrated that the number of facings (i.e., the quantity of the same item that is on the shelf) and the product location on the shelf strongly influence consumer attention, evaluation, and purchase intent (Chandon, Hutchinson, Bradlow, & Young, 2009). Shelf location is also important, with shelves at eye level typically garnering the most attention. Cereal manufacturers, for example, compete to have their adult cereals shelved on the middle shelves (to attract adults who view these items at their eye level) and their children's cereals shelved on the lower shelves (to attract youngsters who view these items at their eye level).

Shelf Labeling

Many consumers value the presence of nutrition labels on store shelves when shopping for food. For a nutritionally focused shelf label to be effective, it is essential that it be implemented at the point of sale in a simple and clear manner. In general, consumers rely on simplifying heuristics, or shortcuts, to assess food labels as part of choosing which foods they will purchase.

Other In-Store Factors: Shopper Education, Sampling, Time in Store

Supermarkets use shopper education and sampling to increase familiarity with unknown products. Retailers know that shoppers are less likely to buy items they have not tried and therefore may end up going to waste.

Time spent in a supermarket is another critical factor with respect to unplanned purchases. Shoppers who spend the most time in-store and shop the most aisles are those with the highest levels of unplanned

(Continued)

(Continued)

purchases (Inman et al., 2009). Purposefully, supermarkets have added nonfood merchandise and services (such as pharmacies, photo labs, and banks) to attract and retain shoppers.

Conclusion

Pricing, in-store design, shelf placement, shelf labeling, shopper education, and food sampling all influence consumer food choice within a supermarket. Savvy marketers have recognized these points of influence for years and have been able to steer consumer decision making toward cost-efficient, well-marketed food brands and food categories.

   Public health researchers and professionals are beginning to catch up. In supermarkets and other grocery stores, programs are being developed that use each of these powerful tools to positively influence consumer choice and consumer behavior toward the purchase and consumption of more healthful foods.

SEGMENTATION AND TARGETING IN FOOD PROMOTION

segmentation
The process of dividing consumers into groups who are likely to respond in the same way to products and promotional (marketing) activity

psychographic
Similar to a demographic group, but based instead on lifestyles and values, which may be shared regardless of demography, geography, or behaviors

An important aspect of modern food marketing is **segmentation**, the process of dividing consumers into groups who are likely to respond in the same way to products and promotional activity. Different promotional campaigns are designed to target these different segments—thus the term *targeted marketing* (Grier & Kumanyika, 2010). Segmentation can be conducted according to demography (e.g., children, adults; high income, low income), geography (e.g., different states, population densities), behavior (e.g., brand loyalty, shopping patterns), and what is termed **psychographic**—lifestyles and values that may be shared by groups regardless of their demography, geography, or behaviors. The idea is that by positioning foods to appeal to and reach these different target groups, the effectiveness of promotional marketing will be significantly enhanced. It recognizes, as put by Grier and Kumanyika (2010, p. 350), that a "one-size-fits-all approach to marketing no longer works among diverse, sophisticated consumers" (see figure 10.2).

   Two demographic segments that have received particular attention are children and ethnic minorities. Children and youth represent an important demographic market because, as one-quarter of the US population, they are a large base of potential customers and influence purchases made by parents and households. They also constitute the future adult market, creating the incentive for manufacturers to instill brand loyalty that will last into adulthood (McGinnis et al., 2006).

   Ethnic minorities are likewise a key target market because of their size, growth, and purchasing power (Grier & Kumanyika, 2010; McGinnis et al., 2006). For example, a content analysis of promotions by Grier and Kumanyika (2008, p. 1626) showed that the evidence was "remarkably consistent" in "demonstrating that advertisements for low-cost, high-calorie, and low-nutrition food and beverage products are more frequent in media targeted to African Americans." The authors suggested that companies are likely to specifically target African Americans because they tend to live in racially segregated neighborhoods, thus facilitating geographical segmentation, their higher use of the media, especially television, and the social and psychological meanings of African American identity, which enhances the ability to create promotions with strong emotional meanings for the target group. Although large demographic segments such as youth or ethnic minorities are important market segments, the process of segmentation extends even further. Advertising by the Coca-Cola Company exemplifies the refined nature of targeting different combinations of customer segments (Sierra Services/SCMC, 2011). For example, the Dasani "Dancing Mom" advertisement (2009) targeted African American mothers aged between twenty-five and thirty-five with the message that "moms can be concerned about health and still be cool." A 2010 advertisement targeted students by showing a student late for an exam being

FIGURE 10.2 Racecar with Red Bull Advertisement Targets Nascar Fans.

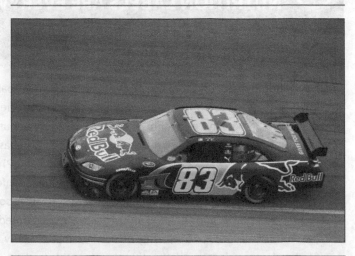

Source: Freewheeling daredevil. "Brian Vickers Red Bull Toyota Camry." (2008). https://www.flickr.com/photos/daredevil26/2264564102/.

awakened by the sound of a Coke being opened. In another example, a 2009 advertisement for Coca-Cola brand Juicy Juice beverages targeted mothers of small children by depicting an emotional moment between mother and child, with a voiceover explaining the brain's development process and how DHA (added to the product) is a building block for brain development.

As indicated by these examples, one of the key trends in segmentation in the 2000s has been targeting consumers concerned about health and wellness. Marketers target this segment (and subsegments) with techniques such as these:

- **Signposts** on the front of food packages that indicate that the product is "better for you," such as the use of a green flag

- **Nutrient claims,** such as "high in calcium" (discussed further in focus 10.2)

- **Health claims,** such as "a diet high in soluble fiber from whole oats and low in saturated fat and cholesterol may reduce the risk of heart disease"

- Using descriptive terms that could be perceived as implying the food is nutritious, such as the word *natural*

- Visuals that give the impression of wellness such as happy children, green fields, or the addition of fruit, or freshness, such as depicting production of the dominant ingredient on a farm

- Claims about the "greenness" of the product, such as "produced using palm oil from sustainable sources"

signposts
Indications such as green flags on the front of food packages to show that a product is better for you

nutrient claims
Claims about the level of a nutrient in a food; used in marketing

health claims
Claims used in marketing, indicating that a food or diet will benefit health

FOCUS 10.2. POP! POINT-OF-PURCHASE NUTRITION LABELS ARE EVERYWHERE: WHO BENEFITS?

Katherine Abowd Johnson

Navigating the grocery store can be overwhelming. Your goal: smart food choices. Your challenge: distinguishing nutritious foods from well-marketed imposters. Obstacles include icons promising a day's worth of whole grains in a cookie and a "healthy star" below one cereal, but not its brand name equivalent. These labels are referred to as point-of-purchase (POP) displays. They primarily consist of labels on the **front of package (FOP)** of the product and shelf labels displayed by retailers that augment regulated information, such as the Nutrition Facts panel (NFP). Since the American Heart Association (AHA) introduced their Heart Smart label in 1987, nonprofits and the food industry have implemented an increasing variety of nutritional POP displays (Institute of Medicine, 2012). They offer an example of how the food industry employs nutrition to sell more food and responds to regulation that threatens this goal.

front of package (FOP)
A location for placing labeling messages

FIGURE 10.3   Facts Up Front FOP System, a Facts-Based Label

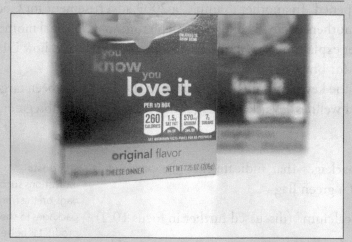

Source: Michael Milli, CLF.

nutrient density
In food, refers to the levels of key nutrients, such as fiber and vitamins, relative to the number of calories; commonly used to describe foods considered to be healthy

You likely recognize the four main types of POP nutrition labels (Schor, Maniscalco, Tuttle, Alligood, & Reinhardt Kapsak, 2010). *Fact-based labels* highlight select information from the NFP, such as the Facts Up Front label in figure 10.3. *Better-for-you systems* identify foods that meet specific nutritional criteria. For example, the AHA's "Heart-Check-Mark" highlights foods that meet their nutritional guidelines, for a fee (American Heart Association, 2013). Figure 10.4 provides an example of a supermarket's healthy foods program. *Graded better-for-you systems* denote foods that meet several tiers of nutritional criteria. For instance, the Guiding Stars shelf label program assigns zero to three stars to each edible product in participating stores, based on its **nutrient density** (Fischer et al., 2011). *Numerical rating systems* are similar, but each product displays a single score. NuVal's system ranks each food using a proprietary algorithm. Broccoli scores a perfect 100, cashews a 25, and Famous Amos Chocolate Chip Cookies a 10 (NuVal LLC, 2013).

The argument for these labels is clear. They enable shoppers to quickly identify nutritious food, which is especially important as NFP use declines sharply (Todd & Variyam, 2008). Studies show even consumers who do use the NFP often only look at one nutrient, but simplified displays that summarize nutrition information help shoppers compare foods based on their overall nutritional quality (Higginson, Rayner, Draper, & Kirk, 2002; Vishwanathan & Hastak, 2002).

As implemented, however, POP labels highlight reasons to buy a food—not avoid it. This promotes sales, but not necessarily health. For instance, Walmart labels nutritious house-brand products with a "Great for You" label, distinguishing them from both unmarked junk food and equally healthful competitors

(Walmart Stores, 2013). Even when stores assess all edible products, less nutritious foods are not labeled "don't buy"; they just remain unmarked. POP labels also frequently only appear on processed foods, suggesting advantages over whole foods. Additionally, summarizing the relative nutrition provided by any one product requires subjective decisions and scientists and consumers cannot evaluate these within proprietary POP systems. Finally, the sheer variety of displays in use also confuses consumers, who struggle to compare them and assess their credibility (British Market Research Bureau, 2009).

The Food and Drug Administration (FDA) began the process of regulating POP labels in 2009, acknowledging these concerns. However, as this book goes to press, no rules have been proposed. In the meantime, the Grocery Manufacturers Association and the Food Marketing Institute have proposed their own fact-based system, "Facts Up Front." Many see this as an industry attempt to preempt regulation by implementing voluntary changes that may be ineffective since these labels do not satisfy many of the Institute of Medicine's evidence-based recommendations to the FDA. Selective use of nutrition as a sales technique and deterring regulation with industry-sponsored voluntary approaches are common tactics of the food industry: watch your grocery aisles for a case study of both.

FIGURE 10.4   Supermarket "Better for You" Advice

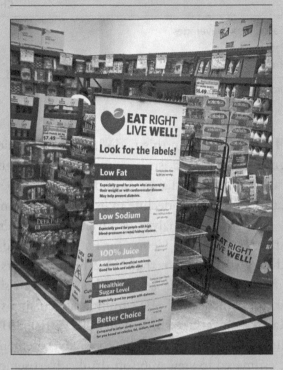

Source: Michael Milli, CLF.

EXTENT OF FOOD PROMOTION

Food is promoted extensively in the United States. Among industry sectors, the food and beverage manufacturing sector spent the seventh largest amount on advertising in 2009 ($7.82 billion), with retailers (including food retailers) spending the most (at $17.15 billion) and automobile manufacturers a close second (US measured ad spending by category, 2009). Of the top ten companies spending the most on advertising in 2010, two were food companies: McDonald's Corporation at number seven (spending $887.8 million) and Walmart at number eight ($873.8 million) (U.S. ad spending totals, 2011). These figures represent an underestimate of spending, because they include only advertising in the measured media.

Expenditure on food advertising and other forms of promotion to children and youth is considerable in the United States. Analysis by the FTC shows that in 2006, forty-eight leading food companies spent approximately $2.1 billion to promote food and beverages to children and adolescents aged two to seventeen in the United States (FTC, 2008), including $1.02 billion for carbonated beverages, restaurant food, and breakfast cereals (see table 10.2). Television advertising dominated the communications channels used to promote foods and beverages to youth, with 46 percent of all reported youth marketing expenditures (FTC, 2008). A follow-up report found that the total amount spent declined to $1.79 billion in 2009, with most of this decrease coming from less spending on television advertisements

TABLE 10.2   The Three Leading Food Categories Marketed to Children and Youth in the United States, 2006

Food Category	Expenditure (in Millions of Dollars)	
	Children	Adolescents
Carbonated beverages	18	474
Fast food	161	145
Breakfast cereals	229	8

Source: FTC (2008).

(FTC, 2012). Yet in this period, food companies increased their spending to market to children and teens in new media, such as online, mobile, and viral marketing, by 50 percent. Given online and viral marketing media are considerably less expensive than television advertising, this may indicate an increase rather than decline in exposure to promotional marketing.

More detailed analysis of advertising to adults and children in measured media using different data sources by the Rudd Center for Food Policy and Obesity at Yale University estimates that the fast food industry spends more than $4.2 billion dollars on advertising (2009 data), the three leading cereal companies spend over $156 million on advertising children's breakfast cereals (2008 data), and beverage companies spend $948 million advertising sugar-sweetened drinks and energy drinks (2010 data) (Harris, Schwartz, & Brownell, 2009, 2010, 2011). Of these advertisements, the average preschooler is estimated as seeing 1,021 fast food advertisements and 642 for cereal per year on television. Teenagers are estimated to view 406 soft drink advertisements per year.

American food companies also conduct extensive promotional marketing outside the United States (Hawkes, 2002). Many low- and middle-income countries are emerging as developing markets with large and growing populations. They thus have growth potential that far exceeds the relatively saturated market of the United States. Europe is also a large market for many American food companies.

WHERE PROMOTIONAL MARKETING FITS INTO THE MODERN FOOD SYSTEM

Promotional marketing has undergone important shifts over time in the United States. It started as a technique to target the "mass market." It then moved toward a greater degree of targeting different population segments, as already described. Today, with the emergence of social media, more and more marketing is tailored to individuals.

Early Promotional Marketing — the Rise of the Mass Market

The onset of modern marketing methods in the United States came in the late nineteenth and early twentieth centuries. This era marked the coming of mass production by big processing giants, such as Kellogg's, Post, Quaker, Birds Eye, and Heinz, mass distribution through the newly developing transport networks, followed by mass retail in the form of supermarkets. Two changes were particularly critical from a marketing perspective. First, mass production created more products than were technically needed by consumers. Second, innovations in packaging (e.g. cans, cardboard) meant that there was a place to stamp a brand that would be viewed by a consumer, unlike the bulk packages used to sell loose, weighed out products of the previous era. Figure 10.5 provides an example.

With these changes came the incentive and the means for food manufacturers to take concerted action to encourage consumers to buy more of their products. Billboards, newspaper and radio advertisements, premium giveaways, and enticing packaging could now be used to convert what had been luxury products into mass-market foods. Essential here was the emergence of the concept of a brand. In this period, iconic American brands came into being, such as Heinz tomato soup and Kraft Mac and Cheese. Brands created a means to advertise products and also provided an incentive. Previously, advertising was considered by many in the food business to be a waste of money. But innovators realized that promoting brands was a means of encouraging consumers to pay more for them: the product inside the package might not be that different between brand *x* and brand *y*, but brand *x* could be perceived as better if marketed differently, and therefore sold at a relatively higher price.

The case of Quaker oats is particularly enlightening. The Quaker Oats Company was a pioneer in advertising in the late nineteenth and early twentieth centuries (Marquette, 1967). Faced with an oversupply of oats, the then-managers of Quaker turned to branding and promotion, believing that, as put by Quaker historian Marquette (1967, p. 67) "oversupply was merely the chronic sickness of underconsumption cured by creation of demand rather than by reduction of supply." They

adopted a single brand—a smiling man in "Quaker garb" on a red and blue setting—and what was then a completely new approach to marketing: **constant exposure**. The Quaker brand was plastered everywhere (see figure 10.6): on billboards, in newspapers and magazines, and as samples on doorsteps. Overall, the strategy was clear: mass marketing a core brand for the mass market using a mass message (Wilkinson, 2002).

Packaging played a key role, too: the ability to market was considerably enhanced by the presence of a boxed carton, which carried not just the brand but also box top offers, collectable coupons for gifts, as well as gifts inside the package. These were to prove highly popular with consumers. In examples provided by Marquette (1967, p. 129) "the big deal in 1901 was a fortune telling calendar

FIGURE 10.5   Jell-O Box Provides an Opportunity for Brand Promotion, 1915.

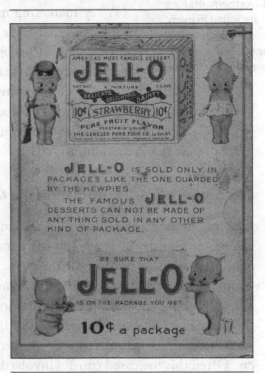

Source: Public domain.

FIGURE 10.6   The Quaker Oats Mascot Quickly Became a Familiar Face Due to Mass Marketing

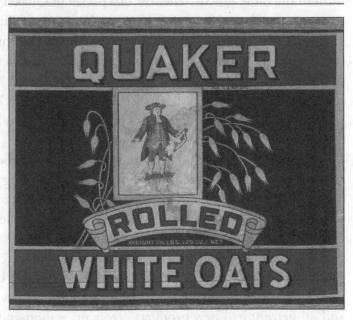

Source: Public domain.

constant exposure
Marketing approach in which advertisements for a product are found in many media such as billboards, newspapers, and magazines, and as samples on doorsteps

in fourteen colors," whereas "by 1928, the annual chinaware premiums had reached 155 carloads of 7,500 sets each."

A key marketing message promoted by Quaker was that oats were healthy. The company started their advertising on the basis that oats "supply what brains and bodies require." Quaker was a pioneer in obtaining scientific endorsements—asking scientists to confirm that the product can promote health (Fitzsimmons, 2012, p. 56).

Even in more recent times, Quaker was the first company to seek, and be granted, Food and Drug Administration (FDA) approval to use a food-specific health claim in their marketing (in 1997). Specifically, they were permitted to state that consuming soluble fiber from oats lowered heart disease risk (Fitzsimmons, 2012).

The Modern Era—Introducing the Market Segmentation

Changes in the nature of supply and demand from the mid-twentieth century onward led to a radical change of industry strategy. On the demand side, the number of consumers grew, became wealthier, and began to value product attributes such as convenience to a higher degree. On the supply side, food companies merged and acquired their competitors, leading to increased levels of industry concentration and the rise of "big food" (i.e., multinational food and beverage companies with huge and concentrated market power; Stuckler & Nestle, 2012). Companies began to exert more control over their suppliers, such as soft drink manufacturers over their bottling operations and supermarkets over food manufacturers. Often this increased control involved imposing "quality standards" to ensure suppliers met specific standards, such as the type and size of potatoes used to make French fries (Henson, 2008; McDonalds, 2008). These changes reflected—and were partly driven by—technological advancements.

With greater control over the supply chain and more modern production technologies, food companies now had more ability to develop highly differentiated products in a cost-efficient manner. They also had the financial incentive to do so. Companies could now, as described by Hatanaka, Bain, and Busch (2006, p. 48), "buy undifferentiated commodities from their suppliers and sell differentiated commodities to their customers," meaning that they could "buy low and sell high(er) while capturing most of the value added." The cost of a packet of Quaker Oats in 1991 was, for example, three thousand times greater than the cost of the oats, despite the falling price of oats over preceding decades (Morgenson, 1991, cited in Cobb-Walgren, Ruble, & Donthu, 1995). The incentive for differentiation also came from the diversity of consumers. Greater product differentiation enabled companies to appeal to a wider and more complex consumer base than the "white housewife" to which companies heavily marketed in the 1940s and 1950s (Hamilton, 2003). Companies could now target different products to ethnic minorities, working class groups, and the wealthier consumer segments willing to pay more for convenience and innovative products.

With this increased ability and incentive for product segmentation, the number of new and rebranded products soared. For example, at its founding Quaker produced basic oats. After broadening out its product portfolio in cereals relatively early, it started to target the children's market with Cap'n Crunch in the 1960s (Marquette, 1967). Their product offerings continued to broaden; in 2012, Quaker sold twenty types of oatmeal, eighteen types of oat cereal, thirty-six types of cereal bars, twenty-one types of rice snacks, and nineteen other cereal products and cookies (Quaker Oats, 2012). This high degree of differentiation applies across the US food system. A survey published in 2004 found that 71 percent of thirty leading food and beverage companies had reformulated products, and 29 percent had new products across three thousand product categories since 2001 (GMA, 2004, cited in McGinnis et al., 2006). For example, in 2012, the Coca-Cola Company had more than 3,500 products in their global portfolio, including 800 low- and no-calorie beverages—reflecting the growing importance of the "health and wellness" segment. In 2011 alone, the company launched more than one hundred low- and no-calorie beverages (Coca-Cola Company, 2012). McDonald's is another example. Long known for its French fries and burgers, the fast food chain has diversified into salads and smaller, lower-calorie menu items (see figure 10.7). The purpose: to discourage mothers concerned about health from saying no to their children when deciding what restaurant to go to—and to encourage them to eat when they get there (Miles, 2010). Generating products for children is another case in point. In the 1990s

FIGURE 10.7 As Health Concerns Grew, McDonald's Introduced Healthy Items, Such as Apple Slices, to Its Menu

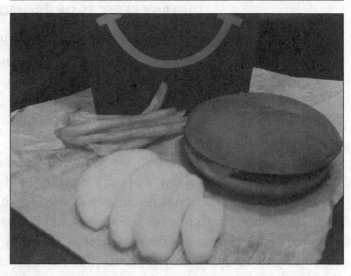

Source: Pamela Berg, CLF.

and early 2000s, the rate of introduction of new products targeted to children exceeded adult-targeted products. The vast majority were for sugar and chocolate candy, snacks, breakfast cereals, and cookies (McGinnis et al., 2006).

Critical here is that segmented products required segmented promotion. Promotion was the process by which information about the newly innovated products could be communicated to different demographic, geographical, behavioral, and psychographic groups. It is not surprising that as the number of new products increased, so did their promotion. Advertising to children began in the 1950s—the same period that child-targeted products began to appear. During the period of most prolific development of children's food in history—the 1990s—there was an estimated twenty-fold increase in spending on child-targeted advertising (McGinnis et al., 2006).

Although the existence of segmented products led to segmented promotional campaigns, even more critical is that the ability to promote these products created the incentive for their development in the first place. Promotion thus became *part* of the product. Today, promotion is used to rebrand products even when no change is made to the products themselves. In 2010, for example, McDonald's developed a promotion for its French fries with the tagline, "Only the best potatoes in the world can make World Famous Fries." The promotion was accompanied with advertising and online videos featuring a farmer with a wholesome image (McDonald's, 2012). This campaign aimed to rebrand McDonald's products as high quality in the context of consumer perception of poor quality (Miles, 2010). The notion of what can be successfully promoted also drives product development. In the case of Cap'n Crunch children's cereal, Quaker first developed a character that would appeal to children—and only after that developed the cereal itself (Marquette, 1967).

Without the ability to promote them, then, a vast array of processed foods that exist in the United States today would not exist. Promotion, combined with product innovation, has become the life blood of the modern US food system (Langlois, Zuanic, Faucher, Pannuti, & Shannon, 2006, p. 19; also Goldman Sachs Group, 2007; Hawkes, Friel, Lobstein, & Lang, 2012). It is not surprising, then, that the costs of marketing as a proportion of the US food dollar have risen rapidly. Between 1980 and 2002, for example, the costs of advertising rose by 380 percent, whereas the farm value increased by just 60 percent (Elitzak, 2004).

DIETARY EFFECTS OF PROMOTIONAL MARKETING

Promotion is used to market all forms of food in the US food system—from oats to frozen vegetables to meat to soft drinks, fast food, and candy. Health concerns have arisen because a large proportion of the marketing reaching food consumers is for foods that dietary recommendations indicate should be consumed in moderation. Content analysis of advertising from the 1950s to the present day shows that foods advertised on television are high calorie and nutrient poor, especially foods promoted to children (McGinnis et al., 2006) (see table 10.3).

It is this concern that led to the identification of food marketing as a negative force for public health. The first outcry about the health effects of food promotion in the United States came about as the results of concerns about dental caries. In 1977, three advocacy organizations—Action for Children's Television, the Center for Science in the Public Interest, and Consumers Union—petitioned the FTC to ban advertisements for sugary foods, following calls several years earlier for restrictions on all advertising to children (Story & French, 2004). Their concern was the large numbers of advertisements for sugary products seen by children (the average child was said to view around seven thousand such ads a year), combined with tooth decay as the number one childhood illness at that time (Westen, 2006). These efforts to restrict advertising by the FTC failed, and in fact caused so much consternation that Congress stripped the FTC of its authority to regulate advertising to children altogether, on the basis of "unfairness" (Pomeranz, 2010).

In response, in 1974, the industry developed a set of "Self-Regulatory Guidelines for Children's Advertising," including a clause on food (Children's Advertising Review Unit, 2012). The

TABLE 10.3   Examples of Studies of the Nutritional Content of Food Advertisements, 1970s–2010s

Year	Result of research study
1950s	45 percent of all advertisements in twenty-four children's programs were for sweetened breakfast cereals, confectionary, or snacks (Alexander, Benjamin, Hoerrner, & Roe, 1998).
1977	64 percent of advertisements in children's television were for cereals, confectionary, snacks, beverages, and fast food (Barcus,1977, cited in McGinnis et al., 2006).
1980s	52 percent of advertisements in children's television were for cereals, confectionary, snacks, beverages, and fast food (Condry, Bence, & Scheibe, 1988).
1994	46.3 percent of foods advertised during Saturday morning television were for fats, oils, or sweet foods, especially breakfast cereals (Kotz & Story, 1994).
2004	Advertising expenditures on food, beverages, candy, and restaurants were $11.26 billion in 2004, versus $9.55 million to promote healthful eating (Consumers Union, 2005)
2005	83 percent of food advertisements during TV programs heavily viewed by children were for fast foods and sweets (Harrison & Marske, 2005).
2008	Compared to cereals marketed to adults, those marketed to children have 85 percent more sugar, 65 percent less fiber, and 60 percent more sodium (Harris et al., 2009).
2010	Consuming a diet based on TV advertisements on Saturday mornings would provide 2,560 percent of the recommended daily servings for sugars, 2,080 percent for fat, but only 40 percent of the recommended daily servings for vegetables, 32 percent for dairy, and 27 percent for fruits. The same diet would substantially oversupply protein, total fat, saturated fat, cholesterol, and sodium, and substantially undersupply important micronutrients (Mink, Evans, Moore, Calderon, & Deger, 2010).

guidelines, which were administered by the especially established Children's Advertising Review Unit (CARU) at the Council for Better Business Bureau, were concerned only with the content of the advertisements—the elimination of phrases that directly encourage excessive consumption such as "the more you scarf the better your chances" (i.e., the more you eat, the better your chances of winning) and storylines that represent healthy food as "dorkish" (Hawkes, 2005). The guidelines did not extend to the quantity of food advertisements, nor to the location of advertising (e.g., in schools), nor to, with some exceptions, most other marketing techniques beyond advertising (Hawkes, 2005).

Concern about food advertising and children's health reemerged in the 1990s in light of rapidly rising rates of obesity, especially among children. An increasing amount of evidence showed that advertising directly influenced food choices (Story & French, 2004). The evidence was brought together for the first time in 2003 in a systematic review of available research published in the United Kingdom (Hastings et al., 2003). The review found that food promotion has an effect on children's food preferences, purchasing, and consumption; that this effect is independent of other factors; and that it operates at brand and category levels (Hastings et al., 2003). This last finding was important because it suggested that the competitive role of food promotion in the modern food system (that is, for one food company to attract consumers away from a competing brand toward their own) was not the only important effect. Rather, advertising increased overall consumption of product categories. For example, Coke advertising not only increases consumption of Coke relative to Pepsi, but also of sugar-sweetened carbonated beverages overall.

These findings were confirmed and refined in a review published by the IOM in 2006. The review concluded that television advertising encourages children to prefer and request high-calorie and low-nutrient foods and beverages (see table 10.4). The findings were then reconfirmed in evidence updates after 2006 by the UK research group responsible for the initial review. The updates, commissioned by the World Health Organization (WHO), confirmed earlier findings on the basis of a substantial

TABLE 10.4 Findings of the IOM Committee on Food Marketing and the Diets of Children and Youth

Indicator	Findings
Preferences and purchase requests	Strong evidence that television advertising influences the food and beverage preferences of children ages two to eleven years*
	Strong evidence that television advertising influences the food and beverage purchase requests of children ages two to eleven years*
	Moderate evidence that television advertising influences the food and beverage beliefs of children ages two to eleven years*
Dietary intake	Strong evidence that television advertising influences the short-term consumption by children ages two to eleven years*
	Moderate evidence that television advertising influences the usual dietary intake of younger children ages two to five years and weak evidence that it influences the usual dietary intake of older children ages six to eleven years; there is also weak evidence that it does not influence the usual dietary intake of teenagers ages twelve to eighteen years
Obesity	Statistically, strong evidence that exposure to television advertising is associated with adiposity in children ages two to eleven years and teenagers ages twelve to eighteen years
	Association between adiposity and exposure to television advertising remains after taking alternative explanations into account, but the research does not convincingly rule out other possible explanations for the association; therefore, the current evidence is not sufficient to arrive at any finding about a causal relationship from television advertising to adiposity.

*Lack of research studies means there is insufficient evidence about the influence of TV advertising on teenagers ages twelve to eighteen years.
Source: McGinnis et al. (2006).

increase in the volume of evidence (Cairns, Angus, & Hastings, 2009; Hastings, McDermott, Angus, Stead, & Thomson, 2006). The only significant change in the evidence base was the growing number of studies finding that television advertising, important though it is, is only one part of an increasingly multifaceted marketing communications mix that typically focuses on building brands and building relationships with consumers.

Another practice that has raised concerns is operating marketing campaigns without clearly disclosing affiliations, as described in perspective 10.1.

Perspective 10.1. Front Groups: Who Is Shaping the Conversation about Health and Wellness?

Anna Lappé

In the 1990s and 2000s, growing evidence about the potential human health impact of the artificial growth hormone (rBST) in dairy production—and evidence about the toll of the hormone on dairy cows—led to mounting pressure to phase out the hormone and label milk produced without it. By the end of 2007, public health advocates and consumer organizations had successfully won the battle to get big chains, such as Starbucks, to go "rBST-free" and many dairy farmers had stopped using the hormone, known by its brand name, Posilac (Mecklenburg, 2007). It was at this time that a new organization was launched, heralding the benefits of rBST. Called American Farmers for the Advancement and Conservation of Technology, or AFACT, its spokespeople and website promoted the benefits of rBST and dismissed any concerns. "Is rBST safe for consumers? Yes, absolutely!" read one section of the site (AFACT, 2009). But although it was presented as a "new producer organization," AFACT was actually a project of a communications firm working for Monsanto—the maker of rBST (Agrimarketing, 2006). This fact was easily missed by visitors to the site or readers of the press about the group.

front groups
Organizations with neutral-sounding names and objective-seeming spokespeople who are actually funded by corporations and work for their interests

AFACT is an example of what are known as **"front groups"**—organizations with neutral-sounding names and objective-seeming spokespeople who are actually funded by corporations and work for their interests. Front groups are a powerful, if misleading, way to influence public opinion: they appear to provide independent voices on complex policy and public health questions. Some front groups are also registered nonprofits, meaning corporate contributors can use donations as tax write-offs. As such, critics contend that these front groups should be seen as lobbying and marketing arms of industry, not tax-free charities.

AFACT is just one of dozens of these organizations working at the intersections of food and public health. The Center for Consumer Freedom (CCF) is another tax-exempt organization active with food and public health issues. With a $2.4 million budget in 2010, CCF receives hundreds of thousands of dollars from the restaurant, alcohol, tobacco, and food industries, and in 2010, its board members included executives with ties to major restaurant chains and big box stores, including P. F. Chang's, TGI Fridays, and Walmart (Center for Consumer Freedom [CCF], 2010).

Though its stated mission is to promote "personal responsibility" and protect "consumer choice," CCF runs media campaigns that fight against organizations, policy makers, and individuals working for public health and animal welfare (CCF, nd). When the New York City Department of Public Health proposed banning sales of sugary drinks larger than sixteen ounces, the Center for Consumer Freedom launched counter-responses including a full-page ad in the *New York Times* attacking the ban (see figure 10.8). The center also attacks specific nonprofit organizations, such as Mothers against Drunk Driving and the Humane Society of the United States. For example, in 2010, the center spent $982,285 on HumaneWatch.org, "a watchdog effort to educate the public about the Humane Society" (CCF, 2010). The Humane Society claims that the center's attacks reflect agribusiness concerns about the society's work to improve farm animal treatment.

Front groups are not always separate legal entities; they can also be initiatives created to push specific agendas, though presented by their creators as reflecting diverse perspectives. Keep Food Affordable, for example, is presented as a public-interest effort with broad-based support, launched in 2011 (Miller, 2012). Its Facebook page includes a picture of a smiling young girl and mom in a supermarket and posts about how to save food and save money. What is not immediately obvious is that this so-called coalition is made up of agriculture groups such as National Pork Producers Council, among other industry trade groups, and was created in response to pressure to reform industrial livestock production to improve conditions for livestock, which producers fear would raise their costs of production.

Critics charge that the deception inherent in a front group—often, but not always, obscuring their financial backers, hiding their bias, and presenting their interests as being in line with the views of the general public—is manipulative: would you feel different about the Center for Consumer Freedom campaign against sugary drinks if you knew beverage companies were funding it? Would you think differently about the Keep Food Affordable coalition if you knew it was being paid for by the pork industry to fight against improvements in conditions inside factory farms? Consumer advocates raise concerns about front groups because these institutions mislead consumers and policy makers and attempt to shape public opinion on key policy questions in the interest of corporations and profit—not public health or consumers' well-being.

FIGURE 10.8   Center for Consumer Freedom Advertisement Targets Ban on Large-Size SSBs, Depicts Mayor Michael Bloomberg as "The Nanny"

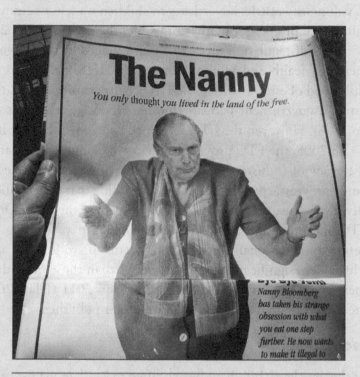

Source: Seth Anderson. (2012). Bloomberg as The Nanny. https://www.flickr.com/photos/swanksalot/7320906998.

RESPONSES FROM GOVERNMENT AND INDUSTRY

The publication of the IOM report proved a turning point in the perception of food marketing to children as a public health issue in the United States. Calls from advocacy groups for more restrictions on food marketing to children became louder. The food industry immediately went on the offensive. From a systems perspective, this would be expected: cutting off promotional marketing means degreasing the wheels that drive the market.

Self-Regulation

The initial policy response from industry was to review the existing CARU guidelines. In 2006, CARU published revised guidelines, which included clauses on advertising targeted to children that is "unfair" as well as misleading and new clauses on advertising "blurred" with editorial content and advergaming (video games that aim to promote a product or service) (Better Business Bureau [BBB], 2006). Coincident with the release of the revised guidelines, the BBB also established the Children's Food and Beverage Advertising Initiative. Under the initiative, signatory food companies agreed for the first time to voluntarily restrict advertising to children on select communications channels on foods not meeting nutritional profiles set by the companies themselves (BBB, 2012).

This self-regulation was actively encouraged by the US government. In 2005, the FTC and Department of Health and Human Services (DHHS) held a workshop on marketing, self-regulation, and childhood obesity, at which the FTC chairperson stated that "based on years of experience with advertising, a government ban on children's food advertising is neither wise nor viable" (Majoras, 2005, pp. 5–6). However, the FTC remained concerned that the industry was not doing enough.

In 2008, the FTC provided a review to Congress of "Marketing Food to Children and Adolescents: A Review of Industry Expenditures, Activities, and Self-Regulation" (FTC, 2008). Though the FTC noted progress, concerns remained, including that the nutritional standards set by the companies themselves were insufficiently strong. Subsequently, the 2009 Omnibus Appropriations Act mandated the FTC and other agencies to set up an Interagency Working Group on Food Marketed to Children to define some national nutritional standards for voluntarily adoption by industry. The draft standards, which were significantly more restrictive than those individual food companies developed to regulate themselves, were published for comment in 2011 (FTC, 2011). The food industry strongly opposed the standards, and a final version was never published.

Legislation

At the state level, bills have been drafted to legislate against certain forms of food advertising to children, including toys provided with fast food meals, advertising on school buses, and advertising in the areas surrounding schools. As of February 2013, all had failed to pass into law (Rudd Center for Food Policy and Obesity, 2013).

Legislation has been developed in other parts of the world, though it remains limited in extent and scope (Hawkes & Lobstein, 2011; WCRF International, 2014). In 2010, the WHO released a set of recommendations on the marketing of foods and nonalcoholic beverages to children (WHO, 2010), which called for "global action to reduce the impact on children of marketing of foods high in saturated fats, trans-fatty acids, free sugars, or salt" (WHO, 2010, p. 5). They stated that "a comprehensive approach has the highest potential to achieve the desired impact" (p. 9). However, no country has to date implemented a comprehensive approach to restricting promotional food marketing to children.

Social Marketing

social marketing
Application of marketing methods developed by the commercial sector to campaigns that promote social benefits including health; does not refer to marketing using social media

Another government response to marketing of less healthy foods has been to adopt **social marketing** techniques to promote "healthy" foods. Social marketing is the application of marketing methods developed by the commercial sector to campaigns that aim to promote social benefits (it does not refer to marketing using social media) (see Hastings, 2007). Evidence suggests that social marketing campaigns involving promoting good nutrition can have positive effects. A review by McDermott et al. (2005) found that out of the twenty-eight studies included, twenty-three reported a significant positive effect for at least one relevant outcome variable, including fruit and vegetable intake, fat intake, other dietary behaviors, and diet-related health variables.

In the United States, social marketing is used to promote fruits and vegetables. In 1991, the National Cancer Institute established a national 5-a-Day Program to promote fruit and vegetable consumption. Conducted in partnership with the fruit and vegetable industry, it promoted the value of fruits and vegetables through "a combination of strategies that leveraged advertising from ... industry partners and developed relationships with media outlets to generate and inform news stories related to the Program" (National Cancer Institute, 2006). Nevertheless, evaluation of the program found that its message was weakened by a lack of regular rebranding and lack of segmentation of messages to lower-income and ethnic minorities—the very

FIGURE 10.9   "More Matters" Social Marketing Campaign Logo

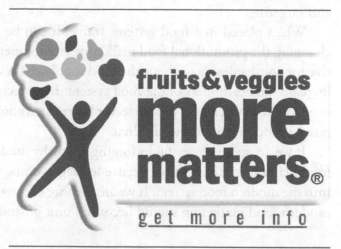

Source: CDC Produce for Better Health Foundation. With permission.

practices that proved essential to the success of commercial marketing in the latter half of the twentieth century. In response, the 5-a-Day program was rebranded in 2007 into the More Matters campaign in order to make the message more compelling (Pivonka, Seymour, McKenna, Baxter, & Williams, 2011) (see figure 10.9). Consumer research was conducted to facilitate the rebranding, finding that the most effective messages appealed to mothers' emotional needs to be responsible. A cross-sectional survey conducted in the year it was launched (2007) found that participants aware of the campaign were more likely to consume more than five servings of fruits and vegetables per day (Erinosho, Moser, Oh, Nebeling, & Yaroch, 2012). However, only 2 percent of the 3,021 adults surveyed were aware of the campaign. Although an indication of the relative newness of the campaign, it also shows the relatively limited reach of social marketing relative to commercial promotions. Indeed, an analysis by the Consumers Union found that the federal and California 5-A-Day spent $9.55 million in 2004 on communications to encourage fruit and vegetable consumption—a significant amount, but tiny compared to the $11.26 billion spent on advertising by the food, beverage, and restaurant industries (Consumers Union, 2005). Whatever its promise, then, the potential (and limitations) of social marketing to promote healthier eating have not yet been fully tested.

CONCLUSION

Promotional marketing has had a profound impact on the US diet, helping to move processed, packaged foods from luxury goods to the mass market. It is now used to drive growth by appealing to market segments and through individualized marketing. A food systems perspective shows just how fundamental promotional marketing is to the functioning of the US food economy—as well as to modern food economies elsewhere.

Yet promotional marketing raises uneasy questions about the risks for public health introduced by the basic functioning of this economic system. These risks are clear from the evidence on the public health impacts of promotional marketing, particularly on vulnerable groups. There have thus far been two approaches to address this: reducing the amount of promotional activity targeting one of these vulnerable groups (children and young people) and using marketing to promote socially productive products.

Neither of the approaches has yet been fully tested, either through a comprehensive restriction on marketing of less healthy foods to children or by extensive social marketing incorporating segmentation and targeting.

When placed in a food systems frame, it can be seen just how profound the effects would be of changing the promotional food marketing environment. Making these changes would create the incentive for companies throughout the food supply chain to change their business models, and in so doing, increase the healthiness of the food system. But precisely because promotion is so fundamental to the modern food system, the private sector has resisted efforts by public health advocates to comprehensively restrict food promotion to children.

If we are to be successful in forging a healthy modern food system, we need action on promotional food marketing. To identify effective leverage points, we need to better understand how marketing fits into the modern food system. If we are to more effectively address modern public health problems, then, modern food marketing should become a unit of study for public health students and practitioners.

SUMMARY

Food promotion is a component of food marketing more generally. It involves any form of commercial communication or message that is designed to, or has the effect of, increasing the recognition, appeal and consumption of the promoted foods. Without advertising and promotion, the US food system would not be what it is today. Promotional activity initially enabled processed foods to move from luxury to mass-market products. Numerous promotional channels and techniques are used in the United States to stimulate demand for all types of food and drinks. These modern marketing methods have their origins in the late nineteenth and early twentieth centuries, when the onset of mass production and the use of packaging created the incentive to develop—and the means to promote—branded foods. In the second half of the twentieth century, the mass market approach to promotional marketing was replaced with a strategy more focused on segmented marketing. Both as a cause and an effect of promotional marketing, product differentiation increased. Three types of strategy are discussed in focus and perspective boxes: within-store marketing, front-of-package labeling, and the misleading use of front groups to promote messages. Public health practitioners and advocates are concerned about the large proportion of promotional food marketing for high-calorie, nutrient-poor foods. Evidence shows that advertising particularly influences children's food preferences, purchase requests, and dietary intakes. There have been only limited actions taken by governments to restrict promotional food marketing, and these face significant opposition.

KEY TERMS

Communications channels	Integrated
Constant exposure	Marketing
Front groups	Measured media
Front of package	Nonmeasured media
Health claims	Nutrient claims
Impulse buys	Nutrient density

Point of sale

Promotion

Psychographic

Segmentation

Signposts

Social marketing

Trade promotion

DISCUSSION QUESTIONS

1. What would the US diet look like if there had never been any food advertising or promotion? What would US food system look like?

2. What difference has the increasing amount of segmentation in modern marketing methods made to the effects of promotional marketing?

3. Is restricting food advertising and promotion desirable or doable today? Is using marketing for promoting healthier eating a preferable approach? What other strategies might be used to alter the marketing environment in order to improve eating behaviors?

4. What kind of full systems change would reduce the incentive for the private food sector to engage in promotional marketing in the first place?

5. To what extent is it a free speech issue to allow marketers to put out whatever messages they wish, targeting whomever they wish, with whatever frequency they wish? What about if they mask their identities?

REFERENCES

AFACT. (2009). *The facts about recombinant bovine somatotropin*. Retrieved from http://itisafact.org/2009/04/the-facts-about-recombinant-bovine-somatotropin-rbst

Agrimarketing. (2006). *Monsanto Dairy, St. Louis, MO, a division of Monsanto Co. specializing in health and breeding products for dairy animals, has selected Osborn & Barr Communications as its agency of record*. Retrieved from www.highbeam.com/doc/1G1-147011117.html

Alexander, A., Benjamin, L., Hoerrner, K., & Roe, D. (1998). "We'll be back in a moment": A content analysis of advertisements in children's television in the 1950s. *Journal of Advertising, 27*(3), 1–9.

American Heart Association. (2013). *Heart-check mark nutritional guidelines*. Retrieved from www.heart.org/HEARTORG/GettingHealthy/NutritionCenter/HeartSmartShopping/Heart-Check-Mark-Nutritional-Guidelines_UCM_300914_Article.jsp

American Marketing Association. (2007). *Definition of marketing*. Retrieved from www.marketingpower.com/AboutAMA/Pages/DefinitionofMarketing.aspx

Barcus, F. E. (1977). *Children's television: An analysis of programming and advertising*. New York: Praeger.

Better Business Bureau. (2012). *Children's food and beverage advertising initiative*. Retrieved from www.bbb.org/us/childrens-food-and-beverage-advertising-initiative

British Market Research Bureau. (2009). *Comprehension and use of UK nutrition signpost labelling schemes*. London: British Market Research Bureau.

Cairns, G., Angus, K., & Hastings, G. (2009). *The extent, nature and effects of food promotion to children: A review of the evidence to December 2008*. Geneva: World Health Organization.

Center for Consumer Freedom. (2010). *Form 990*. Retrieved from www.Guidestar.com

Center for Consumer Freedom. (2012). *The nanny*. Retrieved from www.consumerfreedom.com/wp-content/uploads/2012/06/Bloomberg-nanny_finaldraft.pdf

Center for Consumer Freedom. (nd). *What is the Center for Consumer Freedom?* Retrieved from www.consumerfreedom.com/about

Chandon, P., Hutchinson, J. W., Bradlow, E. T., & Young, S. H. (2009). Does in-store marketing work? Effects of the number and position of shelf facings on brand attention and evaluation at the point of purchase. *Journal of Marketing*, *73*(6), 1–17.

Children's Advertising Review Unit. (2012.). *About the Children's Advertising Review Unit (CARU)*. Retrieved from www.caru.org/about/index.aspx

Cobb-Walgren, C. J., Ruble, C. A., & Donthu, N. (1995). Brand equity, brand preference, and purchase intent. *Journal of Advertising*, *24*(3), 25–40.

Coca-Cola Company. (1995). *Annual report* (pp. 27, 29). Atlanta: Coca-Cola Company.

Coca-Cola Company. (2012). *Products*. Retrieved from www.thecoca-colacompany.com/brands/index.html?WT.cl=1&WT.mm=top-left-menu5-prodinfo-red_en_US

Condry, J., Bence, P., & Scheibe, C. (1988). Nonprogram content of children's television. *Journal of Broadcasting Electronic Media*, *32*(3), 255–270.

Consumers Union. (2005). *Marketing of soda, candy, snacks and fast foods drowns out healthful messages*. San Francisco: California Pan-Ethnic Health Network/Consumers Union. Retrieved from www.consumersunion.org/pdf/OutofBalance.pdf

Elitzak, H. (2004). The consumer food dollar. *Amber Waves*, February.

Erinosho, T. O., Moser, R. P., Oh, A. Y., Nebeling, L. C., & Yaroch, A. L. (2012). Awareness of the Fruits and Veggies–More Matters campaign, knowledge of the fruit and vegetable recommendation, and fruit and vegetable intake of adults in the 2007 Food Attitudes and Behaviors (FAB) Survey. *Appetite*, *59*(1), 155–160.

Federal Trade Commission. (2008). *Marketing food to children and adolescents: A review of industry expenditures, activities, and self-regulation*. A report to Congress. Washington, DC: FTC

Federal Trade Commission. (2011). *Interagency working group on food marketed to children. preliminary proposed nutrition principles to guide industry self-regulatory efforts*. Washington, DC: FTC/CDC/FDA/USDA. Available at http://cspinet.org/new/pdf/IWG_food_marketing_proposed_guidelines_4.11.pdf

Federal Trade Commission. (2012). *Review of food marketing to children and adolescents – follow up report*. Washington, DC: FTC. Available at www.ftc.gov/reports/review-food-marketing-children-adolescents-follow-report

Fischer, L. M., Sutherland, L. A., Kaley, L. A., Fox, T. A., Hasler, C. M., Nobel, J., Kantor, M. A., & Blumberg, J. (2011). Development and implementation of the Guiding Stars Nutrition Guidance Program. *American Journal of Health Promotion*, *26*(2), e55–e63.

Fitzsimmons, R. (2012). Oh, what those oats can do. Quaker Oats, the Food and Drug Administration, and the market value of scientific evidence 1984 to 2010. *Comprehensive Reviews in Food Science and Food Safety*, *11*, 56–99.

Goldman Sachs Group. (2007). *Global: Food and beverages*. London: Global Investment Research.

GMA. 2004. *GMA members: Part of the solution*. Washington, DC: Author.

Grocery Manufacturers Association & Food Marketing Institute. (2011). *GMA and FMI announce "facts up front" as theme for front-of-pack labeling program consumer education campaign* [Press Release]. Retrieved from http://factsupfront.org/Newsroom/2

Grier, S. A., & Kumanyika, S. K. (2008). The context for choice: Health implications of targeted food and beverage marketing to African Americans. *American Journal of Public Health*, *98*(9), 1616–1629.

Grier, S. A., & Kumanyika, S. (2010). Targeted marketing and public health. *Annual Review of Public Health*, *31*, 349–369.

Hamilton, S. (2003). The economies and conveniences of modern-day living: Frozen foods and mass marketing, 1945–1965. *Business History Review*, *77*, 33–60.

Harris, J. L., Schwartz, M. B., & Brownell, K. D. (2009). *Cereal FACTS: Evaluating the nutrition quality and marketing of children's cereals*. New Haven, CT: Rudd Center for Food Policy and Obesity. Retrieved from www.cerealfacts.org

Harris, J. L., Schwartz, M. B., & Brownell, K. D. (2010). *Fast food FACTS: Evaluating fast food nutrition and marketing to youth*. New Haven, CT: Rudd Center for Food Policy and Obesity. Retrieved from www.fastfoodmarketing.org

Harris, J. L., Schwartz, M. B., & Brownell, K. D. (2011). *Sugary drink FACTS: Evaluating sugary drink nutrition and marketing to youth*. New Haven, CT: Rudd Center for Food Policy and Obesity. Retrieved from www.sugarydrinkfacts.org

Harrison, K., & Marske, A. L. (2005). Nutritional content of foods advertised during the television programs children watch most. *American Journal of Public Health, 95*(9), 1568–1574.

Hastings, G. (Ed.). (2007). *Social marketing: Why should the devil have all the best tunes?* Oxford: Elsevier.

Hastings, G., McDermott, L., Angus, K., Stead, M., & Thomson, S. (2006). *The extent, nature and effects of food promotion to children: A review of the evidence*. Geneva: World Health Organization. Retrieved from www.who.int/dietphysicalactivity/publications/Hastings_paper_marketing.pdf

Hastings, G., Stead, M., McDermott, L., Forsyth, A., MacKintosh, A. M., Rayner, M., et al. (2003). *Review of research on the effects of food promotion to children*. London: Food Standards Agency.

Hatanaka, M., Bain, C., & Busch, L., (2006). Differentiated standardization, standardized differentiation: The complexity of the global agrifood system. *Research in Rural Sociology and Development, 12*, 39–68.

Hawkes, C. (2002). Marketing activities of global soft drink and fast food companies in emerging markets: A review. *Globalization, diets, and noncommunicable diseases*. Geneva: World Health Organization.

Hawkes, C. (2005). Self-regulation of food advertising: What it can, could and cannot do to discourage unhealthy eating habits among children. *Nutrition Bulletin, 30*, 374–382.

Hawkes, C., Friel, S., Lobstein, T., & Lang, T. (2012). Linking agricultural policies with obesity and noncommunicable diseases: A new perspective for a globalizing world. *Food Policy, 37*, 343–353.

Hawkes, C., & Harris, J. L. (2011). An analysis of the content of food industry pledges on marketing to children. *Public Health Nutrition, 14*(8), 1403–1414.

Hawkes, C., & Lobstein, T. (2011). Regulating the commercial promotion of food to children: A survey of actions worldwide. *International Journal of Pediatric Obesity, 6*(2), 83–94.

Henson, S. J. (2008). The role of public and private standards in regulating international food markets. *Journal of International Agricultural Trade and Development, 4*(1), 63–81.

Higginson, C. S., Rayner, M. J., Draper, S., & Kirk, T. R. (2002). The nutrition label—which information is looked at? *Nutrition and Food Science, 32*(2–3), 92–99.

Inman, J. J., Winer, R. S., & Ferraro, R. (2009). The interplay among category characteristics, customer characteristics, and customer activities on in-store decision making. *Journal of Marketing, 73*(5), 19–29.

Inman, J. J., Winer, R. S., & Marketing Science Institute. (1998). *Where the rubber meets the road: A model of in-store consumer decision making*. Cambridge, MA: Marketing Science Institute.

Institute of Medicine. (2012). *Front-of-package nutrition rating systems and symbols: Promoting healthier choices*. Washington, DC: The National Academies Press.

Keegan, W. J. (2007). *Global marketing management* (7th ed.). Upper Saddle, River, NJ: Prentice Hall.

Kotz, K., & Story, M. (1994). Food advertisements during children's Saturday morning television programming: Are they consistent with dietary recommendations? *Journal of the American Diet Association, 94*(11), 1296–1300.

Langlois, A., Zuanic, P. E., Faucher, J., Pannuti, C., & Shannon, J. (2006). *Obesity: Re-shaping the food industry*. London: JP Morgan Global Equity Research.

Majoras, D. P. (2005). *FTC/HHS marketing, self-regulation, and childhood obesity workshop*. Comments, July 15. Washington, DC: Federal Trade Commission. Retrieved from www.ftc.gov/speeches/majoras/050715obesityworkshopremarks.pdf.

Marquette, A. F. (1967). *Brands, trademarks and goodwill: The story of the Quaker Oats Company.* New York: McGraw-Hill.

McDermott, L., et al. (2005). *Systematic review of the effectiveness of social marketing nutrition and food safety interventions.* Final Report Prepared for Safefood, University of Stirling. Retrieved from www.management.stir.ac.uk/research/social-marketing/projects/?a=19813

McDonald's. (2008). *McDonald's world famous French fries. McDonald's electronic press pack.* Retrieved from http://mcdepk.com/mqc/trip3/FrenchFry_FactSheet.pdf

McDonald's. (2012). *Supplier stories: Potatoes.* Retrieved from www.mcdonalds.com/us/en/supplierstories.html#/Potatoes

McGinnis, J. M., Gootman, J. A., & Kraak, V. I. (2006). *Food marketing to children and youth: Threat or opportunity?* Washington, DC: National Academies Press.

Mecklenburg, S. (2007). *Letter from Starbucks to Wenonah Hauter.* Retrieved from www.foodandwaterwatch.org/food/food safety/dairy/starbucks-campaign/starbucks-letter-to-fww

Miles, B. (2010). Marketing health conscious. *QSR, 141,* April 12. Retrieved from www.qsrmagazine.com/promotions/marketing-health-conscious?microsite=605+4123

Miller, M. (2012). *New coalition targets food affordability and more.* Pork Network. Retrieved from www.porknetwork.com/pork-news/158010835.html

Mink, M., Evans, A., Moore, C. G., Calderon, K. S., & Deger, S. (2010). Nutritional imbalance endorsed by televised food advertisements. *Journal of the American Dietetic Association, 110*(6), 904–910.

Morgenson, G. (1991). The trend is not their friend. *Forbes, 146,* 114–119.

National Cancer Institute. (2006). *5 a Day for Better Health program evaluation report.* Washington, DC: Author. Retrieved from http://cancercontrol.cancer.gov/5ad_exec.html

NuVal, LLC. (2013). "*The Higher the NuVal^{TM} Score, the Better the Nutrition.*" Retrieved from www.nuval.com/How

Pivonka, E., Seymour, J., McKenna, J., Baxter, S. D., & Williams, S. (2011). Development of the behaviorally focused Fruits & Veggies—More Matters public health initiative. *Journal of the American Dietetic Association, 111*(10), 1570–1577.

Pomeranz, J. L. (2010). Television food marketing to children revisited: The Federal Trade Commission has the constitutional and statutory authority to regulate. *Journal of Law, Medicine and Ethics,* Spring, 98–116.

Quaker Oats. (2012). *Products.* Retrieved from www.quakeroats.com/products.aspx

Rudd Center for Food Policy and Obesity. (2012). Legislation database. Retrieved from www.yaleruddcenter.org/legislation

Schor, D., Maniscalco, S., Tuttle, M., Alligood, S., & Reinhardt Kapsak, W. (2010). Nutrition facts you can't miss: The evolution of front-of-pack labeling; providing consumers with tools to help select foods and beverages to encourage more healthful diets. *Nutrition Today, 45*(1), 22–32.

Sierra Services/SCMC. (2011). *Breaking down the chain: A guide to the soft drink industry.* Oakland, CA: NPLAN/Public Health Law & Policy. Retrieved from http://changelabsolutions.org/sites/phlpnet.org/files/Beverage_Industry_Report-FINAL_20110907.pdf

Story, M., & French, S. (2004). Food advertising and marketing directed at children and adolescents. *International Journal of Behavioral Nutrition and Physical Activity, 1,* 3.

Stuckler, D., & Nestle, M. (2012). Big food, food systems, and global health. *PLoS Med 9*(6), e1001242

Todd, J. E., & Variyam, J. N. (2008). *The decline in consumer use of food nutrition labels, 1995–2006* (Economic Research Report No. 63). Washington, DC: US Department of Agriculture Economic Research Service.

Traveling type nerds check out signs. (2011, March 30). [Blog]. Retrieved from http://letterpressdaughter.blogspot.com/2011/03/traveling-type-nerds-check-out-signs.html

U.S. ad spending totals. (2011). *Advertising Age, 82*(25), 3.

U.S. measured ad spending by category. (2009). *Advertising Age, 80*(43), 16.

Vishwanathan, M., & Hastak, M. (2002). The role of summary information in facilitating consumers' comprehension of nutrition information. *Journal of Public Policy and Marketing, 21,* 305–318.

Walmart Stores. (2013). *Walmart report: "Great For You" food labeling initiative*. Retrieved from http://corporate.walmart .com/global-responsibility/hunger-nutrition/great-for-you

Westen, T. (2006). Government regulation of food marketing to children: The Federal Trade Commission and the kid-vid controversy. *Loyola of Los Angeles Law Review, 39,* 79–92.

Wilkinson, J. (2002). The final foods industry and the changing face of the global agro-food system. *Sociologia Ruralis, 42*(4), 329–346.

World Cancer Research Foundation (WCRF) International. (2014). *Restrict food advertising and other forms of commercial promotion*. Retrieved from http://www.wcrf.org/policy_public_affairs/nourishing_framework/food_marketing_ advertising

World Health Organization. (2010). *Set of recommendations on the marketing of foods and non-alcoholic beverages to children*. Geneva: Author. Retrieved from www.who.int/dietphysicalactivity/marketing-food-to-children/en/index.html

Zachary, D., Palmer, A., Beckham, A., & Surkan, P. (2013). A framework for understanding grocery purchasing in a low-income urban environment. *Qualitative Health Research, 23*(5), 665–678.

Food Supply Chain: From Seed to Sales

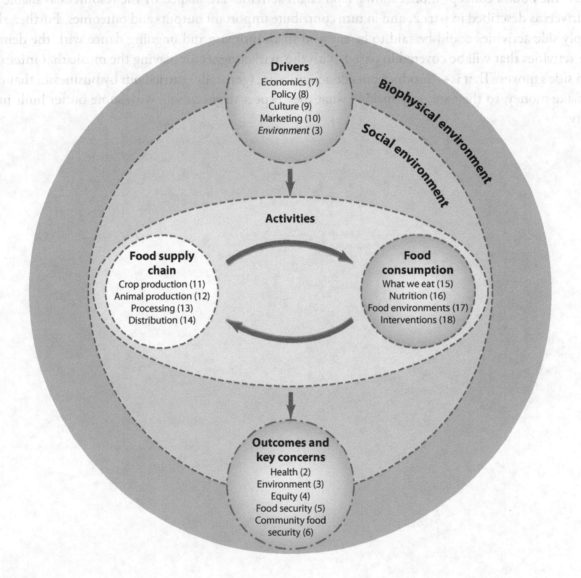

Part 3 Chapters

Chapter 11 Crop Production and Food Systems

Chapter 12 Food Animal Production

Chapter 13 Food Processing and Packaging

Chapter 14 Food Distribution

In part 3, the book takes the reader through the major activities in the food chain up to the point when the food enters consumers' hands. The section includes chapters on crop production (chapter 11), food animal production (chapter 12), food processing and packaging (chapter 13), and food distribution (chapter 14). The chapters describe sector history, structure, and operations. This section also includes some discussion of policy, economic, and industry drivers, as well as impacts on public health, environment, and equity.

As the book's concept model shows, food chain activities are shaped by the resources available and by drivers as described in part 2, and in turn contribute important outputs and outcomes. Further, these supply side activities could be said to be engaged in an intimate and ongoing dance with the demand side activities that will be covered in part 4, with the marketing sector playing the music that intensifies each side's moves. That is—production-side activities are (generally) carried out by businesses that need to make money, so they are only making what they expect they can sell, with some buffer built in for safety.

Chapter 11

Crop Production and Food Systems

Charles A. Francis

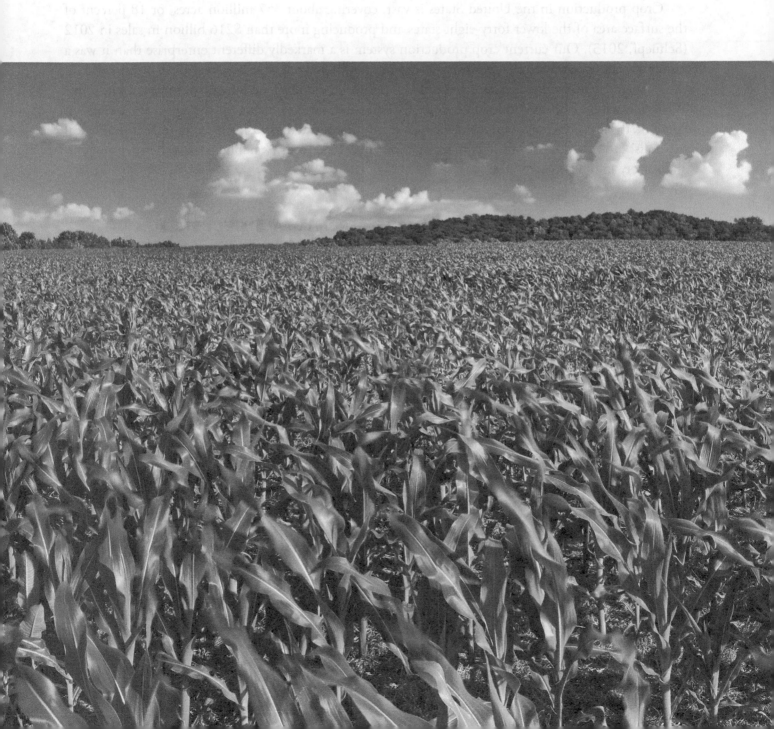

Crop production in the United States is vast, covering about 357 million acres, or 18 percent of the surface area of the lower forty-eight states and producing more than $216 billion in sales in 2012 (Schnepf, 2013). Our current crop production system is a markedly different enterprise than it was a hundred years ago and has changed even more from traditional practices here and around the world. In this chapter the following questions are explored: How did crop production evolve to its current form? What does modern crop production farming look like in farms producing for the national distribution network, those producing for local and regional distribution, and those using organic and agroecological methods? How do these forms of crop production affect food security, public health, the environment, and society in the United States?

HISTORY OF FARMING SYSTEMS—FROM LOCAL TO INDUSTRIAL

Historically, when human populations were relatively small and widely dispersed, slash-and-burn agriculture was the norm. Farmers would cut down foliage and plant crops in an area, then move on when fertility declined. The human food supply increased as people discovered the most productive and desirable strains of crops—those with the largest seeds, nonshattering ears, heads or pods (plants that held their grains until harvest), and those that were palatable, nutritious, and easily stored. These varieties increased productivity, which helped some areas of the world adopt a more organized and sedentary agriculture about twelve thousand years ago (Sauer, 1952).

Early farmers took advantage of mutually beneficial relationships among a variety of plants and domesticated animals (Harris, 1996). The animals provided meat and labor, and fertilized soils with manure while feeding on crops, residues, and pastures. Farmers learned to use rotations (alternating plantings) of cereals and legumes to improve soil fertility and give additional protection against pests, many of which prefer particular crop types and would be less likely to establish

FIGURE 11.1 Farmer Plowing with Horse for Traction

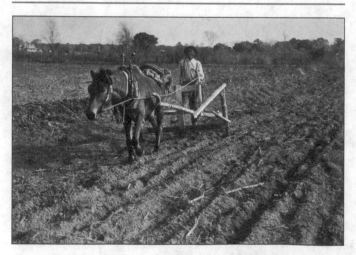

Source: USDA via Flickr Commons. http://www.flickr.com/photos/412840 17@N08/6303010576

if the same crop were not planted continuously. Biodiversity in these systems similarly helped prevent pathogens and insects specific to certain crops from taking over. A diversity of plants also meant that much of the soil profile was saturated with roots that could bring up nutrients from below; soil microbial life converted these nutrients into soluble forms useful to plants. With horses for traction (as in figure 11.1) and a diversity of cattle, hogs, sheep, and poultry for their food supply, family farms needed substantial areas of feed crops to provide for this array of livestock. Growing feed and forage crops further diversified the crop-animal enterprises. Over thousands of years, farmers domesticated wild plants and turned them into domesticated crops, incorporating traits beneficial to agriculture (Balter, 2007). Although the specific methods, plants, and animals varied considerably around the globe, variations in growing conditions stimulated development of agricultural systems that incorporated similar ideas in many different places.

TRADITIONAL SYSTEMS IN THE UNITED STATES

In the United States, early agricultural systems were small scale and **diverse farming systems** (meaning multiple types of plants and animals were grown together), depended on resources internal to the farm, and enabled farm families and communities to achieve a degree of self-sufficiency (Hurt, 2002). Native Americans planted corn, squash, and beans in mixed patterns, often on small flood plains where soils were rich and usually had adequate moisture. The first settlers from Europe likewise cultivated small areas, carving fields out of the forest, planting seeds of the crop species they brought with them, and also adopting the corn and associated crops they found in North America.

diverse farming systems Planting patterns that include two or more species interplanted together, fields that are planted in rotation of different crops, and crop-livestock integration on the farm

Moving westward and clearing more forests, the new immigrants gradually began to enlarge their holdings to plant larger fields and expand into fertile prairies to initiate farming where soils had accumulated organic matter for centuries (see figure 11.2). Using slave labor, Southern farmers planted cotton to feed the waiting mills in England. Much of the food produced was eaten by farm families or sold in nearby communities. Because they relied on horses for preparing and cultivating their land, farmers' output was modest. In the Midwest, there were small communities roughly every ten miles along the rail lines. That meant a farmer could take a horse and wagon with a load of grain five miles to the grain elevator and return home before nightfall.

FIGURE 11.2 Moving Westward: Nebraska Farm Family, 1888

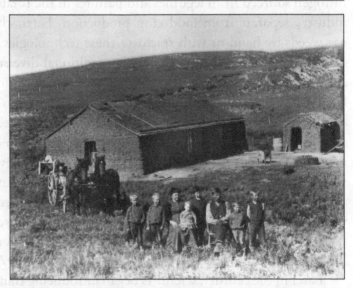

Source: USDA via Flickr Commons. http://www.flickr.com/photos/412840 17@N08/6302886826

EMERGENCE OF AN INDUSTRIAL AGRICULTURE

The nineteenth-century industrial revolution and the advent of chemical fertilizers and pesticides in the twentieth century dramatically changed farming in the United States and many parts of the world.

New implements such as the steel plow, mechanical seeders, and steam-powered threshers drove industrialization in the United States. Because tractors could cover more ground than horses, farmers were able to buy land from neighbors and farms became larger. Steam and then diesel tractors could break open the prairie sod, enabling farmers to plant more wheat and corn. As larger machinery became available and forage crops to feed horses gave way to grains, farms consolidated and many people moved to cities seeking other jobs and higher incomes. These advances made agriculture more efficient, in terms of labor needs, with tractors tilling the land more quickly in preparation for seeding and reducing labor needed for crop cultivation and harvest.

The industrialization of farming made it feasible to plant large monoculture fields, and replacing much of the human labor with machines meant that one farmer could manage ever-larger tracts of land. Other factors enhanced the trend toward larger farms over the twentieth century, such as irrigation systems, larger-scale machinery, favorable commodity prices, and relatively consistent government supports. Abundant natural resources including virgin soils, cheap fossil fuels, fossil water, and relatively stable climates further enabled this expansion. As soils were degraded, increasing use of inputs such as irrigation, fertilizers and energy were essentially necessitated to compensate for the loss.

With large investments in land and equipment came large risks, yet those farmers with an existing land base could use their equity to expand further. As a result, industrialization contributed to farmers with larger farms buying out many smaller ones, fueling a sustained increase in farm size. This has been called a "technological treadmill" in which those who run fast keep buying more land and accessing production inputs, whereas others fall behind or fall off the treadmill (Cochran, 1993). As the farming population shrank, fears of food scarcity strengthened the drive to industrialize so as to produce more food with less human labor.

Chemical use changed as well. In the early twentieth century, the new Haber-Bosch process of synthesizing nitrogen accelerated the development of synthetic fertilizers. Chemical fertilizers replaced the nitrogen sourced from legumes and pastures in the rotation, and raising livestock became a specialized industry separate from food crop production. Later, chemical herbicides reduced the need to manage weeds by hand or with tractors. These technologies made it possible to plant large areas in single crops (monocultures) rather than the traditional diverse crop mixtures. More recently, technological advances have made farming more precise. Global positioning systems now guide equipment and regulate fertilizer and herbicide application. New-generation chemicals have more specific focus on control of particular pests and less environmental impact than earlier ones.

Accompanying these shifts in farm size and management were changes in the crop types and varieties used. For example, irrigation expansion has enabled cultivation of corn, soybeans, and vegetables in areas where rainfall is too limited for successful production in most years without it. Plant breeding efforts accelerated in the twentieth century and became commercialized when breeders developed hybrid seeds with desired traits, such as high yields, pathogen and insect resistance, and tolerance to drought. At the same time, higher yields in many cases led to reduced grain quality (Davis, Epp, & Riordan, 2004; De Vita, Di Paolo, Fecondo, Di Fonzo, & Pisante, 2007).

Later in the century, scientists began introducing transgenic crop varieties, also known as genetically engineered or modified (GE or GMO) crops, which were developed by transfer of genes from one species to another. Most of these traits aim to simplify production by making it easier to manage weeds and insects. To create a transgenic variety, genetic engineers move genetic material from one species to another to insert genes for desired traits. For example, Roundup-ready soybeans are engineered to resist the widely used herbicide Roundup enabling farmers to spray their fields against weeds without killing the soybeans. Other examples are Bt corn, Bt soybeans, and Bt cotton which all contain a transgene that produces a protein from the bacterium Bacillus thuringiensis, which is now integral to their own genomes. GE varieties accounted for 88 percent of all US acreage planted in corn and 93 percent of all soybean acreage in 2012 (US Department of Agriculture [USDA], 2013) (figure 11.3). These technologies have added great convenience to farming, in many cases reducing costs for insecticides and labor, but their costs and benefits and long-term impacts on the environment and food production continue to be the subject of heated debate. Additionally, as discussed in the end of this chapter, in protecting their proprietary seeds through patents, manufacturers have raised costs of seeds and introduced rules for farmers that

FIGURE 11.3 Adoption of GE Crops in the United States, 1996–2013

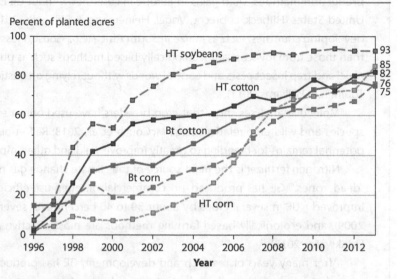

Note: Data for each crop category include varieties with both HT and Bt stacked traits.
Source: USDA.

are perceived as negative, especially in developing countries, where farmers often save seeds from their own harvests to plant again. Now, they cannot legally save their own seeds from these GE varieties and hybrids. Perspective 11.1 presents one assessment of the evidence and perspective on genetic engineering. For another assessment and additional context, students are encouraged to read the USDA's 2014 report, *Genetically Engineered Crops in the United States* (Fernandez-Cornejo, Wechsler, Livingston, and Mitchell, 2014).

Perspective 11.1. The Relevance of Genetically Engineered Crops to Sustainable Agriculture
Douglas Gurian-Sherman

Agricultural technologies must improve sustainability by addressing challenges such as climate change while reducing environmental harm. Genetic engineering (GE) has reduced insecticide use in the United States, but has increased herbicide use by a much greater amount (Benbrook, 2012). Some increases in soil-preserving conservation tillage (reduced plowing for weed control) are attributable to GE crops but most increases in the United States occurred before these crops were commercialized in the mid-1990s (NRC, 2010). Further, resilience to climate change and agricultural pollution have changed little because of GE, and GE is also much more expensive and usually less effective than viable alternatives such as breeding and agroecology.

Minimal Contributions to Productivity and Pollution Reduction

Engineered traits have produced modest productivity gain in corn, and little or none in soybeans in the United States (Gurian-Sherman, 2009). Most productivity improvements come from other breeding and crop

(Continued)

(Continued)

production methods. Yield gains in European countries without GE crops are as high as or higher than in the United States (Hilbeck, Lebrecht, Vogel, Heinemann, & Binimelis, 2013). Yield improvements from Bt traits in developing countries, such as maize in South Africa (e.g., Gouse, Piesse, Thirtle, & Poulton, 2009), often are less than those from low-cost agroecologically based methods such as push-pull, a system using multiple crops to repel and trap insect pests and control weeds without relying on pesticides (Cook, Khan, & Pickett, 2007; Pretty, Toulmin, & Williams, 2011).

Molecular analyses show that crop breeders have used only a small fraction of genetic diversity in crop species and wild crop relatives (e.g., McCouch et al., 2013; Reif et al., 2005). Therefore substantial untapped potential remains for breeding to greatly improve yield and other important traits without using GE.

Nitrogen fertilizer is the main source of the climate change gas nitrous oxide, and causes coastal hypoxic "dead zones." GE has produced no commercial nitrogen-use-efficiency (NUE) trait, whereas breeding has improved NUE in several crops by about 30 to 40 percent over several decades (Gurian-Sherman & Gurwick, 2009), and ecologically based farming methods are most effective at reducing nitrogen pollution (Blesh & Drinkwater, 2013).

After many years of research and development, GE has produced only one drought-resistance trait, in corn, that improves overall productivity by only about 1 percent (Gurian-Sherman, 2012). However, several drought-tolerant corn varieties developed through breeding have been introduced, as well as conventionally bred drought tolerance in several other crop species (Gurian-Sherman, 2012).

Crop breeding is also far less costly than GE and develops traits as rapidly (Goodman & Carson, 2000). Industry puts the cost of a typical successful engineered trait at about $140 million—mostly for R&D, infrastructure, and marketing—compared to about $1 million for typical conventional breeding (Goodman & Carson, 2000; Phillips McDougall, 2011).

Major challenges lie ahead. The few widely successful GE traits are simple—single genes that code directly for insect or herbicide resistance. Traits such as drought tolerance are genetically and physiologically complex, often environment-specific, and controlled by many genes. GE contributions to these traits are likely to be modest for the foreseeable future.

The Broader Context—Industrial Monoculture

GE technology and seed industries are dominated by transnational corporations interested in large commodity markets (Howard, 2009a). Gene patents in many countries, and the high cost of development, enable large companies to control most uses of the technology.

Current GE traits have reduced labor and thereby facilitated the simplification of agroecosystems and increasing farm size. Most GE acreage consists of large and increasing monocultures (Plourde, Pijanowski, & Pekin, 2013) of corn and soybeans in the United States, Brazil, and Argentina. Monocultures are contrary to agroecologically sound farming systems, which reduce pollution and improve resilience while remaining highly productive and profitable (Davis, Hill, Chase, Johanns, & Liebman, 2012).

Monocultures of herbicide-resistant crops have exacerbated herbicide resistant weed development due to overreliance on and poor regulation of these crops. This is leading to a new generation of crops engineered to use older, more toxic herbicides (Mortensen, Egan, Maxwell, Ryan, & Smith, 2012). Also, greatly increased glyphosate herbicide use has resulted in harm to monarch butterfly populations due to reduction of their food sources (Pleasants & Oberhauser, 2013).

In recent years, insects resistant to Bt and secondary insect pests not controlled by Bt are leading to a partial rebound in the use of chemical insecticides and threaten sustainability of some Bt traits (Berry, 2013; Fausti, McDonald, Lundgren, Li, Keating, & Catangui, 2012; Gassmann, Petzold-Maxwell, Clifton, Dunbar, Hoffmann, Ingber, & Keweshan, 2014; Jongeneel, 2013; Tabashnik, Brévault, & Carrière, 2013; Zhao, Ho, & Azadi, 2011). Some newer Bt traits also appear to be harming beneficial insect biodiversity (Stephens, Losey, Allee, DiTommaso,

Bodner, & Breyre, 2012). Bt has led to a laudable reduction in insecticide volume, and some related ecosystem service benefits (Lu, Wu, Jiang, Guo, & Desneux, 2012). However, insecticide sprays have often been replaced by lower-volume insecticide seed coatings, with most acres of corn in the United States treated (Hodgkin & Krupke, 2012). Although Bt has not directly caused this increased seed treatment, it may play an indirect role: the monoculture systems that the predominant GE crops contribute to are vulnerable to pests, which are in turn targeted by treated seeds. The insecticide seed coatings are implicated in harm to honeybees and beneficial insects (Leslie, Biddinger, Mullin, & Fleisher, 2009; Krupke, Hunt, Eitzer, Andino, & Given, 2012).

Some scientists envision that GE crops could be produced by the public sector, designed for use at low cost in sustainable systems. It is unclear how this would be accomplished given the dominance of corporate actors and their products. Although GE may add some value to sustainable systems, it comes at a high cost and is a piecemeal approach to complex problems, for which other systems approaches such as agroecology are better suited. Most public effort should therefore be devoted to more effective and lower-cost approaches that enhance biodiversity and reduce pollution (McIntyre, Herren, Wakhungu, & Watson, 2009), and to breeding. There can be substantial opportunity costs from devoting too much attention to GE at the expense of better options.

The United States currently exhibits a bimodal structure of farming scale, with some very large farms producing much of our food, a growing number of small specialty farms (essentially any property grossing over $1,000 in the United States is classified as a farm), and a shrinking middle group that formerly represented the majority of family farms. Such a distribution makes interpretation of farm size statistics challenging; "average size" does not reveal the growing dichotomy.

Most farms today use industrial methods and produce for mainstream distribution chains. Smaller farm alternatives continue to appear, however, including producing for local and regional markets (see focuses 14.2 and 14.3), and using organic and agroecological methods. In the following, we describe the industrial, local-regional, and organic-agroecological farming sectors, recognizing that there are substantial overlaps and that farms exist along a spectrum of size and degree of industrialization. Because of the industrial sector's dominance, we return in the end to a discussion of its impacts.

INDUSTRIAL CROP FARMING: AN OVERVIEW

Large industrial farms generally include operations on 250 to 5,000 hectares (600 to 12,000 acres), and ownership may involve families, corporations, and outside investors. These farms produce the majority (70 percent) of our food supply, including major cereals such as corn, wheat, rice, and other grains; cotton; and legumes, such as soybeans (collectively referred to as **commodities** because they are commonly sold as undifferentiated products); and fruits and vegetables; nuts; and other noncommodities, collectively referred to as **specialty crops.** Industrial methods are not restricted to large farms; many mid-size and small farms, including family farms, produce commodity crops and use similar conventional production methods, albeit at a different scale. That said, many industrial farms seek to benefit from **economies of scale**, meaning that a farm's larger size enables it to save money by purchasing inputs "in bulk" and managing large fields with ever more expensive and industrial-scale equipment. Mechanization and favorable government-support programs help facilitate such economies. As noted, the industrial model of farming is designed primarily to substitute

commodities
Agricultural crop(s) produced at a large scale; commonly refers to corn, soybeans, wheat, rice, cotton, and animal products

specialty crops
Fruits and vegetables, tree nuts, dried fruits, and other crops that are intensely cultivated and generally demand higher prices in the market than commodity crops

economies of scale
The advantages occuring when quantity of production becomes large and a firm has lower total costs than at lower levels of output; can level off or be reduced after a certain size

capital for labor, meaning that expensive and large machinery substitutes for human and animal energy.

As the industrial model advanced, the number of people directly involved in farming declined substantially since the US farm population peaked between 1910 and 1920 (Dahmann & Dacquel, 1990) Currently, less than 2 percent of the population is active in raising crops and livestock (Dimitri, Effland, & Conklin, 2005). There has been a rural employment shift from farms to industrial and service jobs.

global supply chain
Interconnected system of food exports and imports bringing crops and products to major marketing outlets

comparative advantage
The climatic, labor, or geographic advantage of one area to produce a product more efficiently and at cheaper cost than another

The pattern of consolidating small farms into larger ones fits well with marketing through the **global supply chain**. The milling and export sectors are dominated by a handful of companies operating large-scale processing, distribution, and marketing facilities, and these companies find it easier to deal with fewer farm managers. Similarly, it is easier for them to deal with farms in the same geographic area. Farm location is often driven by the principle of **comparative advantage**, in which crop or animal species are produced in areas seen as particularly well equipped for them. The area's advantage compared to other areas may be its natural conditions, availability of key inputs including workers, concentration of buyers, or proximity to markets. For example, the alluvial soils in the valleys of California provide excellent soil fertility, adequate irrigation water from snow melt from the Sierra Nevada mountains, and close proximity to large populations and markets for food, plus access to national markets with the interstate highway system. To be sure, the system is highly dependent on inexpensive and available fossil fuel for irrigation, because much of the area has limited rainfall during the major growing seasons (California Department of Food and Agriculture, 2013).

Products from industrial farms commonly move into broad distribution systems to be transported away from the local community, destined for livestock feed, production of biofuels, domestic consumption, or export. Little of the economic benefit reaches the local community. Figure 11.4 describes this system, showing the diverse and distant agents involved in growing and distributing commodity crops such as corn and soybeans.

Industrial farming is not primarily rooted in environmental conservation values; however, most industrial farms today do use some methods selected for their environmental benefits. For example, today about 35 percent of US cropland is farmed using no-till methods, which is planting the next year's crop directly into the prior year's crop residue (Horowitz, Ebel, & Ueda, 2010). The method avoids tilling that disturbs and erodes soils, and reduces the number of passes farmers make through a field with farm implements, thus saving substantial energy. Soil erosion on US farms declined by 43 percent between 1982 and 2003, and such methods likely contributed (Huggins & Reganold, 2008). The biggest downside of no-till systems is that they are dependent on herbicides to kill the weeds that were once managed by cultivation. There is research ongoing into organic no-till systems at the Rodale Institute in Pennsylvania and in several universities (Sayre, 2008). But in herbicide usage, too, many farms are downsizing, using integrated pest management strategies to reduce the frequency and quantity of pesticide sprays. Large purchasers, such as McDonald's and Sysco, increasingly require their suppliers to undergo sustainability audits to demonstrate their use of such methods. Other environmentally protective practices are required by law and are thus in widespread use, including using planning tools such as nutrient budgets to minimize fertilizer overuse. Finally, many industrial farms take advantage of conservation subsidies to enhance their conservation practices.

FIGURE 11.4   Typical Relations among Farmers and Other Agents in Corn and Soybean Commodity Crop Growing Networks

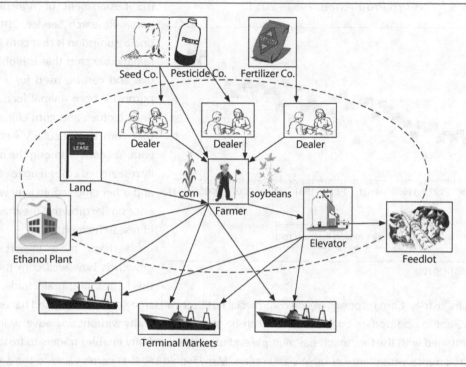

Source: James et al. (2012).

As described in chapters 7 and 8, economic and policy forces have pushed commodity crop prices below the cost of production for several years, although recent price spikes have changed this relationship. Many commodity farms rely significantly on government supports to make up the difference, including insurance and commodity crop subsidies. The sector is also bolstered by other government support, such as for marketing and research. Specialty crop producers and those producing on diversified farms receive far less government support (Hamerschlag, 2009). Focus 11.1 describes the case of corn, one commodity that has received extensive government assistance and much attention for its proliferation and potential contributions to public health problems.

◎ FOCUS 11.1. THE PROLIFERATION OF CORN
Mark Muller

Some consider corn to be an incredible success story, whereas others see the concentration on one major crop as an indication of a food system gone awry (Capehart, 2013). Regardless, corn production in the United States has grown enormously since the middle of the twentieth century, largely due to yield increases, as shown in figure 11.5.

   Many people assume the growth occurs because corn production is profitable and that subsidies and other government interventions have created further incentives for farmers to produce corn. Yet an examination of prices since the 1980s indicates that this is not the case. More times than not corn has been priced below the cost of production, with farm payments simply keeping farmers from going bankrupt rather than creating profits

(Continued)

(Continued)

FIGURE 11.5   US Corn Production, 1961–2011

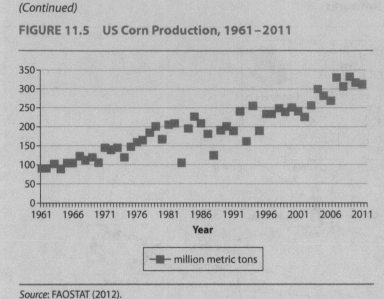

million metric tons

Source: FAOSTAT (2012).

(US Department of Agriculture Economic Research Service, 2013). A second assumption is that corn is simply a remarkable crop that is highly productive and can be used for a variety of purposes, from animal feed to sweetener, biofuel, and corn chips. It is true that corn is particularly easy to work with. Yet corn is among the most heavily researched crops (Fuglie et al., 2011), and other crops could very well experience similar growth if they had this level of research emphasis.

Perhaps most important in its growth is how well corn provides for the farm input, grain trade, and food processing industries. Corn responds well to commercial fertilizer and large-scale planting and harvesting. Further, when kept in appropriate conditions, corn can be stored for months without any adverse impacts on quality. Combined with the fact that it has multiple end uses, this durability enables traders to treat corn very much like a currency with plenty of buyers and sellers. Many would say that corn's value to the agribusiness industry, far more than economic return to farmers, has driven its growth through high and low prices.

FARMS PRODUCING FOR LOCAL AND REGIONAL MARKETS

Since the 1970s, there has been a resurgence of activity by small- and mid-scale farmers interested in producing fruits, vegetables, specialty crops, and livestock for local and regional markets. These farms may focus on direct sale to consumers (through farmers markets, community-supported agriculture, farm stands), farm-to-institution programs, restaurants, or distribution of locally produced foods through conventional grocery channels (Low & Vogel, 2011; Martinez et al., 2010). Some are entrepreneurs from urban areas. Others are conventional farmers or their children, who have decided to farm differently. Others have worked in agriculture and now seek to purchase their own land, and still others never stopped farming in this way. Note that because of the challenges in making a living via farming, the majority of small commercial farms do not fit this local and regional model. Rather, they produce primarily commodity crops and animals that require only part-time effort, so they can stay on the farm while holding off-farm jobs. Although any size farm may produce for local and regional markets, there is an important niche for mid-sized farms, as described in perspective 11.2.

Perspective 11.2. A Bright Future for Farmers in the "Middle"?
Frederick Kirschenmann

Some disturbing trends are taking place in the US farm population, largely unrecognized by the general public. Data seldom conveyed to the public reveal that (as of the 2012 census) 80 percent of our total agriculture sales were produced by just 8 percent of farms. The farms disappearing at the fastest rate are the farms in the "middle"—those that produced between $25,000 and $500,000 annual gross sales. Additionally, almost 29 percent of our farmers were over age sixty-five and only 8 percent under age thirty-five.

The lack of public awareness of these trends is partly because of the current definition of a farm used by USDA—essentially, any place that produces and sells (or usually "would have") $1,000 a year in agricultural products. Using this definition USDA assures the public that we still have slightly more than two million farmers.

The farms we are losing are the very ones in the best position to supply the emerging market demand for highly **differentiated products** produced at a scale that this market requires, as described in the following. Additionally, compared to large, commodity monocultures, medium-sized farms tend to be more diverse and consequently they diversify our food system, thus supporting its security; they also bring more people, money, and life to rural communities, and often they benefit the environment, such as by preventing soil erosion or providing wildlife habitat.

differentiated products
Products that differ from those of competitors, such as based on quality, cultivar, or production method, and thus typically can be sold for higher prices

Conventional wisdom suggests we are losing the farms in the middle because they are not as efficient as the large farms. But on-farm research conducted by Mike Duffy at Iowa State University demonstrated that this was not the case (Duffy, 2009). Efficiencies did improve as farms got larger, but only up to a certain point. Once farms reached a size that exceeds the "middle" definition, no further efficiencies were achieved.

It turns out that what causes farms in the middle to disappear are transaction costs. Given the current concentration in the food industry, food processors need to reduce their costs to meet the price squeeze imposed by the concentrated retail sector. One of the ways that food processors can adjust to that price squeeze is by reducing their transaction costs. It is cheaper for food processors to buy ten thousand hogs from one farmer than to buy one thousand hogs from ten farmers. Consequently the preferred contracts go to the very large farms, and the farmers in the middle become "residual suppliers."

Some mid-sized farmers have found that they can cope with this market reality by jointly selling their products with those from other farms. This market aggregation enables them to differentiate their products (highlight the differences between their products and those in the mainstream) to meet new market demands and reduce their transaction costs (see focus 6.1 on food hubs). Numerous examples of such differentiated, branded market aggregation now exist: Organic Valley of Family Farms, Country Beef, Niman Ranch, Shepherd's Grain, Red Tomato, to name a few (see figure 11.6). One indicator of the success of this aggregation is the average age of the farmers—forty-six and getting younger for Niman Ranch and Organic Valley, versus nearly sixty and getting older for commodity farmers.

FIGURE 11.6   Examples of Agriculture of the Middle Brands

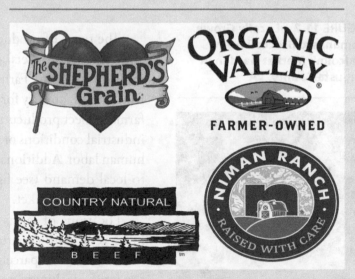

Source: Compiled by CLF.

For decades, few citizens seemed to care about these trends. As long as a constant flow of branded products showed up in local supermarkets at reasonable prices, customers seemed to be satisfied. *Fast, convenient,* and *cheap* appeared to be the only demand in the marketplace.

(Continued)

(Continued)

But that is changing. Ironically, while these grim farm statistics developed, an unprecedented new market emerged—one uniquely suited to the farms in the middle. This new market consists of an increasing demand for highly differentiated food products.

Consumers want fruits and vegetables that are fresh, and therefore often locally grown; beef and dairy products that are grass-fed and raised without subtherapeutic antibiotics or growth hormones; food products that come through a transparent supply chain that provides for complete traceability; and food produced by local family farmers and farm workers who are fairly compensated. Visionary CEOs of food service corporations are beginning to reshape the business culture of their companies to meet these growing demands and take advantage of these new market opportunities.

The emergence of these preferences among some consumers is consistent with sound-free market theory and provides unique opportunities for farmers in the middle. In 1986, Michael Porter of the Harvard Business School argued that there are *two* ways to be competitive in a global economy—being the lowest cost supplier of an undifferentiated commodity or being the supplier of a product that commands higher value by virtue of its differentiation. Each can be equally competitive and therefore successful in the marketplace.

Farmers of the middle have a comparative advantage in producing these highly differentiated products. The small farms that individually bring their products to consumers through direct market channels have neither the capacity nor the distribution efficiency to meet the current demand of restaurants, hospitals, schools, and nursing homes. The mega-farms, designed to mass-produce undifferentiated commodities at the lowest possible price, will find it hard to efficiently produce goods requiring these special features. Furthermore, large commodity farms generally have difficulty producing the kind of food story that consumers want. It is precisely the farmers in the middle who have the productive capacity, the innovative management potential, and the kind of food story that can meet the market demand while simultaneously reducing transaction costs.

FIGURE 11.7 Locally Grown Romanesco Broccoli from Malcolm's Market Garden in Augusta County, VA

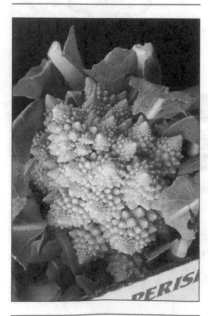

Source: Local Food Hub. (2013).

The types of products coming from farms producing for local and regional markets are usually different from those from the industrial system. Farmers often focus on diverse vegetable and fruit species, poultry for eggs and meat, or pastured livestock. Often farmers select products that are difficult to grow or distribute under industrial conditions or that may require relatively large amounts of human labor. Additionally, heirloom and unusual crops may appeal to local demand (see figure 11.7). Each of these options enters a specific niche market.

Locations of farms producing for local-regional markets follow several distinct patterns. Many are located in and near cities in areas where land parcels are small, and it can be difficult to manage large machinery and protect urban neighbors from chemical drift, where land prices are high and where population centers offer potential markets for locally produced foods. Farm success can be enhanced when there is sufficient geographic concentration of similar farms to enable shared processing, preparation for market, and distribution.

Consumers may assume that products purchased through direct channels were produced with environmentally sound methods; however, this is not a certainty. That said, environmental sustainability and resilience (ability to rebound from negative weather or prices) is often part of *why* these farmers do what they do, and many emphasize such methods even if they do not invest in obtaining organic certification. Some consumers assume that purchasing local products reduces the carbon footprint because the food has traveled less. However, life-cycle analyses find that food miles are not the only nor a consistent predictor of transportation-related emissions, because vehicles such as trains and ships carrying food over thousands of miles can be extremely energy efficient, often more so than trucks traveling a few hundred miles (Weber & Matthews, 2008).

AGROECOLOGY AND ORGANIC FARMING

The third type of farming we discuss is agroecological and organic production (Francis, 2009). *Organic* is a legally defined term with strict criteria governing what products can be certified as organic. Products must be produced without chemical fertilizers or pesticides, transgenic seeds, or sewage sludge for nutrients. Organic farmers depend on careful system design with crop rotations, legumes, and compost for soil fertility (Magdoff & van Es, 2009); diverse plantings to avoid pest attacks (Altieri & Nicholls, 2005); and the use of only approved pest control products to supplement their management practices. Organic certification also requires development of a farm plan and crop rotation, being chemical-free for three years, and having annual on-site inspections. Products must be kept separate from conventionally produced food at all steps from the farm through the market. Many organic farmers describe the system's primary goal as care for the soil, with the insight that healthy soils produce healthy plants (see figure 11.8). Because crops were grown for centuries without chemicals, most

FIGURE 11.8   Earthworms are One Sign of Healthy Soil

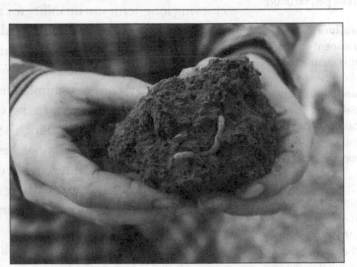

Source: USDA NRCS via Flickr. http://www.nrcs.usda.gov/wps/portal/nrcs/photogallery/ia/newsroom/gallery/?cid=1716&position=Promo#1

indigenous systems were certainly "organic" by today's standards; however, modern organic farming typically combines these traditional principles with evidence from science and uses mechanized equipment.

In 2012 organic food sales were estimated at over $30 billion in the United States (Haumann, 2012) and over $60 billion globally (Organic Market Information, 2010). This represents less than 2 percent of food sales worldwide, but the organic share of vegetable and fruit sales is near 4 percent. In some European countries, for example, Denmark, Austria, and Switzerland, organic food makes up more than 5 percent of all food sales (Willer, Lernoud, & Schaak, 2013).

Originally, organic production was primarily small scale. Because organic products command price premiums, however, some large producers have found organic production to be lucrative. Today, over half of the certified organic food sold in the United States comes from industrial-scale farms and over half the organic food is now sold through six supermarket chains (Organic Trade Association, 2013). Organic food has become widely available from large-scale national retailers. Such mass market products have been controversial, with some criticizing them for their lack of connection to the movement's founding values and others indicating that these products should be encouraged because they have reduced environmental harm compared to conventionally produced foods and have made organic products more widely affordable and accessible.

To further blur the lines between production systems, many smaller farms producing for local markets have dropped the organic label, even as they continue to produce in organic ways. They depend on customer trust and their local reputation, opting not to seek organic certification because of costs of record keeping and the required inspections. According to national organic rules in the United States, farmers may call these products *organic* in the marketplace if sales do not exceed $5,000 per year, although they cannot use the official organic seal. Any farms are allowed to sell products labeled *pesticide free, local,* or *naturally grown,* because use of these terms is not regulated.

Beyond the organic label, **agroecology,** defined as "the integrative study of the ecology of the entire food system, encompassing ecological, economic and social dimensions" (Francis et al., 2003. p. 100), is emerging as an integrative, transdisciplinary approach to agriculture, research, and education. Agroecology encompasses the complexity and challenge of increasing food production (Gliessman, 2007) while achieving long-term sustainability for the food system. Researchers are studying innovative new systems such as **permaculture** (Mollison, 1990), a "permanent agriculture" that combines perennials with annuals and uses integrated planting patterns to reduce soil erosion and increase use water efficiently. **Perennial polycultures** (Jackson, 1980) are systems that mimic the prairie with mixtures of grasses and broadleaf plants and other biodiverse farming strategies, and are designed using lessons from natural ecosystems (Soule & Piper, 1992). These systems are characterized by high species diversity, tight interactions between crops and animals, and dependence on ecological processes for nutrients and plant protection, and are far less expensive than the chemical alternatives. These are among the advances that could solve production, economic, environmental, and social challenges in agricultural systems and food systems.

Despite their often relatively small size, when well managed with adequate labor, many of these farms produce more food per acre than large, mechanized operations (Francis & Porter, 2011). Techniques for maximizing space include intercropping (planting different crops in proximity to each other) and relay cropping (planting a second crop where a not-yet-harvested crop is growing). Research on how to improve multiple-species systems has been limited, thus, there is no adequate measure of their ultimate production and economic potential (Francis, Poincelot, & Bird, 2006).

agroecology

The science and practice of applying ecological principles to agriculture to develop practices that work with nature to mimic natural processes and conserve ecological integrity; other labels for ecological approaches to agriculture include ecological agriculture, agricultural ecology, sustainable agriculture, permaculture

permaculture

The permanent agriculture and stable culture that comes from careful design of integrated annual and perennial crops, livestock, and production practices that contribute to healthy soils, crops, animals, and people

Perennial polycultures

Systems of mixed perennial species that complement each other in the field, exploit natural resources through the entire soil profile, and produce edible grains and forage for livestock; promote their own fertility and pest management and maintain a healthy farm ecosystem

CROP PRODUCTION—IMPACTS ON ENVIRONMENT, FOOD SECURITY, PUBLIC HEALTH, AND SOCIETY

As industrial methods have transformed farming, they have had numerous successes and have contributed to unanticipated problems. An evaluation of current farming and food systems, and thoughtful reflection on what impacts they have on food security, public health, the environment, and society, can help us identify major challenges facing humankind in envisioning and designing action plans to project and enable future desirable systems.

Environmental Impacts

The overall environmental impacts of industrial farming systems are widely variable, with substantial advances evident in soil preservation and protection from erosion as a result of reduced tillage and new equipment to facilitate planting, and substantial negative impacts as a result of resource use, contamination of water and soils, and biodiversity loss.

There is debate about whether new-generation, apparently more benign, chemical pesticides are less harmful to the environment than older ones. Proponents claim that new technologies have reduced the use of pesticides in general and the costs of pest management in specific operations. Those who question the positive impacts of these technologies cite higher costs for new-generation technologies, the growing challenge of pest-resistant organisms—especially weeds and insects, and concerns about the larger farming operations they encourage. Some claim that large industrial farms have lower environmental impact than small conventional farms because of their more frequent use of costly site-specific technologies that place correct amounts of fertilizers and appropriate chemicals where they are needed in the field (see figure 11.9). The alternative, blanket applications of these products, could lead to overapplication and runoff. Additionally, intensive cropping can reduce environmental footprints by reducing land use per amount harvested.

FIGURE 11.9   Frog with Partially Missing Hindlimb

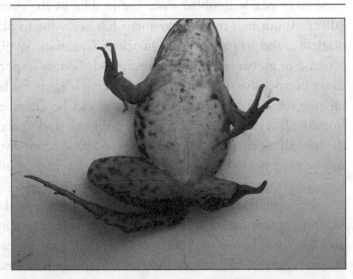

Weed killers, such as atrazine, may increase the risk of deformities of limbs and sex organs in frogs and other amphibians.
Source: US Fish and Wildlife Service, via Flickr. https://www.flickr.com/photos/usfwshq/10820402344/in/set-72157637382485506

As described in chapter 3, however, industrial crop production has been associated with significant environmental harms. Monocrop production substantially reduces biodiversity on farms and can create new management challenges. Among these are dependence on chemicals because of increased pest problems (with the monocultures providing appealing habitat) and need for more costly fertilizers coming from off the farm because animal manure is no longer as available when crops and animals are raised in different locations. Soils with low organic matter levels are far less resilient to drought than healthy soils. Such problems have been addressed by increasing inputs from technology, including use of newer crop varieties, heavier applications of chemical fertilizers and pesticides, and irrigation to support high yields in relatively dry areas. In addition to other limitations of these technologies, they all depend on heavy use of limited natural resources including water, phosphorus, and fossil fuels, resulting in a fragile industrial farming system closely linked to global petroleum sources and prices, and reliant on global political stability and trade (Francis and Porter, 2011; Neff, Parker, Tinch, Kirschenmann, & Lawrence, 2011). So any boost in energy prices means a boost in production costs and can cut into farm profits.

Another concern is the level of chemical use and runoff. Herbicide-tolerant, genetically engineered varieties of corn, soybeans, and cotton are often described as enabling reduced herbicide usage. By some estimates, however, usage has actually increased, because herbicide-resistant weeds developed and farmers used additional and more toxic herbicides to control them (Benbrook, 2012). Nutrient runoff into waterways is another environmental consequence of industrial agriculture, contributing to dead zones with inadequate oxygen to support aquatic life.

Farm policies have enhanced incentives for industrial producers to cover all available land in crops, rather than putting some of their acreage in cover crops or leaving it as prairie. By eliminating natural areas and lines of trees used as windbreaks, for example, such cropping can reduce the biodiversity that makes agriculture more resilient while also contributing to soil erosion.

Food Security

Agricultural technologies have dramatically increased yields of basic cereals and other staple crops, and these have nearly doubled since the middle of the twentieth century (Alston, Beddow, & Cassman, 2008). About half the improvement has been due to plant genetics, and half to increases in fertilizer, pesticide, and irrigation use (Duvick & Cassman, 1999). The ability to create surpluses promoted an increase in global trade and in productivity. More important, this high productivity helped bring relatively inexpensive food to millions, making it easier for families to afford to feed themselves and freeing income for other essential expenses. As will be described, however, some of the affordability derives from the fact that these products are indirectly and directly subsidized by society. Humanity today faces the incredible challenge of doubling food production over the next half-century (Fischetti, 2011). This will be essential to feed a projected population of nine billion people, as human numbers soar, incomes and diets improve, and people's expectations rise.

Yet, agricultural productivity is reaching very real biological limits, as described in chapter 3. Although plant breeders and agronomists have maintained continual crop yield increases over several decades, these boosts to production are leveling off, at least in the major food crops (Cassman, Grassini, & van Wart, 2010). Most land suitable for agriculture, especially that which can be easily irrigated, is already in production (Brown, 1995). The supplies of other key resources, including fossil fuels, phosphorus, and fresh water, are becoming more limited. It is difficult for agriculture to compete when other sectors of society, such as manufacturing and energy generation, can afford to pay a premium for a key input such as water. Data on climate change show that the earth is moving into a period of greater climate instability after enjoying a relatively stable climate during the ten thousand years since the end of the last glacial period, which has been highly favorable for crop growth and productivity (Chehoski, 2006). Most agricultural scientists doubt that doubling our current production is possible, even with technologies that are in the laboratories and experimental fields today and expected tomorrow.

Some observers hold faith that future technological advances will enable us to maintain or even grow our food supply in the face of these challenges. Others suggest that a shift toward more sustainable farming methods and reduced-meat diets is necessary. Regardless, there is a need to explore changes outside food production: in eating habits, grain allocation to nonfood uses such as biofuels, food distribution, family planning availability, and in social changes such as making education available to young women, which tends to result in smaller family size. Additionally, recovering even some of the estimated 30 to 40 percent of food lost in the system from harvest through consumption would provide valuable nutrition (Parfitt, Barthel, & Macnaughton, 2010). Many of these nonproduction topics are explored elsewhere in this text.

Public Health Impacts

As described in chapter 2, although production of an inexpensive food supply has some benefits for food security, industrial crop production is also associated with significant human health impacts of concern.

First, to the extent industrial agricultural practices have contributed to the oversupply of food, they also contribute to a business incentive to get us to eat that food—and thus to obesity and diet-related disease. The balance of crops produced in this country, dominated by commodities used in processed foods and animal feed, plays a role in diet-related diseases including cancer and cardiovascular disease. Corn production, and its role in our diets in the guise of corn-fed beef and high fructose corn syrup, is a particular concern because of its connection to obesity (Bocarsly, Powell, Avena, & Hoebel, 2010). Of course, that balance of crops is substantially shaped by consumer demand. It is likely that low-cost but nutrient-poor foods may alleviate hunger pangs but do little to improve true food security—a concept that includes meeting nutritional needs.

As also described in chapter 2, many pesticides have been linked with health effects, according to the WHO, including effects at low doses for food consumers and communities downstream from farms—and especially effects at high doses received by some farm workers. Health effects of concern include acute effects, such as organophosphate and carbamate poisoning; and chronic effects, such as cancer, reproductive harm, birth defects, and neurological effects. Exposure to nitrates from fertilizer nitrogen runoff is also a concern because of potential effects on infants; and the algal blooms caused by such nutrient overloads in water can cause direct effects from exposure and indirect effects via fish consumption, as described in chapter 12. Many consumers are concerned about public health effects of GE crops. There remains need for additional research independent of industry support; however, to date there is little evidence of direct impacts (Domingo & Bordonaba, 2011).

Other public health effects of concern are more indirect. For example, some industrial agriculture practices contribute to soil erosion and loss of wetlands; in turn, these can lead to flooding, with its attendant risks of drowning, injury, mold exposure, and mental health threats.

Social Impacts

Industrialization has reshaped the rural United States. The reduced agricultural labor needs have led to a shift in rural employment that contributed to population loss in prior decades in many rural areas. Between 1990 and 2000, for example, 25 percent of rural counties experienced population loss; more recently, "nonmetro" county population change has been uneven and not necessarily tied to changes in agriculture (USDA, 2013).

Economic consequences are mixed and complicated, and this is manifested at all levels in the system. For example, the high commodity prices from 2008 to 2012 brought new prosperity and potential to expand the land base and upgrade machinery, with larger corporations or family farms taking most advantage of global food prices at the expense of small operations that are often unable to keep up with needed investments. For some segments of rural communities, these long-term trends have led to a boom in seed, fertilizer, pesticide, equipment, and storage building sales as well as in banking and grain commercialization. Local grain elevators and their employees also benefit, although many of these local farmer-owned businesses have now consolidated and may be controlled by boards of directors far from the local community. When it comes to seed and equipment, larger farms tend to shop for them in a broad marketplace, bypassing local dealers in favor of the best bargains.

The growing concentration in farming and in the industries that process farm products has also had widespread impacts. As farms gain market power they are able to further strengthen their positions versus smaller farms through economies of scale. Concentrated industries often use their market power and political weight to shift conditions in their favor, which is often not aligned with the needs of farmers. As described in Chapter 7, one common measure of market concentration is the CR4 ratio, reflecting the concentration of market shares in an industry's top four firms. A CR4 above 40 percent indicates a consolidated industry. A 2007 report showed that in the soybean-crushing industry, the CR4 was 80 percent, with 71 percent concentrated in the top three firms. The CR4 for flour milling increased from 40 to 63 percent between 1982 and 2005 (James, Hendrickson, & Howard, 2012). Even much of the organic foods market—widely seen as an alternative to large agribusiness—has been consolidated over the past decades (Howard, 2009b).

Another challenge facing small farms is the expansion of intellectual property rights associated with genetically engineered crops. The top seed companies, similar to other agricultural firms, control much of the seed market. Monsanto, the largest seed company, owns the intellectual property of seeds planted on 80 percent of the corn acres and 90 percent of the soybean acres in the United States (Moschini, 2010). Farmers who use seeds that are modified and patented by companies such as Monsanto enter into contracts with the companies. These contracts prohibit growers from reusing the seed year after year, effectively requiring the farmer to annually purchase new seed from the company. Contracts also limit the company's liability in the event of crop failure. One challenge for organic farmers is pollen drift from conventional GMO crop fields, especially for cross-pollinated crops such as maize (corn).

CONCLUSION

Over the millennia of development of agriculture and societies, our food system has evolved from hunting and gathering, to locally oriented and relatively self-sufficient food patterns, to the globalized and highly industrialized food system we observe today. Supermarkets in developed countries are full of products from around the globe, and most people are no longer concerned about seasonality of foods.

There is continuing debate about the positive and negative impacts of an industrial and globalized food production and marketing system. Some tout the industrial system as a modern miracle that provides food to everyone who can afford it, one that uses comparative advantage to maximize production from each climate or soil situation and then exports these products around the globe. Others are concerned about large costs of transportation, overreliance on scarce fossil fuels, and lack of transition toward more sustainable, local food systems. This debate continues. Many are concerned about the apparent change globally toward more unpredictable temperature and rainfall patterns compared to the past two centuries that have favored agriculture and massive population growth. As these changes proceed, concerns may escalate regarding competition for scarce resources and preservation of a livable environment in the future (Chehoski, 2006).

Given the need to greatly increase food production over the first half of the twenty-first century, it will be essential to solve the challenges of each new type of technology. We will need to combine all that science has to offer, with all the best common sense and farmer wisdom, in order to maintain our food supply and preserve the environment and our natural resources.

SUMMARY

Crop production in the United States has evolved over two centuries from a diversified and small-scale system to one that is primarily specialized and industrial scale. The older system that relied primarily on sunlight and natural rainfall plus nutrients derived from the soil organic matter has changed into one dependent on fossil-fuel-based technologies such as chemical fertilizers, pesticides, and extensive irrigation to ensure adequate water for consistent production. One illustration of the tensions between technological and agroecological approaches is the case of genetic engineering. With growing population and increased demand for food, industrial production is considered by some to be essential to maintain our food supply as well as continue to export to other parts of the world. The heavy reliance on nonrenewable inputs, however, introduces a fragility into this system. Greater use of agroecosystems that mimic the natural system and restoration of the biological health of our soils can improve our food system's resilience to climate change and its sustainability for the long term.

The large-scale, labor-efficient farming systems that dominate crop and livestock production have substituted capital for labor. The long-term costs of many technologies are not adequately accounted for in the short-term economic budgets of farming. In the larger food sector, consolidation of processing and marketing brings an efficiency of scale, along with concerns about the quality of food and access by many poor people who cannot get fresh and wholesome produce. There is growing interest in local, small-scale food strategies in which consumers can purchase directly from farmers and reduce the distances in the national and global food system. The niche for organic and agroecological methods is also growing. More than half the organic food sold in the United States comes from industrial-scale farms.

KEY TERMS

Agroecology

Commodities

Comparative advantage

Differentiated products

Diverse farming systems

Economies of scale

Global supply chain

Perennial polycultures

Permaculture

Specialty crops

DISCUSSION QUESTIONS

1. What are the root causes of the major change in farming systems from a diversified, crop-animal integrated model to industrial, specialized methods of producing crops?

2. What are the characteristics of today's high-technology farming systems? How do they efficiently use human labor? Do you think they are essential for feeding a growing global population? Why or why not?

3. The chapter and perspective 11.2 describe how small- and mid-sized farms often seek to produce specialty products marketed primarily to a local and regional consumer base. In what ways do each of these farm types have comparative advantages in these markets?

4. Following are some of the most important emerging issues facing the US farming and food system. Why is each of these important? Are any of them overblown? What other issues would you add to the list?
   a. Potential for higher fossil fuel costs
   b. Diminishing supplies of fresh water for irrigation
   c. Changes in land use away from agriculture and into urban development
   d. Public concerns about safety of transgenic crops and animals
   e. Consolidation of ownership of production, processing, and marketing of food

5. The farming population is getting older. Why do you think this is? What kinds of incentives or programs would help attract more younger and culturally diverse farmers?

REFERENCES

Alston, J., Beddow, J. M., & Cassman, K. G. (2008). Agricultural research, productivity, and food commodity prices. *Giannini Foundation of Agricultural Economics, 12*, 2.

Altieri, M. A., & Nicholls, C. I. (2005). *Manage insects on your farm: A guide to ecological strategies* (Handbook Series Book 7). Washington, DC: Sustainable Agriculture Research and Education Program.

Balter, M. (2007). Seeking agriculture's ancient roots. *Science, 316*(5833), 1830–1835.

Benbrook, C. M. (2012). Impacts of genetically engineered crops on pesticide use in the U.S.—the first sixteen years. *Environmental Sciences Europe, 24*(1), 24.

Berry, I. (2013). *Pesticides gain as corn loses bug resistance.* Retrieved from http://online.wsj.com/news/articles/SB100014241 27887323463704578496923254944066

Blesh, J., & Drinkwater, L. E. (2013). The impact of nitrogen source and crop rotation on nitrogen mass balances in the Mississippi River Basin. *Ecological Applications, 23*, 1017–1035.

Bocarsly, M. E., Powell, E. S., Avena, N. M., & Hoebel, B. G. (2010). High-fructose corn syrup causes characteristic of obesity in rats: Increased body weight, body fat and triglyceride levels. *Pharmacology Biochemistry and Behavior.*

Brown, L. R. (1995). *Who will feed China? Wake-up call for a small planet.* New York: W. W. Norton.

California Department of Food and Agriculture. (2013). *California agricultural statistics review, 2012–2013.* Sacramento: Author. Retrieved from www.cdfa.ca.gov/statistics/pdfs/2013/FinalDraft2012–2013.pdf

Capehart, J. (2013). *Corn—background.* Retrieved from www.ers.usda.gov/topics/crops/corn/background.aspx#.Uo4s ZY2E70h

Cassman, K. G., Grassini, P., & van Wart, J. (2010). Crop yield potential, yield trends and global food security in a changing climate. In C. Rosenzweig & D. Hillel (Eds.), *Handbook of climate change and agroecosystems* (p. 37). London: Imperial College Press.

Chehoski, R. (Ed.). (2006). *Critical perspectives on climate disruption.* New York: Rosen.

Cochran, W. W. (1993). The development of American agriculture: A historical analysis. Minneapolis: University of Minnesota Press.

Cook, S. M., Khan, Z. R., & Pickett, J. A. (2007). Use of push-pull strategies in integrated pest management. *Annual Review of Entomology, 52*, 375–400.

Dahmann, D. C., & Dacquel, L. T. (1990). *Residents of farms and rural areas* (Current Population Reports Series P-20, No. 457). Washington, DC: US Bureau of the Census.

Davis, A. S., Hill, J. D., Chase, C. A., Johanns, A. M., & Liebman, M. (2012). Increasing cropping system diversity balances productivity, profitability and environmental health. *PLOS ONE, 7*(10), e47149.

Davis, D., Epp, M. D., & Riordan, H. D. (2004). Changes in USDA food composition data for 43 garden crops, 1950 to 1999. *Journal of the American College of Nutrition, 23*(6), 669–682.

De Vita, P., Di Paolo, E., Fecondo, G., Di Fonzo, N., & Pisante, M. (2007). No-tillage and conventional tillage effects on durum wheat yield, grain quality and soil moisture content in southern Italy. *Soil and Tillage Research, 92*(1), 69–78. Retrieved from www.sciencedirect.com/science/article/pii/S0167198706000249

Dimitri, C., Effland, A., & Conklin, N. (2005). *The 20th century transformation of U.S. agriculture and farm policy* (Economic Information Bulletin No. 3). Washington, DC: US Department of Agriculture Economic Research Service. Retrieved from www.ers.usda.gov/media/259572/eib3_1.pdf

Domingo, J. L., & Bordonaba, J. G. (2011). A literature review on the safety assessment of genetically modified plants. *Environment International, 37*, 734–742.

Duffy, M. (2009). Economies of size in production agriculture. *Journal of Hunger & Environmental Nutrition, 4*(3–4), 375–392.

Duvick, D. N., & Cassman, K. G. (1999). Post-green revolution trends in yield potential of temperate maize in the north-central United States. *Crop Science, 39*, 1622–1630.

Fausti, S. W., McDonald, T. M., Lundgren, J. G., Li, J., Keating, A. R., & Catangui, M. (2011). Insecticide use and crop selection in regions with high GM adoption rates. *Renewable Agriculture and Food Systems, 27*(4), 295–304.

Fernandez-Cornejo, J., Wechsler, S. J., Livingston, M., & Mitchell, L. (2014). *Genetically engineered crops in the United States*. Economic Research Report E97. Washington, DC: US Department of Agriculture Economic Research Service.

Fischetti, M. (2011). How to double global food production by 2050 *and* reduce environmental damage. *Scientific American*, Oct. 12.

Francis, C. A. (Ed.). (2009). *Organic farming: The ecological system* (Agronomy Monograph, 54). Madison, WI: American Society of Agronomy.

Francis, C. A., Lieblein, G., Gliessman, S., Breland, T. A., Creamer, N., et al. (2003). Agroecology: The ecology of food systems. *Journal of Sustainable Agriculture, 22*, 3.

Francis, C. A., Poincelot, R., & Bird, G. M. (Eds.). (2006). *Developing and extending sustainable agriculture: A new social contract*. Binghampton, NY: Haworth Press.

Francis, C. A., & Porter, P. (2011). Ecology in sustainable agriculture practices and systems. *Critical Reviews in Plant Sciences, 30*, 1–10.

Fuglie, K. O., Heisey, P. W., King, J. L., Pray, C. E. Day-Rubenstein, K., Schimmelpfennig, D., Wang, S. L., & Karmarkar-Deshmukh, R. (2011). *Research investments and market structure in the food processing, agricultural input, and biofuel industries worldwide* (ERR-130). Washington, DC: US Department of Agriculture Economic Research Service.

Gassmann, A. J., Petzold-Maxwell, J. L., Clifton, E. H., Dunbar, M. W., Hoffman, A. M., Ingber, D. A., & Keweshan, R. S. (2014). Field-evolved resistance by western corn rootworm to multiple *Bacillus thuringiensis* toxins in transgenic maize. *Proceedings of National Academy of Sciences, 111*(14), 5141–5146.

Gliessman, S. R. (2007). *Agroecology: The ecology of sustainable food systems*. Boca Raton, FL: CRC Press.

Goodman, M. M., & Carson, M. L. (2000). Reality vs. myth: Corn breeding, exotics, and genetic engineering. *Annual Corn Sorghum Research Conference Proceedings, 55*, 149–172.

Gouse, M., Piesse, J., Thirtle, C., & Poulton, C. (2009). *Assessing the performance of GM maize amongst smallholders in KwaZulu-Natal, South Africa*. Retrieved from www.agbioforum.org/v12n1/v12n1a08-gouse.htm

Gurian-Sherman, D. (2009). *Failure to yield: Evaluating the performance of genetically engineered crops*. Cambridge, MA: Union of Concerned Scientists.

Gurian-Sherman, D. (2012). *High and dry: Why genetic engineering is not solving agriculture's drought problem in a thirsty world*. Cambridge, MA: Union of Concerned Scientists.

Gurian-Sherman, D., & Gurwick, N. (2009). *No sure fix: Prospects for reducing nitrogen pollution through genetic engineering*. Cambridge, MA: Union of Concerned Scientists.

Hamerschlag, K. (2009). *Farm subsidies in California: Skewed priorities and gross inequities*. Environmental Working Group. Retrieved from http://farm.ewg.org/pdf/california-farm.pdf

Harris, D. R. (1996). *The origins and spread of agriculture and pasturalism in Eurasia*. London: University College.

Haumann, B. (2012). *Consumer-driven U.S. organic market surpasses $31 billion in 2011*. Organic Trade Association. Retrieved from www.organicnewsroom.com/2012/04/us_consumerdriven_organic_mark.html

Hilbeck, A., Lebrecht, T., Vogel, R., Heinemann, J. A., & Binimelis, R. (2013). Farmer's choice of seeds in four EU countries under different levels of GM crop adoption. *Environmental Sciences Europe, 25*, 12. Retrieved from www.enveurope.com/content/25/1/12

Hodgson, E., & Krupke, C. (2012). *Insecticidal seed treatments can harm honey bees*. Retrieved from www.extension.iastate.edu/CropNews/2012/0406hodgson.htm

Horowitz, J., Ebel, R., & Ueda, K. (2010). *"No-till" farming is a growing practice* (Economic Information Bulletin No. 70). Washington, DC: US Department of Agriculture Economic Research Service. Retrieved from www.ers.usda.gov/media/135329/eib70.pdf

Howard, P. H. (2009a). Visualizing consolidation in the global seed industry: 1996–2008. *Sustainability, 1*(4), 1266–1287.

Howard, P. H. (2009b). Visualizing food system concentration and consolidation. *Southern Rural Sociology, 24*(2), 87–110.

Huggins, D. R., & Reganold, J. P. (2008). No-till: The quiet revolution. *Scientific American*, July, 70–77.

Hurt, R. D. (2002). *American agriculture: A brief history*. West Lafayette, IN: Purdue University Press.

Jackson, W. (1980). *New roots for agriculture*. Lincoln: University of Nebraska Press.

James, H. S., Hendrickson, M., & Howard, P. H. (2012). *Networks, power and dependency in the agrifood industry* (p. 37). Working Paper. Columbia: University of Missouri Department of Agricultural Economics and Rural Sociology.

Jongeneel, S. (2013). *Expect more soil insecticide used with Bt hybrids*. Retrieved from www.agprofessional.com/news/Expect-more-soil-insecticide-used-with-Bt-hybrids-200626161.html

Krupke, C. H., Hunt, G. J., Eitzer, B. D., Andino, G., & Given, K. (2012). Multiple routes of pesticide exposure for honey bees living near agricultural fields. *PloS One, 7*(1), e29268.

Leslie, T. W., Biddinger, D. J., Mullin, C. A., & Fleischer, S. J. (2009). Carabidae population dynamics and temporal partitioning: Response to coupled neonicotinoid-transgenic technologies in maize. *Environmental Entomology, 38*(3), 935–943.

Low, S., & Vogel, S. (2011). *Direct and intermediated marketing of local foods in the United States*. Economic Research Report 128. Washington DC: US Department of Agriculture Economic Research Service.

Lu, Y., Wu, K., Jiang, Y., Guo, Y., & Desneux, N. (2012). Widespread adoption of Bt cotton and insecticide decrease promotes biocontrol services. *Nature, 487*(7407), 362–365.

Magdoff, F., & van Es, H. (2009). *Building soils for better crops* (3rd. ed.). Handbook Series Book 10, Sustainable Agriculture Research and Education Program. Washington, DC: US Department of Agriculture.

Martinez, S., Hand, M., Da Pra, M., Pollack, S., Ralston, K., Smith, T., Vogel, S., Clark, S., Lohr, L., Low, S., & Newman C. (2010). *Local food systems: Concepts, impacts, and issues*. Economic Research Report 97. Washington, DC: US Department of Agriculture Economic Research Service.

McCouch, S., Baute, G. J., Bradeen, J., Bramel, P., Bretting, P. K., Buckler, E., … Zamir, D. (2013). Agriculture: Feeding the future. *Nature, 499*(7456), 23–24.

McIntyre, B., Herren, H., Wakhungu, J., & Watson, R (Eds.). (2009). *Agriculture at a Crossroads: Global report*. Washington, DC: Crossroads. Retrieved from www.unep.org/dewa/agassessment/reports/IAASTD/EN/Agriculture_at a Crossroads_Global Report %28English%29.pdf

Mollison, B. (1990). *Permaculture*. Washington, DC: Island Press.

Mortensen, D. A., Egan, J. F., Maxwell, B. D., Ryan, M. R., & Smith, R. G. (2012). Navigating a critical juncture for sustainable weed management. *BioScience, 62*(1), 75–84.

Moschini, G. (2010). Competition issues in the seed industry and the role of intellectual property. *Choices, 25*(2).

National Research Council (2010). *The Impact of Genetically Engineered Crops on Farm Sustainability in the United States*. Retrieved from http://dels.nas.edu/resources/static-assets/materials-based-on-reports/reports-in-brief/generically_engineered_crops_report_brief_final.pdf

Neff, R. A., Parker, C. I., Kirschemann, F. L., Tinch, J., & Lawrence, R. S. (2011). Peak oil, food systems and public health. *American Journal of Public Health, 9*, 1587–1597.

Organic Market Information. (2010). Global organic food and drink sales approach $60 billion. Retrieved from www.organic-market.info/web/News_in_brief/World_Trade/Organic_Food/176/199/20/9198.html

Organic Trade Association. (2013, November 28). *Industry statistics and projected growth*. Retrieved from www.ota.com/organic/mt/business.html

Parfitt, J., Barthel, M., & Macnaughton, S. (2010). Food waste within food supply chains: Quantification and potential for change to 2050. *Philosophical Transactions of the Royal Society B: Biological Sciences, 365*(1554), 3065–3081.

Phillips McDougall. (2011). *The cost and time involved in the discovery, development and authorisation of a new plant biotechnology derived trait*. Brussels, Belgium: Crop Life International.

Pleasants, J. M., & Oberhauser, K. S. (2013). Milkweed loss in agricultural fields because of herbicide use: Effect on the monarch butterfly population. *Insect Conservation and Diversity, 6*(2), 135–144.

Plourde, J. D., Pijanowski, B. C., & Pekin, B. K. (2013). Evidence for increased monoculture cropping in the Central United States. *Agriculture, Ecosystems & Environment, 165,* 50–59.

Porter, M. E. (1986). Competition in global industries: A conceptual framework. Boston: Harvard Business School Press.

Pretty, J., Toulmin, C., & Williams, S. (2011). Sustainable intensification in African agriculture. *International Journal of Agricultural Sustainability, 9*(1), 5–24.

Reif, J. C., Zhang, P., Dreisigacker, S., Warburton, M. L., van Ginkel, M., Hoisington, D., … Melchinger, A. E. (2005). Wheat genetic diversity trends during domestication and breeding. *TAG. Theoretical and Applied Genetics. Theoretische und Angewandte Genetik, 110*(5), 859–864.

Sauer, C. O. (1952). *Agricultural origins and dispersal*. Cambridge, MA: MIT Press.

Sayre, L. (2008). *Introducing a cover crop roller without all the drawbacks of a stalk chopper*. The New Farm. Retrieved from www.betuco.be/CA/No-tillage%20-%20rolled-down%20cover%20crop.pdf

Schnepf, R. (2013). *U.S. farm income*. Washington, DC: Congressional Research Service. Retrieved from www.fas.org/sgp/crs/misc/R40152.pdf

Soule, J. D., & Piper, J. K. (1992). *Farming in nature's image: An ecological approach to agriculture*. Washington, DC: Island Press.

Stephens, E. J., Losey, J. E., Allee, L. L., DiTommaso, A., Bodner, C., & Breyre, A. (2012). The impact of Cry3Bb Bt-maize on two guilds of beneficial beetles. *Agriculture, Ecosystems & Environment, 156,* 72–81.

Tabashnik, B. E., Brévault, T., & Carrière, Y. (2013). Insect resistance to Bt crops: Lessons from the first billion acres. *Nature Biotechnology, 31*(6), 510–521.

US Department of Agriculture. (2013). *Population and migration*. Retrieved from www.ers.usda.gov/topics/rural-economy-population/population-migration.aspx#.Upi_xWSeCQ0

US Department of Agriculture. (2014). *Census of agriculture*, 2012. Various tables. Retrieved from www.agcensus.usda.gov/index.php

US Department of Agriculture Environment Research Service. (2013). *Commodity costs and returns: Overview*. Retrieved from www.ers.usda.gov/data-products/commodity-costs-and-returns.aspx

Weber, C. L., & Matthews, H. S. (2008). Food-miles and the relative climate impacts of food choices in the United States. *Environmental Science and Technology, 42*(10), 3508–3513.

Willer, H., Lernoud, J., & Schaack, D. (2013). The European market for organic food, 2011. *FIBL*. Retrieved from http://orgprints.org/22345/19/willer-2013-session-european-market.pdf

Zhao, J. H., Ho, P., & Azadi, H. (2011). Benefits of Bt cotton counterbalanced by secondary pests? Perceptions of ecological change in China. *Environmental Monitoring and Assessment, 173*(1–4), 985–994.

Chapter 12

Food Animal Production

Brent F. Kim, Leo Horrigan, David C. Love, and Keeve E. Nachman

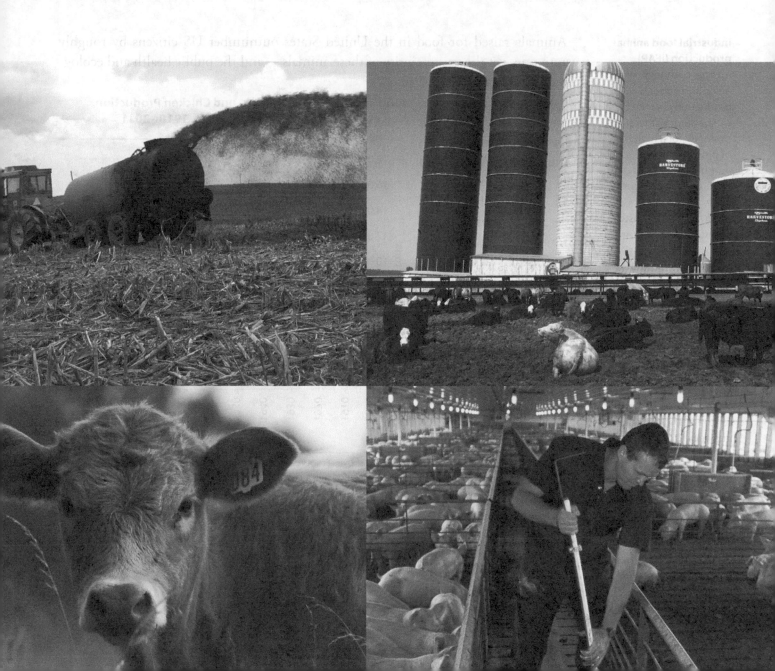

Learning Objectives

- Describe the prevailing approach to food animal production in the United States.

- Summarize major trends in food animal production.

- Give examples of the factors that drove the industrialization of food animal production.

- Describe some of the public health, social, environmental, and animal welfare impacts associated with industrial food animal production.

- Compare industrial and agroecological approaches to food animal production.

- Discuss policy or other interventions aimed at addressing the impacts associated with industrial food animal production, for example, regulating harmful practices or promoting alternatives.

industrial food animal production (IFAP)
An approach to meat, dairy, and egg production characterized by specialized operations designed for a high rate of production, large numbers of animals confined at high density, large quantities of localized animal waste, and substantial inputs of financial capital, fossil fuel, feed, pharmaceuticals, and indirect inputs embodied in feed (e.g., fuel and freshwater)

real consumer prices
Prices as paid by consumers that have been adjusted to account for the changing value of currency (e.g., inflation)

Animals raised for food in the United States outnumber US citizens by roughly seven to one, yet the vast majority of these animals—and the public health and ecological ramifications associated with their production—remain largely out of sight and out of mind for much of the public. Although a small fraction of the nation's poultry, hogs, and cattle are still raised in the pastoral settings traditionally associated with animal agriculture, **industrial food animal production (IFAP)** has emerged as the predominant approach to meat, dairy, and egg production in the US, and increasingly in other parts of the world.

IFAP has been credited with increasing the availability and affordability of animal products in the US food supply (Pew Commission on Industrial Farm Animal Production, 2008). At the end of 2012, US farmers reported an inventory of nearly 2.2 billion food-producing animals (2 billion were chickens); over nine billion were slaughtered over the previous

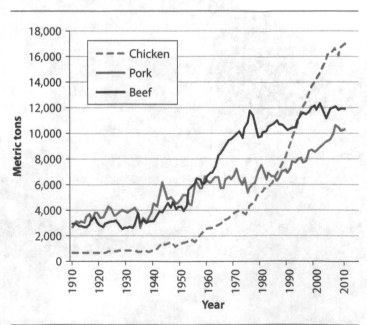

FIGURE 12.1 US Beef, Pork, and Chicken Production, Carcass Weight in Billions of Pounds, 1910–2011

Note: Not shown: From 1930–2011, dairy production increased from 46.7 to 89.0 million tons; egg production increased from 42.9 to 91.8 billion eggs.
Data source: USDA Economic Research Service [ERS] (2013a).

year (US Department of Agriculture [USDA] National Agricultural Statistics Service). The volume of production on US farms (see figure 12.1) is driven in large part by domestic demand; US citizens are among the top per capita consumers of animal products in the world (see figure 12.2), greatly exceeding global averages. The **real consumer prices** of most animal products, meanwhile, are considerably lower than they were in the mid-twentieth century (see figure 12.3).

The abundance and affordability of US animal products is at least partly attributable to industrialization. IFAP's economic success, however, has also been heavily aided by federally subsidized feed crops (Starmer & Wise, 2007), weak enforcement of environmental regulations by federal and state agencies (Graham & Nachman, 2010), tax incentives, research investments, expanded infrastructure, and other supports. Farmers' share of the value from animal product sales, meanwhile, has declined over time (see figure 12.3), reflecting rising costs in processing, transporting, marketing, and retail. Most important, IFAP incurs heavy costs to public health, rural communities, and the environment that are not reflected in the price of animal products. Were these external costs accounted for, the economics of IFAP would reveal themselves to be much less favorable.

Most of this chapter focuses on IFAP because it is by far the predominant approach to meat, dairy, and egg production in the United States, and is associated with such heavy external costs. Although IFAP typically refers to the span of production associated with the animals' life cycle prior to slaughter, including breeding, housing, feeding, and waste management, IFAP is part of an industrialized supply chain that includes growing feed crops, slaughtering animals, and processing carcasses into meat—all of which contribute, to varying degrees, to a related set of public health and ecological concerns.

In contrast to IFAP operators, some farmers take an ecological approach to food animal production, building the strengths of natural ecosystems into agricultural ecosystems in ways that promote sustainable production. They typically raise animals outdoors for all or most of the year, at much lower densities, in diverse systems that include various crops, and with fewer inputs.

Although this chapter focuses on land animals, **aquaculture**—discussed in focus 12.1—is rapidly becoming a more prominent means of food animal production. There are parallels between industrialized forms of aquaculture and its terrestrial counterparts, however, for the sake of brevity *IFAP* is used herein to refer to industrial poultry, pork, beef, dairy, and egg production.

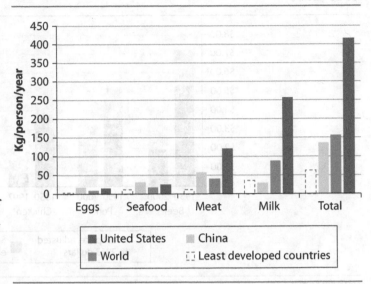

FIGURE 12.2   **Average per Capita Availability of Animal Products, 2009**

Note: Not accounting for food waste. Meat recorded as carcass weight.
Source: Food and Agriculture Organization [FAO] (2013).

aquaculture
Farm-raising fish, crustaceans, shellfish, or aquatic plants, either inland in tanks or ponds, or in enclosures in lakes, rivers, or oceans

FIGURE 12.3
Average Consumer Prices and Farmers' Share of Retail Value for Selected Animal Products, 1950–2000

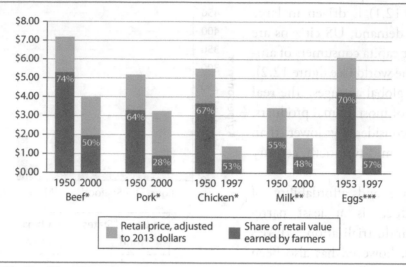

Note: *Per pound, **per half gallon, ***per dozen.
Data sources: USDA ERS (1972, 2013b); Elitzak (1999).

FOCUS 12.1. SEAFOOD HARVEST AND PRODUCTION

David C. Love

wild-capture fisheries
Area of water designated for harvesting fish

wild-caught seafood
Fish or other aquatic animals that are caught in the wild as opposed to farm raised

sustainable harvest levels
For wild-capture fisheries: maximum amount of fish that can be harvested without depleting fish populations below levels necessary to sustain harvests over the long term

natural capital
Living organisms and natural environments that provide goods and services imperative for human survival and well-being; forms the foundation for all economic activity

Seafood is a significant part of the diet for billions of people around the world. In the United States, the average person eats fifteen pounds of seafood per year; most commonly consumed are shrimp, canned tuna, salmon, pollock, tilapia, and catfish (National Fisheries Institute, 2011). Harvesting fish from the wild is still the dominant model, but perhaps not for long. Globally, aquaculture (i.e., aquatic plant and animal farming) contributes sixty-four million metric tons (MTT) of seafood, and **wild-capture fisheries** account for ninety MTT of seafood. Roughly 25 percent of **wild-caught seafood** is small oily fish, such as sardines, herring, and mullet used primarily as animal feed (FAO, 2012).

Fisheries can be a renewable resource similar to timber, wind, and sunlight, but only when the rate harvested per year does not exceed the population growth rate for a particular species. Optimal **sustainable harvest levels** are predicted with mathematical models and used by governments to set fish catch quotas. Unfortunately, overfishing still exists in most fisheries around the world (Worm et al., 2009). It is estimated that large marine predatory fish are at 10 percent of historic levels globally (Meyers & Worm, 2003); therefore, to augment their catch, fishing fleets increasingly harvest fish lower in the food web (Pauly et al., 2002). Meeting a growing demand for seafood without depleting **natural capital** and destabilizing aquatic food webs should be a high priority, which points to an increasingly important role for marine conservation and alternatives to these capture fisheries.

As capture fisheries have stagnated, aquaculture production globally has grown at a remarkable 9 percent per year since the 1970s. Asian countries, including China, India, Indonesia, Thailand, and Vietnam, produce the vast majority of the world's aquaculture, and a significant fraction of their production is sold to the United States, European Union, and other rich nations. Imported farm-raised seafood is highly scrutinized by border inspectors because seafood is susceptible to contamination and spoilage, and overseas producers may not follow the same production or food safety standards as in the United States. Hence, consumer watch groups often consider domestic aquaculture a good alternative to imported aquaculture (for sample recommendations, see www.montereybayaquarium.org/cr/seafoodwatch.aspx).

In the past decade, common types of domestic aquaculture were (1) catfish raised in ponds in the southeastern United States; (2) oysters, mussels, and clams raised in coastal waters along the East, West, and Gulf Coasts; (3) inland farms raising freshwater fish in tanks, ponds, or channelized streams, and (4) salmon raised in netted enclosures or cages in open water, called **open ocean aquaculture**, in the Northeast and Pacific Northwest.

The potential for harmful environmental and human health impacts from aquaculture depends substantially on the farming methods employed and the farm site selection. In open ocean aquaculture, farmed fish can escape, breed, and exchange diseases with wild fish, which weakens the health and genetic diversity of wild populations, and localized pollution from animal waste buildup underneath cages can be carried by water current beyond the farm boundaries (Black, 2008). Other concerns have been raised about feeding fish meal or fish oil to carnivorous farmed species such as salmon, and harvesting juvenile animals from the wild to stock farms, both of which have ecological (Naylor & Burke, 2005) and food security impacts (Tacon & Metian, 2008). As with other IFAP models, animal health is a major challenge for aquaculture because diseases spread easily among aquatic animals raised in high densities. Although most fish pathogens cannot cause disease in humans, the treatment options, such as antimicrobials, antiparasitics, and pesticides, can cause human health risks if residues persist in edible tissues or if antimicrobial use creates antimicrobial resistant bacteria.

Some of the most pressing issues facing aquaculture and fisheries are to find ways to raise fish on nutritious diets that support healthy lipid production without relying solely on wild fish as feed. Governments need to create larger marine reserves as areas off-limits to fishing to allow wild species to rebound, and develop ecosystem-based approaches for siting aquaculture operations that limit harms to aquatic environments. Last, it is recommended that producers transition to more sustainable aquaculture methods. For example, land-based **recirculating aquaculture systems** are water efficient and collect, treat, and recycle wastewater on-site; and in shellfish, aquaculture animals filter-feed on algae from coastal waters, thereby cleaning the waters as they grow (see figure 12.4).

open ocean aquaculture
Offshore (as opposed to inland) fish farms; fish typically raised in netted enclosures or cages anchored to the sea floor or floating on the surface

recirculating aquaculture systems
Indoor or outdoor production systems in which fish are raised in tanks and water is continuously filtered (to remove fish waste) and recirculated through the system

FIGURE 12.4 Aquaponics

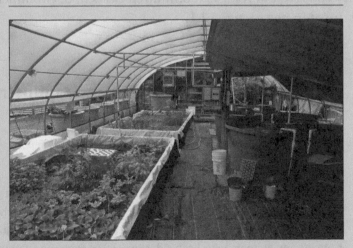

Aquaponics is a form of recirculating aquaculture that applies agroecological principles. Fish (raised in tanks, right) produce waste that fertilizes crops grown in floating media (left); plants, meanwhile, help clean the water. *Source*: Michael Milli, CLF.

INDUSTRIALIZATION OF FOOD ANIMAL PRODUCTION

Prior to industrialization, the way animals were raised for food had remained relatively unchanged since the point at which most farm animals were first domesticated over eight thousand years ago. Poultry, swine, and cattle were primarily raised on small-scale, independently owned farms, with access to the outdoors. Farms were generally diversified, producing a combination of crop and animal species together in complementary ways.

Beginning with poultry production in the 1930s, the twentieth century saw a radical transformation of meat, dairy, and egg production—characterized in part by specialization, mechanization, consolidation, and a drive to increase rates of production over time. Crop production followed parallel trends, discussed at length in chapter 11.

Specialization

Specialization, a hallmark of industrialization, aims to increase efficiency by narrowing the range of tasks and roles involved in production. This approach has been applied across nearly all facets of food animal production. Diversified farms gave way to operations that housed a single breed of animal during a particular period of its lifespan for a singular purpose (e.g., breeding cattle, milking cows, or adding weight to beef cattle before slaughter). Farmers, who were once required to have proficiency in a breadth of trades, fell into more specialized roles. As described in chapter 11, the transition to specialized, routine

mechanization
In agriculture, generally refers to replacement of human and animal labor with machinery

labor allowed for **mechanization**—the replacement of human labor with machinery, such as milking machines, mechanized waste-handling equipment, automated feeders, and computerized monitoring systems. Even the range of genetic diversity among animals in food production has narrowed, particularly among poultry and dairy cattle breeds in the United States (Notter, 1999). One effect of specialized breeding is illustrated by gains in poultry productivity: "broilers," chickens bred and raised exclusively for maximum meat production and the features desired by consumers (e.g., large breast meat), grew to almost twice the weight, in less than half the time, on half as much feed in the 1990s compared to broilers in the 1930s (Striffler, 2005). Genetic selection for productivity also promoted undesirable traits, including increased incidence of heart failure and fractured legs among chickens, and mastitis among dairy cows (Rauw, Kanis, Noordhuizen-Stassen, & Grommers, 1998). Animal welfare harms are further discussed in perspective 12.1.

Perspective 12.1. Husbandry and Industry: Animal Agriculture, Animal Welfare, and Human Health
Alan M. Goldberg and Bernard E. Rollin

Animal agriculture is roughly ten thousand years old. For all but seventy-five of those years, the key to agricultural success was good *husbandry*, which meant taking great pains to meet the animals' physical and psychological natures, augmenting their ability to survive and thrive by providing them with food, protection, water, medical attention, help in birthing, and so on. Thus, traditional agriculture was a fair contract between humans and animals, with both sides benefiting from the relationship. Husbandry agriculture was about placing square pegs into square holes, round pegs into round holes, creating as little friction as possible. Welfare was ensured by the strongest sanction, self-interest, with only the anticruelty ethic needed to deal with sadists and psychopaths unmoved by self-interest. So powerful is the notion of husbandry that when the Psalmist seeks an ideal metaphor for God's relationship to humans, he chooses the shepherd. And, in Christian iconography, Jesus is depicted both as shepherd and sheep.

The rise of confinement agriculture in the twentieth century broke this ancient contract. The industrial values of efficiency and productivity supplanted the core agricultural values of husbandry. With technological "sanders"—hormones, vaccines, antibiotics, air handling systems, mechanization—we could force square pegs into round holes, placing animals into environments where they suffer in ways irrelevant to productivity.

The egg industry was one of the first areas of agriculture to experience industrialization. Traditionally, chickens ran free in barnyards, able to forage and express their natural behaviors—nest-building, dust-bathing, escaping from more aggressive animals, defecating away from their nests, that is, fulfilling their natures as chickens. Industrialization of the egg industry, however, often meant placing chickens with six or more birds in a tiny wire cage, so one animal may stand on top of the others and none can perform their inherent behaviors or even stretch their wings. In the absence of space to establish a dominance hierarchy or pecking order, they cannibalize each other and must be debeaked, producing painful nerve tissue growths. The animal is now an inexpensive cog in a factory machine—the cheapest part at that, and totally expendable. If a nineteenth-century farmer had attempted such a system, he would have gone broke, the animals dead of infections in a few weeks.

The same dismal situation is apparent in all areas of industrialized animal agriculture. Consider, for example, the dairy industry, once viewed as the paradigm of bucolic, sustainable agriculture, with animals grazing on pasture, giving milk, and fertilizing the soil with their manure; the truth is radically different. Most dairy cattle spend their lives on dirt and concrete, never seeing a blade of pasture grass, let alone consuming it.

In a problem ubiquitous across contemporary agriculture, animals have been single-mindedly bred for productivity; for milk production in this case. In 1957, the average dairy cow produced between five hundred and six hundred pounds of milk per lactation. Fifty years later, it is over twenty-one thousand pounds (USDA National Agriculture Statistics Service [USDA NASS], 2012). From 1995 to 2004 alone, milk production per cow increased 16 percent. The result is a milk-bag on legs—unstable legs at that. A high percentage of the US dairy herd is chronically lame (some estimates range as high as 30 percent), and these cows suffer serious reproductive problems. Whereas, in traditional agriculture, a milk cow could remain productive for ten, fifteen, or even twenty years, today's cow lasts slightly longer than two lactations (three years). With such unnaturally high productivity, animals suffer from mastitis. The industry's response to mastitis in portions of the United States has created a new welfare problem by docking cow tails without anesthesia in a futile effort to minimize teat contamination by manure. This procedure, still practiced, has been definitively demonstrated irrelevant to mastitis control or lowering somatic cell count (Stull, Payne, Berry, & Hullinger, 2002).

The intensive swine industry, through a handful of companies, is responsible for 85 percent of the pork produced in the United States; it also is responsible for significant suffering that did not affect husbandry-reared swine. Certainly the most egregious practice in confinement swine industry and possibly, given the intelligence of pigs, in all of animal agriculture, is the housing of pregnant sows in gestation crates or stalls—essentially small cages. Except a few weeks for birthing, the sow spends her entire four-year productive life in these cages. She cannot turn around, walk, or even scratch her rump. A large sow cannot even lie flat but must lie in an arched position on her sternum. Under husbandry conditions, a sow will build a nest on a hillside so excrement runs off; forage a two-kilometer area each day, and take turns with other sows watching piglets, allowing all sows to forage. With the animal's nature thus aborted, she goes mad, exhibiting such bizarre and deviant behavior as compulsively chewing cage bars; she also endures foot and leg problems and lesions from lying on concrete in her own excrement.

Confinement agriculture also has created major problems in environmental despoliation, loss of small farms and rural communities, animal health, human health, and antibiotic resistance. The pioneering review by the

(Continued)

(Continued)

concentrated animal feeding operations (CAFOs) Environmental Protection Agency category for large facility in which animals are confined and fed or maintained for at least forty-five days out of the year, the operation does not produce crops or vegetation, and it meets size thresholds (e.g., 1,000 cattle, 10,000 swine, or 125,000 chickens may classify as a "large CAFO," depending on how animal waste is managed)

Pew Commission on Industrial Farm Animal Production (both of us were commissioners) made clear the negative and important human health consequences of **concentrated animal feeding operations (CAFOs)** (see focus 12.3). Some were well documented, others suggestive and in need of more data, still others were suspect but lacked significant data for full documentation. This has changed in the last few years, but there is clear evidence that poor animal welfare and the associated crowding are causally related to human health consequences.

For example, as described in chapter 2, antibiotic resistance and the consequent proliferation of MRSA (methicillin-resistant *Staphylococcus aureus*), are directly related to nontherapeutic use of antibiotics in farm animal production. Currently, approximately 80 percent of all antibiotics produced in the United States are sold for use in animals. Most antibiotics used in industrial farm animal production are used at subtherapeutic doses, in part to help animals deal with the stress of crowding. MRSA has become a more prevalent, more persistent infection throughout the human population.

Our current methods of industrial farm animal production present significant animal welfare—and related human health—consequences. How can this be reversed and corrected? Clearly, changing the density of animals raised together would be a giant step forward. A more powerful approach would be to change the unacceptable animal welfare standards that are legal but clearly inhumane (for example, battery cages for egg layers). Raising the standards for animal welfare, along the lines of the welfare quality criteria of the European Union, would address most of the negative human health consequences of industrial farm animal production. The added benefits include decreased environmental contamination, improved community relations for industry, and better conditions for the animals raised for food.

Consolidation

Consolidation in agricultural industries is the shift toward fewer and larger farms. In the 1950s, former US Secretary of Agriculture Ezra Taft Benson characterized the drive to consolidate when he called on

consolidation
The shift toward fewer and larger operations in an industry

farmers to "get big or get out" (Zimdahl, 2012). In crop production, this meant scaling up farms and planting from "fencerow to fencerow." Meat, dairy, and egg industries followed in kind, dramatically increasing numbers of animals handled by production and processing facilities. The number of US hog farms, for example, declined from 1,849,000 to 63,000 between 1959 and 2012, and the average number of hogs per farm grew from 37 to 1044 (see figure 12.5) (USDA NASS Census of Agriculture).

Consolidation is in part driven by perceived opportunities to achieve greater economies of scale. Larger animal operations are generally thought to operate at lower per-unit costs of production, edging out smaller competitors. There is a point, however, beyond which increases in scale become economically disadvantageous, partly on account of the need for larger operations to store and transport greater quantities of animal waste. These "diseconomies of scale" would become more salient if IFAP industries were made more accountable for their impacts to water quality and human health (Weida, 2004).

Table 12.1 illustrates the effects of consolidation—the vast majority of US animal products originate in large-scale operations (under federal regulations, these may be classified as CAFOs, depending on their size and practices). In industrial hog and poultry operations, animals are confined in densely stocked indoor facilities. The largest US dairy operations have over fifteen thousand cows, usually in barns or outdoor lots, though farms with one thousand to five thousand cows are more common (USDA ERS, 2006). Beef cattle still spend most of their lives on pasture; under the IFAP model, before slaughter, steers are transported to **feedlots**. Beef feedlots with upwards of thirty-two thousand cattle supply about 40 percent of the market for grain-fed cattle (USDA ERS, 2012) (see figure 12.6).

FIGURE 12.5   Consolidation in Hog Production

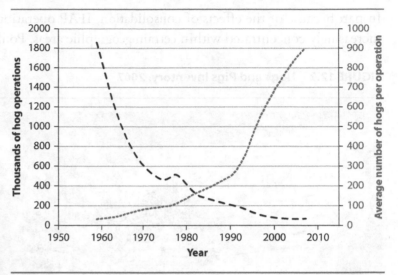

Data Source: USDA NASS Census of Agriculture.

feedlots
Confinement facilities, usually outdoors, where animals (typically cattle) are fed for the purpose of rapid weight gain prior to slaughter

TABLE 12.1   Percentage of US Food-Producing Animals from Large-Scale Operations, 2012

Broiler chicken sales from operations with annual sales of more than 200,000 birds	96%
Hog and pig sales from operations with annual sales of more than 5,000 swine	91%
Hogs and pigs in operations with more than 2,000 animals	90%
Laying hens in operations with more than 50,000 birds	82%

Source: USDA NASS Census of Agriculture.

FIGURE 12.6   IFAP Operations

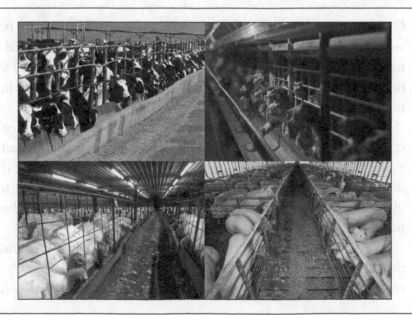

Clockwise from top right: Poultry operation, hog operation, laying hens in battery cages, beef cattle in feedlot.
Sources: (clockwise from top left): NRCS; Mercy for Animals; iStockphoto; Jeff Vanuga, NRCS.

Geography of Production

In part because of the effects of consolidation, IFAP operations and processing facilities have become increasingly concentrated within certain geographic areas. Poultry production operations, for example, cluster in parts of the rural South; in 2011, 58 percent of US chickens were raised in just five states (USDA NASS Census of Agriculture). Figure 12.7 illustrates a similar phenomenon in hog production. IFAP operations tend to cluster in areas with conditions favorable to industry, such as weak environmental regulations, favorable tax policies, and access to feed mills and processing facilities (Herath, Weersink, & Carpentier, 2012; Mallin & Cahoon, 2003). In some regions, IFAP operations are disproportionately sited near low-income communities and communities of color, who may lack the political power to present an effective opposition (Wilson, Howell, Wing, & Sobsey, 2002), placing these populations at greater risk of exposure to IFAP's environmental hazards. The geographic concentration of large numbers of animals—and their waste—further exacerbates public health impacts on surrounding communities.

FIGURE 12.7   Hogs and Pigs Inventory, 2007

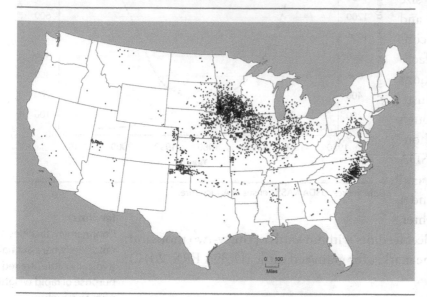

Source: USDA NASS Census of Agriculture. 1 dot = 20,000 animals.

Market Concentration

market concentration
The extent to which market shares in an industry are owned by a small number of companies

horizontal integration
When companies take over or merge with other companies competing in the same enterprise

vertical integration
The merging of two or more businesses involved in different stages of the supply chain for the same product(s) (e.g., the distribution and sales of supermarket goods)

Over time, market shares of meat, dairy, and egg industries have become increasingly concentrated under the ownership of a small number of influential corporations. This **market concentration** (also discussed in chapters 7, 11, and 14) assumes two forms: horizontal and vertical integration. Both raise concerns about the power of a small number of entities to influence how food is produced.

Horizontal integration occurs when companies take over or merge with other companies competing in the same enterprise. As a result of horizontal integration, for example, the four largest meatpacking firms own 82 percent of the market share of the US beef slaughtering and processing industry (James, Hendrickson, & Howard, 2013). Other industries involved in animal production, slaughter, and processing have seen similar trends (see figure 12.8).

Vertical integration occurs when companies gain control of multiple stages along the supply chain of a product. For example, the largest US pork producer and processor, Smithfield Foods, owns the rights to raise a particular breed of hogs, oversees how the animals are raised, slaughters them, processes their meat, and markets the finished products (Martinez, 1999).

In the hog and poultry industries, vertically integrated companies (**integrators**) enter into contracts with **growers**, people who own indoor facilities in which they raise hogs or chickens until they are ready for slaughter, as discussed in perspective 4.4. Integrators typically own the animals, supply specially formulated feed, and specify how animals will be housed and maintained. Growers under contract with integrators lack autonomy over production methods but bear responsibility for handling animal waste and the carcasses of animals that die during production—exposing them to the health risks associated with these hazards.

Market concentration can leave independent farmers with few options for where to bring their animals for slaughter. When processing firms have few competitors in a region, for example, they can demand low prices from farmers, who may have no choice but to accept; shipping live animals to distant processors for competitive prices is rarely feasible. These and other pressures have led many independent farmers to sign contracts with integrators, guaranteeing fixed prices (Wise & Trist, 2010).

IFAP Waste Generation and Management

Swine, poultry, and cattle raised in US IFAP operations collectively produced an estimated 335 million tons of dry **animal waste** in 2005 (USDA AERS, 2005)—more than forty times the amount of human solid waste leaving publicly owned treatment plants (Graham & Nachman, 2010). Waste from cattle and hog operations is often stored as a slurry in outdoor cesspits, euphemistically called **lagoons** (see figure 12.9). A single large IFAP operation can produce as much waste as a small city, but without the benefit of a sewer system or sewage treatment plant; unlike human waste, there is no requirement that animal waste be treated to remove pathogens and chemical contaminants.

The nutrients and organic matter in **manure** promote soil fertility. IFAP waste is typically applied to nearby fields as fertilizer and as a means of disposal. The

FIGURE 12.8 Concentration in Animal Slaughter and Processing Industries

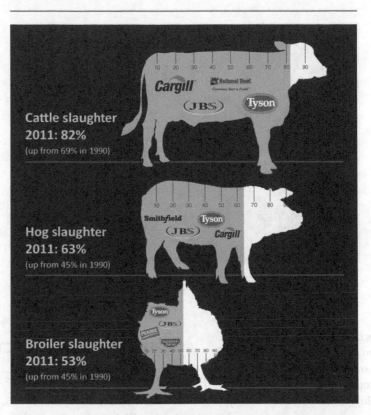

Figure design: Michael Milli and Brent Kim, CLF. Adapted from Anna Lappé and thecoup.org.
Source: James et al. (2013).

integrators
In the hog and poultry industries, refers to the vertically integrated companies that coordinate multiple successive stages of the supply chain

growers
In hog and poultry industries, refers to those contracting with a vertically integrated company to raise animals until they are ready for slaughter

animal waste
Feces, urine, or soiled bedding (e.g., poultry litter)

lagoons
Cesspits used to store liquid cattle or swine waste

manure
Animal waste intended for use as fertilizer

FIGURE 12.9   Waste Storage Pit for a Nine-Hundred-Head Hog Operation in Georgia

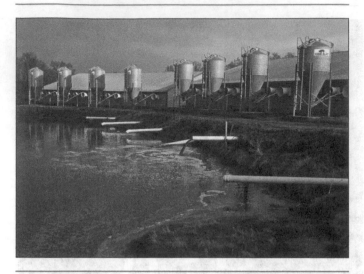

Source: Jeff Vanuga, USDA Natural Resources Conservation Service.

quantities of waste generated at IFAP operations, however, generally far exceed what can be absorbed by surrounding land, and transporting waste farther is often not economically feasible. When IFAP waste is overapplied to land, the excess—along with chemical and bacterial contaminants associated with it—may leach into groundwater and be transported by **runoff** into surface waters. Other potential contamination sources include leakage and overflow from cesspits (e.g., during severe weather) and animal carcasses. The public health and ecological implications of ground and surface water contamination are discussed in the following section.

runoff
The flow of water from rain, irrigation water, and other sources over land; often carries topsoil and contaminants into bodies of water

pathogens
Disease-causing organisms e.g., *Staphylococcus aureus* [bacteria], *Influenza* [virus], and *Cryptosporidium* [parasite]

PUBLIC HEALTH IMPACTS OF IFAP

IFAP operations and processing facilities are associated with a range of health hazards. Exposure to these hazards may be direct, such as among workers at IFAP operations and processing facilities who come in frequent contact with animal waste, carcasses, dangerous equipment, and toxic gases. **Pathogens**, harmful chemicals, and other agents may also be transported to nearby communities and the general public via air, water, soil, and contaminated food. The health effects associated with exposure may include a range of respiratory, gastrointestinal, neurological, and other harms.

Antibiotic Resistance

Antibiotic drugs have been called the health care miracle of the last five hundred years. The routine use of low doses of antibiotic drugs in IFAP, however, threatens to erode the effectiveness of these life-saving—and generally irreplaceable—resources.

Experiments in the 1940s and 1950s found feeding low doses of antibiotics to animals caused them to gain weight faster and on less feed. These findings prompted the introduction of antibiotics to the diets of healthy swine, poultry, and cattle (Gustafson & Bowen, 1997). Although the mechanisms of growth promotion are not fully understood, it has been suggested that continual low doses of antibiotics aid growth by compensating for immune-compromising conditions (Committee on Drug Use in Food Animals, 1999), such as those commonly found in IFAP. An estimated 80 percent of antibiotics sold for human and animal uses in the United States are administered to food-producing animals (US Food and Drug Administration, 2010).

Margaret Chan, director-general of the World Health Organization, warned, "the world is heading toward a post-antibiotic era, in which many common infections will no longer have a cure and, once again, kill unabated" (2011). Dr. Chan's concerns stem from the increasing prevalence of bacterial pathogens that have become resistant to antibiotics, making infections in humans more difficult and expensive to treat (Roberts et al., 2009). Continual exposure to antibiotics at doses below levels needed to treat disease—common to IFAP—favors the selection of these resistant pathogens. In a case of survival of the fittest, bacterial strains that are susceptible to the antibiotic are eliminated, unable to compete with resistant strains, and resistant strains proliferate.

Numerous public health organizations have called on federal agencies to phase out the routine use of certain medically important antibiotics in IFAP. Some industry groups have asserted that restricting antibiotic use would compromise productivity and the health of animals, but evidence suggests otherwise. An economic analysis of poultry producers in the United States demonstrated that the use of antibiotics for growth promotion incurs economic losses to producers (Graham, Boland, & Silbergeld, 2007). After a ban on routine antibiotic use in Denmark, pork and poultry producers maintained high levels of productivity, and long-term animal health was largely unaffected (Aarestrup, Vibeke, Emborg, Jacobsen, & Wegener, 2010). To make it possible to comply with the ban, Danish pork producers improved conditions for animals, including by increasing the amount of space per animal (Government Accountability Office, 2011). Their experience suggests a similar ban in the United States may require parallel measures to maintain animal health.

Occupational Hazards

Crowded conditions in IFAP operations present frequent opportunities for the transmission of viral and bacterial pathogens between animals and between animals and humans. When animals are under stress, they are even more likely to shed pathogens, and are more susceptible to infection. Overcrowding, rough handling (e.g., during transport), feed deprivation, early weaning, and other practices common to IFAP have been shown to induce stress in animals (Rostagno, 2009).

IFAP workers are often in prolonged contact with animals and may be responsible for handling animal waste and large volumes of carcasses (e.g., in processing facilities). These scenarios present opportunities for workers to be infected or **colonized** with pathogens. Colonized or infected workers may spread these pathogens into their homes and communities (Skov & Jensen, 2009).

colonized Carrying pathogenic organism on or inside the body, but showing no signs of illness or infection

IFAP workers may also be exposed to airborne hazards, including ammonia, hydrogen sulfide, and other gases emitted from animal waste; and airborne particulates, which may be composed of dried feces, animal dander, fungal spores, and bacterial toxins. These hazards contribute to a heavy burden of occupational risks; at least one in four workers in indoor IFAP operations are estimated to suffer from respiratory illness (Donham et al., 2007). Exposure to bacterial toxins, for example, has been linked to impaired lung function, inflammation, and asthma (Heederik et al., 2007). Other risks are more acute; hydrogen sulfide emissions from liquid waste cesspits have been implicated in numerous animal and human deaths (Donham, Knapp, Monson, & Gustafson, 1982).

Despite recent improvements, reported injury rates for meat processing facilities workers greatly exceed the average for the US workforce. Workers who incur cuts, burns, or scrapes may be at particular risk of sustaining antibiotic-resistant infections (Mulders et al., 2010). Meat processing facilities frequently hire immigrant workers, who may be less empowered to dispute low wages and hazardous working conditions. In some cases, undocumented immigrants are smuggled into the country by the companies that hire them, and face fears of deportation (Human Rights Watch, 2004). Worker risks are further discussed in chapter 2.

Novel Influenza

Novel influenza viruses present additional concerns related to disease transmission. Hogs, susceptible to both human and avian strains of influenza, can serve as "mixing vessels" in which human, avian, and porcine strains exchange genetic material in a process called **viral reassortment**. The resulting novel virus may then be transmissible from hogs to humans (Ma, Lager, Vincent, Janke, Gramer, & Richt, 2009; Myers, Olsen, & Gray, 2007). Increased contact among large populations of hogs, birds, and humans—increasingly common to areas such as rural North Carolina, where densely stocked hog and turkey operations are in close proximity—offer ample opportunities for viral reassortment. The influenza pandemic of 1918, responsible for more deaths than any other disease outbreak in human history, illustrates the potential implications of novel influenza.

viral reassortment
The exchange of genetic material between different viral strains within the same host

Community Impacts

As noted, workers in IFAP operations and processing facilities may spread pathogens into their communities. People may be exposed to hazards associated with IFAP via air, water, and soil. Proximity to IFAP operations has been associated with multiple adverse health outcomes, including increased risks of methicillin-resistant *Staphylococcus aureus* and other infections (Casey, Curriero, Cosgrove, Nachman, & Schwartz, 2013).

Communities living near to or downstream from IFAP operations may be exposed to a range of waterborne contaminants, including **nitrates**, bacterial and viral pathogens, veterinary pharmaceuticals, heavy metals, and hormones. People may be exposed from drinking contaminated groundwater and from contact with contaminated surface waters. Ingesting high levels of nitrate, for example, has been linked to reproductive harms, diabetes, thyroid conditions, and methemoglobinemia (blue baby syndrome), a potentially fatal condition among infants (Burkholder et al., 2007). Certain varieties of algae—linked to nutrient runoff from IFAP and other sources—produce toxins that can result in neurological impairments, liver damage, stomach illness, skin lesions, and other effects (Van Dolah, 2000).

nitrates
Naturally occurring form of nitrogen, essential for plant growth; formed when microorganisms break down manure, decaying plants, or other organic matter

There is increasing evidence linking airborne contaminants from IFAP to adverse health and social outcomes among nearby residents. Strong odors from nearby IFAP operations, for example, have been known to interfere with daily activities, quality of life, social gatherings, and community cohesion. In addition to the stigma and social disruption they often generate, IFAP odors have been associated with physiological and psychological effects, including high blood pressure, depression, anxiety, and sleep disturbances. Studies have also documented numerous respiratory problems among residents living near IFAP operations.

Health risks and social conflict arising from IFAP operations have contributed to the social and economic decline of rural communities (Donham et al., 2007). Proposals for new IFAP operations, for example, have triggered heated intercommunity conflicts between supporters and opponents—conflicts that can persist or escalate if the facility is built. Focus 12.2 describes a case study from one affected community and stimulates consideration of the multiple stakeholder viewpoints; whereas in perspective 12.2, one community member describes his experiences and concerns.

In many regions, the health and social burdens associated with IFAP fall disproportionately on low-income communities and communities of color—populations already affected by poorer health status and lack of access to medical care (Donham et al., 2007; Wing, Horton, & Rose, 2013). Despite these harms, government policies have had limited success in mitigating waterborne hazards linked to IFAP waste, and IFAP operations are largely exempt from federal regulations on specific air pollutants.

FOCUS 12.2. A CASE STUDY IN RURAL COMMUNITY EXPOSURES: YAKIMA VALLEY, WASHINGTON

D'Ann L. Williams and Meghan F. Davis

Yakima County, located in south-central Washington State, leads the state in dairy production and production of apples, mint, pears, wine grapes, and hops (Yakima County, 2013). Approximately 222,600 people (Yakima County, 2013) and 212,800 cows (including 126,800 dairy cows and beef cattle) live in Yakima County (USDA NASS Census of Agriculture); the highest dairy concentration is between Prosser and Yakima City (Washington State Department of Ecology, 2009).

The proximity of these industrial facilities to rural communities creates the potential for airborne and waterborne exposures. Airborne contaminants, such as ammonia, an irritating gas released from cow waste; allergens; and **endotoxin**, a bacterial toxin, are known to affect health. Nutrients, such as nitrates, also may be released in waste water from dairies. In high concentrations, these contaminants can be toxic to humans, animals, and plants. To learn more about such exposures, research was conducted that measured particulate matter, ammonia, and a cow allergen (Bos d 2) in samples taken inside and outside homes (Williams, Breysse, McCormack, Diette, McKenzie, & Geyh, 2011). Cow allergen and endotoxin were chosen as markers indicating exposures from cows and fecal wastes (Williams et al., 2011). Bos d 2 comes only from cows, so quantifying its concentrations helps researchers understand the extent to which other contaminants, identified and unidentified, might come from dairies. Researchers found concentrations of these markers were higher in homes near dairies versus homes greater than three miles away.

endotoxin
Toxin present in outer membrane of certain bacteria (whether the bacteria are alive or dead); released when bacterium dies; human exposure has been associated with adverse health effects including inflammation and fever

Groundwater has been evaluated for thirty years in the region. In 2012, the US Environmental Protection Agency (EPA) estimated that six large dairies in Yakima County leak between 3,300,000 to 40 million gallons of liquid waste annually, contaminating groundwater. Manure pollution occurs at higher concentrations closer to dairies and decreases further away from the facilities along a concentration gradient. Tetracycline, an antibiotic drug administered to cows and used by people, was found in down-gradient wells, but not in wells up-gradient of the dairy facilities, suggesting that the dairies and irrigation crop fields contribute to groundwater contaminants (EPA, 2012). However, no studies have evaluated the impact of these discharges on human health.

Yakima has a history of environmental activism centered on the dairy industry. Many residents are Hispanic or Native American, making environmental exposures in this area an environmental justice issue. In 1999, the Community Association for the Restoration of the Environment (CARE) sued a Yakima Valley dairy for discharging pollutants into US waters. Subsequently, CARE has filed multiple lawsuits against other dairies for noncompliance with water monitoring, failure to implement **best management practices (BMPs)**, and against the Washington Department of Ecology for failure to protect groundwater.

best management practices (BMPs)
Agricultural practices designed to minimize adverse environmental effects

Responding to community concerns about airborne emissions, dust, waste, and odor from dairy facilities, the Yakima Regional Clean Air Agency proposed a "Dairy Scorecard" in 2011 (Yakima Regional Air Quality Agency, 2012). The Dairy Scorecard lists BMPs that Yakima dairies must use to effectively manage manure, air emissions, and odors. Community activists question the validity of this program because it allows dairies to select only those BMPs currently in use on their farms, the monitoring program is funded primarily by the dairy industry, only dairy industry stakeholders were involved in program development, and monitoring relies solely

(Continued)

(Continued)

on visual inspection. The debate, involving many stakeholders, is ongoing about whom to measure, how to measure, and how to address emissions from industrial dairy facilities.

Thinking about Yakima Valley

- Imagine you are one of the following stakeholders in this debate. If you attended a county meeting proposing to increase the number of dairy facilities in Yakima County, would you argue for or against the increase, and why?

  - Resident, concerned with your own health and property values, living within a mile of an industrial dairy facility

  - Dairy producer, concerned with the success of the business, running a seven thousand cow dairy

  - Grass-fed dairy owner with six hundred cows, concerned with maintaining organic status in the face of chemical contamination from nearby industrial dairies

  - EPA official or health department official investigating elevated nitrate levels in wells of residents

  - County official concerned with the economic stability of Yakima

  - Tree fruit producer, concerned with food safety, whose orchard is adjacent to a large dairy that sprays manure on fields nearby

  - Winemaker, concerned with dairy odors, who caters to tourists

- Yakima is one of the few places where exposure assessments have been performed in communities near industrial dairies. Researchers did not measure health effects and other exposures (e.g., pathogens, pesticides). If you were a researcher with limited funding, what would you measure and why?

- Dairy facilities argue that information about how many animals they raise, chemical and drug use, and management practices are proprietary. Would access to this information benefit researchers? If so, how?

Perspective 12.2. Living in Duplin County
Devon J. Hall, Sr. (as told to Leo Horrigan)

I've lived in Duplin County, North Carolina, pretty much all of my fifty-seven years. Growing up I remember hogs, chickens, and a garden in almost everyone's yard. Everyone grew food, and you'd always have enough to share with neighbors.

It wasn't until about twenty-five years ago that you started to see the industrialized farms being built in our neighborhoods. Tobacco was the cash crop then, but tobacco was being phased out, so it made sense to raise hogs instead. Back then, I didn't see any problem with the big hog barns.

In early 2005, though, I met Dr. Steve Wing from UNC-Chapel Hill, and that's when my eyes began to be opened to the negative effects of these CAFOs. There were many people, myself included, who could no longer use their shallow wells for drinking water because of contamination.

Initially, we didn't want to blame industry for these problems, but a lot of water sampling has found DNA markers that indicate these contaminants are linked to hog waste, poultry waste, etc., from these industrial farms. Researchers have found *E. coli*, traces of MRSA, and other harmful bacteria in their sampling. We know some of that pollution is carried through the air, too.

PUBLIC HEALTH IMPACTS OF IFAP • 305

It was in early 2005 that I realized there was a place for me as an activist. It touched my heart to hear stories from my neighbors about problems they were having with CAFOs, and I said to myself, if someone had to speak up, if someone had to address this issue, why not me?

The most common health complaints in the community are burning eyes and scratchy throats, which people blame on the ammonia-type smell from hog urine, and people gag from the manure smell. Workers in the confinement buildings talk about a chronic cough—one that persists until they get out of that facility and into some fresher air.

With other respiratory illnesses, such as asthma, it's hard to prove that CAFOs aggravate it, but common sense might tell you that the stench in the air and the particulate matters could trigger an asthma attack. The industry should be working with the community to research these kinds of questions and find solutions.

No one complained about smells when it was just a few hogs being raised on the ground—even if they were close by. But, nowadays, you might be able to get a whiff of a CAFO that's a mile and a half away—where they could be raising as many as five thousand hogs on one farm—and it can affect your quality of life.

I had some out-of-town visitors recently, and when it was nice outside and you'd expect the smaller children to go out and play, they said, "What's that awful smell?" It all comes home to you then. We adults have become immune to it. You wake up in the morning with it and you go to sleep at night smelling it.

Another problem that concerns me is what we call "dead boxes," which are like large, uncovered dumpsters that are sometimes overflowing with dead animals from those big barns. They're waiting to be picked up and trucked to a rendering plant, but in the meantime those rotting animals are attracting buzzards. Imagine having one of these boxes sitting maybe seventy-five feet from your driveway—or having one of those uncovered "dead trucks" rolling through your neighborhood? I believe anything that smells so bad that it makes you want to puke cannot be healthy.

Some people would like to leave Duplin County to get away from these problems. But, who would they sell their property to? Any potential buyer might ask: "What's that odor? Does it always smell like that?"

Personally, I don't want to move away. Duplin County is home to me, and all six of my siblings. Five of us live within two hundred yards of each other, on land that's been passed down from our grandparents.

On the other hand, I'd be hesitant to invest in land here. There are 522 hog CAFOs in this county, and we're told they're raising 2.2 million hogs each year. I've heard the actual number might be even higher. That's more than thirty-five hogs for every person in Duplin.

Mind you, I don't want these contract growers to be put out of business. I feel an obligation to protect them, too, because many of them live within walking distance of those confinement buildings. I even believe they are sympathetic to their neighbors and would do things differently if the industry would let them. But, I also believe industry intimidates growers, just like it has intimidated some community members who have criticized industry practices.

My bottom line is, the current method of disposing of hog waste is harming our environment and our health, and we need changes. Let them make their money. If they want to raise hogs in confinement buildings, let them do it. As long as they can clean it up. And companies like Smithfield should bear some of the cost of the technologies that could clean up the waste.

If you're sitting in Smithfield's corporate offices, it's easy to say that the smell is "not that bad," because you are just looking at the profit side of it. But, what kind of price tag do you put on people's lives and their health and well-being?

Microbial Hazards in Animal Products

Disease-causing microorganisms originating in IFAP operations, including antibiotic-resistant pathogens, can enter the food supply at various points along the supply chain. Contaminated food prepared or handled improperly poses risks to exposed persons, including fever, nausea, diarrhea, chronic illness, and death.

Many of the pathogens associated with food-borne illness, such as *Salmonella* and *E. coli,* reside in animals' digestive tracts and can contaminate food via animal waste. Fertilizing food crops with IFAP manure that has not been properly treated to eliminate pathogens, for example, can contaminate produce; this is often how fresh produce becomes contaminated. When IFAP waste contaminates water sources, contaminants can also be transferred to food crops if fields are irrigated using the contaminated water. Some contaminants can enter plant tissues through roots, increasing food safety concerns because washing produce does not remove internalized contaminants (Solomon, Yaron, & Matthews, 2002).

Contaminants can also spread into the food supply at meat processing facilities. Motivated by slim profit margins and the desire to achieve economies of scale, facilities typically process large quantities of carcasses per shift—increasing the potential for widespread cross-contamination. At poultry processing facilities, for example, a single processing line can legally operate at 140 birds per minute, offering ample opportunity for pathogens to spread between carcasses via processing equipment and facility workers—particularly if the animals' digestive tracts are accidentally severed. The geographic area over which processing facilities distribute products has become broader, increasing the risk of widespread exposure to contamination from any one incident (Woteki & Kineman, 2003).

An estimated one-half of US food-borne illnesses caused by seafood are attributable to algal toxins. The algae and other marine microorganisms responsible for seafood contamination are naturally occurring; however, nutrient pollution from IFAP operations can spur the proliferation of certain species of algae linked to food-borne illness (Van Dolah, 2000).

Chemical Hazards in Animal Products

Some of the health concerns associated with consuming animal products stem from inputs used in

arsenical drugs
Drugs containing the element arsenic; added to some animal feeds to increase feed efficiency, promote weight gain, and prevent infection

IFAP, such as added hormones used in beef and dairy production and animal feed ingredients (see also chapter 2).

IFAP feeds are formulated to maximize meat, dairy, and egg yields at minimal cost, and may contain antibiotics, preservatives, waste materials, fillers, and a host of other ingredients. The implications of antibiotic use in IFAP have already been discussed; a number of other additives also pose public health concerns. Certain **arsenical drugs**, for example, are approved for use in poultry production. Arsenic has been found to accumulate in poultry meat (Nachman, Baron, Raber, Francesconi, Navas-Acien, & Love, 2013) and is associated with elevated risks of certain cancers, cardiovascular disease, diabetes, and cognitive defects in children. In 2013, the FDA withdrew approvals for three of the four arsenical drugs used in US meat production.

IFAP feed may also contain products of animal origin, including fats, bones, blood, feathers, excreta, and whole rendered carcasses (Sapkota, Lefferts, McKenzie, & Walker, 2007). In some cases, the use of these ingredients may "recycle" contaminants such as heavy metals, dioxins, and prions into the human food supply (Love, Halden, Davis, & Nachman, 2012), increasing contaminant concentrations in animal tissues and raising exposure risks among consumers.

In the United States, growth-promoting hormones are administered to an estimated two-thirds of all beef cattle, 90 percent of feedlot cattle (Johnson & Hanrahan, 2010), and one-third of dairy cattle

(California Breast Cancer Research Program, 2007). The use of these hormones is suspected as a possible contributor to cancer risk and other negative human health effects. The potential risks, however, are difficult to assess, in part because beef and dairy intake may contribute to cancer risk independent of added hormone use.

GLOBAL AND ECOLOGICAL CONCERNS

Food animal production (industrial and otherwise) affects ecosystem change at regional and global scales, as discussed in chapter 3. Depending on production practices, it can promote biodiversity and soil fertility, as well as degrade aquatic ecosystems, erode topsoil, contribute to global climate change, and deplete freshwater supplies. Such environmental effects are deeply connected to public health.

Climate Change

A rapidly changing climate is among the greatest threats to human health and ecosystems. Human activities, including food production, are overwhelmingly responsible for the rise in atmospheric greenhouse gas emissions that contribute to global warming. Beef, pork, and dairy production account for almost half of the emissions associated with US food supply chains (Weber & Matthews, 2008). Major agricultural emission sources include cattle belching and animal waste. Much of the greenhouse gas emissions from crop production—including emissions from synthetic fertilizer use and fossil fuel combustion—are attributable to growing feed for animals.

Impacts on Aquatic Ecosystems

The contamination of waterways with animal waste can dramatically alter aquatic ecosystems by introducing excess nutrients, which contribute to rapid accumulations of algae (**algal blooms**) and, subsequently, a hypoxic (low-oxygen) **dead zone**, where most aquatic organisms cannot survive (Mallin & Cahoon, 2003) (see also chapter 3).

algal blooms
A rapid accumulation of algae

Aquatic nutrient pollution has also been linked to the growth of *Pfiesteria*, a toxin-producing microorganism. Manure spills from hog operations in North Carolina have been implicated in *Pfiesteria* outbreaks that resulted in massive fish kills. Concerns over toxic human exposure to *Pfiesteria* have prompted numerous closings of beaches and commercial fishing areas (Mallin & Cahoon, 2003).

dead zone
Area of water with insufficient oxygen to support most organisms

Land Use and Global Food Security

Keeping pace with population growth, rising meat consumption, and biofuel demands would require raising global food production by an estimated 70 percent by 2050, compared to 2005 to 2007 levels (Food and Agriculture Organization, 2009a). Crop yield increases through technology, however, appear to be reaching their limit, and nearly 40 percent of the earth's landmass is already covered by cropland and pasture with little room to expand without clearing forests. These limitations are compounded by a host of environmental concerns linked to food production, including climate change, deforestation, biodiversity loss, soil degradation, and declining reserves of fossil fuels, fresh water, and mineral fertilizers. In light of these challenges, feeding the world will likely require changing how existing agricultural

agroecology
The science and practice of applying ecological principles to agriculture to develop practices that work with nature to mimic natural processes and conserve ecological integrity; other labels for ecological approaches to agriculture include *ecological agriculture, agricultural ecology, sustainable agriculture, permaculture*

agroecosystems
Communities of organisms in an agricultural setting (e.g., plants, animals, fungi, bacteria), their environment (e.g., soil, water), and the interactions among them

pasture-based system
A model of food animal production in which animals are primarily raised outdoors for all or most of the year, and are free to graze or forage (even if diets are supplemented with feed, as is common with hogs and poultry)

land is used (and, concomitantly, what people eat). Livestock production uses roughly three-quarters of the world's agricultural land, making it a prime candidate for these changes (Foley et al., 2011).

The use of cropland to produce animal feed represents a net drain on the world's food supply. Only 40 percent of North American cropland is devoted to growing food for direct human consumption (Foley et al., 2011); the bulk of the remainder is devoted to feed crops. Contrary to claims that IFAP is efficient, the vast majority of calories and protein in feed crops are lost when they are converted to animal products (Smil, 2002). Beef production is particularly inefficient; per unit of meat, cattle consume on average three times as many calories from feed compared to swine and poultry.

AGROECOLOGICAL APPROACHES TO FOOD ANIMAL PRODUCTION

In contrast to IFAP, some farmers take an ecological approach to food animal production. **Agroecology**, as discussed in chapters 3 and 11, is a science and a practice; as a practice, it aims to build the strengths of natural ecosystems into agricultural ecosystems (**agroecosystems**) in ways that promote sustainable production.

Agroecological approaches to food animal production typically involve raising animals outdoors for all or most of the year, at much lower densities, in diverse systems that include various crops, and with fewer inputs (see figure 12.10). Such a model is often referred to as a **pasture-based system**.

Although agroecology represents a small fraction of food animal production in the United States, more farmers are adopting longstanding pasture-based practices and refining them, merging traditional wisdom with current science-based evidence on sustainable practices.

FIGURE 12.10   Clagett Farm Produces Grass-Fed Beef and a Variety of Organically Grown Vegetables

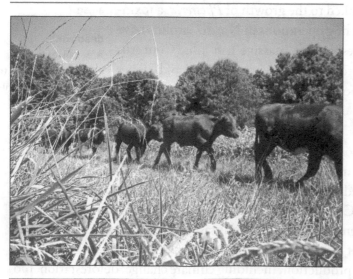

Source: CLF.

When managed properly, animals raised in pasture-based systems can confer numerous health and ecosystem benefits, in part because their manure is a form of organic matter that helps build fertile soil. In contrast to industrial operations, the manure generated by pastured animals poses fewer concerns related to air, water, and soil contamination. This is largely because manure is deposited (by the animals themselves) in smaller quantities, over a wider expanse, and generally does not exceed amounts the land can absorb. For cattle, their natural diet of grasses may reduce food safety concerns; feeding them grain alters the pH of their digestive systems in ways that foster proliferation of bacterial pathogens (Callaway, Elder, Keen, Anderson, & Nisbet, 2003). Well-managed pasture-based operations also keep animals away from waterways to further limit pollution and limit the number of animals grazing in any one area to prevent soil erosion. Regularly moving animals to new areas of pasture (**rotational grazing**) further minimizes erosion, promotes pasture growth, and spreads manure more evenly over land. Additionally, agroecology generally eschews the use of antibiotics, hormones, and other inputs that remain in animal waste; among USDA organic-certified farms, these additives are prohibited.

rotational grazing
Practice of regularly moving animals to new areas of pasture

Agroecology requires considerable knowledge, skills, and management on the part of farmers. In return, farmers gain greater autonomy over how to raise their animals, compared to IFAP operators on contract with integrators. Pasture-based farmers also generally earn greater profits per animal, in part because of lower feed costs and the fact that some consumers are willing to pay a premium for pasture-raised products (Clancy, 2006).

Animals on pasture have greater freedom to express natural behaviors and are not subject to many of the physical, social, and emotional harms associated with IFAP. In some cases, alleviating animal stress may also reduce risks to human health (see "Occupational Hazards").

POLICY AND DIETARY CHANGE

Various policy measures have been proposed to help mitigate the harms of IFAP, including strengthening restrictions on antibiotic use and waste application, improving enforcement of air- and water-quality standards, mandating greater monitoring and transparency on the part of industries, increasing the involvement of communities near existing or proposed IFAP operations, and raising animal welfare standards (Pew Commission on Industrial Farm Animal Production, 2008). Furthermore, a shift in policy incentives toward supporting ecological alternatives could lessen the predominance of IFAP. Focus 12.3 describes the Pew Commission on Industrial Farm Animal Production and its policy recommendations.

The future of food animal production will also be driven, to a large degree, by consumer choices. Because US citizens consume animal products at roughly three times the global average (Food and Agriculture Organization, 2009b)—far more than necessary, by any nutritional standard—they are uniquely positioned to effect change to industry practices by shifting toward more plant-based diets and by supporting agroecological approaches when choosing animal products. Policy measures, working in parallel with behavior change, could help make these dietary shifts more affordable.

FOCUS 12.3. THE PEW COMMISSION ON IFAP: POLICY RECOMMENDATIONS AND BARRIERS TO REFORM
Robert P. Martin

In 2005, the Pew Charitable Trusts and the Johns Hopkins Center for a Livable Future established the Pew Commission on Industrial Farm Animal Production. The commission's charge was to develop consensus recommendations to solve the problems created by IFAP operations in the areas of public health, the environment, animal welfare, and rural communities. Commissioners were asked to bring their expertise to the discussion but to check their biases at the door.

(Continued)

(Continued)

The commission comprised fourteen leaders and luminaries of their respective fields, including experts in animal health, the institutional food service industry, medicine, nutrition, production agriculture, ethics, state and federal policy, and infectious disease. Over the course of two and a half years, the commissioners met with a wide range of stakeholders, including industry representatives, affected populations, farmers, consumer advocates, animal welfare advocates, federal regulators, environmental activists, and diverse academics. The commission also visited industrial swine, dairy, cattle, egg, and broiler chicken production facilities. The industrial agriculture sector in the United States is not monolithic; their reaction to the commission's inquiry ranged from open hostility to wary cooperation.

The commissioners deliberated for more than 250 hours, reviewing eight technical reports drafted for their study and more than 170 peer-reviewed reports on relevant topics. Their final report, *Putting Meat on the Table: Industrial Farm Animal Production in America* (Pew Commission on Industrial Farm Animal Production, 2008) was released in April 2008. Commissioners found the industrial system was not sustainable. It represented an unacceptable level of threat to public health, an unacceptable level of damage to the environment, was harmful to the animals confined in the most restrictive confinement operations, and was detrimental to the economy of communities where they are located.

Specifically, the commission developed twenty-four consensus recommendations to deal with the problems found in the four major study areas. Twelve of those recommendations addressed public health problems and five of those twelve concerned the routine use of antibiotics in the industrial system to compensate for overcrowding, lack of natural movement, and poor waste handling.

The top five recommendations were as follows:

nontherapeutic antibiotic use
Antibiotic use in the absence of clinical disease, as diagnosed by a licensed veterinarian (e.g., for growth promotion or disease prevention)

- Phase out and ban **nontherapeutic antibiotic use** in food animal production, ban new approvals of nontherapeutic use of antimicrobials for food animals, and retroactively investigate previously approved antimicrobials

- Require permitting of a larger number of operations

- Phase out and ban liquid waste management systems

- Ban gestation crates in swine production, battery cages in egg production, and restrictive veal crates

- Aggressively enforce all existing antitrust laws

The original Pew Commission report release was a landmark event because the report cataloged the primary problems caused by industrial food animal production for the first time in one publication. It generated new interest among nongovernmental organizations and policy makers at the local, state, and federal levels to solve the important problems outlined.

Since the release of the report, several organizations have undertaken efforts to implement the commission's recommendations, but many problems persist. A five-year follow-up report released in 2013 by the Center for a Livable Future (CLF, 2013) determined that state and federal policy makers had failed to address the problems outlined in the Pew Commission report and had, in some cases, acted regressively on this reform agenda. Further, it found that although the original Pew Commission report was welcomed by reform advocates, the industrial animal sector and pharmaceutical industry had opposed change, thus stalling reform efforts.

SUMMARY

In the context of the more than eight thousand years since most farm animals were first domesticated, the industrialization of food animal production represents a rapid, widespread, and unprecedented shift in the scale and practices used in raising animals for food. The resulting model is characterized by specialized, densely stocked operations that rely heavily on a declining pool of synthetic and natural resources, and harbor animal waste in enormous quantities. A small number of transnational corporations control a majority of the production and marketing of animal products, and they dictate many of the production practices that were once under the stewardship of farmers and communities. The IFAP model is enabled and supported by weak environmental regulations and by economic incentives that have been codified into federal and state legislation.

The public health, social, occupational, environmental, and animal welfare challenges that stem from IFAP are complex and widespread. Many of these stem from the inputs involved in production, waste management practices, and the scale of operations. Mitigating these harms may involve shifting to more ecological approaches to food animal production, enacting policy change, and changing diets.

KEY TERMS

Agroecology	Manure
Agroecosystems	Market concentration
Algal blooms	Mechanization
Animal waste	Natural capital
Aquaculture	Nitrates
Arsenical drugs	Nontherapeutic antibiotic use
Best management practices (BMPs)	Open ocean aquaculture
Colonized	Pasture-based system
Concentrated animal feeding operation (CAFO)	Pathogens
Consolidation	Real consumer prices
Dead zone	Recirculating aquaculture systems
Endotoxin	Rotational grazing
Feedlots	Runoff
Growers	Sustainable harvest levels
Horizontal integration	Vertical integration
Industrial food animal production (IFAP)	Viral reassortment
Inputs	Wild-capture fishery
Integrators	Wild-caught seafood
Lagoons	

DISCUSSION QUESTIONS

1. How do the strengths and limitations of IFAP compare to those of agroecological approaches?

2. What are the most influential drivers of the scale and practices associated with IFAP?

3. What policies or interventions might be effective in addressing the harms associated with IFAP? Which problems should be prioritized, and why? Who are the stakeholders who should be involved? What barriers might need to be overcome?

4. How realistic is it to expect that Americans will change their appetites for animal products? Are there similar examples in which entrenched cultural behaviors and attitudes changed? How were those changes brought about?

5. What will the production, processing, retailing, and consumption of animal products look like in twenty years? In one hundred years? Why? Ideally, how should these practices evolve?

6. Perspective 12.1 states that "raising the standards for animal welfare ... would address most of the negative human health consequences of industrial farm animal production." How would one lead to the other?

7. Why are animal products from more sustainable operations generally more expensive than products from the prevailing industrial system? Should they necessarily cost more?

ACKNOWLEDGMENTS

The authors thank Shawn McKenzie and Dr. Christopher Heaney for comments and suggestions, and Claire Fitch and Ginny Weinmann for research assistance.

REFERENCES

Aarestrup, F. M., Vibeke, J. F., Emborg, H.-D., Jacobsen, E., & Wegener, H. (2010). Changes in the use of antimicrobials and the effects on productivity of swine farms in Denmark. *American Journal of Veterinary Research*, 71(7).

Black, K. D. (2008). Environmental aspects of aquaculture. In K. Culver & D. Castle (Eds.), *Aquaculture, innovation and social transformation* (pp. 97–113). Dordrecht, The Netherlands: Springer.

Burkholder, J., Libra, B., Weyer, P., Heathcote, S., Kolpin, D., Thorne, P. S., & Wichman, M. (2007). Impacts of waste from concentrated animal feeding operations on water quality. *Environmental Health Perspectives*, 115(2), 308–312.

California Breast Cancer Research Program. (2007). *Identifying gaps in breast cancer research*. Retrieved from www.cbcrp.org/sri/reports/identifyinggaps/gaps_full.pdf

Callaway, T. R., Elder, R. O., Keen, J. E., Anderson, R. C., & Nisbet, D. J. (2003). Forage feeding to reduce preharvest *Escherichia coli* populations in cattle, a review. *Journal of Dairy Science*, 86(3), 852–860.

Casey, J. A., Curriero, F. C., Cosgrove, S. E., Nachman, K. E., & Schwartz, B. S. (2013). High-density livestock operations, crop field application of manure, and risk of community-associated methicillin-resistant *Staphylococcus aureus* infection in Pennsylvania. *JAMA Internal Medicine 21205*(21), 1980–1990.

Center for a Livable Future. (2013). *Industrial food animal production in America: Examining the impact of the Pew Commission's priority recommendations*. Retrieved from www.ncifap.org

Chan, M. (2011). *Combat drug resistance: No action today means no cure tomorrow*. World Health Organization. Retrieved from www.who.int/mediacentre/news/statements/2011/whd_20110407/en/index.html

Clancy, K. (2006). *Greener eggs and ham: The benefits of pasture-raised swine, poultry, and egg production*. Cambridge, MA: Union of Concerned Scientists.

Committee on Drug Use in Food Animals, Panel on Animal Health, Food Safety, and Public Health, N.R.C. (1999). *The use of drugs in food animals: Benefits and risks*. Washington, DC: National Academies Press.

Donham, K., Knapp, L., Monson, R., & Gustafson, K. (1982). Acute toxic exposure to gases from liquid manure. *Journal of Occupational Medicine*, 24(2), 142–145.

Donham, K., Wing, S., Osterberg, D., Flora, J. L., Hodne, C., Thu, K. M., & Thorne, P. S. (2007). Community health and socioeconomic issues surrounding concentrated animal feeding operations. *Environmental Health Perspectives*, 115(2), 317–320.

Elitzak, H. (1999). *Food cost review, 1950–97*. Agricultural Economic Report No. 780. Washington, DC: US Department of Agriculture Economic Research Service.

Foley, J. A., Ramankutty, N., Brauman, K. A., Cassidy, E. S., Gerber, J. S., Johnston, M., ... Zaks, D.P.M. (2011). Solutions for a cultivated planet. *Nature.*

Food and Agriculture Organization. (2009a). *Global agriculture towards 2050.* Rome: Author.

Food and Agriculture Organization. (2009b). *The state of food and agriculture: Livestock in the Balance.* Rome: Author.

Food and Agriculture Organization. (2012). *State of the world fisheries and aquaculture.* Rome: Author. Retrieved from www.fao.org/docrep/016/i2727e/i2727e.pdf

Food and Agriculture Organization. (2013). *FAOSTAT.* Retrieved from http://faostat3.fao.org

Government Accountability Office. (2011). *Antibiotic resistance: Agencies have made limited progress addressing antibiotic use in animals.* Washington, DC: Author.

Graham, J. P., Boland, J. J., & Silbergeld, E. (2007). Growth promoting antibiotics in food animal production: An economic analysis. *Public Health Reports 122*(1), 79–87.

Graham, J. P., & Nachman, K. E. (2010). Managing waste from confined animal feeding operations in the United States: The need for sanitary reform. *Journal of Water and Health* December, 646–670.

Gustafson, R. H., & Bowen, R. E. (1997). Antibiotic use in animal agriculture. *Journal of Applied Microbiology, 83*(5), 531–541.

Heederik, D., Sigsgaard, T., Thorne, P. S., Kline, J. N., Avery, R., Bønløkke, J. H., ... Merchant, J. A. (2007). Health effects of airborne exposures from concentrated animal feeding operations. *Environmental Health Perspectives, 115*(2), 298–302.

Herath, D., Weersink, A., & Carpentier, C. L. (2012). Spatial dynamics of the livestock sector in the United States: Do environmental regulations matter? *Journal of Agricultural and Resource Economics, 30*(1), 45–68.

Human Rights Watch. (2004). *Blood, sweat, and fear: Workers rights in U.S. meat and poultry plants.* New York: Author.

James, H. S., Hendrickson, M. K., & Howard, P. H. (2013). Networks, power, and dependency in the agrifood industry. In H. James (Ed.), *The ethics and economics of agrifood competition* (pp. 99–126). Dordrecht: Springer Science-Business Media Press.

Johnson, R., & Hanrahan, C. E. (2010). *The U.S.-EU beef hormone dispute.* CRS Report R40449. Washington, DC: Congressional Research Service.

Love, D. C., Halden, R. U., Davis, M. F., & Nachman, K. E. (2012). Feather meal: A previously unrecognized route for reentry into the food supply of multiple pharmaceuticals and personal care products (PPCPs). *Environmental Science & Technology 46*(7), 3795–3802.

Ma, W., Lager, K. M., Vincent, A. L., Janke, B. H., Gramer, M. R., & Richt, J. A. (2009). The role of swine in the generation of novel influenza viruses. *Zoonoses and Public Health 56*(6–7), 326–337.

Mallin, M. A., & Cahoon, L. B. (2003). Industrialized animal production—a major source of nutrient and microbial pollution to aquatic ecosystems. *Population and Environment, 24*(5), 369–385.

Martinez, S. W. (1999). *Vertical coordination in the pork and broiler industries: Implications for pork and chicken products* (Agricultural Economic Report No. AER-777). Washington, DC: US Department of Agriculture.

Meyers, R. A., & Worm, B. (2003). Rapid worldwide depletion of predatory fish communities. *Nature 423* 280–283.

Mulders, M. N., Haenen, A. P., Geenen, P. L., Vesseur, P. C., Poldervaart, E. S., Bosch, T., ... Van De Giessen, A. W. (2010). Prevalence of livestock-associated MRSA in broiler flocks and risk factors for slaughterhouse personnel in The Netherlands. *Epidemiology and Infection, 138*(5), 743–755.

Myers, K. P., Olsen, C. W., & Gray, G. C. (2007). Cases of swine influenza in humans: A review of the literature. *Clinical Infectious Diseases: An Official Publication of the Infectious Diseases Society of America, 44*(8), 1084–1088.

Nachman, K. E., Baron, P. A, Raber, G., Francesconi, K. A, Navas-Acien, A., & Love, D. C. (2013). Roxarsone, inorganic arsenic, and other arsenic species in chicken: A U.S.-based market basket sample. *Environmental Health Perspectives*, *121*(7), 818–824.

National Fisheries Institute. (2011). *Top 10 consumed seafoods*. Retrieved from www.aboutseafood.com/about/about-seafood/top-10-consumed-seafoods

Naylor, R., & Burke, M. (2005). Aquaculture and ocean resources: Raising tigers of the sea. *Annual Review of Environment and Resources*, *30* 185–218.

Notter, D. R. (1999). The importance of genetic diversity in livestock populations of the future. *Journal of Animal Science*, *77*, 61–69.

Pauly, D., Christensen, V., Guénette, S., Pitcher, T. J., Sumaila, U. R., Walters, C. J., Watson, R., & Zeller, D. (2002). Towards sustainability in world fisheries. *Nature 418*, 689–695.

Pew Commission on Industrial Farm Animal Production. (2008). *Putting meat on the table: Industrial farm animal production in America*. Baltimore: The Pew Charitable Trusts and the Johns Hopkins Bloomberg School of Public Health.

Rauw, W. M., Kanis, E., Noordhuizen-Stassen, E. N., & Grommers, F. J. (1998). Undesirable side effects of selection for high production efficiency in farm animals: A review. *Livestock Production Science*, *56*(1), 15–33.

Roberts, R. R., Hota, B., Ahmad, I., Scott, R. D., Foster, S. D., Abbasi, F., ... Weinstein, R. A. (2009). Hospital and societal costs of antimicrobial-resistant infections in a Chicago teaching hospital: Implications for antibiotic stewardship. *Clinical Infectious Diseases: An Official Publication of the Infectious Diseases Society of America*, *49*(8), 1175–1184.

Rostagno, M. H. (2009). Can stress in farm animals increase food safety risk? *Foodborne pathogens and disease*, *6*(7), 767–76.

Sapkota, A. R., Lefferts, L. Y., McKenzie, S., & Walker, P. (2007). What do we feed to food-production animals? A review of animal feed ingredients and their potential impacts on human health. *Environmental Health Perspectives*, *115*(5), 663–670.

Skov, R. L., & Jensen, K. S. (2009). Community-associated meticillin-resistant *Staphylococcus aureus* as a cause of hospital-acquired infections. *The Journal of Hospital Infection*, *73*(4), 364–70.

Smil, V. (2002). Worldwide transformation of diets, burdens of meat production and opportunities for novel food proteins. *Enzyme and Microbial Technology*, *30*(3), 305–311.

Solomon, E., Yaron, S., & Matthews, K. (2002). Transmission of *Escherichia coli* 0157:H7 from contaminated manure and irrigation water to lettuce plant tissue and its subsequent internalization. *Applied and Environmental Microbiology*, *68*(1), 397–400.

Starmer, E., & Wise, T. A. (2007). *Feeding at the trough: Industrial livestock firms saved $35 billion from low feed prices* (GDAE Policy Brief No. 07–03). Medford, MA: Tufts University.

Striffler, S. (2005). *Chicken: The dangerous transformation of America's favorite food*. New Haven, CT: Yale University Press.

Stull, C. L., Payne, M. A., Berry, S. L., & Hullinger, P. J. (2002). Evaluation of the scientific justification for tail docking in dairy cattle. *Journal of the American Veterinary Medical Association 220*(9), 1298–1303.

Tacon, A.G.J., & Metian, M. (2008). Aquaculture feed and food safety: The role of the food and agriculture organization and the Codex Alimentarius. *Annals of the New York Academy of Sciences 1140*, 50–59.

US Department of Agriculture Agricultural Economic Research Service. (2005). *National program 206: Manure and byproduct utilization*. Washington, DC: Author.

US Department of Agriculture Economic Research Service. (1972). *Farm-retail spreads for food products*. Washington, DC: Author.

US Department of Agriculture Economic Research Service. (2006). *Profits, costs, and the changing structure of dairy farming*. Washington, DC: Author.

US Department of Agriculture Economic Research Service. (2012). *Cattle: Background*. Retrieved from www.ers.usda.gov/topics/animal-products/cattle-beef/background.aspx#.UWJ-wKKJhYU

US Department of Agriculture Economic Research Service. (2013a). *Food availability (per capita) data system*. Retrieved from www.ers.usda.gov/Data/FoodConsumption/FoodAvailIndex.htm

US Department of Agriculture Economic Research Service. (2013b). *Price spreads from farm to consumer*. Retrieved from www.ers.usda.gov/data-products/price-spreads-from-farm-to-consumer.aspx#.UtAJ5NJWrTp

US Department of Agriculture National Agricultural Statistics Service. The Census of Agriculture.

US Department of Agriculture National Agriculture Statistics Service. (2012). *Milk: Production per cow by year, US*. Retrieved from www.nass.usda.gov/Charts_and_Maps/Milk_Production_and_Milk_Cows/cowrates.asp

US Environmental Protection Agency. (2012): *Relation between nitrate in water wells and potential sources in the lower Yakima Valley, Washington* (EPA-910-R-12–003). Washington, DC: Author.

US Food and Drug Administration. (2010). *Letter to the Honorable Louise M. Slaughter: Sales of antibacterial drugs in kilograms*. Washington, DC: Author.

Van Dolah, F. M. (2000). Marine algal toxins: Origins, health effects, and their increased occurrence. *Environmental Health Perspectives, 108*(Suppl. 1), 133.

Washington State Department of Ecology. (2009). *Lower Yakima Valley groundwater report—preliminary assessment and recommendations document* (#10–10–009). Retrieved from https://fortress.wa.gov/ecy/publications/publications/1010009.pdf

Weber, C. L., & Matthews, H. S. (2008). Food-miles and the relative climate impacts of food choices in the United States. *Environmental Science and Technology, 42*(10), 3508–3513.

Weida, W. J. (2004). Considering the rationales for factory farming. In *Environmental health impacts of CAFOs: Anticipating hazards—searching for solutions* (pp. 1–45). Iowa City, IA. Retrieved from www.worc.org/userfiles/file/Weida-economicsofCAFOs.pdf

Williams, D. L., Breysse, P. N., McCormack, M. C., Diette, G. B., McKenzie, S., & Geyh, A. S. (2011). Airborne cow allergen, ammonia and particulate matter at homes vary with distance to industrial scale dairy operations: An exposure assessment. *Environmental Health, 10*(1), 72.

Wilson, S. M., Howell, F., Wing, S., & Sobsey, M. (2002). Environmental injustice and the Mississippi hog industry. *Environmental Health Perspectives*, April (110 Suppl.), 195–201.

Wing, S., Horton, R. A., & Rose, K. M. (2013). Air pollution from industrial swine operations and blood pressure of neighboring residents. *Environmental Health Perspectives, 121*(1), 92–166.

Wise, T. A., & Trist, S. E. (2010). *Buyer power in U.S. hog markets: A critical review of the literature*. Medford, MA: Tufts University.

Worm, B., et al. (2009). Rebuilding global fisheries. *Science 325*(5940), 578–585.

Woteki, C. E., & Kineman, B. D. (2003). Challenges and approaches to reducing foodborne illness. *Annual Review of Nutrition, 23*, 315–344.

Yakima County. (2013). *About Yakima County*. Retrieved from www.yakimacounty.us/about.asp

Yakima Regional Air Quality Agency. (2012, March 8). Air quality management and best management practices for dairy operations. Prepared by Gary Pruitt. Yakima Valley, WA: Yakima Regional Clean Air Agency.

Zimdahl, R. R. (2012). *Agriculture's ethical horizon* (2nd ed.). Waltham, MA: Elsevier.

Chapter 13

Food Processing and Packaging

George A. Cavender

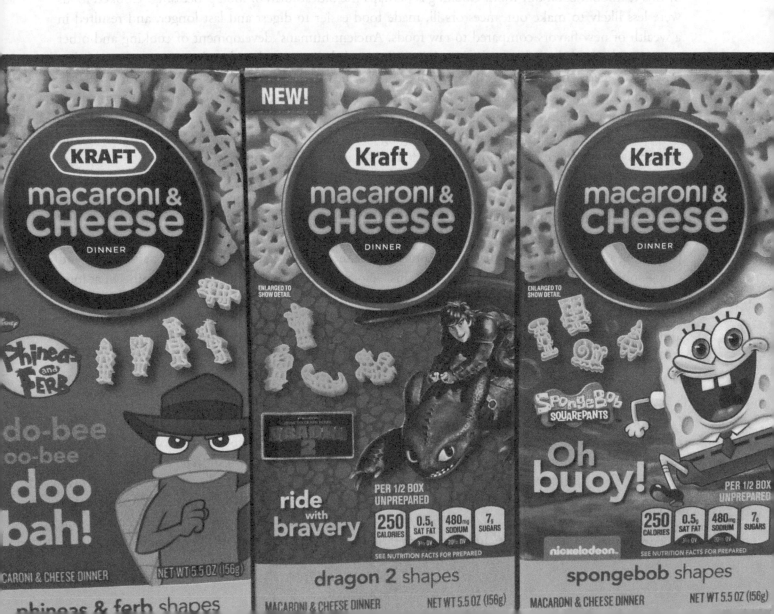

Learning Objectives

- Understand the reasons why foods are processed and how processing can change foods, both positively and negatively.

- Identify the four major methods of processing foods.

- Understand the functions of food packages, materials used, and how packages can affect the food inside.

- Appreciate the complex ways in which the food industry interacts with the environment and consider ways this interaction can be improved.

- Discuss historical, social, cultural, and economic factors contributing to how foods are processed.

It all started with fire. Fire is often heralded as one of humankind's greatest discoveries. It enabled us to fend off predators, make improved tools, live in inhospitable places, and most important, in context of this textbook, cook our food. Cooking is perhaps the oldest form of food processing. Cooked foods were less likely to make our ancestors ill, made food easier to digest and last longer, and resulted in a wealth of new flavors compared to raw foods. Ancient humans' development of cooking and other processes changed their diets, which in turn influenced their descendants' evolution: jaws become less developed, teeth changed, and the appendix became the vestigial organ that it is today (Emes, Aybar, & Yalcin, 2011). Food also became more portable and longer lasting, and with those changes came the need for packaging to contain and protect the food. As civilization has advanced through history, many methods of food processing and packaging have been developed to address emerging needs and concerns—with success and some unintended health and ecologic impacts.

Today, most foods have been processed in some fashion and nearly all are distributed using some form of packaging. Concerns are common regarding the nutritional impacts of food processing and the environmental impacts of food packaging. But processing and packaging can have benefits as well, including for food safety, food security, and the feasibility of distributing food. To many people, food processing and packaging are "black box" topics, with the actual mechanisms behind what is done—and why—obscured behind the factory door. In this chapter we aim to open the box, to examine what food processing and packaging are, why and how they are performed, and how they affect the foods we eat. We will also describe how processing and packaging affect public health and the environment. Focus and perspectives boxes provide critical approaches to complement this descriptive overview.

FOOD PROCESSING

Food processing can be defined in multiple ways. Put simply: *food processing is everything that happens to a food between the farm and fork.* Advocates of whole or natural foods might well offer a more negative definition, such as, *food processing is a catchall term for the various ways food is modified to make it more profitable, typically at the expense of the consumer's health, the product's quality, or both.* A more neutral definition, however, is, *the application of* **unit operations** *(e.g., steps within processes) to effect desired changes in food.* Note that this definition includes unit operations performed by the consumer, such as chopping

unit operations
Steps within processes; used to describe the tasks involved in food processing

and cooking. In this chapter, however, we limit ourselves primarily to commercial food processing—processes performed prior to consumer contact. We will discuss physical methods such as cutting, homogenization, or shaping; thermal methods such as blanching and pasteurization; temperature-lowering methods such as freezing; and formulation methods such as adding flavors, colors, or nutrients. The next section provides a general overview of food processing, focusing on two principal questions: why are foods processed and what methods are used?

In general, processing is used to improve one or more properties of the food, with the underlying reasons falling into one (or more) of four categories: safety, quality, value, and convenience.

Safety

One of the most important reasons for processing food is to prevent illness or even death. Food safety hazards can be chemical—for example, pesticide residues, **adulterants** such as melamine, and even **naturally-occurring compounds** such as those found in unprocessed cassava root (see figure 13.1). Hazards can also be physical in nature, presenting a choking hazard or a risk of dental trauma because of the food's size, shape, or texture. Finally, hazards can be biological. Biological hazards likely receive the most press in the United States, and rightly so; according to the US Centers for Disease Control and Prevention (CDC), approximately forty-eight million people in the United States become ill due to microorganisms in their food annually, and three thousand will die from those illnesses (CDC, 2012). Organisms such as *Clostridium botulinum* (which causes botulism), *E. coli* O157:H7, *Salmonella,* and *Listeria monocytogenes* pose significant food safety threats. Although sound food production and processing methods can help prevent contamination, once a food item is contaminated, processing and handling can be used to control these organisms.

adulterants
Compounds that contaminate food

naturally-occurring compounds
Chemical compounds that occur naturally in plants (in contrast to those that are manufactured)

FIGURE 13.1 Cassava Tuber

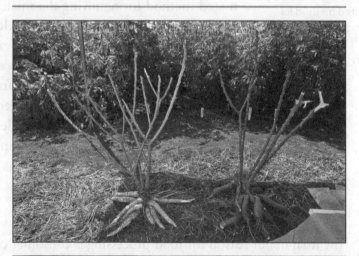

Although cassava is an important foodstuff for much of the developing world, the starchy tubers naturally contain cyanogenic (cyanide-producing) compounds, which can lead to the development of goiter, neurological problems, or even death. Proper processing eliminates these compounds.
Source: José Cruz—ABr, Wikimedia Commons. http://commons.wikimedia .org/wiki/File:Embrapa_news_sp_of_cassava_%28Jos%C3%A9_Cruz_ABr% 29_25jan2008.jpg

Quality

Loss of quality can transform a safe and desirable food into something that almost no one would be willing to eat. Whether due to minor changes in appearance, texture, and flavor or to full-on spoilage, the end result is wasted food and economic losses to consumers and producers. Cultural factors also play into our openness to eating imperfect products. **Shelf life** refers to the length of time a food takes to become undesirable; extending shelf life is one of the major reasons why food is processed. There are multiple mechanisms by which shelf life can be shortened. Foremost in the minds of most consumers is microbial spoilage. We have all encountered moldy bread, sour

shelf life
The length of time a food takes to become undesirable

milk, and meat that just smells "off." Unless controlled by processing, the organisms responsible for this kind of spoilage, which are typically different from those that lead to illness, can multiply rapidly and render a product unappealing to consumers. Of course, even without the action of microorganisms, foods can degrade to the point they are undesirable. Fruits brown, oils go rancid, and meats lose their red color all without the aid of yeast and bacteria. These types of changes are chemical in nature, and controlling or preventing them requires rapid consumption or careful processing. Change to the moisture content of food rounds out the list of important degradation mechanisms. Although changes in the total amount of water in a food can result in quality losses, such as soggy crackers or wilted greens, a more important property is **water activity**, which measures the amount of water in the food that is available to participate in chemical reactions and microbial growth, and it also influences the texture of the food. With proper packaging, storage, and other unit operations, however, changes in moisture content and water activity can be minimized and their impact on shelf life lessened.

water activity
Measure of the amount of water in a food available to participate in chemical reactions and microbial growth; influences food texture

Increasing Value

Processing can also increase the usefulness and yield of a food, extracting extra value from a given product. Processing to add value ranges from fairly simple operations such as pregelatinizing starch so that it can be used in instant pudding and gravy mixes, thereby simplifying preparation for the consumer, to complex physical techniques such as **advanced meat recovery** (an automated method for removing the small pieces of meat left behind during deboning), which enables meat processors to produce more product at a lower price than before. Other ways processors seek to add value include enhancing flavors or colors and adding vitamins. Although these processes can greatly affect convenience and price, many of them worry consumers focused on nutrition and safety and can lead to heated public debate (e.g., the 2012 controversy over the use of finely textured lean beef trimmings in ground beef in order to reduce product cost and fat content, or as it was called in the media, the "pink slime" controversy) (Greene, 2012). The controversy also highlights the complex challenge of understanding when a line has been crossed—when "beef" is no longer "beef"—as described in figure 13.2.

advanced meat recovery
Automated method for removing small pieces of meat left behind during deboning

Convenience

The final major reason for food processing is consumer convenience. Food processing enables the consumer to enjoy a food without having to undergo sometimes-laborious preparation. One does not need to thresh and grind wheat or pasteurize and churn cream in order to bake a cake, because processing has given us packaged flour, butter, and cake mixes. If a person desired, they could even forgo the actual baking, instead purchasing a packaged or frozen cake. Even foods that we usually do not think of as having been processed, such as shell eggs, have often been subjected to several unit operations, such as washing, grading for quality, and sorting (in addition to consumer convenience, these processes aid in marketing and food safety).

Food processing and food technology are often used for the best of reasons, as previously described; and they are also often used in ways consumers would be less happy to understand. Perspective 13.1 explores positive reasons for processing, while perspective 13.2 shares information about industry optimization of flavors to create products that are challenging to resist.

FIGURE 13.2 When is Beef not Beef?

When is Beef not Beef?

In 2012 the US became aware of a "lean finely textured beef" (or as the media dubbed it- "Pink Slime") and its use in ground beef. During the ensuing media storm, many accusations were made against the food industry, and great amounts of misinformation were spread about, particularly on the internet. Opponents of the product claimed that it was a disgusting, Frankensteinian product made from unwholesome ingredients and unfit for human consumption. Proponents countered that it was simply beef which had been treated to make it more safe for consumption. The final outcome of the controversy is still unclear, with the largest manufacturer bringing suit against the media in order to recover massive damages. What is clear, however, is that there is no clear common definition of "beef". Take a look at the list below and ask yourself where you would draw the line and why.

Dressed Carcass: The body of an animal after slaughter, draining of blood, removal of skin and other unwanted parts (head, hooves, feet, etc)

Side: One half of a dressed carcass that has been sawn in half along the spine. Typically done in the case of large animals like cattle and pigs.

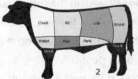

Primal Cuts: The name given to the major portions of a dressed carcass, typically removed from a dressed carcass or side by sawing or cutting. The name and specific location tend to vary by country, due to historical and cultural differences.

2

Sub-primal Cuts: In the case of large primals (e.g the Round primal in the US system), smaller cuts are sometimes made to make handling and processing easier.

Retail Cuts: Smaller cuts of meat taken from either the primal or sub-primal cuts, and intended for sale to and preparation by consumers. Common terms include roasts, steaks, chops and racks (of ribs)

3

Ground Beef: Beef which has been cut into tiny pieces by means of a grinder. In the US this beef must come from primal cuts or trimmings, and may be no more than 30% fat. While ground beef can be made from any primal cut, if the beef is labeled using the name of a specific primal, it may only contain meat/fat from that cut (e.g ground chuck must be made only from the chuck primal).

Trimmings: Small pieces of meat remaining after the processing of primal/ sub-primal cuts into retail cuts.

Lean Finely Textured Beef: Beef trimmings which have been finely chopped and subjected to a specialized process to reduce their fat content and control potentially dangerous bacteria.

4

5

Mechanically Separated Meat: An edible meat product created by a specialized machine that uses high pressure to remove the attached edible meat from bones. The actual product has a paste-like consistency and must be labeled according to the species from which the meat comes (e.g beef, pork, chicken)
Note: In the US, Mechanically Separated Beef is not allowed in any food product due to concerns over Variant Creutzfeldt-Jakob disease (Mad Cow disease).

Image IDs and credits:
1. Sides of Beef (USDA), 2 US Primal Cuts (Wikimedia), 3 Steaks (USDA), 4. Beef Trimmings (Beef Products, Inc.),
5. Frozen Lean Finely Textured Beef (Beef Products, Inc.)

Source: G. Cavender

Perspective 13.1. Food Technology: Equal Partner for a Healthy Future

Fergus M. Clydesdale

To improve their lives, consumers worldwide grasp at new technologies like a drowning person to a raft. In the United States and the developed world, we routinely work on PCs or Macs, listen to our MP3 players, and search out "apps" on our handheld devices. When going out to dinner, we use a GPS system to find the restaurant. And in developing countries, many of these technologies also are used; all are envied and sought after.

(Continued)

(Continued)

Now consider the extraordinary case of food technology. President Obama's wife, Michelle, tends a White House vegetable garden, which is a wonderful activity to show people where food comes from. But she contends that doing so enables us to avoid processed foods. In effect, she is telling us to avoid food technology.

Food technology is not a pejorative term. Why is it that consumers and many health professionals in the developed world treat it that way and all other technologies are viewed as a boon to humankind? Imagine the uproar if we insisted on the use of manual typewriters, overheads, 2 × 2 slides, chalkboards, and 78 rpm records.

There is a yearning for the world that author Michael Pollan so eloquently describes in his books *The Omnivore's Dilemma* and *In Defense of Food*. Please understand that no one is going to argue the nutritional virtues of fruits and vegetables picked in your own backyard, rushed to the kitchen, and eaten. However, most consumers don't have a garden or year-round growing climate and must depend on the supermarket.

Fresh produce takes about twenty-one days to travel from the field to the supermarket (one shudders at the carbon footprint) but only hours to get from the field to the processing plant for freezing or canning. As a result, the processed products are often superior in nutrition and flavor to what we call fresh in the supermarket.

It is an often overlooked fact that the food industry produces the food we eat. This leaves us with the inescapable conclusion, though a revelation to many, that in order to change the food supply, we must work with the food industry to produce the most nutritious and best-tasting, healthy foods possible.

FIGURE 13.3   Honey: Nature's Food Processing

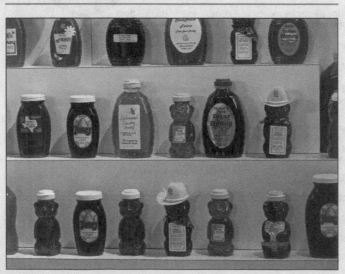

Source: Andreas Praefcke, Wikimedia Commons.

Technology at its best is an optimization of what we do in the kitchen and in nature. Consider the process for making honey (see figure 13.3). The bee ingests nectar, adds invertase (a nonnutritive food additive) in its gut, and then regurgitates the resultant mixture in the hive. Other bees ingest and further refine it in their guts prior to regurgitating the final product into the honeycomb. There is nothing wrong with honey, although it is recommended that toddlers not eat it as it may contain spores of *Clostridium botulinum,* a deadly pathogen. But modern technologies would never use such a process, nor be allowed to by regulatory agencies, for many reasons including food safety.

A lack of understanding of food technology and its many contributions is even evident in the Dietary Guidelines Advisory Committee, which I was privileged to serve on in 2005. There is generally only one food scientist selected for the committee who is thought of mainly as a contributor to food safety. This is shortsighted at best. The committee should have more food scientists and undergo a structural change involving a different charge from Congress. Because the guidelines aren't followed by most people, the committee could be charged to recommend more appealing foods and diets achieved, in part, by using technology. We must emphasize nutrition, sensory quality, food safety, convenience, acceptance, and cost, whether food is whole from nature or processed and formulated.

How can technology achieve this? Safety, flavor and taste, convenience, and cost may be self-evident. However, nutrition may not be as obvious. Technology could increase nutrient density through breeding and fortification, create fats with the proper functional qualities and nutritional profiles, use the proper balance of macronutrients, decrease caloric density, create fresh foods in new forms, and use food as a vehicle to carry physiologically significant bioactives in a stable and bioavailable form. And, finally, through research at the genetic, molecular, and technological levels, we may be able to bring personalized nutrition to consumers in the future.

Why limit the bounties of technology only in the area of food? After all, in Massachusetts a hundred years ago, there was not much else but salt cod and beans to eat in winter. We have certainly improved our diet by using technology.

The earth is adding 146 persons every minute and we owe these new global citizens the benefits of technology to provide enough food. Instead of deriding technology, let's take advantage of it so that we can have a modern food supply for a modern world that includes fresh and processed healthy foods at a price that people can afford and in a form that's appealing, convenient, and safe.

Perspective 13.2. Ten Food Secrets You Need to Know
Michael Moss

10. The inventors of processed food refer to their work as "engineering" because it involves an incredible amount of laboratory time and high math. When Howard Moskowitz, a legend in the industry, recently engineered a new soda flavor for Dr. Pepper, he tested out sixty-one formulations of the sweet flavoring, each only slightly different from the next, and put these through 3,904 consumer tastings, then applied regression analysis to find the perfect formula guaranteed to be make the soda a hit.

9. Every one of our ten thousand taste buds is wired for sweet taste, but even we can get too much sugar in our food. So what Moskowitz and other food scientists seek out is called the "bliss point," which is the perfect amount of sweetness, not too little, not too much. With sugar being added to more and more items in the grocery store, there are now calculated bliss points for pasta sauce, bread, frozen pizza, and on and on.

8. In many ways, fat is even more powerful than sugar as an additive to processed foods. It has twice the calories as sugar, but it will sneak up on the brain when you don't realize you are eating a fatty food. Even more problematic for consumers, the kind of fat that is bad for you, known as saturated fat, is typically solid and really fools the brain. Scientists refer to it as the "invisible fat" because it slips into your diet and body unseen. But boy does it add to the allure. The attraction of fat is known to food companies as "mouthfeel," like the warm gooey sensation of melted cheese.

7. Salt is valued for what companies call its "flavor burst," hitting the tongue straight away with a salty taste that races to the pleasure zone of the brain, which in turn compels you to eat more. And salt manufacturers have learned to manipulate the physical shape of salt to most perfectly suit the needs of processed foods, from powdery salts for soups to chunks shaped like pyramids with flat sides that stick to the outside of food and interact quickest with your saliva.

6. Beyond salt, sugar, and fat, the snack food companies have perfected other aspects of their snacks to maximize their allure and irresistibility. Take chips. Research shows that noisier chips taste better, so every effort is made to increase the crunch. The industry also refers warmly to the phenomenon known as "vanishing caloric density," epitomized by Cheetos. When they melt in your mouth, they fool the brain into thinking

(Continued)

(Continued)

the calories have disappeared, as if you were eating celery. No calories, no reason for the brain to tell you to stop eating already.

5. There is a growing consensus among nutritionists that as far as calories and weight gain go, sugar is sugar is sugar, no matter if it is derived from beets or cane (table sugar), from corn (high fructose corn syrup), or from the latest craze in processed food sweeteners: fruit concentrate. This term applies to fruits—mostly grapes and pears because they are least expensive—that are condensed and processed, in some cases stripped of everything but the sugar molecules. Beware of foods that tout "made with real fruit" on the front, not to be confused with fresh fruits, which have the fiber and bulk that is so highly valued by nutritionists.

4. Beware of other touts on the front of packages, such as "low fat" or "all natural." They can easily fool you into overlooking the other reality. As the small print in the nutrition facts box often shows, a low-fat yogurt can have as much sugar as ice cream, and all natural products can be fully loaded in sugar, fat, and salt.

3. The largest single source of saturated fat in our diet now is cheese, and this is by no accident. When we started drinking low-fat and skim milk in the 1960s to reduce our intake of saturated fat, the dairy industry, with help from the government, started slipping that fat back into our diets in the form of cheese. Cheese was turned into an additive—stuffed into pizza crusts, added to peanut butter crackers, and reformed as cubed, stringed, diced, grated, and tubbed for easier cooking at home. In all, this helped triple our average consumption of cheese to as much as thirty-three pounds a year.

2. The food giants are more hooked on sugar, fat, and especially salt than we are. We're not even born liking salt. We develop a taste for it at six months, and recent studies suggest that diets high in processed foods will have kids licking the salt shaker by preschool. But you can get off salt merely by avoiding processed foods for six weeks or so, and then everything in the store will taste way too salty. Not so, the food giants. They need lots of salt to preserve their products so they can sit on the shelf for weeks at a time. They need salt to avoid using more costly ingredients such as fresh herbs and spices. And they need salt to cover up bad flavors inherent to food processing, such as the one known as warmed-over flavor caused by the oxidation of fat in meat.

1. This bodes ill for the latest vows of food companies to cut back on their loads of salt, sugar, and fat. But there are some things you can do as a consumer to fight back. First, educate yourself. It will hopefully leave you feeling more empowered, simply by knowing all that the food companies do to lure you in and keep you coming back for more. Spend more time on the fringes of the grocery store, where the fresh fruits and vegetables are kept. And when you hit the center aisles, beware of the items at eye level. Industry research (they put devices on shoppers' heads to monitor their eye movements) shows that we look mostly toward the middle sections, at eye level, so that's where the biggest selling items—those most loaded with salt, sugar, and fat—are placed. Reach low and reach high for better health.

Source: Moss, M. (2013). Michael Moss is the author of *Salt, Sugar, Fat*. Random House, 2013.

HOW DO WE PROCESS FOODS?

The goal of food processing is to create one or more desired changes in food, and there are many unit operations that contribute to this goal; they can be broadly classified as physical methods, thermal methods, temperature-lowering methods, and formulation. By understanding these we can better address potential unwanted side effects.

TABLE 13.1 Selected Physical Unit Operations

Process	Description	Purpose	Product Examples
Grinding	Particles of food are chopped, smashed, or crushed.	Creation of a uniform or reduced particle size	Coffee, flour, hamburger
Forming	Pressure is used to force a product into a mold or die.	Development of a desirable shape prior to further processing	Formulated chicken nuggets, fish sticks, sausage and burger patties
Advanced meat recovery	Pressure and abrasion are used to remove residual meat and connective tissue from bones, which must not be broken or crushed during the process.	To maximize the amount of protein recovered from a given animal carcass	Lean finely textured beef trimmings (used as an ingredient in many other meat products)
Homogenization	Liquid or semisolid foods are forced through a valve that creates a high shear condition, disrupting certain structures within.	To prevent the separation of a product	Milk, salad dressing, mayonnaise
High-pressure processing	Products, typically packaged, are exposed to pressures in excess of 100 MegaPascals (MPa) (roughly 100,000 times atmospheric) for a predetermined length of time.	Inactivation of dangerous microbes with minimal loss of product quality; shellfish exposed to this process are also removed from their shells	Some luncheon meats, guacamole, and oysters
Extraction	The product is exposed to a fluid that dissolves certain compounds within it. This fluid is then separated from the product, and either or both may be processed further.	Removal of undesirable compounds or creation of a concentrated source of desirable ones	Decaffeinated coffee, natural flavor extracts, natural colors

Physical Methods

Physical processing methods, listed in table 13.1, rely on pressure and force to yield a desired change in a food. These methods can be applied to change the size of a food, such as dividing a beef carcass into smaller portions, shredding cheese, and even reducing the diameter of microscopic fat globules in milk through homogenization. Physical processes can be used to remove undesirable parts of a food—for example, deboning fish, shelling nuts, peeling coconuts, and pitting fruits. Shaping and texture can be changed, producing formed patties, nuggets, and the like. Pressures and forces can even inactivate microbes and enzymes, as evidenced by some of the more modern methods such as high-pressure processing (see figure 13.4).

FIGURE 13.4 High-Pressure Processing Apparatus

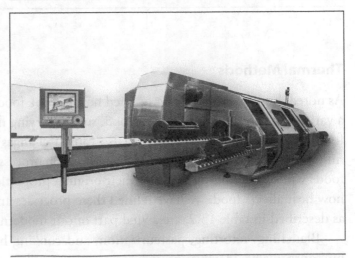

Using extremely high pressures (greater than those found at the bottom of the ocean), processors can inactivate dangerous bacteria and preserve food quality without heating the food.
Source: Hiperbaric.

TABLE 13.2   Selected Thermal Unit Operations

Process	Description	Purpose	Products
Retorting	Sealed containers of product are heated under pressure to temperatures in excess of the boiling point of water.	The inactivation of thermally resistant pathogens, such as *C. botulinum* spores	Canned foods, foods in pouches, some food in jars
Blanching	Fruits and vegetables are exposed to hot water or steam for a brief period.	The destruction of certain enzymes responsible for a loss in quality, primarily polyphenol oxidase	Most frozen and retorted vegetables
Pasteurization	Liquid foods are heated to a certain temperature and held there for a predetermined time.	Inactivating vegetative microbes, destroying certain enzymes	Milk, juices, some beers and wines
Hot smoking	Foods are exposed to the uncooled products of incomplete combustion of wood. Additional heat may also be supplied.	Elimination of pathogenic and spoilage organisms, development of characteristic flavors and colors	Beef jerky, smoked cheeses, other smoked meats
Extrusion	Ingredients are mixed and heated, building up pressure before being forced through a small opening. This rapid change in pressure causes flash boiling in the product, resulting in an open, "puffy" texture.	Development of desirable texture and structure	Puffed rice cereal, cheese puffs, pet foods
Steam peeling	Fresh produce is exposed to high-pressure steam inside of a sealed vessel for long enough to heat the skin but not cook the rest of the product. When the pressure is released, flash boiling occurs just under the skin, causing it to rip off.	Removal of undesirable peels	Tomatoes, peaches, and other produce

Thermal Methods

As noted, human societies have applied heat to cook food since prehistoric times. Societies also adopted a variety of techniques to preserve food, such as drying fruits and smoking meats; these methods made foods safer and longer lasting, but also caused changes in texture and flavor. Beginning in the mid-nineteenth century, as canning and pasteurization processes were developed, people were able to preserve foods while maintaining many of their original properties. As our understanding has grown regarding how heat affects food, we have refined these processes and created new ones. Today thermal processes, as described in table 13.2, are a vital part of our modern food supply.

Blanching, retorting, pasteurization, and cooking have benefits including eliminating a range of microorganisms, inactivating enzymes, improving flavor, and changing food texture (see figure 13.5).

Temperature-Lowering Methods

Today, a variety of processing methods, listed in table 13.3, enable us to eat "fresh" foods year-round, and to eat frozen foods with quality that surpasses canned goods and rivals fresh foods. By lowering the temperature of a food, we can limit the growth of undesirable microorganisms, slow down the rate of most chemical and biochemical reactions, and, if the temperature is low enough, halt nearly all degradative processes. With the exceptions of certain types of (typically tropical) fresh fruit that lose quality when chilled, the more one lowers the temperature of a food, the longer its shelf life will be extended (Fellows, 2000). Low-temperature methods of processing typically fall into one of two categories—freezing, which involves applying temperatures low enough to solidify the liquids in a food—and chilling, which involves

FIGURE 13.5 Food Retort

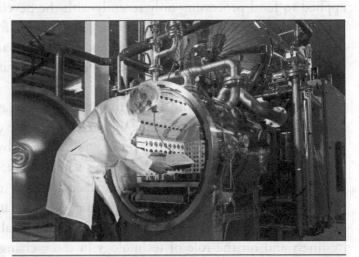

Retorts, such as the one pictured here, are used to produce canned or other shelf-stable foods. Careful control of temperature and pressure enables food processors to heat packaged foods to temperatures well above the normal boiling point of water to inactivate pathogens such as the spores of *Clostridium botulinum*.
Source: David Kamm, US Army.

TABLE 13.3 Selected Temperature-Lowering Operations

Process	Description	Purpose	Product Examples
Blast freezing	Foods are exposed to high-velocity streams of extremely cold air until the water within them solidifies.	To freeze products rapidly, ensuring minimal damage and maximum preservation of quality	Frozen meats and fish
Spray cooling	Warm or hot products are sprayed with cooler water.	To reduce product temperature quickly; often done immediately after a thermal process in order to preserve quality	Meats, fresh vegetables, fresh fruits, single-use condiments, canned foods
Vacuum tunnel chilling	Freshly rinsed produce is placed into a sealed chamber and a vacuum is created. This vacuum causes moisture on the product surface to evaporate, lowering the product temperature.	Simultaneously chilling and drying	Many fresh fruits and vegetables
Cryogenic freezing	Products are immersed in or sprayed with liquefied gases, such as liquid nitrogen or carbon dioxide.	Rapid freezing of high-quality products	Ice cream pellets, foods intended for long-term commercial storage
Freeze drying	Frozen products are exposed to a vacuum, resulting in the sublimation of the ice into vapor.	Creating dried products that maintain the shape, structure, and colors of the original product and that, when rehydrated are of a much higher quality than those made by other drying methods	Instant meals made for backpackers

temperatures above the food's freezing point. Although some may assume that these processes were applied to food processing only recently with the development of refrigeration technology, in reality humans have been using cooling methods to process food since the dawn of our existence in some cases. Early temperature-lowering processes relied on naturally occurring ice or cold water, sometimes supplemented by salts to lower the temperature even further. These processes were limited by climate and the availability of ice.

Thriving industries arose during the late nineteenth and early twentieth centuries, centering around supplying ice year round. After being harvested in the cold months, large slabs of ice were stored in insulated buildings for later use. Businesses and wealthy individuals could have smaller pieces of ice delivered to meet their needs. Even with such a system, our forebears remained dependent on nature to provide the ice. All of this changed when modern refrigeration came to prominence in the early twentieth century, first as a means to produce ice, and later to refrigerate and freeze foods for transport (Marsh & Olivo, 1979). Focus 13.1 provides a historical perspective on our changing attitudes toward freshness and on the role of technology in those changes. Today's food processors have a variety of refrigeration methods at their disposal, from water sprays used to cool packages of nearly all thermally processed foods, to blast freezers that use massive fans to blow extremely cold air (−20° C or lower) over food, freezing meats and vegetables solid in less than an hour, to cryogenic freezers that use liquefied gases such as liquid nitrogen to freeze delicate foods such as individual berries or premium meats in minutes.

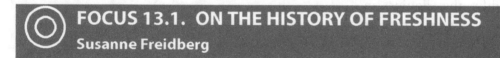

FOCUS 13.1. ON THE HISTORY OF FRESHNESS
Susanne Freidberg

I had spent years studying the modern history of fresh food trades without considering that freshness itself might have a history. But the controversies surrounding early refrigeration showed that although people in the late nineteenth and early twentieth centuries clearly valued freshness, as we do now, they had quite different ideas about where it could come from, how long it could last, and what could be done to it. How, then, have the meanings of this ephemeral food quality changed along with the technologies that are supposed to protect it? This was the question I aimed to answer in my book, *Fresh: A Perishable History* (2009).

The plural matters here. Not only has the term *fresh* meant different things in different times, places, and foods; it has also come to connote a range of other qualities generally valued by consumers in modern industrial societies: natural, healthful, pure, youthful, even simply new. In order to highlight this variety, I decided to draw on the histories of several fresh foods. I also used these histories to show how much the varied meanings of freshness owe to marketing as well as broader changes in daily rhythms of work and leisure, especially for women.

I started by learning about the science of food preservation and spoilage. I wanted to understand why, for example, beef can age for weeks but most kinds of fish degrade within hours. I wanted to understand how cold temperature changes different foods at the molecular level, and how those changes affect (or don't) taste and texture. And then I wanted to see how and how much the biochemistry of different foods has shaped their role in the larger history of freshness.

The fact that chilled beef lasts for weeks, for instance, partly explains why it was the primary cargo of the refrigerated steamships that first began crossing oceans in the late 1870s. But only partly: red meat's long-time association with wealth and power was one of the main reasons why these ships were even built. In the mid-nineteenth century, prices for fresh beef were rising in the industrializing cities of Europe and especially Britain, as the working classes aspired to eat more like the elite. Medical opinion was also turning against salted meats, especially as a staple for soldiers. Securing an affordable, reliable fresh beef supply thus became a political and even military concern.

Cattle abounded in the Americas, but animals imported live could bring disease. What was clearly needed was a means to keep a boatload of meat cool for up to a month. Many engineers worked on this problem on both sides of the Atlantic. The first to solve it, the Frenchman Charles Tellier (later known as France's "père du froid" [father of cold]) received a hero's welcome in cattle-rich Argentina, which went on to develop the world's largest chilled meat export trade. In short, as one early historian of the trade wrote in 1908, "the desire to export fresh meats was the father of all ideas of refrigerating transportation, both by land and sea." By land, of course, it was the iced rail car, popularly known as the "reefer," that the Chicago meatpackers developed in order to carry their products to coastal markets.

Refrigeration's invention hardly ensured the commercial success of refrigerated food. On the contrary, it took aggressive marketing. Trade journals provided insights into the marketing strategies used by different producers' groups. The California orange growers who founded Sunkist emphasized the flawless beauty of their fruit—a beauty that ordinary East Coast consumers could now enjoy daily and year round. Advertisements for iceberg lettuce made what would now seem outrageous claims about the vitamin content and fat-melting qualities of this nutritionally vapid vegetable (see figure 13.6). Many of these ads appeared in women's magazines such as *Ladies Home Journal* and *Good Housekeeping*, as did ads for iceboxes and later electric refrigerators.

Women's magazines also offer clues about how broader socioeconomic and scientific changes influenced consumers' food shopping and cooking priorities. Middle-class American housewives in the 1920s, for example, were expected to make do with less domestic help than previous generations while maintaining

FIGURE 13.6   1930 Iceberg Lettuce Advertisement

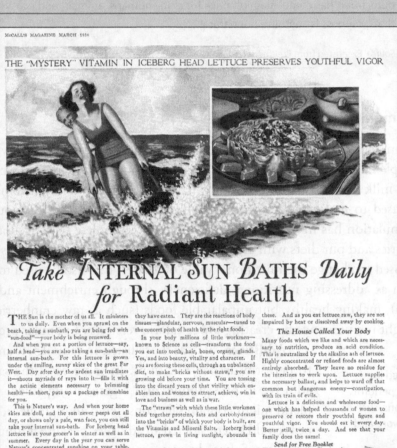

Women were urged to "take internal sun baths daily for radiant health," and were told the "mystery" vitamin in iceberg head lettuce preserved youthful vigor.

(Continued)

(Continued)

busier social schedules. For them, an electric fridge offered multiple conveniences: it got rid of the frequent visits from the iceman; it saved on shopping trips; it could even be used to prepare fashionable new dishes, such as Jell-O salads. Growing popular awareness of first bacteria and later calories and vitamins, similarly, helped sell consumers on the value of both "protective" fresh foods (fruits and vegetables, eggs and dairy products) and the appliance needed to protect their freshness.

As in the past, part of the appeal lies in the distinction associated with fresh food, at least in times and places where relatively few people have access to it. But history also shows that freshness is a profoundly paradoxical quality. It appears preindustrial, yet its wide availability—whether in supermarkets or farmers markets—depends on a host of industrial technologies, from refrigeration to the Internet. "Fresh" may connote pure, but it has come at a high price for many humans, animals, and ecosystems. Its history shows, ultimately, that freshness is anything but natural.

Source: Excerpted from Freidberg (2011).

Formulation Methods

Formulation is the act of combining ingredients to create or improve a food. This is the process most people think of when referring to "processed food." Formulation is what turns ground meat into sausage and milk into ice cream mix, and what helps slow cooking oil from going rancid. It is also what can be used to make desserts more indulgent and snacks more delicious, leading to the bad name that formulation has in some public health circles, complete with accusations of filling foods with empty calories and our diets with artificial chemicals. But formulation is just a tool—although it may indeed be used to change the nutritional value of food, it can also be used to provide valuable health benefits, such as addressing nutritional deficiencies through enrichment and fortification (e.g., vitamin A or iron), making healthy but unpalatable foods (such as raw cranberries) taste better, and helping with weight maintenance by creating lower-calorie versions of popular products.

additives
Ingredients used in formulation to perform desired functions, such as emulsifiers, flavors, and colorants

Additives, such as those listed in table 13.4, are ingredients used in formulation to perform desired functions. In some cases the same item could be considered an additive in one product and a general ingredient in another. For example, a spice blend might contain salt, considered an ingredient, whereas the salt added to a can of peas could be considered an additive, because it functions as a preservative and a flavor enhancer. Salt and sugars are the most-used additives in processed foods, helping to control microbial growth and improve flavor. That said, their position as "most used" is primarily because of the actual amounts needed to produce desired effects, similar to most less-traditional additives such as artificial sweeteners and preservatives, can impart flavor or preserve foods at much lower levels. For example, it takes two to three hundred times as much sugar as Sucralose to reach the same level of sweetness, and almost five hundred times as much salt as sodium nitrite to inhibit botulism. There are also other reasons for the common use of salt and sugar, including price (sugars and salt are relatively inexpensive compared to some artificial additives), consumer preferences for the taste of foods containing salt or sugar (especially because many artificial sweeteners have a pronounced aftertaste), and the more recent desire of some consumers to purchase products with a "clean label" (i.e., one containing only natural and identifiable ingredients). Perspective 16.2 discusses concerns that have been raised about safety of some common additives and the potential role of FDA in regulation.

TABLE 13.4 Common Additives and Their Functions

Additive Type	Purpose	Natural Examples	Human-Made Examples
Colorants	Provide desirable colors to formulated food	Carmine, beet juice extract, saffron, annatto, lycopene, carotene, riboflavin	Caramel color, tartarazine (yellow #5), indigotine (blue #2)
Emulsifiers	Used to prevent the separation of oil and water in food	Lecithin, egg yolks	Polysorbate 80, brominated vegetable oil, glycerol ester of wood rosin
Flavors	Impart various flavor notes to a food	Vanilla extract, orange oil, oleoresin capsaicin	Ethylvanillin, diacetyl
Preservative	Extends shelf life by either making chemical reactions less likely or inhibiting the growth of microorganisms	Salt, sugar, α-tocopherol, nisin, lactic acid	Butylated hydroxytoluene (BHT), potassium sorbate, ascorbic acid, sodium benzoate, "sulfites"
Flavor enhancers	Increase the perception of certain tastes	Soy sauce, hydrolyzed yeast extract, disodium inosinate	Monosodium glutamate
Stabilizers	Help to prevent separation of ingredients and impart a more substantial structure	Gelatin, guar gum, pectin, carrageenan, various proteins	
Intensive sweeteners	Provide sweet taste at very low usage levels, resulting in caloric reduction	Stevia extract	Aspartame, sodium saccharine, cyclamate, acesulfame K, some sugar alcohols
Nutrients	Fortification and enrichment of foods	Various vitamins and minerals	
Humectants	Prevent moisture loss in foods and enable a moist texture in shelf-stable foods	Sugar, glycerol, fructose, various sugar syrups	Propylene glycol, mannitol, sorbitol

FOOD PACKAGING

In the simplest terms, packaging is a unit operation that places food (or other items) into a container of some sort. This makes it a part of food processing—a very important part—because in developed countries, a majority of foods sold to the consumer are packaged in some form of container. Consumers generally prefer to purchase foods protected from the environment. Even foods commonly purchased loose or in bulk, such as fresh produce, have typically been transported to the market in boxes or crates, and are sometimes wrapped in plastic (see figure 13.7). Many people place these foods in disposable bags before putting them in their shopping carts. Packaging is so prevalent that we often refer to the package when speaking of foods in common speech: for example, "I placed a pack of crackers in your lunch box," or "he

FIGURE 13.7 Many Consumers Prefer to Purchase Foods Wrapped in Protective Packaging

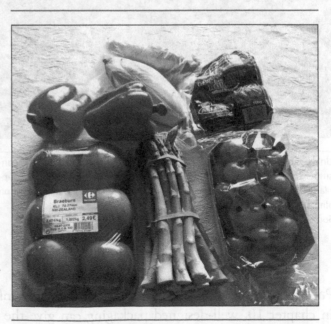

Source: KVDP Wikimedia commons.

gave us a nice bottle of wine." Packaging also affects how we perceive a product even before we purchase it. For example, some people eschew products in cans, believing they must be of lower quality than those in glass jars, even though both might have the same ingredients and have been processed similarly.

In the next section we will examine the many reasons for packaging foods, as well as the types of packages used in the food industry. We will address the effects packaging can have on the food inside, the people who eat it, and the world they live in in subsequent sections as part of processing as a whole.

Why Are Foods Packaged as They Are?

Technically, every food in the world could be packaged in a steel can, a glass jar, or a paperboard box, but looking at the shelves of the local market reveals plastic bags, metallized pouches, foam trays, transparent films, and bottles of various types. So why do we see so many different types of packages?

Product Protection   A primary reason for packaging is product protection: we package foods to prevent them from losing quality because of physical damage, contamination with foreign matter (including microorganisms), and spoilage. The type of package used depends on the product itself and how likely it is to be damaged or contaminated. Beyond the packaging materials, even the method of packaging can be protective; for example, snack chips are often packaged in polymer bags much larger than the volume of chips, not necessarily to deceive the consumer, but to create space for air (or another gas) to be added to cushion the chips and reduce breakage.

FIGURE 13.8   Old Soda Cans

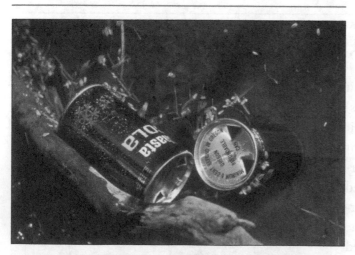

Unlike modern beverage cans, these cans from the 1970s required the consumer to have a specialized tool to open and drink. This design was supplanted by the more convenient pull-tab and later the stay-tab found on almost all beverage cans today.
Source: David Falconer, US EPA.

Convenience Modern packaging systems are designed with an eye toward consumer convenience, in terms of portioning and ease of use. Large and small packages meet consumer needs in different ways, offering product portions catered to where and how the consumer will use them. Consider the various ways milk is packaged: in eight-ounce bottles for people on the go, in gallon jugs for home use, and in twenty-liter flexible bags for the restaurant industry. Of course, even with a package of optimal size, convenience is compromised if the consumer cannot easily access the food inside. Although many older packages were more difficult to open (see figure 13.8), most modern packages incorporate features aimed at ease of use, such as screw caps, pull tabs, pop tops, and zipper closures. Even heating is now made more convenient with microwavable packaging.

Packaging and Marketing Packaging can also influence our shopping behaviors. As described in chapter 10, well-designed packaging can give the appearance of a higher-quality product, link a product with certain emotions or messages, and help us to identify a favored brand. Packaging also provides us with product details, such as nutritional information, ingredients, preparation instructions or suggestions, whether or not the package can be recycled, or the brand's philosophy. A product's package also provides a canvas for the marketing department. Marketing plans can also be affected by package choice, because the ability to produce undistorted artwork affordably can vary between different packaging materials and designs. The type of package chosen can also influence the product's final price, with heavier materials increasing transportation costs, fragile materials increasing the risk of product loss due to breakage, and newer, more advanced packaging materials, often made from plastics, typically costing more to adopt. A successful package design addresses all of these concerns, balancing the consumer perspective and environmental concerns with the financial realities of the market.

Packaging Materials

The search for new and better packaging materials has been going on for as long as people have been putting food into containers. Some of the oldest methods used wrappings of leaves, woven baskets, or bags made from animal skins and organs. These gave way to clay vessels and wooden casks (barrels) for wine and beer, which in turn were supplanted by tin-plated steel cans and glass jars. These packages, and countless others, were chosen for the same reasons we have just examined: product protection, consumer convenience, and matters of commerce. Table 13.5 examines the main types of packaging materials used in the United States today, and figure 13.9 presents examples of common polymer packages.

TABLE 13.5 Common Packaging Materials in the United States Today

Glass	
Manufacturing: Sand (silica) is fused together under high temperatures, with various minerals typically added to improve properties, and then molded into the desired shape while molten.	
Benefits: • Impermeable to moisture and oxygen • Essentially inert chemically • Transparent—enables consumer to see inside • Easily recycled • Can be made in vibrant colors for aesthetics or product protection (e.g., beer)	Drawbacks: • Heavy • Prone to breakage

Metals	
General	*Manufacturing:* Metals are combined and melted together before rolling or pressing to produce standardized flat shapes. Flat shapes are cut and formed into the desired form, including rigid containers such as cans and closures (lids) for other containers, as well as foils and coatings designed to improve the performance of other materials. Benefits: • Virtually impervious to oxygen and moisture • Capable of blocking out all light • Unparalleled ability to transfer heat • Easily recycled Drawbacks: • Vary with specific metal—see the following

(Continued)

TABLE 13.5   Common Packaging Materials in the United States Today (*Continued*)

Steel	***Manufacturing:*** Especially used in cans and closures, commonly lined with chromium plating and polymer coatings to improve corrosion resistance

Benefits:

- Virtually impervious to oxygen and moisture
- Capable of blocking out all light

- Unparalleled ability to transfer heat
- Easily recycled

Drawbacks:

- Reactive, especially with acidic foods, so must be protected with lining

Aluminum	***Manufacturing:*** Most commonly used for beverage cans, foils, and as a coating material to improve the properties of flexible materials such as paper and plastics

Benefits:

- Lighter weight than steel or glass
- More easily worked than other metals
- More resistant to certain types of corrosion

- Can be formed into extremely thin shapes (as low as 4.4 μm, roughly one-fifteenth the diameter of a human hair)

Drawbacks:

(Compared with steel):

- Increased expense
- Decreased package strength
- Increased reactivity with acidic foods versus steel

Other

Paper and Paperboard	***Manufacturing:*** Wood (or rarely other types of plant material) are ground into pulp, mixed with water and other chemicals, formed into the desired shape, and dried. Virtually all are then coated with one or more materials to improve the properties of the container or label.

Benefits:

- Ability to be printed
- Ease of combining with other materials to create tailor-made packages

- With proper coating and precise folding to protect exposed edges can even be used to store liquids for prolonged periods

Drawbacks:

- Prone to damage via moisture, either from the food inside or the environment

Polymer Packaging Materials	Although polymers can and do occur often in nature (e.g., cellulose in plants and chitosan in shellfish exoskeletons), the vast majority of polymers used to package foods are human-made. Pellets of a given polymer are obtained from a manufacturer and are formed using heat and pressure into the desired shape (e.g., bottles, jars, closures, and films).

Benefits:

- Lighter weight than comparable glass or metal packages
- Less likely to shatter or become dented
- Can be combined with other materials (including other types of polymers) to improve the physical, barrier, and chemical resistance properties of a package
- Some kinds microwavable

- Many types capable of being heat sealed, creating tamper-evident seals and stronger closures
- Can be engineered to withstand extreme temperature ranges, from freezing to the heat of retorting

Drawbacks:

- Inferior barrier properties compared with metal or glass
- Lack of widespread recycling programs for some types

FIGURE 13.9 Some Common Polymer Packages

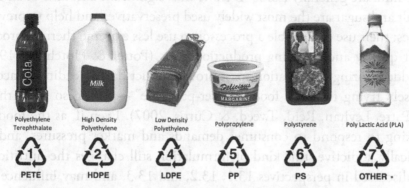

Polyethylene Terephthalate	High Density Polyethylene	Low Density Polyethylene	Polypropylene	Polystyrene	Poly Lactic Acid (PLA)
1	2	4	5	6	7
PETE	HDPE	LDPE	PP	PS	OTHER •

* - Recycling code 7 is used for any polymer that is not one of the other 6 or if a package is made of 2 or more polymers, thus not all bottles with this code are made from PLA

Source: G. Cavender.

FOOD PROCESSING AND PACKAGING: CHALLENGES

Although the overall goal of processing is to effect desired changes in food, and the overall goal of packaging is to protect products, undesired impacts can occur as well, with ramifications for health and the environment. The processing and packaging industries face a considerable challenge to maintain benefits in areas such as safety, convenience, and waste prevention, and address these concerns.

Canned or dried fruits do not have the same taste, texture, or nutritional value as fresh ones. Orange juice from concentrate does not taste the same as fresh. Milk that has been thermally processed to eliminate pathogens (pasteurized) also suffers vitamin losses. Packaging can cause changes such as absorbing and trapping flavor compounds or causing a metallic taste. In the following section we will look at some of the undesirable changes that a food can experience, primarily unrelated to the primary goal of a unit operation. We will look at quality and nutritional changes, and try to understand how they happen and what is done to help prevent or lessen them.

Nutritional Changes in Food through Processing and Packaging

Processing can alter the nutritive and healthful qualities of foods in several ways. Nutrients can be lost or they can be made more available to our bodies; formulation can increase sugars, fats, and salts, and harmful compounds can migrate from the package into our food. Similar to colorants and flavors, some nutrients can be readily damaged during thermal processing—but even those fairly resistant to damage sometimes end up being physically removed during production. Vitamins and minerals are lost when the bran is removed from wheat during milling and when cream is removed from skim milk. In many cases these losses are well known and easily predicted, enabling processors to enrich or fortify the products to offset (at least partially) the loss. Sometimes this fortification is part of a larger public health strategy, for instance, enriching flour with folic acid to improve birth outcomes. Although thermal and physical methods can lower the nutritive value of foods, sometimes they actually improve them. Vegetables such as spinach contain a large amount of calcium, but the human body cannot fully process all of it because it is bound in the plant matter. During thermal processing, the structure of the food is altered, and the nutrients become more easily absorbed.

Though increases in vitamins and minerals are typically desirable, in developed nations, increases in sugars, fats, and sodium are generally less so. Despite this, significant amounts of all three are added to many products. Salt and sugar are the most widely used preservatives and help to prevent the growth of dangerous microbes; their use can enable a processor to use less extreme thermal processes, potentially increasing product quality and reducing production costs (Potter & Hotchkiss, 1998). Salt, sugars, and fats are also added during formulation to improve product flavor, leading to accusations that the industry is purposely trying to make foods "hyper-palatable"—tasting so good they are essentially addictive (Davis, Patte, Levitan, Reid, Tweed, & Curtis, 2007). Even if, as the food industry claims, they are only seeking to respond to consumer demands and market pressures, and that their products are not physically addictive, this kind of formulation still changes the nutritional properties of a food as further discussed in perspectives 13.1, 13.2, and 13.3, and may influence consumer eating patterns.

The introduction of foreign compounds to food during contact with processing equipment or packaging has been given media attention because of concerns over Bisphenol-A (BPA) and other estrogenic endocrine-disrupting compounds (Howdeshell, Hotchkiss, Thayer, Vandenbergh, & vom Saal, 1999). These are compounds that can disrupt the delicate balance of hormones that regulate our bodies, potentially leading to problems with reproductive organs and other systems, particularly in infants and children (Vogel, 2009), as described in focus 2.3. Although these compounds have not yet been banned in the United States, increasingly manufacturers are substituting other packaging materials; some question the safety of the substitute materials, claiming that they have not been adequately tested either. Before BPA, there were concerns over heavy metals such as lead and tin leaching into canned foods from cans' inner plating or soldered seams (Robertson, 1998). Although tin is fairly inert in the human body, lead has been linked with impacts from impaired mental development in children to reproductive harm to mental and psychological problems and even, at high levels, to organ failure and death (Blunden & Wallace, 2003; CDC, 2007). In the 1970s, concern over potential liver damage or cancer and neurological effects because of vinyl chloride led to changes in the use of polyvinyl chloride packaging for foods and spirits (CDC, 2006). Even as far back as ancient Rome, production of a popular condiment called *sapa* or *defrutum* in lead vessels is thought to have led to widespread health and reproductive issues (Reddy & Braun, 2010). With increased understanding of how foods interact with their containers and how containers might affect consumers, processors are able to prevent or lessen the dangers involved through changes in packaging, food, or both.

Quality Changes in Food through Processing and Packaging

The unit operations used to extend shelf life, increase safety, improve utility, improve flavor, and provide added convenience can sometimes affect the quality characteristics of the food—textures, colors, and flavors. This problem is typically most severe in foods processed with heat or cold, but other processes also can contribute to some degree.

A food's texture is largely determined by biological compounds, such as proteins and complex carbohydrates, and structures, such as cells. These compounds and structures are also remarkably similar to the targets of most thermal processes—the enzymes and microorganisms that cause a loss of quality or safety. Thus when we apply heat to inactivate enzymes and kill microorganisms, proteins coagulate, reducing flexibility, and cells rupture, providing less support. Because these changes increase with temperature and process time, thermal processes are typically designed to expose foods to the minimum heat needed to achieve the process goal; they are also coupled with rapid post-process cooling.

Freezing, too, can cause undesirable texture changes in food by damaging cellular structures, in this case due to the formation of ice crystals. These crystals cause cell membranes and walls to rupture and drive water from cells. The more slowly a food is frozen, the larger the crystals become and the greater the damage to the food (see figure 13.10). On thawing, the foods are less firm and may release liquids. Rapid freezing avoids much of this change, because it produces smaller ice crystals less likely to damage the food's cellular structure; however, rapid freezing is costly (Pardo & Niranjan, 2006).

Food color is primarily determined by complex organic chemicals called pigments. As we have seen, complex organic chemicals can be damaged or altered during processing,

FIGURE 13.10 Freezing Can Cause Undesirable Texture Changes in Foods Such as These Frozen Vegetables

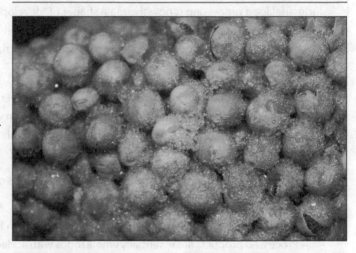

Source: Paul Wilkinson, Flickr.

particularly thermal processing, and pigments are no exception. Some pigments are fairly stable, such as the lycopene in red tomatoes; others can easily be destroyed by thermal processing, such as the oxymyoglobin responsible for the red color of fresh beef (Potter & Hotchkiss, 1998). When these color changes are considered detrimental, processes are often altered to prevent or mask them—either by changing the conditions of an existing unit operation or through the use of preservatives and colorants.

Substantial changes in food taste or aroma may be the most off-putting to consumers. No one wants to bite into a piece of food and find it flavorless, or even worse, detect an undesirable foreign flavor. Most flavor compounds are fairly complex molecules, and similar to pigments, they can be destroyed, created, or released. Flavor compounds are also typically volatile—they evaporate even at relatively low temperatures. Although necessary for our perception, this volatility is also responsible for the evaporation and loss of many compounds during heating. And though this loss can be limited with sealed packaging, care must be taken in choosing the package, lest it absorb and trap some of the flavor compounds in a phenomenon known as *flavor scalping* (Sajilata, Savitha, Singhal, & Kanetkar, 2007).

The creation of new flavors during processing is common. Although these can be desirable, such as the caramel notes in sweetened condensed milk, more often they are not. Examples include sulfurous compounds in canned vegetables, oxidized fats in canned meats, poultry, and seafood, and the "scalded milk" flavor of shelf-stable milk. Undesirable flavors can also be caused by food packaging because compounds migrate from the external environment or the package itself.

Sometimes processing additives change food flavors in ways that are strongly preferred by consumers, leading to a different set of undesirable consequences—those stemming from overconsumption, as described in perspectives 13.2 and 13.3.

Perspective 13.3. Ultra-Processing and a New Classification of Foods

Carlos Monteiro, Geoffrey Cannon, Renata Bertazzi Levy, Rafael Moreira Claro, and Jean-Claude Moubarac

Industrial food processing is now the main shaper of "developed" or "mature market" food systems and thus of dietary patterns and related states of disease, health, and well-being. The food classification we have developed takes into account the nature, extent, and purpose of industrial food processing. It classifies foodstuffs into the following three groups:

- A first group of *unprocessed foods and foods that are either minimally processed*, such as dried and packaged brown rice, pasteurized and refrigerated milk, and frozen vegetables; *or moderately processed*, such as packaged white rice or white wheat flour. The purpose of this processing is essentially to prolong the duration of foods.

- A second group of *processed culinary ingredients*, such as oils, fats, sugar, and salt, used in combination with foods to make freshly prepared dishes and meals

- A third group of *ready-to-consume food products*, which include processed and ultra-processed products. Processed products are essentially whole foods with added salt or sugar, such as salted meats, cheese made from fermented milk and salt, bread made from fermented whole wheat flour, water and salt, and fruits canned in syrup. The purpose is to prolong duration of foods and modify their palatability.

Ultra-Processed Products

Ultra-processed food and drink products are formulations made from substances derived from foods to which preservatives and cosmetic and other types of additive are added, with no or little whole food. The purpose is to create durable, accessible, convenient, and highly palatable, ready-to-drink, ready-to-eat, or ready-to-heat products typically consumed as snacks or desserts or as fast meals which replace dishes prepared from scratch.

Some ingredients of ultra-processed products are extracted from foods, such as oils and fats, starches and sugars, soy protein and milk whey, and remnants of meat. Others involve further processing of food constituents, as for example by hydrogenation or hydrolysis. Numerically, most of the ingredients of ultra-processed products are additives, such as preservatives, emulsifiers, solvents, bulkers, sweeteners, flavors, and colors.

Ultra-processed products include chips and many other fatty, sweet, or salty snack products; cola and other soft and "energy" drinks; burgers, hot dogs; ice cream, chocolates, candies; margarines; poultry "nuggets," fish "sticks"; industrial breads, breakfast cereals, "energy" bars, cakes, pastries, cookies, desserts; and canned, dehydrated, and "instant" soups and noodles.

Several characteristics of ultra-processed products are associated with higher risk of obesity and other chronic noncommunicable diseases:

- *Nutritionally unbalanced:* Their average nutrient profile is substantially inferior to that of foods and culinary ingredients combined. They are usually fatty, sugary, or salty, and depleted in fiber, micronutrients, and other bioactive compounds. They are often high in saturated fats and trans fats.

- *Energy-dense:* Their average energy density is around 60 percent higher than that of foods and freshly prepared meals. This makes them liable to disturb processes in the digestive system and brain that signal satiety and control appetite.

- *Hyper-palatable:* Many are formulated to be habit-forming and even quasi-addictive, and thus also liable to disturb regulation of energy balance and cause overconsumption and obesity.

- *Mindless eating:* Most are snacks, drinks, or ready-to-consume dishes. They are typically designed to be consumed anywhere—in catering outlets, from drive-ins and takeaways, at home while watching television, at a desk, or in the street. Tables, and often plates and implements, are not needed.

- *Aggressively advertised:* Many are branded products of transnational and other very large corporations that buy and make processed industrial ingredients very cheaply. Such corporations have vast advertising and marketing budgets to make their products seem attractive and even glamorous, especially to vulnerable consumers such as children. Many are formulated with added vitamins, minerals, and other compounds, which allow manufacturers to make or imply health claims.

The Rise of Ultra-Processed Products

The rapidly increased sophistication of food technology has made ultra-processed products cheap to manufacture, often intensely palatable, and very profitable. The trend away from traditional, usually family-based, ways of life and toward immediate individual gratification encourages snacking on these fast food products. Colossal, lightly-regulated transnational corporations aggressively penetrate lower-income countries in the global South. As the production and consumption of ultra-processed products rises, the preparation and consumption of dishes and meals freshly made from foods and culinary ingredients falls, and rates of obesity and related chronic diseases increase.

Legislation Is Needed

The impact of ultra-processed products on human health is an example of market failure, to which the rational and ethical solution is legislation. Public health and public goods are protected by legislation that limits availability, affordability, and use of, for example, guns and drugs, cigarettes and alcohol. Legislation that makes unprocessed and minimally processed foods more available and affordable, and restricts advertising and marketing of ultra-processed products and taxes them at point of sale, is needed now.

Further Reading

Canella, D. S., Levy, R. B., Martins, A. P., Claro, R. M., Moubarac, J.-C., Baraldi, L. G., Cannon, G., & Monteiro, C. A. (2014). Ultra-processed food products and obesity in Brazilian households (2008–2009). *PLoS One, 9*(3), e92752.

Monteiro, C. A., & Cannon, G. (2012). The impact of transnational "big food" companies on the South: A view from Brazil. *PLoS Medicine, 9*(7).

Monteiro, C., Gomes, F., & Cannon G. (2010). The snack attack. *American Journal of Public Health, 100*(6), 975–981.

Monteiro, C. A., Moubarac, J.-C., Cannon, G., Ng, S. W., & Popkin, B. (2013). Ultra-processed products are becoming dominant in the global food system. *Obesity Reviews, 14*(Suppl. 2), 21–28.

Moodie, R., Stuckler, D., Monteiro, C. A., et al. (2013). Profits and pandemics: Prevention of harmful effects of tobacco, alcohol, and ultra-processed food and drink industries. *Lancet, 380* (February 12).

Moubarac, J.-C., Martins, A. P., Claro, R. M., Levy, R. B., Cannon, G., & Monteiro, C. A. (2012). Consumption of ultra-processed foods and likely impact on human health. Evidence from Canada. *Public Health Nutrition, 16*(12), 2240–2248.

Moubarac, J.-C., Parra, D., Cannon, G., & Monteiro, C.A.M. (2014). Food classification systems based on food processing: Significance and implications for policies and actions; A systematic literature review and assessment. *Current Obesity Reports* (*10*).1007/s13679–014–0092–0.

FOOD PROCESSING AND THE ENVIRONMENT

Food processors take in raw material and put out packaged finished products. In doing so they require energy and water, as well as methods of disposing of their waste. Without an eye toward conservation and sustainability, these requirements can negatively affect our environment.

Energy Use

Every unit operation in a food process requires energy, and as technology is increasingly modernized and automated, the amount of energy used by municipal sources may only increase. According to the USDA, the food system accounts for approximately 15 percent of the total energy used by the nation (an amount increasing over time), with food processing and packaging accounting for a significant portion of that amount (Canning, Charles, Huang, Polenske, & Waters, 2010). In monetary terms, though, this expenditure accounts for a meager 2 to 3 percent of the cost of food production, predictably making it easily dismissed by many processors (Mishra, Bakr, & Niranjan, 2006). Processors may find it difficult to justify the purchase of expensive new equipment and systems when the resultant cost savings—initially and over the long term—are so low. As energy costs rise, however, these incentives may shift.

Water Use

Access to adequate water has always been vital to the food industry, resulting in many processing plants first being built in clusters along lakes and rivers, and then later being located in low-population areas that would have less competition for water supplies. Today, food processors require vast amounts of potable water—to rinse produce, clean the processing plant, use as an ingredient, and use in heating and cooling baths and sprays. These uses add up, and the average food processor actually uses much more water than raw ingredients, so much so that a plant that produces chicken nuggets can require over one gallon of water for every eighteen nuggets made (Carawan & Waynick, 1996; Wilbey, 2006). As the burden on our water resources continue to grow, and our populations become more centralized, the cost of acquiring that water can only increase.

Waste Production: Industry

Processing and packaging generate significant amounts of solid and liquid wastes. Although the actual rate of edible product lost during processing is quite low (10 percent or less in Europe and North America, depending on the type of food, and in some cases much less), the total amount is still in the millions of tons, and that doesn't include the inedible portions and most liquid wastes (Gustavson, Cederberg, Sonesson, van Otterdijk, & Meybeck, 2011). Surprisingly, the modern food industry has a generally good record for processing its own waste streams to lessen environmental impacts. For example, although there are thousands of food-processing plants in the United States, from 1991 to 1997, there were only seventy-eight EPA cases brought against food processors, and violations of the Clean Water Act and Clean Air Act made up slightly more than half of those (US Environmental Protection Agency [EPA], 1999)—although, as chapter 12 indicates, agency enforcement is not necessarily a reliable indicator of environmental impact.

Commonly, packaging wastes at the factory level are avoided and those that are unavoidable are typically recycled. Most of the solid wastes from undesirable portions of food items, such as bones, entrails, seeds, and peels, are turned into saleable products, such as compost, animal feed, leather, pillow stuffing, or fuel (Potter & Hotchkiss, 1998); otherwise, processors would need to pay to have them removed. Liquid wastes are much more problematic, potentially containing dangerous microorganisms and compounds that could be detrimental to the local ecosystem. All but the smallest processors in the most remote locations cannot merely flush such liquid wastes down the drain (Wilbey, 2006); modern laws and regulations such as the Clean Water Act and analogous state laws limit what can be discharged where, either through prohibition or through punitive fee schedules. As a result, many of the larger food processors have on-site wastewater treatment systems capable of reducing the strain on the local municipal sewer system and the environment (Potter & Hotchkiss, 1998; Wilbey, 2006).

Postconsumer Waste

Although some food processors might not have fully embraced waste reduction, most are making progress, and some are quite conscientious. Some do continue to use more packaging than is necessary, often for marketing purposes. The most conscientious of food processors, however, can create sustainable plants that generate little waste and are highly energy efficient; they can select packaging materials for recyclability and even donate money to environmental charities, but if their consumers choose not to or are unable to continue this pattern, it could well make little difference. One of the biggest ways consumers can lessen the environmental impact of processed food is by recycling. Although recycling is something we all know about, and most packaging materials can be recycled, many materials that could be recycled are not. Metal and glass are among the easiest packaging materials to recycle, yet in 2010, only approximately 67 percent of steel cans, 50 percent of aluminum beverage cans, and 41 percent of glass bottles in the United States were recycled by consumers, the rest ending up in landfills (Anonymous, 2010, 2011; EPA, 2012a). Paper and paperboard saw similar recycling rates (over 67 percent), but it is important to remember that this includes non-food-related items, and also that many recyclers do not accept paper products that have been laminated, coated, or contaminated with food (Cole, 2012; EPA, 2011). Perhaps the lowest recycling rates are those of polymer packages: plastic bottles and jars made from HDPE and PETE were both recycled less than 30 percent of the time, and plastics in general (again, including nonfood uses) saw a recycling rate of 8 percent in 2010 (EPA, 2012b). Reasons for these low rates of recycling are many, but include consumer confusion as to what can and cannot be recycled, differences in the ease of recycling, and—particularly for plastics—differences in the availability of recycling programs (based on geography and material type).

SUMMARY

This chapter presents an overview of food processing and packaging, explaining how and why different procedures are performed. Food processing involves the use of one or more unit operations to alter some property of the food, either to preserve it, to make it safer, to increase its value, or to make it more convenient for the consumer. Processing can include heating, cooling (including freezing), physical manipulation, and combining multiple ingredients. Packaging choices are motivated by the nature of the food, the properties of the materials, the opinions of consumers, and the needs of the market. Throughout the chapter, we have seen the origins of both processing and packaging and have gained some insight into the development of today's modern system, in which almost all food is processed to some degree. We have also explored some of the ways these methods affect the food itself, with positive and negative impacts for health, environment, and quality. Energy-dense processed foods and foods with certain additives pose particular public health concerns.

Through the perspectives and focus pieces, this chapter has described historical, social, cultural, and economic factors that affect processing decisions, and in turn, how our food processing decisions in some ways provide a window into society. This exploration should foster an appreciation for the amount of work that goes into maintaining the modern food system and generate some thoughts on ways to improve the system's impacts on nutrition and environment, further strengthening its food safety and other benefits.

KEY TERMS

Additives	Shelf life
Adulterants	Unit operations
Advanced meat recovery	Water activity
Naturally-occurring compounds	

DISCUSSION QUESTIONS

1. One of the difficulties in discussing food processing, particularly between different sectors (e.g., public health versus the food industry versus the public), is the lack of common ground regarding what processing is. After reading this chapter, what product or products did you come to realize were processed more than you had previously thought?

2. Many in the public health sector blame the processed food industry for contributing to the increase in obesity and diet-related disease, whereas the industry typically responds that they are only responding to customer demand. Some blame government for not regulating industry more directly. Where do you think the primary responsibility lies? Based on that, what do you think should be done?

3. Which is worse: a small (based on overall weight) package that cannot be recycled or a larger one that can?

4. Many times processing is undertaken to address a serious concern (such as dangerous microorganisms or short shelf life). Yet, that same processing can cause new concerns (such as increases in sodium levels or loss of nutrients). What do you consider to be a fair trade-off?

5. Rank the following items according to how likely you are to purchase them when shopping for groceries: fresh peas, peas in a can, "no salt added" peas in a can, peas in a glass jar, frozen peas. What factors influenced your ranking? Are they scientifically based? (If you don't eat peas, feel free to substitute a vegetable you do eat.)

6. Refer to figure 13.2: "When Is Beef Not Beef?" Where would you draw the line? Similarly, perspective 13.3 categorizes foodstuffs from "unprocessed foods" to "ultra-processed food products"—implying the latter are not foods. Where would you draw that line?

7. Foods that have been processed with preservatives and well packaged can take longer to spoil than fresh foods. Do the resultant reductions in food waste mean purchasing such foods should be considered environmentally preferable to purchasing fresh foods? Even if the packaging creates its own waste? How would your answer differ by food type?

REFERENCES

Anonymous. (2010). *Recycling and the environment*. Retrieved from www.gpi.org/recycle-glass/environment

Anonymous. (2011). *Steel recycling information*. News and resources. Retrieved from www.recycle-steel.org

Blunden, S., & Wallace, T. (2003). Tin in canned food: A review and understanding of occurrence and effect. *Food and Chemical Toxicology, 41*(12), 1651–1662.

Canning, P., Charles, A., Huang, S., Polenske, K. R., & Waters, A. (2010). *Energy use in the U.S. food system*. Washington, DC: US Department of Agriculture Economic Research Service.

Carawan, R. E., & Waynick, J. B. (1996). *Reducing water use and wastewater in food processing plants: How one company cut costs* (CD-35). Raleigh: North Carolina Cooperative Extension Service.

Centers for Disease and Control. (2006). *Toxicological profile for vinyl chloride*. Atlanta, GA: Agency for Toxic Substances and Disease Registry. Retrieved from www.atsdr.cdc.gov/toxprofiles/tp20-c6.pdf

Centers for Disease and Control. (2007). Lead toxicity. In US Department of Health and Human Services (Ed.), *Case studies* (Vol. *2012*). Atlanta, GA: Author. Retrieved from www.atsdr.cdc.gov/csem/csem.asp?csem=7&po=0

Centers for Disease and Control. (2012). *Estimates of foodborne illness in the United States*. Retrieved from www.cdc.gov/foodborneburden/index.html

Cole, G. (2012, March 25). The mid-valley recycling cycle. *Albany Democrat-Herald*. Retrieved from http://democratherald.com/news/local/the-mid-valley-recycling-cycle/article_59e51ef0–7635–11e1-af22–0019bb2963f4.html

Davis, C., Patte, K., Levitan, R., Reid, C., Tweed, S., & Curtis, C. (2007). From motivation to behaviour: A model of reward sensitivity, overeating, and food preferences in the risk profile for obesity. *Appetite, 48*(1), 12–19.

Emes, Y., Aybar, B., & Yalcin, S. (2011). On the evolution of human jaws and teeth: A review. *Bulletin of the International Association for Paleodontology, 5*(1), 37–47.

Fellows, P. (2000). *Food processing technology: Principles and practice*. Boca Raton, FL: CRC Press.

Freidberg, S. (2009). *Fresh: A perishable history* (pp. 1, 4–10). Cambridge, MA: Belknap Press.

Freidberg, S. (2011). *On the history of freshness*. American Council of Learned Societies. Retrieved from www.acls.org/news/8–9–11/.

Greene, J. L. (2012). *Lean finely textured beef: The "pink slime" controversy* (R42473). Washington, DC: The Library of Congress. Retrieved from www.fas.org/sgp/crs/misc/R42473.pdf

Gustavson, J., Cederberg, C., Sonesson, U., van Otterdijk, R., & Meybeck, A. (2011). *Global food losses and food waste*. Rome: Food Agricultural Organization. Retrieved from w.fao.org/docrep/014/mb060e/mb060e00.pdf

Howdeshell, K. L., Hotchkiss, A. K., Thayer, K. A., Vandenbergh, J. G., & vom Saal, F. S. (1999). Environmental toxins: Exposure to bisphenol-A advances puberty. [10.1038/44517]. *Nature, 401*(6755), 763–764.

Marsh, R. W., & Olivo, C. T. (1979). *Basics of refrigeration* (2nd ed.). New York: Van Nostrand- Reinhold.

Mishra, N., Bakr, A.A.E.-A., & Niranjan, K. (2006). Environmental aspects of food processing. In J. G. Brennan (Ed.), *Food processing handbook* (pp. 385–399). Weinheim, Germany: John Wiley & Sons.

Monteiro, C. A., Cannon, G., Levy, R. B., Claro, R. M., & Moubarac, J.-C. (2012). The food system. Processing. The big issue for disease, good health, well-being. *World Nutrition, 3*(12), 527–569. Retrieved from www.wphna.org

Moss, M. (2013).10 food secrets you need to know. *Publishers Weekly*.

Pardo, J. M., & Niranjan, K. (2006). Freezing. In J. G. Brennan (Ed.), *Food processing handbook* (pp. 128–146). Weinheim, Germany: John Wiley & Sons.

Potter, N. N., & Hotchkiss, J. H. (1998). *Food science*. Berlin: Springer.

Reddy, A., & Braun, C. L. (2010). Lead and the Romans. *Journal of Chemical Education, 87*(10), 1052–1055.

Robertson, G. L. (1998). *Food packaging: Principles and practice*. New York: Marcel Dekker.

Sajilata, M. G., Savitha, K., Singhal, R. S., & Kanetkar, V. R. (2007). Scalping of flavors in packaged foods. *Comprehensive Reviews in Food Science and Food Safety, 6*(1), 17–35.

US Environmental Protection Agency. (1999). *Multimedia environmental compliance guide for food processors* (EPA 305-B-99–005). Washington, DC: Author.

US Environmental Protection Agency. (2011). *Paper recycling: Frequent questions*. Retrieved from www.epa.gov/osw/conserve/materials/paper/faqs.htm

US Environmental Protection Agency. (2012a). *Aluminum. Wastes—Resource conservation—Common wastes & materials*. Retrieved from www.epa.gov/osw/conserve/materials/alum.htm

US Environmental Protection Agency. (2012b). *Plastics*. Retrieved from www.epa.gov/osw/conserve/materials/plastics.htm

Vogel, S. A. (2009). The politics of plastics: The making and unmaking of Bisphenol-A "safety." *American Journal of Public Health, 99*(S3), S559–S566.

Wilbey, R. A. (2006). Water and waste treatment. In J. G. Brennan (Ed.), *Food processing handbook* (pp. 399–428). Weinheim, Germany: John Wiley & Sons.

Chapter 14

Food Distribution

Edward W. McLaughlin and Miguel I. Gómez

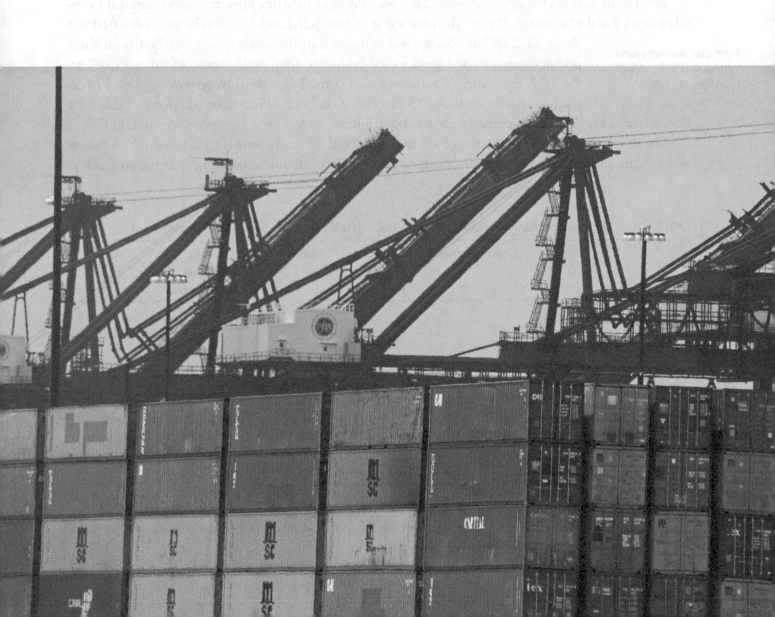

LEARNING OBJECTIVES

- Understand the history of the US food distribution system and its evolution into the contemporary structure of expanded vertical integration and consolidation at virtually all levels.

- Describe the nature of distribution channels and explain why marketing intermediaries are used.

- Understand the different marketing intermediaries available to the food industry and the benefits each of these offers.

- Review the emerging direct market channels and their role in the overall food distribution system.

- Describe a range of positive and negative impacts stemming from Walmart's size and practices.

- Elaborate channel behavior and organization, including segmentation of distribution channels and growth of private label products.

Food is the nation's largest industry, and has been for more than one hundred years (National Commission on Food Marketing, 1966). The total value of food purchases by US consumers in 2010 was about $1.2 trillion. Most food consumed in the country is purchased from three primary sources: food service establishments, food retail stores, and direct markets. By 2007, the principal entities of the US **food distribution system** employed 19.65 million people, or about 13 percent of the total US civilian workforce. Table 14.1 demonstrates the dramatic increase in the food distribution system's size between 1954 and 2007.

food distribution system
System that brings food from farms to tables

The distribution system that brings food to the tables of US consumers is characterized by a variety of segments and diverse practitioners. It begins with supply companies providing farm inputs (such as

TABLE 14.1   US Food Distribution System, 1954–2007: Establishments, Sales, and Employment

	Farms	Manufacturers	Wholesalers	Retailers	Eating, Drinking Establishments	TOTAL
Number of Establishments						
1954	4,782,416	42,374	49,728	384,616	319,657	5,578,791
1982	2,240,976	22,130	44,894	176,219	319,873	2,804,092
2007	2,204,792	29,333	42,430	247,852	571,621	3,096,028
Sales ($1,000)						
1954	24,644,477	45,703,975	51,900,246	39,762,213	13,101,051	175,111,962
1982	131,900,223	280,529,300	330,780,782	240,519,746	101,722,808	1,085,452,859
2007	297,220,491	677,645,440	955,662,150	712,224,807	433,404,527	3,076,157,415
All Employees						
1954	4,296,694	1,647,204	553,350	1,025,849	1,352,828	8,875,925
1982	4,855,857	1,487,700	815,051	2,347,603	4,665,830	14,172,041
2007	2,636,509	1,598,718	959,455	4,790,507	9,630,090	19,615,279

Source: US Department of Agriculture (1956,1984, 2009); US Census Bureau (1957, 1984, 2012); US Department of Commerce (1956a, 1956b, 1985a, 1985b, 2007a, 2007b, 2012).

seeds and pesticides) and their farmer customers. It continues via various means of transport to initial assembly, processing, and manufacturing facilities, often for conversion of raw commodities to different food products. From there it travels to sales destinations, primarily food service (restaurants, cafeterias) and retail outlets. Figure 14.1 provides a simplistic representation of the major distribution channels of the US food distribution system, including approximate dollar values of sales in the main distribution segments for 2010.

marketing channel intermediaries
Businesses that participate in the food distribution channel beyond the farm gate

This chapter outlines the major segments of the food distribution system and discusses the role of **marketing channel intermediaries**. It summarizes the evolution of this multilevel system, leading to a discussion of the current ownership structures of food distribution industries and the system performance. Complementing a discussion of the mainstream food system is a description of the direct marketing sector for local and regional foods. Finally, we share projections from industry executives as one lens into the future of the food distribution system.

distribution channel
Path through which food products travel from farm to consumer; the food distribution system is composed of various channels, such as the supermarket channel and the food service channel

The public health implications of our food distribution system may not be immediately apparent. Yet a **distribution channel** fundamentally shapes our food system, including the types of foods available to consumers and their prices, as well as the

FIGURE 14.1   Major Distribution Channels for US Food Products and Flows

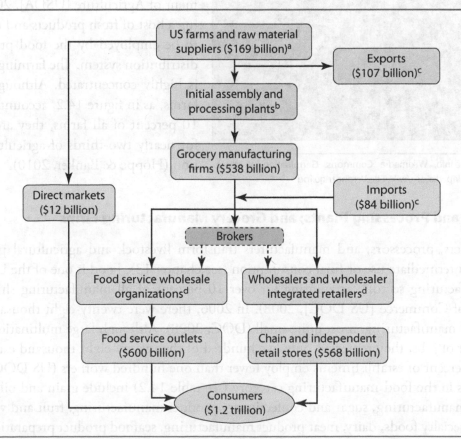

Note: Dollar values provided where available (2010).
Source: Chapter authors' calculation from various sources cited in the text, unless indicated. [a]US Department of Agriculture Economic Research Service (2010). [b]Only involved in selected categories. [c]US Census Bureau (2012). [d]The total value of wholesale sales for food service wholesale organizations and wholesalers and wholesaler integrated stores combined is $673 billion. Disaggregated values are not available.

ability of farmers, food companies, and others to influence what we eat and how food is produced. We encourage students to think about these connections as they read this descriptive overview of the US food distribution system.

PRIMARY SEGMENTS OF THE FOOD DISTRIBUTION SYSTEM

Distribution of agricultural and food products in the United States is a complex and often fragmented system composed of many pathways and channels. From initial sources of agricultural production or ports of importation, products make their ways through the distribution system in both fresh and processed forms until they reach their ultimate sales destination at food service and retail outlets.

FIGURE 14.2   Large-Scale Wheat Farm

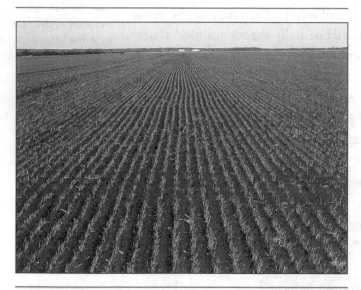

Source: Soil-Science.info, Wikimedia Commons. Germination of Winter Wheat. http://en.wikipedia.org/wiki/File:Veranotrigo.jpg

Agricultural Production

As described in chapters 11 and 12, the agricultural production sector includes the cultivation of animals, plants, and other life forms for food, fiber, and other products. In the United States there were over nine hundred million cropland acres in 2007 (US Department of Agriculture [USDA], 2009), providing a host of fresh products and raw materials to be employed by the food processing and distribution system. The farming sector today is highly concentrated. Although large-scale farms, as in figure 14.2, account for less than 10 percent of all farms, they are responsible for nearly two-thirds of agricultural production (Hoppe & Banker, 2010).

Assembling and Processing Plants; and Grocery Manufacturing Firms

Food assemblers, processors, and manufacturers transform livestock and agricultural products into products for intermediate use or final consumption (see chapter 13). Food is one of the United States' largest manufacturing sectors, accounting for over 10 percent of all manufacturing shipments (US Department of Commerce [US DOC], 2008). In 2006, there were twenty-eight thousand establishments in food manufacturing, most quite small (DOC, 2008). Although large multinationals account for 36 percent of jobs, they represent only five hundred of the twenty-eight thousand establishments. Eighty-nine percent of establishments employ fewer than one hundred workers (US DOC, 2008).

Subsectors in the food manufacturing category (see table 14.2) include grain and oilseed milling, animal food manufacturing, sugar and confectionary product manufacturing, fruit and vegetable preserving and specialty foods, dairy, meat product manufacturing, seafood product preparation and packaging, and bakeries, among others (US DOC, 2008).

TABLE 14.2   Distribution of Employment in Food Manufacturing

Industry	Employment, 2007		Value of Shipments, 2010	
	(in Thousands)	%	$ Billions	%
Food Manufacturing	**1,482**	**100**	**1,243**	**100**
Animal slaughtering and processing	507	34	346	28
Bakeries and tortilla manufacturing	278	19	113	9
Fruit and vegetable preserving and specialty	173	12	125	10
Other food products	165	11	164	13
Dairy products	129	9	176	14
Sugar and confectionary	74	5	57	5
Grain and oilseed milling	61	4	156	13
Animal food	51	3	86	7
Seafood product preparation and packaging	44	3	20	2

Sources: Bureau of Labor Statistics (2008); US Department of Commerce (2011).

Food Brokers

Food brokers act as food manufacturer representatives and facilitate sales between manufacturers and retailers. They do not take ownership or physical possession of products. There were over six thousand food broker companies in the United States in 2007 (US DOC, 2007a). Food brokers' customers usually include a mixture of retail stores as well as independent and chain wholesalers. Hiring a food broker to get products on the market is sometimes more cost-effective for food manufacturers than paying an internal company salesperson. Typically, food brokers earn commissions of approximately 3 to 5 percent on branded food products.

Food Wholesalers

Food wholesale firms take charge of goods from food manufacturers, usually in large amounts, and in turn sell them to retail establishments (both food service and food retail firms) at marked up prices. Broadly speaking, there are two types of food wholesalers (Martinez, 2007). One type includes **merchant wholesalers**, who typically buy and resell food, assemble it for distribution, load it for transport, and deliver it to an array of customers (e.g., supermarkets, food service establishments, or the export market). Merchant wholesalers also purchase food from, and deliver to, other wholesalers. Merchant wholesalers account for over three-quarters of all grocery and related product sales for a total of $487 billion in 2007 (US DOC, 2007a). The other type of wholesaler is manufacturers' sales branches and offices, which comprised about 22 percent of total wholesale food sales in year 2007 (US DOC, 2007a). Such branches and offices are typically separate from manufacturers' plants and are focused on marketing their own products at wholesale (see figure 14.3). Food wholesalers are also sometimes classified according to the product lines they carry, such as specialty (e.g., produce and dairy), miscellaneous (e.g., soft drinks and baked goods), and general line (e.g., primarily dry groceries).

merchant wholesalers
A type of wholesaler who typically buys and resells food, assembles it for distribution, loads it for transport, and delivers it to an array of customers (e.g., supermarkets, food service establishments, or the export market)

FIGURE 14.3   Wholesale Food Warehouse

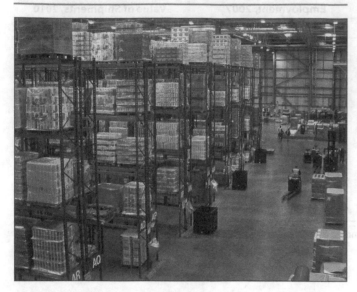

Source: Distribution centre, J. Sainsburys. Nick Saltmarsh. Flickr commons.

Food Retailer Stores

As retail food stores evolved into supermarkets and became a permanent part of the economic landscape of most developed countries, they splintered into numerous store types, each targeted at separate consumer segments. One contemporary typology separates US retail grocery stores into three channels: traditional, nontraditional, and convenience stores. Although once accounting for nearly 80 percent of all retail food store sales and still the dominant format today, conventional (or traditional) supermarkets have lost considerable market share. By 2010, traditional supermarkets accounted for only about 40 percent of retail grocery store sales (see table 14.3). The difference today is mostly accounted for by a variety of so-called nontraditional formats that tend to be much larger and price-oriented, such as supercenters (17.2 percent of grocery store sales) and wholesale clubs (8.5 percent), or smaller and limited assortment, such as what once were considered "alternative channels": drug stores (5.5 percent), dollar stores (2.2 percent), and convenience stores (15.1 percent).

TABLE 14.3   Retail Store Numbers, Dollar Share and Sales, Grocery and Consumables, 2011

Format	Number of Stores	Dollar Share	Annual Sales ($ Millions)
Total Traditional Grocery Stores	**40,229**	**46.7%**	**$500,972**
Traditional supermarkets	26,345	40.1	429,993
Fresh format	911	1.0	10,367
Limited assortment	3,730	2.7	28,609
Super warehouse	542	1.9	19,876
Other (small grocery)	8,701	1.1	12,126
Total Convenience Stores	**154,373**	**15.1%**	**$162,351**
Convenience (w/ gas)*	125,333	12.9	138,807
Convenience (w/o gas)	29,041	2.2	23,544
Total Nontraditional Grocery Stores	**55,683**	**38.2%**	**$410,315**
Wholesale club	1,331	8.5	91,100
Supercenter	3,609	17.2	184,248
Dollar store	24,512	2.2	24,031
Drug	22,534	5.5	58,659
Mass	3,518	4.4	47,222
Military	179	0.5	5,054
Total All Formats	**250,285**	**100%**	**$1,073,639**

*Does not include gasoline sales
Source: Bishop (2012).

Food Service Outlets

The food service sector is a broad, diversified industry that deals with the preparation and service of food outside the home (see figure 14.4). Restaurants, school cafeterias, and catering services are all forms of food service. US food service outlets reached about $600 billion in sales in 2011 at nearly one million locations and employed nearly thirteen million people (National Restaurant Association, 2012). Food from food service establishments comprises just over 50 percent of total food spending, marginally higher than from retail stores.

In the food service channel, **segmentation** of format has been the rule for many decades because restaurants and eating places are designed to appeal to different consumers based on menu styles, preparation methods, and pricing. The US food service industry is often divided into two categories: commercial (e.g., restaurants, retail, travel, and leisure), accounting for perhaps 80 percent of all food service sales; and noncommercial or institutional (e.g., education, health care, military), accounting for the remainder (see table 14.4). Those major categories are further split into subgroups targeted at different consumer needs. For example, restaurants have two major subcategories, full service and limited service; in turn, limited service is divided into fast food and fast casual, the latter generally offering a more complex quality-price combination than the former.

FIGURE 14.4   Subway Is the Largest Fast Food Chain in the US Food Service Sector

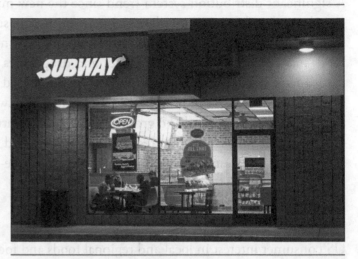

Source: Dwight Burdette, Wikimedia commons. en.wikipedia.org/wiki/File:Subway_restaurant_Pittsfield_Township_Michigan.JPG

segmentation
The process of dividing consumers into groups who are likely to respond in the same way to products and promotional (marketing) activity

TABLE 14.4   2011 US Food Service Industry Retail Sales

Segment	2013 Retail Sales Equivalent	
	($ Billions)	**(Share)**
Total Restaurant and Bars	**417.5**	**67.0**
Limited-service restaurants	229.0	36.9
Full-service restaurants	185.2	29.8
Bars and taverns	3.3	0.5
Other Foodservice Segments	**203.3**	**32.7**
Retail hosts (in premises of retailers)	38.8	6.3
Travel and leisure	53.1	8.6
Business and industry	14.2	2.3
Education	33.6	5.4
Health care	24.3	3.9
All others	39.2	6.3
Total Food Service	**620.8**	*100*

Source: Technomics (January 2014).

Blurring Boundaries

A significant distribution system trend since the new millennium has been the blurring of these various channel and format boundaries. A generation ago, supermarkets, mass merchandising stores, drug stores, and even restaurants mostly each sold different merchandise; that is, supermarkets sold chiefly food, mass merchants chiefly nonfood, and drug stores chiefly pharmaceutical and health care products. Today, retailers of all formats understand that food is a regular need and thus will drive customer traffic to their stores—and that, while there, customers will make several secondary, nonfood purchases along with their fresh food and groceries. Evidence of further blurring between store types is the rapidly growing sales of in-retail store restaurants and prepared meals for take-out from supermarkets—and, at the same time, restaurants are also offering more take-out food for at-home consumption.

Direct Markets

US consumer interest in local and regional foods and foods sold in markets directly from the producer has increased sharply in recent years. About half of local foods are sold through retail and food service outlets and half through direct-to-consumer marketing (e.g., farmers markets, u-pick operations, and community-supported agriculture [CSA] programs) (Low & Vogel, 2011a). Sales of local and regional products have grown substantially in recent years and were estimated to be approximately $12 billion in 2011 (Low & Vogel, 2011b). The number of farmers markets increased from less than two thousand in 1994 to 8,144 in 2013 (USDA Agricultural Marketing Service, 2013). At the end of this chapter, we return to a discussion of the role of direct marketing in the food distribution system. About half of local foods are sold through direct consumer marketing such as farmers markets.

EVOLUTION OF US FOOD DISTRIBUTION

Depicting the development of the food distribution system over the past century involves tracing the transformation from small, privately owned entrepreneurial entities to the larger, corporate enterprises that are common today. In the early twentieth century, almost all buyers and sellers—farmers, shippers, grain elevator operators, canners, brokers, truckers, various wholesalers, retailers, eating places—were independently run and poorly coordinated. The family farm and the family firm dominated. But farm and firm size, numbers, and ownership were to change dramatically during the ensuing decades.

input firms
Firms selling inputs to farmers

vertical integration
The merging of two or more businesses involved in different stages of the supply chain for the same product(s) (e.g., the distribution and sales of supermarket goods)

Today, the majority of agribusiness **input firms** selling to farmers (e.g., purveyors of seed, feed, fertilizer, equipment), as well as many of the firms to which farmers ultimately sell their food products (e.g., branded food manufacturers, food service, and retail customers) are national companies, guided by stock shares publicly traded on open exchanges. Thus producers frequently must buy inputs from large companies with selling power and then, at the time of sale, face even larger, publicly held, sometimes even global, food manufacturers and retailers with **vertical integration** who wield enormous bargaining leverage. Agricultural producers are caught in the middle. This structural dilemma is perhaps best illustrated by one statistic: in 2007, 2.2 million commercial farmers existed in the United States (USDA, 2007), but there were only an estimated 138 supermarket chains (University California Davis and Cornell University's Food Industry Management Program estimates, 2012). When sellers outnumber buyers sixteen thousand to one, it is not surprising that negotiation of price and other terms can appear one-sided.

economic concentration
Extent to which a market is dominated by relatively few firms

Among the many changes in the US food distribution system, none is more important than increasing **economic concentration**. From produce farms to restaurant chains and virtually everything in between, today fewer firms control a greater share of the overall business than at any time in the past. In 2002, there were 33 percent fewer fluid milk–processing plants than a decade earlier, processing 46 percent more milk per plant (US Census Bureau, 2007). The number of US hog farms dropped from 260,000 in 1990 to 60,000 by 2010 (USDA Economic Research Service, 2011), following the **consolidation** trend common among all US livestock producers. Concentration of food manufacturers has steadily increased over the past thirty years: in 1972, the top fifty food processors accounted for 39 percent of sales but by 2007 they accounted for 51 percent of sales (US Census Bureau, 2007). Likewise, the retailing sector has experienced unprecedented concentration increases in recent years.

consolidation
The shift toward fewer and larger operations in an industry

Walmart: Two Angles

Below are two perspectives on Walmart to illustrate some of the potential social benefits and damages of this concentration. One is from the chapter authors, the other is an excerpt from the 2012 book *Foodopoly* by Wenonah Hauter, executive director of Food & Water Watch. Although the two essays differ in their implied valuation of Walmart's impacts, they are not directly contrasting, but rather approach the store from different angles. Indeed, Walmart's vastness makes it not only the elephant in our refrigerator but also the proverbial elephant that is experienced differently by each observer. Walmart's dominance is such that most people have opinions about it. And when Walmart becomes the country's largest seller of organic foods or of healthy, low-priced produce, is that beneficial? What do you think?

Perspective 14.1. The Impact of Walmart
Edward McLaughlin and Miguel Gómez

Arguably the most remarkable development in the food distribution system over the past several decades is the emergence of Walmart as a food retailer and the resulting impacts on the organization of the entire distribution system. The company was incorporated in 1969 by Sam Walton, its iconic founder, as a discount mass merchandiser (Walmart, 2013). It grew rapidly. In 1988, Walmart entered the food business with a new **food retail format** that was to transform retailing: the "supercenter." To facilitate "one-stop shopping," the supercenter combined Walmart's traditional lines of apparel and general merchandise with grocery products and fresh foods all under one roof (see figure 14.5). Through disciplined operating practices and aggressive investments in supply chain efficiencies, the supercenter became Walmart's engine for growth over the next two decades, delivering spectacular results: by 2011, Walmart had passed the multinational oil companies to become the world's largest company (2012 revenues: $444 billion) (CNNMoney, 2011a) with more than 4,400 stores in the United States and another 5,600 around the globe.

food retail format
Type of retail outlet, in terms of range of products and services, pricing, promotional programs, operating style, or store design and visual merchandising (e.g., traditional supermarkets, specialty food shops)

(Continued)

(Continued)

FIGURE 14.5   Fresh Produce Section in Walmart

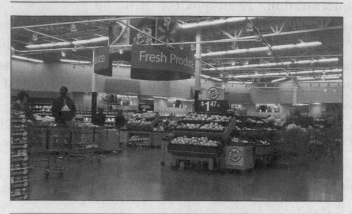

Source: Maryland   Pride,   Wikimedia   Commons.   http://commons
.wikimedia.org/wiki/File:Laurel_Walmart_Produce_Section.jpg

Some observers have found the saga of Walmart's unprecedented growth to be an inspiring commercial success story: a small town entrepreneur, through economy and hard work, manages to build a global institution offering safe and low-priced foodstuffs and merchandise to consumers around the world while providing much needed jobs in rural areas. Indeed, with more than 2.2 million associates (CNN Money, 2011b), Walmart is the largest employer and one of the largest taxpayers in the United States. Perhaps most important, Walmart's success is not simply the financial gain of one company in the private sector. Walmart has been recognized repeatedly for providing more effective relief to victims of natural disasters than the government (Horwitz, 2009).

Independent research studies have estimated that considerable portions of the productivity gains for the entire US economy come from efficiencies created by Walmart alone: the management consulting firm McKinsey reported that from 1987 to 1999 about a quarter of all US productivity increase came from the retailing sector and "about a sixth of the improvement in retail productivity came … directly or indirectly from Walmart" (Postrel, 2002). Many Walmart suppliers and retail competitors acknowledge that meeting Walmart's expectations or competing with its distribution system innovations has made them better and leaner operators, enabling those companies to lower prices to consumers: after entry by Walmart, existing supermarkets typically reduce their prices and many studies have demonstrated that food at Walmart is 8 percent to 27 percent lower priced than at large supermarkets (Hausman & Leibtag, 2007). But others don't share such unbridled enthusiasm for Walmart.

FIGURE 14.6   Walmart Critics State That Substandard Wages Keep Many Employees below the Poverty Line

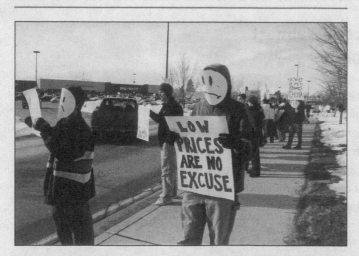

Source: Brave New Films, Flickr Commons. https://www.flickr.com/photos/
walmartmovie/25962894/

Walmart's many critics have claimed economic and social abuse, including, among many other examples, substandard wages keeping many employees below the poverty line; limited health insurance coverage, in effect shifting that sizable burden to taxpayers (Dube & Jacobs, 2002); and discrimination in pay and promotion based on gender or race. Although the Supreme Court ultimately (after eleven years) ruled in favor of Walmart in perhaps the most famous of the gender discrimination suits against the company (*Walmart v. Dukes*), the verdict has been said to be less because of the Court's ideological agreement with Walmart's civil rights practices than it was with the Court's inability to deal with the staggering number of a million female plaintiffs in the suit (Toobin, 2011). Certain community groups and labor unions further contend that Walmart's entry into new markets destroys community fabric and vitality because many local small businesses are forced to close down and, moreover, wages are driven down in other local businesses. In a recent sweeping review of more than fifty studies, the authors concluded that Walmart entry eliminates three local jobs for every two it creates, reduces the sales of existing supermarkets and variety stores by 10 to 40 percent, and sends most of its revenues out of the community (Angotti, Paul, Gray, & Williams, 2010). These are not trivial assertions.

The policy challenge of increasing economic concentration is balancing the trade-offs between consumer benefits produced by new system efficiencies (e.g., low food prices and job creation), workers' welfare created by new employment conditions (e.g., job numbers versus job quality), and community economic vitality (e.g., sales and property tax revenue versus diminished local business vitality) (see figure 14.6).

Perspective 14.2. Walmarting the Food Chain
Wenonah Hauter

When Americans shop for food, they are likely to visit one of the big grocery giants. No part of the food industry has more influence over the US diet than Walmart and the other three large grocery chains: Kroger, Costco, and Target. Together, these companies comprise about 50 percent of all grocery sales in the United States (SN's top 75 retailers for 2011, 2010; North American food retailers, 2011). In the one hundred largest US markets, they dominate over 70 percent of sales—leaving consumers with few choices (Martinez, 2007).

In the 1990s, the grocery industry began consolidating when large grocery store chains merged or bought out other regional retailers and large warehouse clubs, and Walmart expanded into grocery products. The large grocery store chains have focused on consolidation, mergers, and takeovers since then in an effort to compete with the giant food warehouses.

Although Walmart opened its first supercenter—in which food is sold alongside other retail products—only in 1988, within twelve years the chain became the largest food retailer in the United States (Martinez, 2007). Today over half of Walmart's business comes from grocery sales (Walmart, 2011), and one in three dollars spent on groceries in this country goes to Walmart (Clifford, 2011). When there is a single player as large as Walmart, individual consumers are no longer the food manufacturing industry's most important customer; Walmart is.

Because Walmart is the largest purchaser of food and agricultural products, it exerts considerable influence over which foods are available, how they are produced, and the prices farmers receive. Walmart is now the biggest customer for many of the top food companies, but each of these suppliers represents only a sliver of Walmart's total business, meaning that suppliers cannot choose to forgo demands made by Walmart.

The company continually pressures its suppliers to cut costs, and food companies have no choice but to comply. When Walmart makes a decision to change the way it does business, the entire industry shifts to keep up. And despite what Walmart would have the public believe, these decisions are made with profits in mind. The company's public relations campaigns about helping people live better belie the negative impact it has had on our food system.

More than just size and market share have enabled Walmart to exercise such considerable control over suppliers. Walmart's success is the result of several specific ways in which it does business. Most important is the way it manages its supply chain (Irwin & Clark, 2006; Martinez, 2007) by shifting costs and responsibilities to its

(Continued)

(Continued)

suppliers. Walmart requires suppliers to adopt supply-chain management, logistics, and data-sharing programs and to manage their own inventory, even on store shelves (Leonard, 2005; Martinez, 2007).

Additionally, contracts with Walmart are nonnegotiable: if a supplier wants to do business with the world's largest retailer, they must accept Walmart's terms without modification (Schmitt, 2009). Walmart has shifted the liability for supply disruptions to suppliers. If there are perceived discrepancies with an order or even if not enough product is sold, Walmart can charge the supplier a fine, known as a "chargeback." These fees, which have become more common in other retail industries as well, can be significant—sometimes in the hundreds of thousands of dollars (Hays, 2001).

Walmart demands volume. For instance, Walmart buys one billion pounds of beef each year (Codey, 2005; Lutey, 2008). For a company obsessed with increasing efficiencies in its supply chain, it makes considerably more sense for it to get this meat from a few large meatpackers rather than from numerous small, local suppliers. Smaller producers are also less likely to be able to meet and afford Walmart's technological requirements, unlike the bigger players in the industry.

The demand from Walmart and other grocery chains for large volumes of supplies has driven consolidation all the way down the food chain as each part of the food system grows in size to fill the demand at the lowest price. Today, the twenty largest food manufacturers produce 60 percent of all the brands sold in grocery stores. The largest three food processors, PepsiCo, Nestlé, and Kraft, manufacture packaged foods that are so ubiquitous in the US diet that most people eat their products every single day. Walmart's business model is a large part of the problem, so it can never be a meaningful part of the solution for the dysfunctional food system.

Farms

FIGURE 14.7   Number of Farms and Average Farm Size, 1900–2007

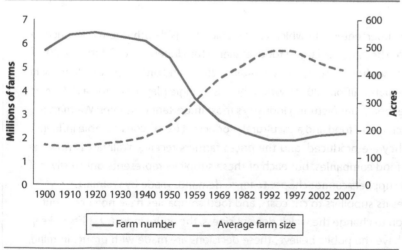

Source: National Agricultural Statistics Service (2009).

As described in chapters 11 and 12, by the middle of the twentieth century, dramatic structural changes and consequences of technological advances could be observed in all phases of the food distribution system. Rapid increases in agricultural productivity occurred as new farming methods led to a move away from fragmented, multiple enterprise farms to larger and more specialized operations focusing on a limited number of commodities. Figure 14.7 demonstrates the steady decline in farm numbers over the twentieth century as the average farm became larger. This trend stabilized in the 1990s, and even began to reverse, because production was maintained through efficiency increases instead of additional acreage.

Greater farm output was achieved with ever-smaller labor investments: the percentage of the US labor force working on farms declined from approximately 40 percent in 1900 to less than 2 percent by 2007 (see figure 14.8). Even as food supplies rose, the change came with profound implications for family farms and rural communities, as well as producing environmental and public health impacts (see chapters 3, 12, and 13).

As farm productivity rose, the increased volume of food entering the distribution system created new challenges in achieving efficiencies—in transport, refrigeration, storage, packaging, and selling techniques—and in the reduction of distribution system waste.

FIGURE 14.8   Percent of US Labor Force Working on Farms, 1900–1990

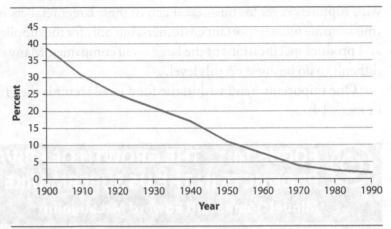

Source: National Agricultural Statistics Service (2009).

Retail Stores

In the early twentieth century, "service grocery stores"—where clerks filled each order separately—were the predominant food markets. But as labor became more expensive and consumers began to demand "one-stop shopping," a revolutionary type of store was conceived. In time, it would be called the *supermarket* and was among the most important developments in the US food distribution system in the past one hundred years.

Supermarkets grew rapidly, increasing from roughly 13,600 square feet in size in the 1950s to more than 200,000 square feet in some so-called supercenters in the 2000s. Naturally, these larger stores were able to accommodate new products, categories, departments, and services undreamed of by the service grocery pioneers: Walmart Supercenter, for example, carries a staggering one hundred thousand different products, roughly half of which are food.

Unlike many other parts of the food distribution system, where consolidation ruled the day, concentration of US food retailing was stable over much of the twentieth century. Between 1929 and 1993, the share of the total food retailing market occupied by the top eight chains remained about 26 percent. However, new retailing consolidation began in the early 1990s in response to favorable stock markets, easy financing availability, and the push to ever larger companies and stores driven in part by the success of Walmart. By 2008, the top eight grocery chains, excluding Walmart, accounted for approximately 45 percent of all food sold in the United States (see figure 14.9). This share has

FIGURE 14.9   Market Shares for US Grocery Chains, 1929–2008

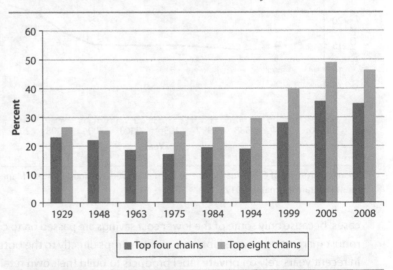

■ Top four chains   ■ Top eight chains

This chart depicts relative stability in food retailing concentration from 1929 to the mid-1990s and a substantial increase afterward.

Source: USDA ERS calculations using data from US Census Bureau; Monthly Retail Trade Survey, 1992–2009; and company annual reports.

been forecast to reach as high as 65 percent by 2015 (Cornell Food Executive Program, unpublished data, 2012). If only eight buyers control two-thirds of the entire US retail market, they wield enormous leverage with suppliers eager for business. Each of these larger retailers requires enormous quantities of food and thus become more important customers, but only for the suppliers large enough to meet the volume needs and product specifications of the large retail companies. Many small- and medium-sized suppliers find it difficult to do business on this level.

One important trend within the food retail sector is the growth of private label products, described in focus 14.1.

FOCUS 14.1. THE GROWTH OF PRIVATE LABEL PRODUCTS IN THE US SUPERMARKET SECTOR
Miguel Gómez and Edward McLaughlin

Private label (or "own" label) products usually display a retailer's own brand label instead of the brand of the supplier. They are generally sourced from small or regional processors, or occasionally even the same brand manufacturer, and marketed and distributed by the retailer. Such products have existed at least since the 1880s when retail pioneer, The Great Atlantic & Pacific Tea Company, began to put its "A & P" label on certain foods such as teas, coffees, baking powders, and spices (Levinson, 2011). Throughout most of the 1990s, US retailers' private label sales averaged about 15 percent of overall sales but by 2010, retail private label sales accounted for nearly 20 percent of overall store sales, constituted a growing share of retail profits, and were projected to grow further (see figure 14.10). Every major supermarket company has its own private brand, for example, *Safeway Select* and *O Organics* (figure 14.11), *Kroger Big K, Publix Greenwise Produce,* and *Whole Foods 365.*

FIGURE 14.10   Private Label Penetration in the US Supermarket Sector

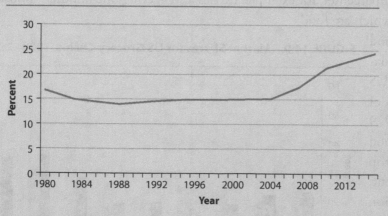

Source: University of California Davis and Cornell University's Food Industry Management Program estimates (2012).

Underscoring growth of private label products is the dynamic interplay of the differing distribution strategies of food manufacturers and retailers. Retailers have a legion of motivations to justify their entry into selling products under their own name. First, because private label manufacturers have limited advertising and R&D activity, their goods cost less: they are willing to sacrifice margin in exchange for volume and predictability from retail customers. Second, retailers are in turn able to offer these lower cost goods at lower retail prices, thus conveying a value message to their consumers. Third, in most cases, because only some of the lower cost savings are passed on to consumers, retailers are able to enjoy more robust margins on private label sales, which drops directly to the bottom line. Fourth, many retailers, especially in recent years, rely on private label products to build their own retail brand image: private label can reinforce uniqueness, innovation, special quality, and healthful positioning that generally, because the complexity of integrating all private label program elements with other unique features of a retailer, cannot easily be imitated by competitors.

Private label sales growth has a number of consequences for distribution system participants. One, consumers are able to gain access to a wide variety of consistent quality foods at prices ranging from 20 percent to as much as 50 percent lower than national brand equivalents. Private label products meet the same exacting food regulations as branded products, and, indeed, many consumers report that they perceive no quality difference between retailers' main private label offering and the equivalent product from the national (or international) brand. Two, generally, retailers are able to increase sales, profits, and, often, consumer loyalty to brands that are not available elsewhere.

FIGURE 14.11   O Organics Is a Private Label of Safeway

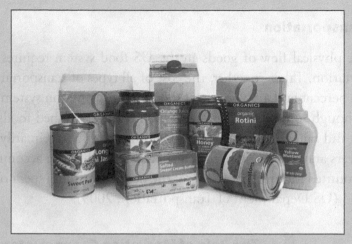

Source: Michael Milli, CLF

The consequences of private label goods on suppliers are not clear. On the one hand, much like the 1880s, today's national brand manufacturers view retail private label initiatives as a threat to their better-established brands: if a shopper opts for a retailer's private label offering, the national brand is bypassed. This is a frequent source of distribution system tension. Ironically, on the other hand, the leading manufacturer brands are often not the most threatened. The strength of the leading brand in a category is often such that its retail shelf position and merchandising does not change in the face of rising private label sales, because retailers are reluctant to reduce exposure of a leading product that attracts shoppers. Instead, more commonly, it is the second- and third-tier manufacturer brands that are more often deleted as private label sales grow. Thus, certain suppliers actually benefit from retailers' private label sales growth: the leading manufacturer brands and the small processors who produce the private label products for the retailer.

Food Service

Another development that paralleled the growth of the supermarket was the enormous expansion of the food service branch of the food distribution system. In the early 1900s, food consumption outside of the home accounted for only about 10 percent of all consumer food expenditures (see figure 14.12). One hundred years later, as noted previously, consumers spent about equal percentages on food from food service and retail sources. (Of course, although expenditures are roughly equivalent, because restaurant and institution prices are considerably

FIGURE 14.12   Allocation of Food Expenditures by Channel, 1910–2010

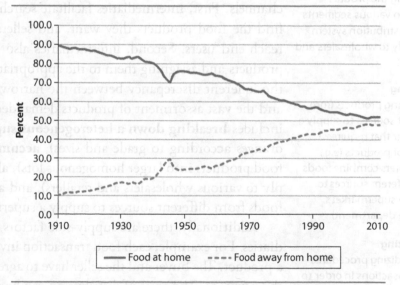

Source: US Department of Agriculture Economic Research Service (2013). Food Expenditure Tables.

higher to cover the additional service and labor provided in such establishments, the actual volume of food moving through food service channels is still much less than in retail stores.)

Transportation

The physical flow of goods in the US food system requires the support of multiple modes of transportation. Taken together, the cost of all types of transportation, excluding energy, fluctuated between 3.5 percent and 4.5 percent of total food distribution system costs from 1993 to 2008 (USDA, 2011). Although some agricultural commodities and finished foodstuffs move to market by means of water, air, and rail, trucks are by far the dominant mode primarily because of the flexibility they provide to buyers and sellers and to the smaller size lots they can accommodate. In 2007, truck shipments of food accounted for over 90 percent of the nearly $1 trillion spent on all modes of transportation for domestic food (US Department of Transportation, 2009).

The Role of Marketing Channel Intermediaries

breaking down a heterogeneous supply
A sorting function of the distribution system that separates products with different prices or for different buyers (e.g., a citrus packing plant sorts oranges by grade and size)

accumulation
Aggregation of a product to make transportation and other functions economical

allocation
Rerouting the product supply to various segments of the distribution system (primarily to wholesalers and retailers)

assorting
Combining products from different sources to supply a customer that requires a variety of products (e.g., wholesalers combine foods from different sources to supply a supermarket's produce department)

routinizing
Standardizing procedures and transactions in order to minimize costs in the food distribution system

Most food suppliers do not sell their products directly to consumers, even within the local and regional food sectors; they rely instead on the specialized expertise of other distribution system members. Figure 14.1 shows the major intermediaries in the food distribution system between producers and consumers, including, for example, manufacturers and wholesalers. Having more intermediaries often adds complexity (for instance, see focus 7.1 on the varied retail price response[s] to changes in farm gate prices). So, if the system is made more complex by intermediary distribution channels, what advantage do they provide? Why, for example, do not all food manufacturers sell their products directly to consumers? According to Coughlan et al. (2006), there are two sets of factors that influence the structure of the distribution channel: demand side and supply side.

Several demand factors (related to the needs of end users such as retailers, food service workers, and consumers) explain the existence of intermediary distribution channels. First, intermediaries facilitate searching. End users are uncertain where to find the food products they want, and sellers such as farms are uncertain how to reach end users. Second, intermediaries also perform the function of sorting food products and assigning them to the appropriate channels. This adds value because of the inherent discrepancy between the narrow range of products made by suppliers and the vast assortment of products demanded by consumers. This sorting function includes **breaking down a heterogeneous supply** (e.g., a citrus packing plant sorts oranges according to grade and sizes), **accumulation** (e.g., a wholesaler aggregates food products into larger homogenous lots), **allocation** (e.g., rerouting product supply to various wholesalers and retailers), and **assorting** (e.g., wholesalers combining foods from different sources to supply a supermarket's produce department).

Additionally, there are supply-side factors that support the existence of intermediaries. For example, each food transaction involves ordering, valuing, and paying for a product. The buyer and the seller have to agree on the mode, amount, and timing of the payment. The costs of distribution can be minimized by **routinizing** these transactions. Routinization also contributes to standardization of food products so that their characteristics can be compared and assessed with ease. Another supply-side factor is reduction in the number of contacts during the process of food distribution, because without intermediaries, every food producer would have to interact with all potential buyers, adding substantial cost to the distribution system.

In short, intermediaries participate in the food distribution system because they add value and help reduce costs. This does not mean that direct contact between producer and consumer is not desired for particular markets. For example, farmers markets and CSA enterprises are successful in meeting the demand for certain segments of consumers who value attributes such as proximity to the source of the foods they consume, to the people that produce them, and the methods employed in food production and distribution.

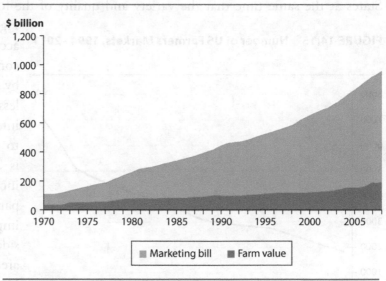

FIGURE 14.13   Allocation of US Consumer Food Expenditures 1970–2008

Source: US Department of Agriculture Economic Research Service (2013). Marketing Bill for US-Grown Food.

SYSTEM TRENDS IN CONSUMER EXPENDITURES

As the food distribution system has evolved over time, the portion of consumer expenditures returned to the farm producer has declined. For example, in 1970 farmers received roughly $0.32 of every consumer food dollar. By 2011, the number had fallen to $0.15.5 (see figure 14.13). The explanation for this trend is found in the much expanded role of "marketing activity," defined by the USDA as including all post-farm-gate functions such as transportation, packaging, financing, energy, labor, processing, advertising, wholesaling, and retailing. It may be argued that the value added by such activity and new technologies has contributed to the quality of the final food product and the efficiency with which it moves through the supply chain. Nonetheless, it remains true that farmers who have not added other "marketing" activities, such as packing, cooling, and advertising, retain less of the consumer dollar than they did in decades past.

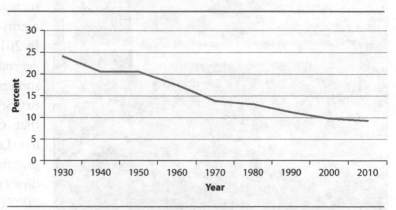

FIGURE 14.14   US Food Expenditures 1930–2010 (as a Percentage of Disposable Income)

Source: US Department of Agriculture Economic Research Service (2013).

An important index of food distribution system performance is the percentage of income that consumers allocate for food. Many economists use this measure as an indicator of the overall efficiency of a country's food distribution system. That is, the smaller the share of their incomes that consumers need to spend on food, the larger is the share that they have left to improve the quality of their lives in other areas. During the twentieth century, this number has fallen dramatically in the United States at the same time that the variety and quality of the food consumed has improved markedly.

FIGURE 14.15   Number of US Farmers Markets, 1994–2011

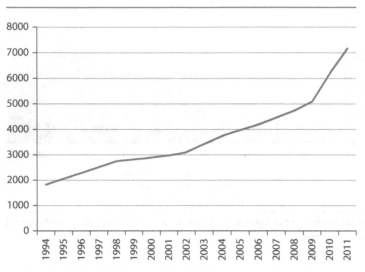

Source: US Department of Agriculture Agriculture Marketing Services Division (2013).

Figure 14.14 shows that food expenditures accounted for almost one-quarter of US consumers' disposable incomes in 1930 but by 2010 food expenditures accounted for less than 10 percent of their incomes. In interpreting these changes, it is important to point out that this efficiency measure is a relative term. That is, the share of income spent on food has been reduced in part because real household incomes have improved with more women working outside the home and greater shares of income are now spent on energy and health care. Finally, it may argued that reducing the share of income spent on food wrongly encourages policies that are low cost at the expense of the environment, food safety, and health.

Direct Marketing and Locally and Regionally Grown Foods

FIGURE 14.16   Seasonal Produce at the Market

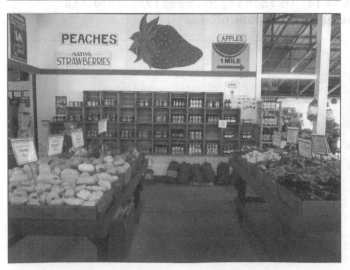

Source: Infrogmation of New Orleans, Wikimedia Commons. Burris Farm Market, Loxley Alabama. http://commons.wikimedia.org/wiki/File:Loxley_Farm_Market_interior.JPG

Sales of locally and regionally grown food account for only about 1 percent of total domestic food sales (see figure 14.1); however, such sales are one of the fastest growing segments of the US food system (see figure 14.15). In 2010 about half of locally grown fruit and vegetable sales were marketed directly to consumers (e.g., farmers' markets, roadside stands, or CSAs) and half to "intermediated channels," that is, to various retail and food service outlets (Low & Vogel, 2011a). The USDA reports that the sales of agricultural products through direct marketing outlets reached $1.2 billion in 2007 (USDA, 2009). Many supermarkets seek to satisfy new customer demand for local foods as an opportunity to increase customer loyalty. Such local buying has begun to have impacts on mainstream fruit and vegetable supply chains in the major growing areas during the months when seasonality enables local production to become a viable supply source (King et al., 2010). Focus features 14.2 and 14.3 provide a broader overview of local and regional food systems. Perspective 4.2 also considers issues of justice in local food systems.

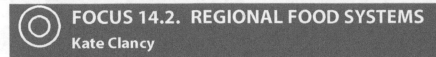

FOCUS 14.2. REGIONAL FOOD SYSTEMS
Kate Clancy

The idea of regional food systems is relatively new; it has been the subject of little research and attention compared to local (Kneafsey, 2010). A region incorporates multiple scales of food governance, such as cities, counties, or multiple counties, and states or multiple states. Ideally, a regional food system would operate at various scales and geographies to supply some significant portion of the food needs of its population (Clancy & Ruhf, 2010). To this end researchers have begun to calculate the capacity of the twelve-state Northeast region to produce a number of different foods.

Although many people make no distinction between the terms *local* and *regional*, they do not mean the same thing and the concepts are not interchangeable. Regions have fluid boundaries and are larger geographically and in terms of functions, including their role in meeting the population's food needs, volume of food produced, biodiversity, supply chain numbers, markets, land use, and policy (Clancy & Ruhf, 2010). Local food systems are of course part of regional food systems; the former being defined by groups applying various geographic boundaries, such as one hundred miles.

A region may be an appropriate and more relevant scale for implementing rural and urban development than a local area because it affords more marketing opportunities for farms of all sizes. Regional efforts also may be more relevant for agriculture and food strategies because they operate at a larger scale and can encompass a diversity of crops, cropping systems, and distribution models (Kneafsey, 2010; Ruhf & Clancy, 2010).

Strengthening regional governance structures, such as multistate planning commissions, could assist with developing regional links between food producers and consumers through, for example, the growth of regional public sector institutional procurement and land-use planning decisions (Kneafsey, 2010). At this time most land-use decisions are in the hands of local political bodies, which do not have knowledge of the food production needs of the larger region of which they are a part, thus hampering their ability to compare trade-offs between development pressures and the long-term food security of their region (Clancy & Ruhf, 2010).

A regional food system is a desired vision, as is a local food system. Neither one should seek or claim food self-sufficiency—but rather, self-reliance. Self-reliance is the ability to produce as much food as possible regionally, without undue harm to the environment. For the foreseeable future, self-reliance also includes engaging in trade with others at all levels of food procurement from local to global. We now understand that this nested-scales structure is what makes the resilience of a complex system possible. Resilience, described in perspective 1.1, is the ability to return to usual function after a disturbance; with regard to food, resilience is present when there are complementary and redundant food system components at different scales that, as an example, can provide food when other parts of a region are experiencing drought. In the Northeast this occurs, for example, when hay is delivered from different states in the region to cattle in drought-ridden areas.

FOCUS 14.3. LOCAL FOOD SYSTEMS
Kate Clancy

Local food, generally identified as being produced within a specific geographic boundary such as one hundred or four hundred miles, has been of interest for some time, but only recently has hit most big cities and small towns. The earliest interest in local food dates back to the 1970s when the oil crisis caused people and

(Continued)

(Continued)

states to consider what would happen if global and national food supplies were disrupted. In the last fifteen years, the phenomenon has grown much larger for many reasons including environmental concerns, a focus on community food security, the unwanted dominance of large food corporations, and interest by consumers in supporting local farmers and in better understanding the origins of food (Martinez et al., 2010).

FIGURE 14.17   CSA Weekly Share Items

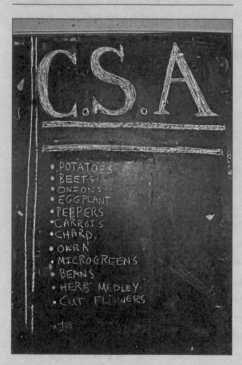

Source: CLF.

Although the phenomenon is growing, sales overall remain small. In 2008, farmers who only made direct sales to consumers (through farmers markets, roadside stands, on-farm stores, and CSAs [see figure 14.17]) made $877 million. More than twice that amount of sales, $2.7 billion, was intermediated, that is, local and regional farms selling only to distributors and grocery stores, restaurants, and other retailers. Finally, sales for farms that sold directly and intermediated were $1.2 billion. The total of $4.8 billion, however, only comprised 1.9 percent of total gross farm sales in 2008 in the United States (Low & Vogel 2011a). Sales continue to grow: industry estimates are that local food sales were close to $7 billion in 2011 (USDA Agricultural Marketing Service, 2013).

In 2010 a USDA Economic Research Service study summarized many of the key elements of local food systems (Martinez et al., 2010). They found that the production of locally marketed foods is more likely to occur on small farms located in or near metropolitan counties. Although small, medium, and large farms participate in farmers markets and other direct market venues, 81 percent of all farms reporting local food sales in 2008 were small (less than $50,000 in gross annual sales). These farms averaged $7,800 in gross local food sales per farm in 2008 (Low & Vogel 2011b). Second, they report that people who value high-quality foods produced with low environmental impact are willing to pay more for them. Many locally produced foods are not organic or sustainably produced, but many consumers incorrectly conflate the two, as noted in the main text. As consumers learn more about the differences, this confusion may resolve. Third, federal, state, and local government programs increasingly support local food systems. This includes the *Know Your Farmer, Know Your Food* initiatives at USDA and many efforts conducted by local food policy councils. Local food policy efforts target issues including farmland protection, food production, retail markets, food sales, food waste, institutional changes, and planning (Clancy, 2011). Finally, Martinez et al. (2010) found that as of early 2010 there were few empirical studies on the impact of local food marketing on environmental quality or health. Most research has looked at the economic impacts of local food production and sales, and most studies focused on farmers markets. More research will enable advocates and policy makers to understand not only the predicted economic impacts and benefits of food produced for local consumption but also the issues around seasonality, infrastructure, and economic costs of building larger local systems.

Advantages and Disadvantages

Some analysts argue that local and regional food supply chains provide certain advantages over the mainstream chains that supply products to supermarkets (O'Hara, 2011). Such advantages include preserving local landscapes and family farms, strengthening local and regional economies, knowing the origin of one's food, building relationships with farmers and neighbors, reducing environmental impacts, providing fresher food products, increasing variety, and reducing prices (Martinez et al., 2010). Additionally, some farmers are able to obtain greater gross revenue by selling their goods via direct marketing in local outlets than by selling to mainstream channels (e.g., wholesalers and retailers), even though these additional revenues must often cover the farmers' own additional marketing costs (King et al., 2010). Moreover, some researchers suggest that farmers often receive a larger share of the retail value by participating in local and regional food distribution systems (King et al., 2010).

Other studies point to the disadvantages and challenges faced by direct marketing and local and regional food distribution. King et al. (2010), for example, suggest that direct markets appear destined to remain only a small portion of the food supply chain, for several reasons. First, the contemporary food distribution system has evolved over more than a century to deliver goods across vast distances, at all times of the year, in a highly efficient manner. Part of the reason for this "efficiency" is likely the result of all factors—environmental and health costs, to cite only two—not being included in the costs that consumers pay for food. Nevertheless, it is not clear that consumers would be willing to pay greater food prices for a more complete cost accounting of their food distribution system. Second, patronizing numerous local food outlets (e.g., farmers markets or CSAs) rather than a smaller number of supermarkets to meet food needs may result in greater systemwide energy use. This greater energy use is not simply because of less efficient fuel usage but particularly, often, to the lower energy requirements in more optimally suited production locales (Desrochers & Shimizu, 2012). For instance, because of scale economies, the challenges of logistics, and, often, lower production costs, it can be more costly to deliver produce that comes from the East Coast, such as Virginia to Washington, DC, than it is to deliver apples from a major production area, such as Yakima, Washington (*The Packer*, 2013). Third, production seasonality often limits year round availability of local and regional food, particularly of fresh fruits and vegetables. In New York State, for example, local strawberries are in season for about only three weeks in early summer (King et al., 2010). Finally, at least in the short term, locally marketed food frequently lacks the public and private infrastructure required for orderly and coordinated food distribution: price reporting, market transparency, food safety regulation, and volume requirements to meet consumer demand (O'Hara, 2011).

THE FUTURE OF RETAIL FOOD DISTRIBUTION

Extrapolating trends from many of the tables and figures in this chapter is one common means to arrive at the "food distribution system of the future." Although a good start, such a method is necessarily reliant on historical data only. Another means to forecast possible future scenarios is to ask the people responsible for shaping industry decisions: company executives. For twenty-five years, Cornell University Food Executive Program (FEP) has conducted an annual survey in which senior-level food manufacturers and retailers are asked to provide projection of the future based on their experience and their knowledge of their companies' likely plans and strategies. (We note that the sample does not include restaurateurs and those involved in local and regional food systems.) Participants are presented with a series of future scenarios and given three choices about the likelihood of each scenario developing: "by 2015, after 2015, or never." Recognizing the limitations of any attempt to forecast the future—and the fact that some key stakeholder groups are not included in this survey—table 14.5 (Cornell Food Executive Program, unpublished data, 2012) presents selected responses from sixty-five food executives from the 2012 FEP. These executives projected that marketing health and nutrition will

TABLE 14.5 2012 Food Industry Forecast (Percentage of Food Executive Respondents)

Industry Issues	By 2015	After 2015	Never
Industry Structure			
The top ten food chains in the United States will account for 75 percent of retail food sales (2011: about 60 percent).	42.9	51.8	5.4
Dollar stores will represent a significant threat to conventional supermarkets when they begin to carry fresh foods.	67.9	23.2	8.9
Store size has already peaked; new formats will be smaller but with higher sales productivity.	75.0	19.6	5.4
Specialty food stores will begin to reemerge as supercenter sizes appear too large to shop for many consumers.	50.0	45.4	3.6
One-half of all supermarkets will have restaurants or some sit-down eating area.	19.6	57.1	23.2
Sixty percent of supermarket sales will be perishable foods (2011: about 45 percent).	19.6	62.5	17.9
Advertising and Promotion			
Grocery suppliers will shift relatively more marketing funds to promotions and relatively less to brand advertising in major media.	52.7	25.5	21.8
Retailers will shift to targeted electronic messages to distribute their ads for greater effectiveness and efficiency as inserts in fewer newspapers become rare.	61.8	38.2	0.0
Branding			
Food safety concerns will increasingly shift in-store food preparation to suppliers.	50.0	35.7	14.3
Market share of private label products will increase to 25 percent in the United States (2011: about 18 percent).	66.1	26.8	7.1
Retailers demand supplier-funded promotional activity to support their own marketing strategies rather than media advertising to support brands.	76.8	19.6	3.6
Food Policy Trends			
Supermarkets will begin to market health and nutrition as obesity becomes more prevalent.	92.9	7.1	0.0
Supermarkets will increase wages and benefits to workers as consumers become more sympathetic to the plight of low-paid store employees.	12.5	26.8	60.7
Strategies of conventional supermarkets will increasingly diverge from Walmart as they concede a very different approach is needed.	60.7	35.7	3.6
Demand for "local foods" will significantly change the location and structure of food production and processing.	38.2	36.4	25.5
Local or state governments will ban sales of certain foods deemed "harmful" or "unhealthful."	33.9	42.9	23.2

Source: University California Davis and Cornell University's Food Industry Management Program estimates (2012).

become ubiquitous for supermarkets by 2015. Most also agreed that, by 2015, new food retail formats will be smaller with higher sales productivity; and that dollar stores will be the most significant threat to conventional supermarkets when they begin to carry fresh foods. Another important trend is that retailers will demand more supplier-funded promotions (e.g., funds for in-store advertising and off-invoice allowances) as opposed to media advertising to support brands.

SUMMARY

This chapter focused on the distribution system that brings food to the tables of US consumers. The complex system is characterized by a variety of segments and diverse practitioners beginning with farms; continuing via various means of transport to assembly, processing, and manufacturing facilities; and ultimately arriving at food service establishments and retail outlets. The chapter describes the history of the food distribution system, explaining the forces driving the move from small, privately owned entrepreneurial entities to the larger, corporate enterprises that we know today. Among the many changes in the US food distribution system, one of the most important has been increasing economic concentration. From produce farms to restaurant chains and virtually everything in between, today fewer firms control a greater share of the overall business than at any time in the past. A significant distribution system trend since the new millennium has been the blurring of various channel and format boundaries. Horizontal and vertical integration have brought formerly separate, distinct businesses together as fewer but larger entities, often encompassing far greater product variety, economic, and geographic scope.

Food comes to consumers through three primary channels: food service establishments, chain and independent food retail stores, and direct markets. The dollar value of food purchased from food service establishments and retail stores is roughly the same, but the latter is the primary source of food purchases in terms of volume. The dollar value of food sold through direct market channels is growing rapidly but is quite small—but it is an important low-volume, high-value channel for certain food producers selling to consumer segments that value the attribute "local" or "regional." The food distribution system today is highly differentiated to meet needs for the many types of consumers.

Members of the food distribution system—farmers and food companies alike—influence the types of food available to consumers, the prices, and the methods of production, processing, and distribution. Accordingly, they affect public health and the environment.

KEY TERMS

Accumulation

Allocation

Assorting

Breaking down a heterogeneous supply

Consolidation

Distribution channel

Economic concentration

Food distribution system

Food retail format

Input firms

Marketing channel intermediaries

Merchant wholesalers

Routinizing

Segmentation

Vertical integration

DISCUSSION QUESTIONS

1. The authors focus primarily on describing the structure of the food distribution system. They then encourage students to consider the public health implications. What do you see as the main ways the organization of today's food distribution system affects public health? What sorts of changes might improve health outcomes?

2. List and describe the main food distribution channels in the United States and the intermediaries that participate in each. Why do intermediaries exist in the food distribution system?

3. What explains the small share of direct market channels in the total dollar value of sales in the food distribution system?

4. Why are food retail prices less volatile than prices at the farm gate?

5. Describe the principal forces that have shaped the evolution of the US food distribution system in the past one hundred years.

6. What are the consequences of the consolidation of food companies into fewer but larger firms on consumers and farm producers? What, if anything, should be done to address such consolidation?

7. Discuss the predictions for the future of food distribution made by food industry executives. Do you agree or disagree? Are there other potential changes that should be on the list? How might this list differ if different groups had been asked, including those in the direct marketing industry?

8. Perspectives 14.1 and 14.2 present two different angles on Walmart's impacts. Which resonates more for you and why?

REFERENCES

Angotti, T., Paul, B., Gray, T., & Williams, D. (2010). *Walmart's economic footprint: A literature review prepared by Hunter College Center for Community Planning & Development and New York City Public Advocate Bill de Blasio*. Retrieved from http://advocate.nyc.gov/files/Walmart.pdf

Bishop, W. (2012). The future of food retailing. *Competitive Edge*, June.

Clancy, K. (2011). *Digging deeper into some of the issues confronting local food policy and councils*. Seminar for Ohio State University Agroecosystems Management Program, November 16. Retrieved from amp.osu.edu/wp-content/uploads/2013/05/Kate-Clancy-OSU-11–16–11.pdf

Clancy, K., & Ruhf, K. (2010). Is local enough? Some arguments for regional food systems. *Choices*, *25*(1).

Clifford, S. (2011). Walmart tests service for buying food online. *New York Times*, April 24.

CNNMoney. (2011a). *FORTUNE 500: Our annual ranking of America's largest corporations*. Retrieved from http://money.cnn.com/magazines/fortune/fortune500/2011/index.html

CNNMoney. (2011b). *Global 500: Wal-Mart stores*. Retrieved from http://money.cnn.com/magazines/fortune/global500/2011/snapshots/2255.html

Codey, C. (2005). With sizzling sales, Wal-Mart wants say in beef production. *Arkansas Democrat-Gazette*, June 26.

Coughlan, A., Anderson, E., Stern, L. W., & El-Ansary, A. I. (2006). *Marketing channels* (7th ed., p. 578). Upper Saddle River, NJ: Prentice-Hall.

Desrochers, P., & Shimizu, H. (2012). *The localvore's dilemma: In praise of the 10,000-mile diet*. New York: PublicAffairs Books.

Dube, A., & Jacobs, K. (2002). *Hidden cost of Wal-Mart jobs*. Retrieved from http://laborcenter.berkeley.edu/retail/walmart.pdf

Hausman, J., & Leibtag, E. (2007). Consumer benefits from increased competition in shopping outlets: Measuring the effect of Wal-Mart. *Journal of Applied Econometrics*, *22*(7), 1157–1177.

Hauter, W. (2012). *Foodopoly: The battle over the future of food and farming in America*. New York: The New Press.

Hays, C. L. (2001). Big stakes in small errors: Manufacturers fight retailer "discounts" in shipping disputes. *New York Times*, August 17.

Hoppe, R. A., & Banker, D. E. (2010). *Structure and finances of U.S. farms: Family farm report, 2010 edition* (Economic Information Bulletin 66, p. 72). Washington, DC: US Department of Agriculture Economic Research Service.

Horwitz, S. (2009). Wal-Mart to the rescue: Private enterprise's response to Hurricane Katrina. *Independent Review*, *3*(4).

Irwin, E. G., & Clark, J. (2006). *The local costs and benefits of Wal-Mart*. Columbus, The Ohio State University, Department of Agricultural, Environmental, and Development Economics.

King, R. P., Hand, M. S., DiGiacomo, G., Clancy, K., Gómez, M. I., Hardesty, S. D., Lev, L., & McLaughlin, E. W. (2010). *Comparing the structure, size, and performance of local and mainstream food supply chains* (Economic Research Report No. 99). Washington, DC: US Department of Agriculture Economic Research Service.

Kneafsey, M. (2010). The region in food-important or irrelevant? *Cambridge Journal of Regions, Economy and Society, 3*, 177–190.

Leonard, C. (2005). Wal-Mart tightens distribution to increase stock. *Arkansas Democrat-Gazette*, June 19.

Levinson, M. (2011). *The great A&P and the struggle for small business in America* (p. 341). New York: Hill and Wang.

Low, S., & Vogel, S. (2011a). *Direct and intermediated marketing of local foods in the United States* (Economic Research Report No. 128). Washington, DC: US Department of Agriculture Economic Research Service.

Low, S. A., & Vogel, S. (2011b). Local foods marketing channels encompass a wide range of producers. *Amber Waves, 9*(4), 18–22.

Lutey, T. (2008). "State ranchers watch Wal-Mart's beef demands." *Billings Gazette*, February 1.

Martinez, S. W. (2007). *The U.S. food marketing system: Recent developments 1997–2006* (Economic Research Report No. 42). Washington, DC: US Department of Agriculture Economic Research Service.

Martinez, S., Hand, M., Da Pra, M., Pollack, S., Ralston, K., Smith, T., Vogel, S., Clark, S., Lohr, L., Low, S., & Newman, C. (2010). *Local food systems: Concepts, impacts, and issues* (Economic Research Report No. 97). Washington, DC: US Department of Agriculture Economic Research Service.

McLaughlin, E. W. (2004). The dynamics of fresh fruit and vegetable pricing in the supermarket channel. *Preventive Medicine, 39S2*, 81–87.

National Commission on Food Marketing. (1966). *Organization and competition in food retailing* (Technical Study No. 7, p. 1). Washington, DC: US Government Printing Office.

National Restaurant Association. (2012). *Facts at a glance.* Retrieved from www.restaurant.org/research/facts

O'Hara, J. K. (2011). *Market forces: Creating jobs through public investment in local and regional food systems.* Union of Concerned Scientists. Retrieved from www.ucsusa.org/marketforces

Postrel, V. (2002). Lessons in keeping business humming, courtesy of Wal-Mart U. *New York Times*, February 28. Retrieved from www.nytimes.com/2002/02/28/business/28SCEN.html

Ruhf, K., & Clancy, K. (2010). *It takes a region: Exploring a regional food systems approach.* Northeast Sustainable Agriculture Working Group. Retrieved from http://api.ning.com/files/nRTEesYytUshUdiU-IEPLW6lFFE3Zgcz44LFacsKlo5K6 P0X43KSuSZOkwFHiTQF6a0t5O9mAXuWNb0HbP7GZjgKVUkE7gVY/NESAWGRegionalFoodSystemFINAL Sept2010.pdf

Schmitt, E. (2009). The profits and perils of supplying to Wal-Mart. *Business Week*, July 14.

Securities and Exchange Commission. (2011). *Wal-Mart Stores Inc. form 10-K filing.* Retrieved from www.sec.gov/Archives/ edgar/data/104169/000010416913000011/wmt10-k.htm

SN's top 75 retailers for 2011. (2010). *Supermarket News*, December 1. Retrieved from http://supermarketnews.com/top-75-retailers-amp-wholesalers/sns-top-75-retailers-2011

The Packer. (2013). Walmart banks on scale to leverage local produce, CXX(9). Retrieved from www.thepacker.com/fruit-vegetable-news/193308171.html

Technomics. (2014 January). U.S. foodservice industry forecast. Retrieved from www.technomic.com/Resources/Industry_ Facts/dynUS_Foodservice_Forcast.php

Toobin, J. (2011). *Betty Dukes v. Walmart. New Yorker,* June 20.

North American food retailers. (2011). *Supermarket News*, January 24.

US Census Bureau. (1957). *United States census of manufactures: 1954* (Vol. 2). Washington, DC: Author.

US Census Bureau. (1984). *United States census of manufactures: 1982* (Vol. 2). Washington, DC: Author.

US Census Bureau. (2007). *Economic census. Manufacturing: Subject series.* Retrieved from http://factfinder2.census.gov/ faces/tableservices/jsf/pages/productview.xhtml?pid=ECN_2007_US_31SR12&prodType=table

US Census Bureau. (2012). *Statistical tables 2012.* Retrieved from www.census.gov/compendia/statab/2012/tables/12s1312.pdf

US Department of Agriculture. (1956). *1954 census of agriculture* (Vol. 2, General Report). Retrieved from http://agcensus.mannlib.cornell.edu/AgCensus/censusParts.do?year=1954

US Department of Agriculture. (1984). *1982 census of agriculture: Summary and state data* (Vol. 1, Part 51). Retrieved from http://usda.mannlib.cornell.edu/usda/AgCensusImages/1982/01/51/1982–01–51.pdf

US Department of Agriculture. (2007). *2007 census of agriculture: Farm numbers.* Retrieved from www.agcensus.usda.gov/Publications/2007/Online_Highlights/Fact_Sheets/Farm_Numbers/farm_numbers.pdf

US Department of Agriculture. (2009). *2007 census of agriculture: Summary and state data* (Vol. 1, Part 51). Retrieved from www.agcensus.usda.gov/Publications/2007/Full_Report/usv1.pdf

US Department of Agriculture Agricultural Marketing Service. (2013). *Farmers markets and direct to consumer marketing.* Retrieved from www.ams.usda.gov/AMSv1.0/farmersmarkets

US Department of Agriculture Economic Research Service. (2011). *A revised and expanded food dollar series* (Economic Research Service Report No. 114). Washington, DC: Author.

US Department of Agriculture Economic Research Service. (2013). *Food expenditure series.* Retrieved from www.ers.usda.gov/amber-waves/2013-august/price-inflation-for-food-outpacing-many-other-spending-categories.aspx#.U1a1Wvk7u-1

US Department of Agriculture Economic Research Service. (2014). *Food dollar series 2011.* Retrieved from www.ers.usda.gov/data-products/food-dollar-series/food-dollar-application.aspx#.U1BUvvldVzY

US Department of Agriculture National Agricultural Statistics Service. (2009). *Trends in US agriculture.* Retrieved from www.nass.usda.gov/Publications/Trends_in_U.S._Agriculture/Farm_Population/index.asp

US Department of Commerce. (1956a). *Census of business: 1954* (Vol. 4, Wholesale Trade—Area Statistics). Retrieved from https://archive.org/stream/1954censusofbusi04unse#page/n3/mode/2up

US Department of Commerce. (1956b). *Census of business: 1954* (Vol. 2, Retail Trade—Area Statistics). Retrieved from https://archive.org/stream/1954censusofbusi21unse#page/n3/mode/2up

US Department of Commerce. (1985a). *Census of business: 1982* (Vol. 4, Wholesale Trade—Area Statistics). Washington, DC: Author.

US Department of Commerce. (1985b). *Census of business: 1982* (Vol. 2, Retail Trade—Area Statistics). Washington, DC: Author.

US Department of Commerce. (2007a). *Economic census: 2007. Census of wholesale trade.* Retrieved from www.census.gov/newsroom/releases/archives/economic_census/2009–05–07_economic_census.html

US Department of Commerce. (2007b). *Economic census: 2007. Census of retail trade.* Retrieved from www.census.gov/econ/isp/sampler.php?naicscode=44–45&naicslevel=2#

US Department of Commerce. (2008). *Industry report food manufacturing NAICS 311* (p. 13). Retrieved from www.trade.gov/td/ocg/report08_processedfoods.pdf

US Department of Commerce. (2011). *American FactFinder 2010 Value of product shipments.* Retrieved from http://factfinder2.census.gov/faces/tableservices/jsf/pages/productview.xhtml?pid=ASM_2010_31VS101&prodType=table

US Department of Commerce. (2012). *Economic census*: 2007. Census of accommodation, food service, and other services. Retrieved from www.census.gov/prod/2011pubs/12statab/services.pdf

US Department of Transportation. (2009). *Freight Facts and Figures 2009.* Retrieved from http://www.ops.fhwa.dot.gov/freight/freight_analysis/nat_freight_stats/docs/09factsfigures/index.htm

Wal-Mart Stores, Inc. Securities and Exchange Commission. 10K Filling. January 31, 2011 at 6, 10.

Wal-Mart Stores Inc. (2007). *The nation's first Wal-Mart Supercenter receives modern design conversion.* Press release, January 12.

Walmart. (2013). *History timeline.* Retrieved from www.walmartstores.com/aboutus

Food in Communities and on Tables

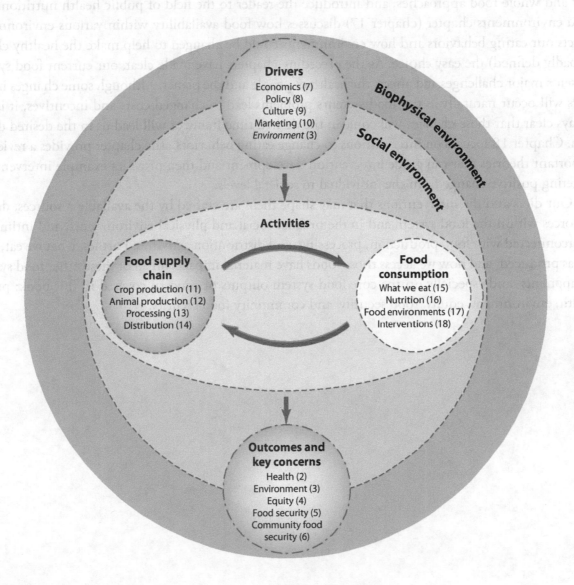

Drivers
Economics (7)
Policy (8)
Culture (9)
Marketing (10)
Environment (3)

Biophysical environment

Social environment

Activities

**Food supply
chain**
Crop production (11)
Animal production (12)
Processing (13)
Distribution (14)

**Food
consumption**
What we eat (15)
Nutrition (16)
Food environments (17)
Interventions (18)

**Outcomes and
key concerns**
Health (2)
Environment (3)
Equity (4)
Food security (5)
Community food
security (6)

Part 4 Chapters

In Part 4, the journey through the food chain continues with four chapters on the consumer subsystem. This section details what we eat and what happens when food of different types reaches our tables and communities. Chapter 15 provides an overview of current US diets, covering not only the "what" but also the "when" and "where," and some of the diversity in diets, the "who." The nutrition chapter (chapter 16) then explains what happens to this food inside our bodies, what we should eat from a health standpoint and why. We discuss key macronutrients and micronutrients as well as total diet and whole food approaches, and introduce the reader to the field of public health nutrition. The food environments chapter (chapter 17) discusses how food availability within various environments affects our eating behaviors and how environments could be changed to help make the healthy choice (broadly defined) the easy choice. As the preceding chapters have made clear, our current food system presents major challenges and affects the health of people and the planet. Although some changes in our diets will occur naturally as the food system's problems lead to changed costs and incentives, it is not always clear that those changes will come in the desired time frame or will lead us in the desired direction. Chapter 18 focuses on interventions to change eating behaviors. The chapter provides a review of important theories that can guide intervention development and then provides example interventions targeting positive change from the individual to societal levels.

Our diets and the interventions that may shape them are crafted by the available resources, driven by forces within the food system and in the broader social and physical environments, and intimately interconnected with food production, processing, and distribution activities. Further, what we eat, how it was produced, and how we access those foods have material impacts on all of these other food system components, and especially on the core food system outputs of concern covered in this book: public health, environment, equity, food security, and community food security.

Chapter 15

Food Consumption in the United States

Alanna Moshfegh

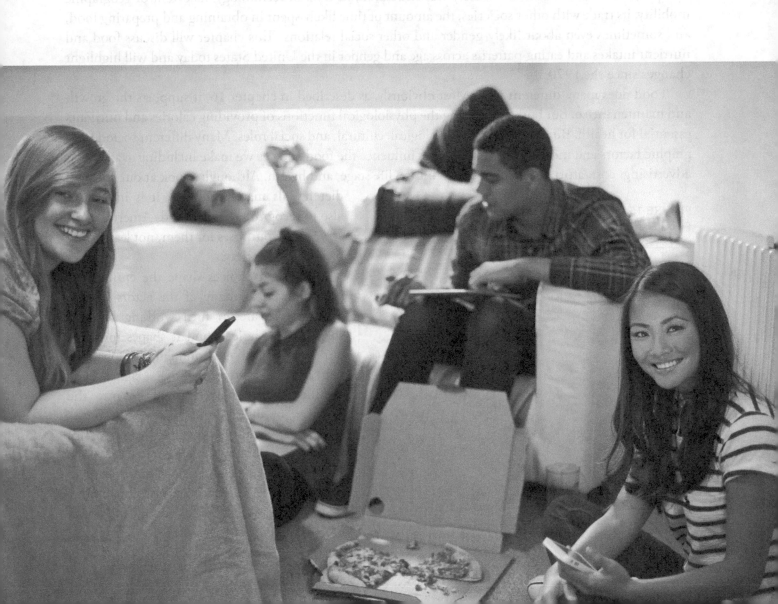

Learning Objectives

- Describe food intakes and eating patterns in the United States and major trends in intake since the 1970s.

- Identify nutrients of concern for Americans.

- Understand the utility and background of national dietary surveys conducted in the United States.

- Assess food waste and its implications in the United States.

When archaeologists seek to understand long-ago societies or fossilized remains, some of their greatest insights come from analyzing clues about what was eaten. The nutritional content of likely diets, combined with skeletal and other findings, can give much insight into people's likely health status. Other useful information includes: was the food cultivated, gathered, or hunted; was it cooked or otherwise processed, and if so, how and with what tools? Based on such details, archaeologists can create rich projections about how the society was structured, its level of technology, its extent of geographic mobility, its trade with other societies, the amount of time likely spent in obtaining and preparing food, and sometimes even about likely gender and other social relations. This chapter will discuss food and nutrient intakes and eating patterns across age and gender in the United States today and will highlight changes since the 1970s.

Food does many different jobs. Most obviously, as described in chapter 16, it supports the growth and maintenance of our bodies, fulfilling the physiological functions of providing calories and nutrients essential for health. But it also plays psychological, cultural, and social roles. Many different sociodemographic factors and individual characteristics influence the food choices we make including availability, advertising, cost, attitudes, habits, taste, culture, life stage, and health. Although a look at our national diet reveals many concerns, it is important also to recognize that the foods Americans eat serve many purposes for them, not least being pleasure and satiety.

Our food choices shape the entire food system (even as many of the actors in that food system are in turn working hard to shape those choices) and it shapes much of our society and environment. The banana you bought yesterday sent a signal back up the supply chain and played into the activities of distributors, marketers, processors, and producers in the United States and internationally (see figure 15.1). The summed bananas and other food choices made by Americans have a powerful impact on our food system's land, energy and water use, its greenhouse gas emissions, workers,

FIGURE 15.1   Bananas: Our Food Choices Shape the Food System

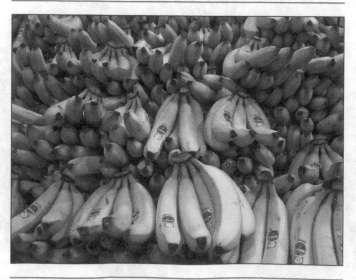

Source: Rinse, Flickr Commons, https://www.flickr.com/photos/rinses/3602799397/

communities, biodiversity, and so on. They further radiate out into society, affecting the economy, politics, and social relations in a variety of ways explored elsewhere in this textbook.

This chapter places particular emphasis on the nutritional implications of our food choices. We all want long and productive lives, and the foods we eat can be a powerful tool in achieving that. Every day, we make choices about food. Some eating patterns contribute to diet-related conditions, such as overweight, high blood pressure, elevated serum cholesterol levels, and osteoporosis, and these conditions increase the risk of certain chronic diseases and health outcomes—coronary heart disease, some types of cancer, stroke, gallbladder disease, diabetes, and bone fracture. Other eating patterns may reduce those risks. In public health, it's important to be able to assess risk for these conditions, and knowing what people eat and drink and the nutrient content of the food provides clues for the assessment. In this way, understanding food intake is fundamental for addressing nutrition and health.

National dietary data, such as those provided in this chapter, summarize these collective food choices and are essential for many public policy activities and evaluations to ensure the public's health, safety, and well-being. Experts use food intake data to make recommendations about what constitutes a healthy diet and to evaluate diets compared to these recommendations. These recommendations include the 2010 **Dietary Guidelines for Americans (DGA)** (US Department of Agriculture [USDA] and US Department of Health and Human Services [DHHS], 2010) and **ChooseMyPlate** (USDA Center for Nutrition Policy and Promotion, 2011), the educational program to promote healthy eating to consumers based on the 2010 Dietary Guidelines for Americans (see figure 15.2); the nutrition objectives of **Healthy People 2020** (DHHS, 2010); and the nutrient requirements established by the National Academy of Sciences' **dietary reference intakes (DRIs)** (Institute of Medicine Food and Nutrition Board, 2000). Federal food assistance programs also rely on food consumption data to establish their program standards and to assess program effectiveness in meeting the nutritional needs of the poor.

FIGURE 15.2 Times Have Changed!

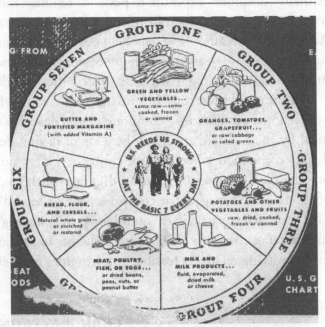

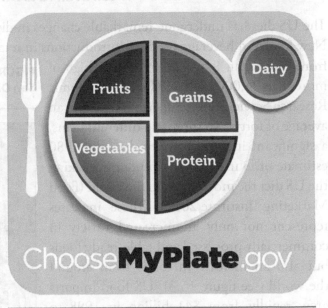

USDA's 2010 ChooseMyPlate dietary guidelines and the 1943 Nutrition Chart creating the "Basic Seven" food groups (including butter and margarine).
Sources: USDA; Office for Emergency Management, National Archives.

Dietary Guidelines for Americans (DGA)
The health and nutrition guidelines reviewed by an expert panel and produced by the US Department of Agriculture and US Department of Health and Human Services that govern all federal nutrition policy and programs

Beyond making dietary recommendations, we can use food intake data to estimate consumers' exposure to pesticide residues, food additives, and contaminants, and to develop food fortification, enrichment, and food labeling policies. Additionally, because these data help describe the demand for food and agricultural products, they are useful in establishing plans and policies relevant to food production, processing, packaging, distribution, marketing, and disposal.

In order to share this information in a comprehensive way, this chapter breaks down our diets into components and describes what we eat item by item, meal by meal. There are many benefits of having detailed information about dietary components. Yet, in some contexts, it is far more meaningful to examine broader dietary patterns. A "**total diet approach**" focuses on the combination of foods and beverages that comprise people's total diets on average over time. This approach is particularly useful for understanding how dietary components sum to reflect patterns of exposures, whether to nutrients or contaminants, and for identifying relatively feasible opportunities for dietary change.

CHANGING EATING PATTERNS

The US diet has undergone remarkable changes in diversity since the 1970s. New food and beverage product introductions in retail outlets have increased from more than 9,500 in 1992 to a high of more than 24,000 in 2007 (USDA Economic Research Service, ndb). Supermarkets carry an average of forty-two thousand different items, a significant increase compared to the 1980 estimate of fourteen thousand items, making the US diet the most varied in the world (Food Marketing Institute, 2012). These increases represent not only an increased variety in commercially processed and table-ready foods but also an increase in foods from around the world (see figure 15.3). US food imports grew rapidly, from $41 billion in 1998 to nearly $78 billion in 2007, with the greatest growth among value-added products (foods that have increased in value through processing or packaging). Although raw commodity imports grew at a rate of 14 percent between 1998 and 2007, consumer-ready food products grew over 100 percent (Brooks, Regmi, & Jerardo, 2010).

ChooseMyPlate
An educational program and visual "plate" developed by the US Department of Agriculture to promote healthy eating to consumers based on the 2010 Dietary Guidelines for Americans

Healthy People 2020
The US ten-year goals and objectives that guide national health promotion and disease prevention efforts (US Department of Health and Human Services)

dietary reference intakes (DRIs)
Evidence-based nutrient standards set by the Institute of Medicine and the National Academy of Sciences for estimating optimal intakes in healthy individuals

total diet approach
Dietary pattern that focuses on the combination of foods and beverages that comprise people's total diets on average over time

FIGURE 15.3 Dole Honduras Ship Unloading Imports in San Diego

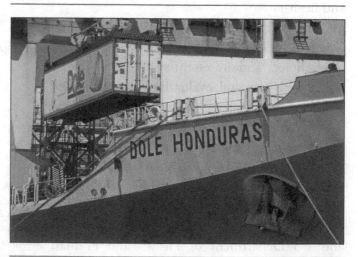

About 95,000 twenty-foot containers of Dole fruit pass through this port annually.
Source: Dale Frost, Port of San Diego.

Methods for Assessing Food Consumption

There are a variety of ways to assess food consumption, from global measures of food availability to detailed measures of individual food intake. **Food availability assessment** involves measuring the food supply—the availability of basic commodities, such as wheat, beef, and eggs, at the farm level or an early stage of processing. It does not measure use of highly processed foods—such as bakery products, frozen dinners, and soups—in their finished form. In general, the amount of food available for human consumption is calculated as the difference between available commodity supplies summed from data sources on production, imports, and stocks of food at the beginning of the year, minus exports and nonfood uses such as animal feed. Data are often presented on a per capita basis. Two of the most important food availability measures are the US Department of Agriculture's **food availability data series** and the Food and Agriculture Organization's **food balance sheets** (USDA, nd; Food and Agriculture Organization, nd). Although food availability data are sometimes used as a proxy for food intake, they cannot account for sociodemographic and individual characteristics that affect food intake or account for specific types of foods or beverages. Further, they overestimate consumption because they do not account for losses such as from meat trimming, cooking, plate waste, and spoilage (Kantor, Lipton, Manchester, & Oliveira, 1997); in the United States approximately 40 percent of food produced is wasted (Hall, Guo, Dore, & Chow, 2009) (see focus 15.3).

Nutrition experts generally recognize that it is best to assess diets and dietary patterns at the individual level because of the variability of food intake across individuals. There are four primary individual level methods: the **food record**, the **diet history method**, the **food frequency questionnaire**, and the **twenty-four-hour dietary recall**. Of the four methods, which are explained further in focus 15.1, the twenty-four-hour dietary recall has been demonstrated as the preferred method for monitoring and studying diets of the population because they provide high-quality dietary intake data with minimal bias (Kipnis et al., 2003; Moshfegh et al., 2008; Schatzkin et al., 2003; Subar et al., 2012).

food availability assessment
Assessment measuring use of basic commodities, such as wheat, beef, and eggs at the farm level or an early stage of processing

food availability data series
Time series data measuring food supplies available for domestic consumption (USDA Economic Research Service)

food balance sheets
Provide a comprehensive picture of a country's food supply patterns by showing availability of food items for human consumption for a specified time period (Food and Agriculture Organization)

food record
Detailed record of foods and beverages an individual consumes over a given period of time

diet history method
Information collection, usually by a trained interviewer, about intake frequencies of various foods and the typical makeup of meals

food frequency questionnaire
Assessment tool asking about usual frequency of consumption of a select group of foods for a specific period of time

twenty-four-hour dietary recall
A quantitative research method in which individuals are asked to recall types and amounts of all foods and beverages eaten in the prior twenty-four hours

FOCUS 15.1. METHODS FOR ASSESSING DIETS OF INDIVIDUALS
Alanna Moshfegh

Nutrition and health professionals and researchers use four data collection methods to assess diets, as described in the following (Pao & Cypnel, 1996). There is considerable variation in use of these methods, from the means of collection, to details about foods and portions, to the length of time the method is to cover.

- **Food record.** The food record is kept by the individual or designate (for example, a mother for her child) for a specified time period, usually one to seven days. Each food is weighed or estimated by use of household measures or typical portions when the food is consumed or shortly thereafter.

- **Diet history method.** The diet history method commonly uses a trained interviewer to compile information about how frequently subjects eat particular foods, as well as the typical makeup of meals. It may include a food record for a select number of days. Diet histories may cover varying topics, including the type,

(Continued)

(Continued)

frequency, preparation, consumption practices, and amount of foods consumed. Most variations attempt to capture usual eating patterns for an extended period of time.

- **Food frequency questionnaire.** The food frequency questionnaire asks the individual about usual frequency of consumption (and sometimes portion size) for a select list of foods for a specific period of time, such as the past month or past year. The types of foods on the list vary depending on interest, such as specific nutrients, the total diet, or specific types of foods.

- **Twenty-four-hour dietary recall.** The individual is asked to recall and describe the kinds and amounts of all foods and beverages consumed during the prior twenty-four-hour period. The recall, administered by a trained interviewer or self-administered using an automated questionnaire, includes probing questions and strategies to encourage and help organize the individual's memories about eating events, food details, and amounts consumed.

What We Eat in America (WWEIA)
Two-day dietary intake interview component of the annual National Health and Nutrition Examination Survey; the only nationally representative dietary survey in the United States (US Department of Agriculture and US Department of Health and Human Services)

The following sections present a portrait of the calories, nutrients, meals, snacks, and specific foods and beverages we consume in the United States. They are based on 2007–2008 data about mean daily intake from the US Department of Agriculture's **What We Eat in America (WWEIA)**, the dietary interview component of the National Health and Nutrition Examination Survey (NHANES) (DHHS, 2014; Raper, Perloff, Ingwersen, Steinfeldt, & Anand, 2004). Focus 15.2 provides a brief summary of surveys used to collect dietary data. The survey is currently the US government's primary way of capturing information about what we eat.

FOCUS 15.2. NATIONAL DIETARY SURVEYS IN THE UNITED STATES

Alanna Moshfegh

The USDA and the DHHS have conducted periodic nationwide surveys to collect national information on food consumption since the 1930s. The most recent survey, What We Eat in America (WWEIA), is the dietary interview component of the National Health and Nutrition Examination Surveys (NHANES), which is a program of studies assessing the health and nutritional status of adults and children in the United States (DHHS, 2014).

Sample

- Approximately five thousand individuals of all ages are interviewed annually on two nonconsecutive days about their food and beverage intakes.

- These persons are located in counties across the country, fifteen of which are visited each year.

- Data are weighted to be representative of the US population for the years of collection.

Dietary Data

- Two twenty-four-hour dietary recalls are collected on each individual: one in person, one by telephone.

- A standardized interview method, the USDA Automated Multiple-Pass Method, is used for collecting the dietary recalls by trained interviewers.

- The five steps—(1) quick list, (2) forgotten foods list, (3) time and occasion, (4) detail and review, and (5) final probe—include multiple passes through the twenty-four hours of the previous day, during which respondents receive cues to help them remember and describe foods and beverages they consumed.

- Results include the types and amounts of foods and beverages (including all types of water) consumed during the twenty-four-hour period prior to the interview and the amount of energy and sixty-four nutrients and food components from those foods and beverages.

- Nutrient values for the foods and beverages reported were determined using the USDA Food and Nutrient Database for Dietary Studies, which is updated to reflect the food supply to correspond with the two years of data publicly released.

- For dietary data see www.ars.usda.gov/ba/bhnrc/fsrg and www.nhanes.gov.

- It goes without saying that diets in the United States are enormously heterogeneous, based on geography, demography, and culture. Although this chapter focuses on the broad contours of US diets, it does present some information by demographic groups, particularly whites, blacks, and Hispanics. Other ethnic groups are included in the survey; however, sample size limitations prevent reporting data for other groups. Resources on diets of Asian Americans are provided in the online supplement for this textbook. See chapter 9 for additional context on cultural aspects of diet.

Intakes of Calories and Key Nutrients

For Americans, the mean daily caloric intake is 2,070 calories. Compared to 1977–1978, this number represents an increase of about 200 calories per day (see figure 15.4). Over time, the sources of these calories have changed. Fats now provide one-third of our calories compared to 43 percent in 1977–1778, and carbohydrates account for half, compared to 40 percent back then. Calories from protein have remained fairly constant during this period, at about 15 percent of the total.

As described in chapter 16, the 2010 Dietary Guidelines for Americans highlight the need for Americans to consume more of the following nutrients: potassium, dietary fiber, calcium, and vitamin D. In addition, some specific population groups need to raise consumption of other nutrients. Females capable of becoming pregnant should consume more iron and folate, and people age fifty years and above should get more vitamin B_{12}.

FIGURE 15.4   Changes in Calories and Sources of Calories in American Diets: 1977–1978 to 2007–2008

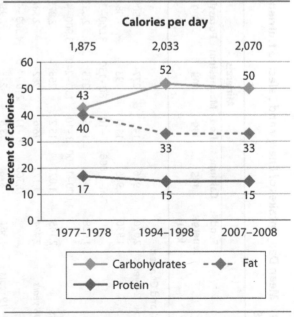

Source: USDA.

Table 15.1 summarizes the mean daily intakes of calories and selected nutrients by age groups and sociodemographic variables.

TABLE 15.1 Mean Daily Intakes of Energy and Selected Nutrients by Age and Gender, Race and Ethnicity, and Income Status in the United States, 2007–2008

	Food energy kcal	Minerals					Folate	C mg	A	Vitamins			Sugars gm	Dietary fiber g	Cholesterol mg
		Calcium mg	Iron mg	Magnesium mg	Potassium mg	Sodium mg				D	B12	E			
Age (years) and Gender:															
All individuals, 2+ years	2,070	946	14.7	277	2,509	3,330	527	84.2	607	4.6	5.19	7.2	120	15.2	276
2–5 years	1,536	985	11.0	193	1,984	2,230	415	96.2	590	6.3	4.32	4.5	110	10.9	184
RDA*		700–1,000	7–10	80–130	3,000–3,800	1,000–1,200	150–200	15–25	300–400	15	0.9–1.2	6–7		19–25	300
6–11 years	1,928	956	13.5	215	2,053	2,933	499	80.9	567	5.0	4.85	6.0	131	12.8	213
RDA*		1,000–1,300	8–10	130–240	3,900–4,500	1,200–1,500	200–300	25–45	400–600	15	1.2–1.8	7–11		25–31	300
12–19 years	2,145	1,027	15.2	253	2,275	3,505	560	80.3	604	4.8	5.42	6.9	135	14.1	262
Males, 12–19 years	2,424	1,173	16.6	282	2,587	3,990	610	86.6	680	5.9	6.68	7.7	152	14.9	312
RDA*		1,300	8–11	240–400	4,500–4,700	1,500	300–400	45–90	600–900	15	1.8–2.4	11–15		31–38	300
Females, 12–19 years	1,861	878	13.8	223	1,957	3,013	509	73.8	528	3.8	4.14	6.0	116	13.3	212
RDA*		1,000–1,200	8–18	310–320	4,700	1,200–1,500	400	75	700	15–20	2.4	15		21–25	300
20+ years	2,115	929	15.1	294	2,637	3,430	534	84.2	613	4.4	5.26	7.5	117	15.9	292
Males, 20+ years	2,507	1038	17.5	334	3,026	4,043	613	91.3	649	5.0	6.32	8.3	133	17.7	362
RDA*		1,000–1,200	8	400–420	4,700	1,200–1,500	400	90	900	15–20	2.4	15		30–38	300
Females, 20+ years	1,766	833	13.0	258	2,290	2,884	463	77.9	580	3.8	4.32	6.9	103	14.3	230
RDA*		1,000–1,200	8–18	310–320	4,700	1,200–1,500	400	75	700	15–20	2.4	15		21–25	300
Race/Ethnicity:															
White	2,107	983	15.1	286	2,600	3,402	537	77.9	636	4.7	5.37	7.6	122	15.4	274
Black	2,021	800	13.6	234	2,128	3,178	465	103.2	539	3.5	4.75	6.5	122	12.7	281
Hispanic	2,027	945	14.5	273	2,449	3,114	518	94.2	540	4.9	5.08	6.2	114	15.9	287
Income Status:†															
Under 131% of poverty	1,999	888	13.8	251	2,309	3,086	493	85.7	542	4.4	4.32	6.2	126	13.8	264
131–185% of poverty	2,012	940	14.1	262	2,377	3,289	5151	80.9	566	4.5	4.85	6.5	122	14.2	295
Over 185% of poverty	2,112	973	15.2	289	2,603	3,454	543	83.9	639	4.7	5.42	7.6	119	15.7	279

*Values presented are Recommended Dietary Allowances (RDA) taken from Dietary Reference Intake reports published by the National Academy of Sciences, www.nap.edu, except for cholesterol based on 300mg recommended in the 2010 Dietary Guidelines forAmericans, www.nutrition.gov.

†Income status defined as percent of poverty level based on family income, family size, and composition using US Census Bureau poverty thresholds. The poverty threshold categories are related to Federal Nutrition Assistance Programs, www.fns.usda.gov.

Source: What We Eat in America, NHANES 2007–2008, one day, all individuals two-plus years (n = 8,529), excluding breast-fed children.

Despite of the diversity of foods available, most Americans have diets falling below recommended minimums for certain nutrients and above recommended maximums for others (Drewnowski, Maillot, & Rehm, 2012; Troesch, Hoeft, McBurney, Eggersdorfer, & Weber, 2012). In 2005–2008, almost all individuals regardless of age had diets below the DRI recommendations for potassium, dietary fiber, and vitamins D and E, and above the DRI for sodium. Further, one-third to one-half of individuals failed to meet their DRI recommendations for magnesium, calcium, vitamins A and C, and folate. Although only 10 and 4 percent of individuals, respectively, did not meet the recommendations for folate and iron, for females, the proportion was much greater. For folate, 20 percent of females fourteen years and older did not meet the recommendation; and for iron, 15 percent of females fourteen to fifty years of age did not. Although over a third of the population consumed inadequate cholesterol, an additional third exceeded the threshold of 300 mg of cholesterol, as recommended in the 2010 Dietary Guidelines for Americans and by numerous other scientific groups.

It should be noted that this evaluation covers dietary intake only, without consideration of use of **dietary supplements**. Use of dietary supplements has increased since the early 1990s (Gahche et al., 2011). However, Fulgoni and others (2011) have evaluated nutrient intakes from food and dietary supplements and reported that even after their supplement use, a significant proportion of individuals still did not get enough of vitamins A, C, D, and E, among others. Dietary supplements are not a substitute for a healthy diet—an important message emphasized in the 2010 Dietary Guidelines for Americans. Healthy food choices that are nutrient dense contain not only the essential vitamins and minerals but also dietary fiber and other naturally occurring substances not contained in dietary supplements, which may have additional positive health effects.

> **dietary supplements**
> Products intended to supplement the diet by providing vitamins, minerals, herbs, or other substances

Eating Away from Home

Americans are eating out more today than ever before. Food consumed away from home in 2007–2008 accounted for twice the proportion of average daily calories compared to that in 1977–1978: 34 percent versus 17. This increase is associated with the increase in total caloric intake, as further explored in perspective 15.1. A number of factors contributed to the trend of increased dining out, including a larger share of women employed outside the home and more convenient fast food outlets. Americans have more than five hundred thousand food service and drinking places to choose from when making away-from-home food choices (US Bureau of Census, 2009; USDA, 1984). The popularity of eating out presents a challenge for Americans. Studies have shown that food selections made away from home are higher in nutrients that Americans overconsume (e.g., fat and saturated fat) and lower in nutrients that Americans underconsume (e.g., calcium, fiber, and iron). Further, eating out is positively associated with body weight, a concern given that the prevalence of obesity has doubled between the 1970s and 2008 (Boumtje, Huang, Lee, & Lin, 2005; Guthrie, Lin, & Frazao, 2002; USDA & DHHS, 2010).

Perspective 15.1. The Supersizing of America: A Time for Action
Lisa R. Young

In 2002, my colleague Marion Nestle and I found that food portions available away from home had increased since the 1970s, and had done so in parallel with rising rates of obesity (Young & Nestle, 2002). Our 2012 follow-up paper found that portions of many foods available outside the home had continued to increase (Young &

(Continued)

Nestle, 2012) and are well beyond federal serving sizes used as standards for dietary guidance and food labels (Young & Nestle, 2003).

Large food portions may encourage people to consume more food (Rolls, Roe, & Meengs, 2006) and to underestimate calories consumed (Wansink & Chandon, 2006). Americans spend nearly half their food budgets on—and consume about one-third of their daily calories from—foods prepared outside the home, where portions have increased (US Department of Agriculture Economic Research Service [ERS], 2010).

Recent Changes in Food Portions

FIGURE 15.5   Parallel Trends in Rates of Overweight and Obesity, Calories Available in the Food Supply, and Introduction of New Large Size Portions, United States, 1960–2009

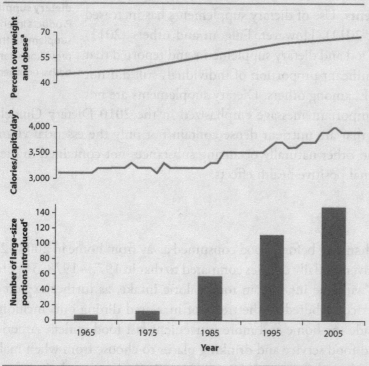

Source: USDA.

([a]US adults over age 20 BMI > 25). NHANES surveys from 1960–2008 (CDC, 2008).
[b]*USDA food availability series*: www.ers.usda.gov/Data/FoodConsumption
[c]Large portions introduced by decade; bars display midpoint year.

Portions of many foods have continued to increase, among them hamburgers, pizza, burritos, candy bars, and beverages. For example, McDonald's introduced an Angus Third Pounder (850 kcal) and Wendy's introduced larger-sized burgers including a Triple Baconator burger (~1,300 kcal). Burger King introduced a Quad Stacker sandwich (1,000 kcal) and a king-size forty-two-ounce soda (410 kcal). Its Original Whopper contained 670 kcal, but the more recent Triple Whopper provides 1,230 kcal with cheese. Subway introduced "Footlong" recession specials containing nearly 1,200 calories each. Hardee's debuted Thickburgers with two-thirds of a pound of beef; its Monster Thickburger contains 1,420 calories. For context, most Americans require 2,000 to 3,000 kcal per day to maintain weight. As shown in figure 15.5, this trend coincides with the availability of calories in the US food supply and the increasing prevalence of overweight among US adults.

Because the cost of food is low relative to the costs of labor and processing, competition has encouraged the food industry to offer larger portions as a way to expand market share. Food companies price larger portions favorably as a means to stimulate sales. At a local New York City Kentucky Fried Chicken (KFC), the smallest twenty-ounce soda costs twice as much per ounce as the sixty-four-ounce Mega Jug.

Food companies are reluctant to eliminate larger-size portions. When offering smaller sizes, they typically introduce new larger-size items concurrently. McDonald's dropped the term *Supersize*, but continues to sell large portions under different names. TGI Friday's offers a Right Portion Right Price promotion but also sells many larger portions, including a ten-ounce steak and a full rack of ribs.

A Call to Action

To address the problem with growing portion sizes, four approaches should be considered (discussed in greater detail in our 2012 article).

Education and Public Health Campaigns Aimed at Individuals

Health professionals should continue to advise patients to eat less by choosing smaller portions and eating only when hungry. Physicians and nutritionists should advocate portion-control strategies when advising patients who need to lose weight. Such approaches can be effective. Obese adults are more likely to report achieving meaningful weight loss if they consume smaller portions rather than by following fad diets (Nicklas, Huskey, Davis, & Wee, 2012).

Uniform and Reality-Based Serving-Size Standards

Serving size definitions need to be more consistent and comprehensible. The FDA establishes serving size standards for food labels and USDA uses a different set of standards for dietary guidance. Both sets are smaller than the amounts people typically eat and can be confusing, because the standards differ in size and units of measurement (Young & Nestle, 2012). Furthermore, FDA standards can be twice as large as USDA standards for common foods such as pasta, juice, and peanut butter. Neither agency intends its standards as recommendations for how much food individuals should consume at one time. One uniform system is needed to advise the public and explain the relationships among portion size, calories, and body weight.

Price Incentives for Smaller Portions

Offering price breaks and encouragement to reduce portion sizes may lead consumers to buy smaller portions. One study involved offering customers the option to order a half-size portion. Although only 1 percent of diners asked for smaller portions on their own, one-third accepted offers to downsize. They then consumed fewer calories and did not compensate by ordering more (Schwatz, Riis, Elbel, & Ariely, 2012).

Limits on Portion Sizes in Food Service Establishments

If voluntary efforts by food companies to reduce portion sizes continue to prove ineffective, policy approaches should be considered. A good starting point might be to insist on clear serving-size definitions and limitations on the amount of food allowed to be marketed as single servings. These could be limited to no more than twice the standard size given on food labels, or sixteen ounces for a soda, for example.

Health professionals and policy makers should be urged to consider these and other such approaches and work together to alleviate the effects of large food portions on weight gain.

MEAL PATTERNS—WHEN WE EAT

Meal patterns and snacking frequency are important dietary characteristics. In 2007–2008, two-thirds of individuals reported the standard three-meal pattern of breakfast, lunch, and dinner. Whites compared to blacks and Hispanics, and those in higher-income households compared to those in lower-income households, were more likely to eat three meals a day. Very young children (age two to five years) were most likely to report the three-meal pattern, and teens were the least likely. As

FIGURE 15.6   Contribution of Meal and Snacks to Energy, Sources of Energy, 2007–2008

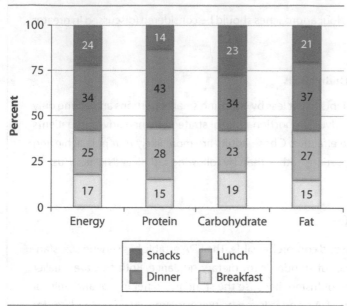

Source: USDA.

FIGURE 15.7   McDonald's McGriddle Is Eggs, Bacon, and Cheese Sandwiched between Two Pancakes

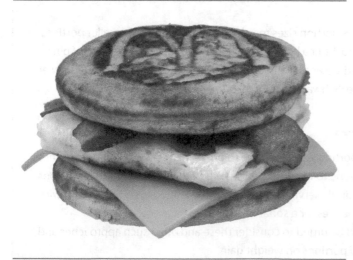

Source: Evan-Amos.

for snacks, regardless of age, at least half of the population reported eating snacks on three or more occasions per day. Figure 15.6 shows the contribution of meals and snacks to daily calories. About one-third of our daily calories were consumed at dinner, followed by one-fourth each at lunch and snacks, and 17 percent at breakfast.

Breakfast

In a study about breakfast in America in 2001–2002, the most frequently reported foods at breakfast included ready-to-eat cereals; breads, bagel, rolls, and English muffins; eggs; and fruits. The most frequently reported beverage was coffee followed by fruit juice, milk, and soda (USDA, 2007). Americans ate about one-fourth of breakfasts away from home, compared to 7 percent in the late 1970s. At these meals compared to those at home, respondents more frequently reported drinking soda and eating bacon and sausage, sweet rolls, fried potatoes, breakfast sandwiches, and eggs. These choices reflect the offerings at fast food establishments and convenience stores, the most frequently reported sources of away-from-home breakfast foods (see figure 15.7). By contrast, when eating at home, Americans more frequently reported eating ready-to-eat cereal, milk, fruits, and juice.

On any given day, 83 percent of Americans report eating breakfast (often referred to as the "most important meal of the day"). Nearly all of the very young (two to five years of age) report eating breakfast. Skipping breakfast is particularly common among teens and young adults, blacks, and those with lower family income. Compared to thirty years ago, the groups with the largest decline in eating breakfast are children and adolescents, with a greater decline for the latter than for any other age group. Then, at least 95 percent of children ate breakfast compared to now where 89 percent of children six to eleven years and 71 percent of teens eat breakfast. The decline in breakfast by adolescents may be positively associated with obesity, likely due to a mistaken belief that regular morning fasting is an effective weight loss strategy (Seiga-Riz, Popkin, & Carson, 1998).

TABLE 15.2   Percent of Daily Mean Intakes of Select Nutrients Provided by Meals and Snacks in the United States, 2007–2008

Nutrient	Breakfast %	Lunch %	Dinner %	Snacks %	Contribution for day %
Calories	17	25	35	24	100
Protein	15	28	43	14	100
Fat	18	27	37	21	100
Calcium	23	22	30	25	100
Iron	27	23	33	17	100
Magnesium	19	22	32	26	100
Potassium	20	23	35	22	100
Sodium	15	30	41	14	100
Folate	29	22	32	17	100
Vitamin C	22	20	30	28	100
Vitamin A	29	21	33	18	100
Vitamin D	36	18	28	18	100
Vitamin E	17	24	34	25	100
Total sugars	20	19	23	37	100
Dietary fiber	18	25	36	21	100
Cholesterol	28	25	37	10	100

Source: What We Eat in America, NHANES 2007–2008, one day, all individuals two-plus years (*n* = 8,529), excluding breast-fed children. Totals for contribution of meal and snack may not equal 100 due to rounding.

FIGURE 15.8   Cereal Label Showing Nutrients

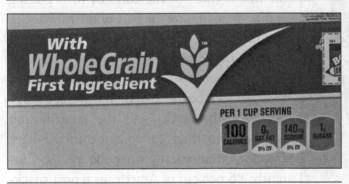

Source: CLF

Skipping breakfast means losing out on critical nutrients. Breakfast typically provides a big payoff in nutrients for the calories. Although breakfast contributes 17 percent of total daily caloric intake, it adds disproportionately to meeting recommended total daily nutrient intakes including for vitamin D (36 percent), folate and vitamin A (29 percent), iron (27 percent), calcium (23 percent), potassium (20 percent), and dietary fiber (18 percent) (see table 15.2). The greater contribution to nutrients from breakfast is not surprising since one-third of Americans report eating breakfast cereals and cereal bars, which are generally fortified with vitamins and minerals. As for nutrients Americans need to limit, breakfast contributes 20 percent of total sugars, 18 percent of fat, and 15 percent of sodium. (Figure 15.8 shows a breakfast cereal with a far better nutrient profile.)

Lunch

Lunch is just as important as breakfast, because it replenishes our bodies from the morning activities and gets us through the afternoon until dinner. Unlike breakfast, the percentage of Americans consuming lunch on any given day—80 percent—has not declined since the 1970s. Those who do skip lunch are more likely to be males seventy-plus years of age, blacks, Hispanics, and those from lower family income.

Lunch contributes a smaller proportion of total dietary intake now (one-fourth of calories on average) than it did in the 1970s (one-third). Generally speaking, the levels of needed nutrients in lunches tend to be reasonably proportional to the percent of daily calories. For nutrients Americans need to limit, lunch provides about 30 percent of the sodium, 27 percent of fat, and 19 percent of total sugars (see table 15.2).

Dinner

Dinner, the meal consumed at the end of the day, is rarely skipped. Almost all individuals (92 percent) report eating dinner. Of all meals and snacks, dinner provides the largest portion of daily calories—an average of about a third for adults and older children and about a fourth for very young children (two to five years). In the 1970s, dinner provided about 45 percent of the daily calories. Dinner also provides the largest proportion for many nutrients with two exceptions: vitamin D provided by breakfast and total sugars provided at snacks (see table 15.2).

Snacking

FIGURE 15.9   Vending Machines Facilitate Snacking

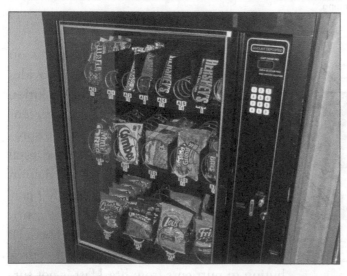

Source: Nenyedi.

We are a nation of snackers. For years, nutrition experts have advised that we eat small portions and eat frequently, in order to keep up our energy and as a strategy to avoid overeating unhealthy foods. A popular term for this is *grazing*. The concern with grazing is that many ignore the part of the message to eat only a little, yet pay attention to the part about eating often.

Prominence of snacking in the US diet today cannot be overstated. The average number of daily snacks and the contribution of snacks to total daily caloric intake have increased dramatically since the 1970s. Currently, 96 percent of Americans report snacking on any given day, and many are snacking extensively. Forty percent report three to four snacks per day and 16 percent report at least five or more snacks. In the mid-1990s about three-fourths of Americans reported snacking, up from a little over half in 1977–1978.

Snacks comprise on average about 25 percent of total daily caloric intake for adults and children compared to about 12 percent in the late 1970s. The calories from snacks are more likely to be coming from fat and carbohydrate than from protein (as in the snacks that can be obtained from the vending machine in figure 15.9). There is limited evidence supporting a positive relationship between snacking and nutrient intakes. Snacks provide at least 25 percent of the daily intakes of calcium, magnesium, and vitamins C and E. At the same time, they provide more than one-third of daily intake of total sugars, one-fifth of fat, and 14 percent of sodium.

In studies reported by Sebastian and others (2010, 2011), teens and adults who ate four or more snacks in a day consumed about one and a half times as many calories as those who reported no snacks.

That said, even though those who snacked more frequently had higher daily calorie intakes, their body mass index scores did not differ from their nonsnacking counterparts, possibly because they were more physically active.

WHAT WE EAT

The preceding section described what we eat based on *when* we eat it. Next, we take a closer look at *what* we eat specifically based on food groups. Tables 15.3 and 15.4 summarize, respectively, daily food and beverage intakes in grams for twelve major groups of foods and beverages and selected subgroups, and the percent of calories, protein, carbohydrates, sugars, and fats in US diets from these groups. Amounts

TABLE 15.3 Daily Mean Food Intakes* and Their Contribution to Daily Energy and Sources of Energy in the United States, 2007–2008

Major Food Groups and Selected Subgroups†	Reporting %	Intake/Day g	Food energy %	Protein %	Carbohydrate %	Sugars %	Fat %
Grains	95	172	25	14	32	16	19
Breads and Rolls	60	43	6	5	8	2	2
Sweet Bakery Products	43	34	6	2	7	9	6
Savory Snacks and Crackers	46	20	5	2	5	#	6
Mixed Dishes	70	258	20	29	16	5	24
Pasta, Macaroni, Rice Mixed Dishes	21	58	4	4	4	1	4
Meat, Poultry, Seafood Mixed Dishes	22	53	4	7	2	1	4
Soups	13	51	1	2	1	1	1
Pizza	13	29	4	5	3	1	5
Protein Foods	81	140	16	35	3	1	26
Poultry	27	32	4	10	1	#	5
Cured Meats and Poultry	36	27	3	6	#	#	6
Legumes and Nuts/Seeds	9	12	1	1	1	#	1
Eggs and Egg Dishes	19	21	2	3	#	#	1
Seafood	9	11	1	3	#	#	1
Dairy	83	244	11	14	8	16	14
Milk, whole and reduced fat	32	101	3	4	2	4	3
Milk, lowfat and nonfat	15	49	1	2	1	2	#
Flavored milk	6	20	1	1	1	2	1
Ice cream	17	21	2	1	2	4	2
Vegetables and Fruits	79	206	8	4	11	10	6
Vegetables	67	118	5	3	6	2	6
Fruits	44	88	3	1	5	8	#
Other Foods	86	61	7	2	8	13	10
Candy	29	11	3	1	4	5	2
Total		1,081	87	98	78	100	99

*Food group quantities represent average intakes of both consumers (users of that group) and nonconsumers on the survey day. Quantities for consumers alone can be calculated by dividing the average intake of a food group by percentage of individuals using foods from that group.
†Foods included in the major food groups and subgroups based on the What We Eat in America Food Categories available at www.ars.usda.gov/ba/bhnrc/fsrg.
#Indicates a nonzero value too small to print
Source: What We Eat in America, NHANES 2007–2008, one day, all individuals two-plus years (*n* = 8,529), excluding breast-fed children.

TABLE 15.4 Daily Mean Beverage and Water Intakes* and Their Contribution to Daily Energy in the United States, 2007–2008

Major Beverage Groups and Selected Subgroups[†]	Reporting %	Intake/Day g	Food Energy	Protein %	Carbohydrate %	Sugars %	Fat %
Sweetened Beverages	52	358	7	1	14	27	#
Soft drinks	36	243	5	#	9	19	#
Fruit drinks	18	79	2	#	3	6	#
Diet Beverages	18	129	#	#	#	#	#
Diet Soft Drinks	16	129	#	#	#	#	#
Alcoholic Beverages	18	140	3	1	2	1	#
Beer	11	117	2	1	1	#	0
Wine	5	13	1	#	#	#	#
100% Juice	24	81	2	#	4	6	#
Citrus Juices	14	41	1	#	2	3	#
Fruit juices, other than citrus	11	36	1	#	2	3	#
Coffee and Tea							
Coffee	40	249	#	1	#	1	#
Tea	25	175	1	#	2	3	#
Water	77	937	#	#	#	#	0
Tap and Plain Bottled Water	76	913	0	0	0	0	0
Flavored/enhanced Water	3	25	#	#	#	0	#
Total		1,132	13	3	22	38	1

*Beverage group quantities represent average intakes of both consumers (users of that group) and nonconsumers on the survey day. Quantities for consumers alone can be calculated by dividing the average intake of a food group by percentage of individuals using foods from that group.
[†]Beverages included in the major beverage groups and subgroups based on the What We Eat in America Food Categories available at www.ars.usda.gov/ba/bhnrc/fsrg.
#Indicates a nonzero value too small to print
Source: What We Eat in America, NHANES 2007–2008, one day, all individuals two-plus years (*n* = 8,529), excluding breast-fed children.

are based on the foods and beverages as consumed. The sections following describe intakes by major groups in descending order of contribution to daily calories.

Grains and Grain Products

Grains and grain products make up one-fourth of Americans' calories and almost one-third of the carbohydrates we eat. Of the grain products in our diets, breads and rolls make up about one-fourth and sweet bakery products, including cakes, pies, cookies, brownies, doughnuts, and pastries, are also substantial at 20 percent.

Mixed Dishes

Mixed dishes include multi-ingredient foods such as stew, meatloaf, pizza, soup, pasta, and rice dishes. These types of foods have become increasingly popular and today they comprise about one-fifth of our daily calories and nearly one-third of our daily protein. We eat more than double the amount of mixed dishes today compared to the 1970s. Three main categories of mixed dish foods each account for about a fifth of our consumption: pasta- and rice-based dishes; meat-, poultry-, and seafood-based dishes; and soups.

Pizza is an example of the growing popularity of these types of foods. Compared to the 1970s, the percentage of Americans reporting eating pizza on any given day has tripled from 4 to 13 percent. Children six to eleven years of age are the group most likely to report pizza at 22 percent. Averaged across the whole population, pizza contributed 4 percent of calories. However, for those who reported eating pizza on a given day, it accounted for more than one-fourth of their calories that day (at 27 percent) (Rhodes, Adler, Clemens, LaComb, & Moshfegh, 2014). The amount of pizza consumed has also increased over time, from roughly the equivalent of one slice (one-eighth of a large cheese pizza) to the equivalent of more than two slices.

Protein Foods

Although many foods have protein in them, the category of protein foods refers to foods chiefly composed of protein, including separate pieces of meat, poultry, or seafood; cured meat and poultry products; eggs; legumes and nuts and seeds. We eat about six ounces of such foods on average per day. These foods contribute the largest proportions of daily protein and fat in our diets at 35 and 26 percent, respectively, and 16 percent of daily calorie intake. Despite dietary guidance to replace protein foods that are higher in solid fats with choices that are lower (USDA and DHHS, 2010), animal sources account for about two-thirds of the protein foods by weight. Today we eat slightly more poultry than red meat; thirty years ago we ate about three times as much red meat as poultry.

Dairy

Americans consume an average of eight ounces of dairy products each day. We drink over 70 percent of this (six fluid ounces) as milk. Despite the 2010 Dietary Guidelines recommendation to consume low-fat or nonfat milk, over half of the milk consumed is whole or reduced-fat milk (USDA and DHHS, 2010).

A study of 2005–2006 national survey data found that children two to eleven years of age consumed the most milk—about twice as much as adults (Sebastian, Goldman, & Wilkinson Enns, 2010). Milk intake was related to race or ethnicity but not income. Blacks consumed less milk than whites and Mexican Americans, potentially related to the high rates of lactose intolerance among African Americans. Milk intake is associated with intakes of vitamin D, potassium, and calcium, nutrients most Americans need to consume more of. Those who drink milk had intakes of vitamin D, calcium, and potassium 180, 49, and 16 percent higher, respectively, than those who did not report drinking milk (Sebastian et al., 2010).

Cheese is an ingredient in many mixed dishes and is eaten by itself. In a study assessing cheese intake from all food sources in 2001–2002, more than two-thirds of individuals reported eating cheese and foods containing cheese on any given day (Martin, Carlson, Bowman, Clemens, & Moshfegh, 2012). The average daily intake of cheese from all food sources was just over an ounce at thirty-one grams. Most cheese (81 percent) was consumed as part of a mixed dish or in combination with another food item. Sandwiches represent the top source of cheese in the diet. As with milk, whites consumed significantly more cheese than blacks, thirty-four grams and twenty-two grams, respectively.

Vegetables

FIGURE 15.10   Change in Percentage Reporting Fruits and Vegetables

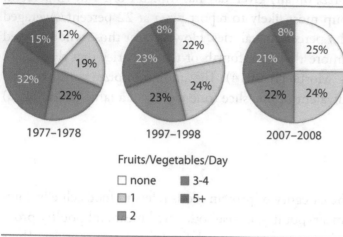

1977–1978   1997–1998   2007–2008

Fruits/Vegetables/Day

☐ none   ◼ 3-4
▦ 1   ◼ 5+
▦ 2

Source: USDA.

A key dietary message to Americans is to consume adequate amounts of vegetables and fruits. In messages for consumers based on the 2010 Dietary Guidelines for Americans, it was recommended that vegetables and fruits should make half your plate (USDA Center for Nutrition Policy and Promotion, 2011). Despite these messages, one out of every four Americans reports eating no vegetable or fruit (excluding juices) on any given day, twice that compared to three decades ago (see figure 15.10). Further, nearly half of Americans (46 percent) report eating only one to two vegetables or fruits per day.

Produce consumption varies by socioeconomic background. By income status, those in lower-income households consumed the least vegetables. Kirkpatrick and others (2012) have also reported that race and ethnicity and income are associated with vegetable intake. Hispanics consumed significantly fewer vegetables compared to whites and blacks.

Mean intake of vegetables is 118 grams per day. For context, a small fast food order of French fried potatoes weighs about 85 grams, a medium baked potato weighs about 170 grams, and one cherry tomato, two raw baby carrots, or two cooked broccoli florets weigh about 20 grams. White potatoes, the most frequently reported vegetable, are eaten by one-third of Americans on any given day. They represent one-third of all vegetable consumption (40 grams). About half of the white potatoes eaten are in the form of fried potatoes. Americans consume low levels of nutrient-packed red and yellow and dark-green vegetables despite guidance to do otherwise. Men twenty years of age and older consume an average of twenty-six grams of red and yellow and dark-green vegetables per day, and women consume an average of thirty-two grams.

Fruits

Just under half of Americans report eating fruit (excluding juices) on any given day. Mean intake is eighty-eight grams per day. For context, a medium three-inch apple weighs about 180 grams. Very young children two to five years of age consume the most fruits on any given day and teens twelve to nineteen years of age consume the least, 116 and 69 grams, respectively. Given how much more teens weigh than two- to five-year-olds, this disparity in fruit intakes is even greater. The most frequently reported fruits include apples and bananas, followed by oranges, melons, and berries.

Snack Foods

Snack foods, including savory snacks (e.g., potato and corn chips), crackers, sweet bakery products (e.g., cookies, cakes, and pies), ice cream, and candy, provide more than one out of every five calories eaten by Americans each day. Although these types of snack foods can make some positive contributions to intake of key nutrients, several studies have found that more frequent snacking was associated with higher total energy intake and a higher proportion of energy provided by added and total sugars (Larson & Story, 2013). These types of foods are very popular and widely available in various diverse settings where Americans spend their time. Sweet bakery products are eaten by half of Americans each day and savory snacks and crackers and candy are each eaten by about a third.

Beverages and Water

Americans consume an average of just over five cups (forty-three fluid ounces) of beverages (drinks other than water) each day. Intakes of the subgroups "coffee and tea" and "sweetened beverages" each make up about one-third of beverage intake (fourteen and twelve fluid ounces, respectively). All other drinks, including milk, unsweetened juices, diet beverages, and alcohol, comprise the last third. Americans drink about one-third the amount of diet beverages as they do sweetened beverages. Children age six to eleven years drink slightly more soft drinks and fruit drinks combined (ten fluid ounces) than milk (nine fluid ounces), and teens aged twelve to nineteen years drink twice as much (fourteen and seven fluid ounces, respectively). Three-fourths of Americans report drinking water on any given day. Mean daily intake is four cups (thirty-two fluid ounces). All beverages including water are consumed several times during the day.

Beverages are a significant source of calories and nutrients. Overall, beverages contribute 13 percent of daily calorie intake and more than one-third (38 percent) of daily total sugar intake. Sweetened soft drinks are the largest contributor to total sugars in the diet. Numerous studies examining the association between increased intake of sugar-sweetened beverages and later weight change are supportive of an association suggesting that a high intake of sugar-sweetened beverages increases the risk of obesity and diabetes. Some scientists have stated that sufficient evidence exists for public strategies to discourage consumption of sugary drinks as part of a healthy lifestyle. As well, local and state policies to limit sales of soft drinks in schools or sales of larger sizes of soft drinks in public establishments are emerging in an effort to curtail excessive intake.

In a study on beverage choices of adults, beverages (not surprisingly) provided all the alcohol and most of the caffeine—they also contributed considerable amounts of nutrients including vitamins C and D (LaComb, Sebastian, Wilkinson Enns, & Goldman, 2011). Consumption of beverages by adults differed by race and ethnicity. Whites consumed more beverages overall relative to blacks and Hispanics. Whites and Hispanics consumed more milk and milk drinks than blacks. Whites also consumed more coffee, tea, and diet soft drinks than blacks or Hispanics.

The Food We Do Not Eat

The preceding sections have provided an overview of what we eat. It is important also to consider what we *do not* eat. Food is wasted all along the chain from production to consumption, as described in focus 15.3, with profound implications for our food system and environment.

FOCUS 15.3. WHAT ABOUT THE FOOD THAT'S NOT EATEN? FOOD WASTE IN AMERICA AND ITS ECOLOGICAL IMPACTS

Dana Gunders

Imagine leaving the grocery store with five bags filled to the brim with your favorite foods. As you walk through the parking lot, two slip out of your hand. You look at them, shrug, and just keep walking. Seems ridiculous, right? But that is essentially what is occurring throughout our food system.

How Much Food Is Wasted?

In the United States, about 40 percent of all edible food goes uneaten (Hall et al., 2009). A large portion of that waste is caused by consumers. Potatoes are left on a breakfast platter, lettuce goes bad hidden in the back of the fridge, and chips remain on the nacho plate because who can really eat *that* many chips, particularly the ones without cheese?

What Does Wasting Food Cost Us?

The cost of wasted food is enormous. The average American throws away $31 per month, in the form of about twenty-four pounds of food (Buzby, Wells, & Hyman, 2014). Nationally, we toss around $162 billion per year in consumer- and retail-level food waste (Buzby, Wells, & Hyman, 2014).

The needless resource use is also staggering. First, there are the water, energy, chemicals, and greenhouse gas emissions that go into producing, packaging, and transporting discarded food. Then, nearly all food waste ends up in landfills where it decomposes and releases methane, a greenhouse gas at least thirty-four times more potent than carbon dioxide. Consider these resource estimates used to produce all the food that never gets eaten in the United States:

- 25 percent of all freshwater used in the United States (Hall et al., 2009)

- 4 percent of total US oil consumption (Hall et al., 2009)

- 35 million tons of landfill waste (and related greenhouse gas emissions) (US Environmental Protection Agency, 2012)

Nutrition is also lost. Even today, about one in six Americans lacks a secure supply of food. Reducing wasted food in the United States by 30 percent would amount to enough food to feed all fifty million food-insecure Americans their total diet, if it were distributed appropriately (assuming 2,500 kcal per capita per day and an annual total of 150 trillion calories in losses, as reported in Hall et al. [2009]).

Why Is Food Wasted?

Addressing wasted food is not as straightforward as taking fewer potatoes on your breakfast plate (though that is a good start). Food is lost all along the supply chain, and the reasons vary. On farms, entire fields are sometimes left unharvested because the price farmers would receive is too low for them to recoup even the costs of harvesting. Inventory can be left over at distribution centers. Grocery stores overstock their shelves in the hopes that abundant food displays will inspire more sales. In restaurants, long menus and large portions—often two to eight times government recommended serving sizes—can lead to waste. And then there's us, consumers, tossing half a sandwich because we don't feel like carrying it home.

At the heart of this problem are two basic realities. First, food represents a small portion of many Americans' budgets, both individuals and businesses, making the financial cost of wasting food too low to outweigh the convenience. Second, the more food consumers waste, the more those in the food industry can sell. This is true throughout the supply chain in which waste downstream translates to higher sales for anyone upstream. Overcoming these and other drivers of food waste will require raising the issue's priority to the level it merits.

What Can Be Done about It?

The good news is, it doesn't have to be this way. In fact, we weren't always this wasteful. Today, we discard 50 percent more food in the United States than we did in the 1970s (Hall et al., 2009).

Much can be learned from work underway in Europe. Both the United Kingdom (UK) and the European Union have conducted research to outline drivers and identify potential solutions to food waste. In January 2012, the European Parliament adopted a resolution to reduce food waste by 50 percent by 2020 and designated 2014 as the "European year against food waste" (Parliament calls for urgent measures to ban food waste in the E.U., 2012). An extensive British campaign called "Love Food Hate Waste" has since 2006 raised awareness through advertisements, information on food storage and preparation, and in-store education. In just five years, avoidable household food waste in the UK decreased 21 percent through a combination of that campaign and higher food prices (WRAP, 2012). In addition, more than fifty leading food retailers and brands in the UK jointly committed to reduce waste in their own operations, as well as upstream and downstream in the supply chain. As part of this effort, companies have reengineered processing methods, streamlined product delivery systems, and developed innovative packaging that enables reuse and longer shelf life.

There will always be some food waste, but composting is a much preferred disposal solution over landfill because it can recycle nutrients and reduce greenhouse gas emissions. Anaerobic digestion is another option, which generates energy out of food and then enables what's left to be composted.

We can all be part of the solution. As you go about shopping, cooking, and eating in your everyday life, remember that even the most sustainably farmed food does us no good if it is never eaten.

CONCLUSION

This chapter provides a descriptive overview of US diets in aggregate: when we eat and what we eat. Americans have become increasingly aware of the importance of diet to maintain health and reduce the risk of chronic diseases; however, we still underconsume some nutrients and overconsume others. Further, there remain disparities in diet healthfulness. Chapter 16 will put this information into clearer context by explaining the core principles of nutrition. It should be emphasized that despite the utility of discussing diets in a granular way based on specific nutrients, a total diet approach gives a richer perspective on what we eat across meals and on the types of opportunities for making change. Additional richness also comes from examining the great differences in diets across the United States by demography, geography, and other factors; however, that is beyond the scope of this chapter.

Major shifts in where and when we eat have occurred since the 1970s. Snacking has become a way of life, with a majority of Americans snacking at least three or more times a day compared to nearly half of Americans not snacking at all in the late 1970s. Today, snacking provides one-fourth of our total daily calories. There has also been a shift in where we eat: we now consume a third of our calories from away-from-home sources such as restaurants and fast food establishments, a doubling from the late 1970s. This overview of "what we eat" provides key grounding for understanding the food system as it exists today. What we eat determines what we produce (and the reverse as well). This chapter describes a food system substantially balanced toward producing grain and animal protein products and requiring a vast food processing industry to turn raw products into the consumed foodstuffs. Further, although the survey, What We Eat in America, does not distinguish by season or geography, we can infer from the eating patterns that the chapter is describing a food system far removed from the rhythms of nature, when the types of foods we eat would necessarily vary by season and region. Accordingly, this system requires an extensive distribution network, including not only transportation but also a well-developed sector of intermediaries engaged in brokering domestic and international trade. By describing what—and how much—we eat, this chapter also provides some insights into how our dietary choices may play out in diet-related disease and environmental impacts.

This chapter can help us develop a positive vision for the US diet of the future: what trends are most important to encourage? To reverse? Based on what we know today, what are the most important overall directions for change?

SUMMARY

Understanding what we eat can provide insights into the impact of diet on health outcomes, disease risk, food system shifts, agricultural production, and environmental issues. Americans' food and beverage choices are dynamic and reflect an ever-changing food supply. Because foods and beverages and their nutrient content are fundamental to maintaining optimal health and preventing chronic disease, timely and accurate information on what Americans are eating and drinking is essential. Dietary data collected through nationwide surveys provide useful benchmark data and are valuable for assessing the impact of public food and health programs, determining food policies and regulations, and providing a primary data source for applied nutrition research including disease risk assessment, nutrition and health issues, food safety, economics, and environmental issues. The data are also used to formulate dietary recommendations for the population. The US diet has diversified immensely since the 1970s, but many people still fail to meet dietary recommendations. On average, Americans consume too many calories and sodium, and too little potassium, dietary fiber, calcium, and vitamin D. Americans, on average, consume more two hundred calories more per day than in 1977–1978. One-third of calories come from fat today compared to 43 percent in 1977–1978 and 50 percent from carbohydrates compared to 40 percent then. The contribution of protein remained at 15 percent of calories. Snacking, eating away from home and portion sizes have increased substantially over time. Finally, about 40 percent of edible food is thrown out.

KEY TERMS

ChooseMyPlate	Food balance sheets
Dietary Guidelines for Americans (DGA)	Food frequency questionnaire
Dietary reference intakes (DRIs)	Food record
Dietary supplements	Healthy People 2020
Diet history method	Total diet approach
Food availability assessment	Twenty-four-hour dietary recall
Food availability data series	What We Eat in America (WWEIA)

DISCUSSION QUESTIONS

1. If future archaeologists read this chapter, what might they infer about the food system and society based on the description of what we eat?

2. What are some of the most important changes to the US diet since the 1970s? Why have they occurred? What trends in US diets are most important to encourage? To reverse?

3. What are some of the ways our diets influence the broad US food system and ways the food system influences our diets?

4. Sodium consumption far exceeds recommended levels. Should the responsibility for decreasing sodium levels in foods be shifted to food manufacturers or should we as individuals be more aware of our sodium consumption? Or should both occur? Explain your reasoning.

5. Based on the information in this chapter, which groups are most at risk for nutrient deficiencies? What else would you like to know about diets in those groups to help identify ways to reduce those risks?

6. What are strengths and limitations of each of the four methods of dietary assessment?

7. What can be done to reduce the trend toward large portions in restaurants? Will consumers patronize restaurants that shrink portion sizes?

8. What do you think can be done on your campus to reduce the amount of food that gets wasted?

9. Why do you think we are wasting more food now than in the 1970s?

ACKNOWLEDGMENTS

The author acknowledges and thanks John C. Clemens, statistician, and Arminda Kovalchik, nutritionist, Food Surveys Research Group, Beltsville Human Nutrition Research Center, US Department of Agriculture, for data programming and statistical analyses and technical assistance, respectively.

REFERENCES

Boumtje, P. I., Huang, C. L., Lee, J.-Y., & Lin, B.-H., et al. (2005). Dietary habits, demographics, and the development of overweight and obesity among children in the United States. *Food Policy*, 30, 115–128.

Brooks, N., Regmi, A., & Jerardo, A. (2010). *U.S. food import patterns, 1998–2007 (FAU-125)*. Washington, DC: US Department of Agriculture Economic Research Service.

Buzby, J. C., Wells, H. F., & Hyman, J. (2014). The estimated amount, value, and calories of postharvest food losses at the retail and consumer levels in the United States. US Department of Agriculture Economic Information Bulletin 121. Retrieved from www.ers.usda.gov/publications/eib-economic-information-bulletin/eib121.aspx#.U4k0xi9upVs

Centers for Disease Control and Prevention. (2008). *Prevalence of overweight, obesity and extreme obesity among adults: United States, trends 1960–62 through 2005–2006*. Retrieved from www.cdc.gov/nchs/data/hestat/overweight/overweight_adult.htm

Drewnowski, A., Maillot, M., & Rehm, C. (2012). Reducing the sodium-potassium ratio in the US diet: A challenge for public health. *American Journal of Clinical Nutrition*, 96, 439–444.

Food and Agriculture Organization. (nd). *Food balance sheets*. Retrieved from http://faostat.fao.org/site/354/default.aspx

Food Marketing Institute. (2012). *Supermarket facts: Industry overview 2012*. Retrieved from www.fmi.org/research-resources/supermarket-facts

Fulgoni, V. L., Keast, D. R., Bailey, R. L., & Dwyer, J. (2011). Foods, fortificants, and supplements: Where do Americans get their nutrients? *Journal of Nutrition, 141*(10), 1847–1854.

Gahche, J., Bailey, R., Burt, V., Hughes, J., Yetley, E., Dwyer, J., Picciano, M. F., McDowell, M., & Sempos C. (2011). *Dietary supplement use among U.S. adults has increased since NHANES III (1988–1994)* (NCHS Data Brief No. 61), 1–8. Retrieved from www.cdc.gov/nchs/data/databriefs/db61.pdf

Guthrie, J., Lin, B., & Frazao, E. (2002). Role of food prepared away from home in the American diet, 1977–78 versus 1994–96: Changes and consequences. *Journal of Nutrition Education, 34*, 140–150.

Hall, K. D., Guo, J., Dore, M., & Chow, C. C. (2009). The progressive increase of food waste in America and its environmental impact. *PLOS ONE, 4*(11), e7940.

Institute of Medicine Food and Nutrition Board. (2000). *Dietary reference intakes: Applications in dietary assessment*. Washington, DC: National Academies Press.

Kantor, L., Lipton, K., Manchester, A., & Oliveira, V. (1997). *Estimating and addressing America's food losses (Food Review No. FR-20–1)*. Washington, DC: US Department of Agriculture Economic Research Service.

Kipnis, V., Subar, A. F., Midthune, D., Freedman, L. S., Ballard-Barbash, R., Troiano, R. P., Bingham, S., Schoeller, D. A., Schatzkin, A., & Carroll, R. J. (2003). Structure of dietary measurement error: Results of the OPEN biomarker study. *American Journal of Epidemiology, 158*(1), 14–21.

Kirkpatrick, S. I., Dodd, K. W., Reedy, J., & Krebs-Smith, S. M. (2012). Income and race/ethnicity are associated with adherence to food-based dietary guidance among US Adults and Children. *Journal of The Academy of Nutrition and Dietetics, 112*, 624–635.

LaComb, R. P., Sebastian, R. S., Wilkinson Enns, C., & Goldman, J. D. (2011). *Beverage choices of U.S. adults: What we eat in America, NHANES 2007–2008* (Food Surveys Research Group Dietary Data Brief No. 6). Retrieved from www.ars.usda.gov/SP2UserFiles/Place/12355000/pdf/DBrief/6_beverage_choices_adults_0708.pdf

Larson, N., & Story, M. (2013). A review of snacking patterns among children and adolescents: What are the implications of snacking for weight status? *Childhood Obesity, 9*, 2.

Martin, C., Carlson, J., Bowman, S. A., Clemens, J., & Moshfegh, A. J. (2012). *Cheese in the American diet: Foods contributing to cheese intake in WWEIA, NHANES 2001–2002*. Poster presented at the 36th National Nutrient Databank Conference, March, Houston.

Moshfegh, A. J., Rhodes, D. G., Baer, D. J., Murayi, T., Clemens, J. C., Rumpler, W. V., Paul, D. R., Sebastian, R. S., Kuczynski, K. J., Ingwersen, L. A., Staples, R. C., & Cleveland, L. E. (2008). The US Department of Agriculture automated multiple-pass method reduces bias in the collection of energy intakes. *American Journal of Clinical Nutrition, 88*, 324–332.

Nicklas, J. M., Huskey, K. W., Davis, R. B., & Wee, C. C. (2012). Successful weight loss among obese US adults. *American Journal of Preventive Medicine, 42*(5), 481–485.

Pao, E. M., & Cypel, Y. S. (1996). Estimation of dietary intake. In E. E. Ziegler & L. J. Filer (Eds.), *Present knowledge in nutrition*. (7th ed.). Washington, DC: ILSI Press.

Parliament calls for urgent measures to ban food waste in the E.U. (2012). *European Parliament News*, January 19.

Raper, N., Perloff, B., Ingwersen, L., Steinfeldt, L., & Anand, J. (2004). An overview of USDA's dietary intake data system. *Journal of Food Composition and Analysis, 17*, 545–555.

Rhodes, D. G., Adler, M. S., Clemens, J. C., LaComb, R. P., & Moshfegh, A. J. (2014). *Consumption of pizza: What we eat in America, NHANES 2007–2010* (Food Surveys Research Group Dietary Data Brief No. 11). Retrieved from www.ars.usda.gov/SP2UserFiles/Place/12355000/pdf/DBrief/11_consumption_of_pizza_0710.pdf

Rolls, B. J., Roe, L. S., & Meengs, J. S. (2006). Large portion sizes lead to a sustained increase in energy intake over 2 days. *Journal of the American Dietetic Association, 106*(4), 543–549.

Schatzkin, A., Kipnis, V., Carroll, R. J., Midthune, D., Subar, A. F., Bingham, S., Schoeller, D. A., et al. (2003). A comparison of a food frequency questionnaire with a 24-hour recall for use in an epidemiological cohort study: Results from The Biomarker-based Observing Protein and Energy (OPEN) study. *International Journal of Epidemiology*, *32*(6), 1054–1062.

Schwatz, J., Riis, J., Elbel, B., & Ariely, D. (2012). Inviting consumers to downsize fast-food portions significantly reduces calorie consumption. *Health Affairs*, *31*(2), 399–407.

Sebastian, R. S., Goldman J. D., & Wilkinson Enns, C. (2010). *Snacking patterns of U.S. adolescents: What we eat in America, NHANES 2005–2006* (Food Surveys Research Group Dietary Data Brief No. 2). Retrieved from www.ars.usda.gov/SP2UserFiles/Place/12355000/pdf/DBrief/2_adolescents_snacking_0506.pdf

Sebastian, R. S., Goldman, J. D., Wilkinson Enns, C., & LaComb, R. P. (2010). *Fluid milk consumption in the United States: What we eat in America, NHANES 2005–2006* (Food Surveys Research Group Dietary Data Brief No. 3). Retrieved from www.ars.usda.gov/SP2UserFiles/Place/12355000/pdf/DBrief/3_milk_consumption_0506.pdf

Sebastian, R. S., Wilkinson Enns, C., & Goldman, J. D. (2011). *Snacking patterns of U.S. adults: What we eat in America, NHANES 2007–2008* (Food Surveys Research Group Dietary Data Brief No. 4). Retrieved from www.ars.usda.gov/SP2UserFiles/Place/12355000/pdf/DBrief/4_adult_snacking_0708.pdf

Siega-Riz, A., Popkin, B., & Carson, T. (1998). Trends in breakfast consumption for children in the United States from 1965 to 1991. *American Journal of Clinical Nutrition*, *67*(Suppl.), 748S–765S.

Subar, A. F., Kirkpatrick, S. I., Mittl, B., Zimmerman, T. P., Thompson, F. E., Bingley, C., Willis, G., et al. (2012). The automated self-administered 24-hour dietary recall (ASA24): A resource for researchers, clinicians, and educators from the National Cancer Institute. *Journal of the American Academy of Nutrition and Dietetics*, *112*(8), 1113–1296.

Troesch, B., Hoeft, B., McBurney, M., Eggersdorfer, M., & Weber, P. (2012). Dietary surveys indicate vitamin intakes below recommendations are common in representative western countries. *British Journal of Nutrition*, *108*, 692–698.

US Bureau of the Census. (2009). *2007 economic survey. Sector 72: EC077211: Accommodation and food services: Industry series: Preliminary summary statistics for the United States: 2007*. Retrieved from www.quora.com/How-many-restaurants-are-there-in-the-US

US Department of Agriculture. (1984). *Nutrient intakes: Individuals in 48 states, year 1977–78*. Retrieved from www.ars.usda.gov/SP2UserFiles/Place/12355000/pdf/7778/nfcs7778_rep_i-2.pdf

US Department of Agriculture. (2007). *Breakfast in America, 2001–2002*. Retrieved from www.ars.usda.gov/SP2UserFiles/Place/12355000/pdf/DBrief/1_Breakfast_2001_2002.pdf

US Department of Agriculture Center for Nutrition Policy and Promotion. (2011). *ChooseMyPlate*. Retrieved from www.choosemyplate.gov

US Department of Agriculture Economic Research Service. (2010). *Food marketing system in the U.S.: Food service*. Retrieved from www.ers.usda.gov/Briefing/FoodMarketingSystem/foodservice.htm

US Department of Agriculture Economic Research Service. (nda). *Food availability (per capita) data system*. Retrieved from www.ers.usda.gov/data-products/food-availability-(per-capita)-data-system.aspx

US Department of Agriculture Economic Research Service. (ndb). *New product introductions of consumer packaged goods, 1992–2009*. Retrieved from http://search.ers.usda.gov/search?affiliate=ers&query=New%20Product%20Introductions%20of%20Consumer%20packaged%20Goods,%201992–2009

US Department of Agriculture and US Department of Health and Human Services. (2010). *Dietary guidelines for Americans, 2010* (7th ed.). Washington, DC: US Government Printing Office. Retrieved from www.ers.usda.gov/Data/FoodConsumption/

US Department of Health and Human Services. (2010). *Healthy people 2020*. Retrieved from www.healthypeople.gov

US Department of Health and Human Services. (nd). *National health and nutrition examination survey 1999–2014 survey content*. Retrieved from www.cdc.gov/nchs/data/nhanes/survey_content_99_14.pdf

US Department of Health and Human Services, Centers for Disease Control and Prevention. (2014). *National Health and Nutrition Examination Survey*. Retrieved from http://www.cdc.gov/nchs/nhanes.htm

US Environmental Protection Agency. (2012). *Municipal solid waste generation, recycling, and disposal in the United States: Facts and figures for 2012*. Retrieved from www.epa.gov/waste/nonhaz/municipal/msw99.htm

Wansink, B., & Chandon, P. (2006). Meal size, not body size, explains errors in estimating the calorie content of meals. *Annals of Internal Medicine, 5*(5), 326–332.

WRAP. (2012). *Household food and drink waste in the U.K. 2012* Retrieved from www.wrap.org.uk/content/household-food-and-drink-waste-uk-2012

Young, L. R., & Nestle, M. (2002). The contribution of increasing portion sizes to the obesity epidemic. *American Journal of Public Health, 92*(2), 246–249.

Young, L. R., & Nestle, M. (2003). Expanding portion sizes in the US marketplace: Implications for nutrition counseling. *Journal of the American Dietetic Association, 103*(2), 231–234.

Young, L. R., & Nestle, M. (2012). Reducing portion sizes to prevent obesity: A call to action. *American Journal of Preventive Medicine, 43*(5), 565–568.

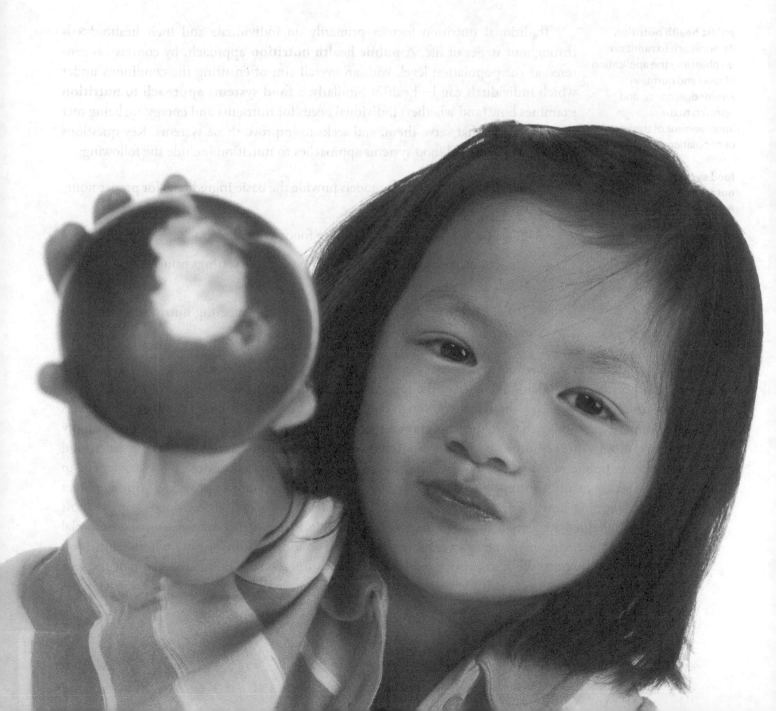

Chapter 16

Nutrition

Courtney A. Pinard, Amy L. Yaroch, and Teresa M. Smith

Learning Objectives

- Understand the science of nutrition within the broader context of food systems and the public health nutrition approach.

- Describe nutrient composition, additives, dietary recommendations, and how whole foods can achieve necessary nutrition.

- List potential impacts on the human body when there is an oversupply or undersupply of specific nutrients.

- Understand how the current state of the food system affects Americans' dietary habits.

public health nutrition
An approach to nutrition emphasizing the application of food and nutrition knowledge, policy, and research to the improvement of the health of populations

food systems approach to nutrition
Approach that considers the impacts of food on human health and the processes involved in producing, transforming, distributing, accessing, consuming, and disposing of food

Traditional nutrition focuses primarily on individuals and their health needs throughout stages of life. A **public health nutrition** approach, by contrast, is centered at the population level, with an overall aim of ensuring the conditions under which individuals can be healthy. Similarly, a **food systems approach to nutrition** examines how (and whether) individual needs for nutrients and energy are being met by the systems that serve them, and seeks to improve those systems. Key questions for public health and food systems approaches to nutrition include the following:

- Do current agricultural models provide the basic ingredients for proper nourishment?

- Do supermarkets make nourishing foods available?

- Do schools, workplaces, homes, and health care settings prioritize good nutrition?

- Do government policies and programs aid in meeting nutrition needs of all citizens?

To understand the answers to these questions, it is necessary first to know something about the nuts and bolts of human nutrition—of how the food we eat affects our bodies. The goal of this chapter is to focus in on the basics, although we do touch on broader public health nutrition topics. We address two primary questions: what are the important nutrients? What are their impacts, both in undersupply and oversupply, on the human body? We also briefly discuss how nutrition relates to the broader food system in a public health approach. Because the quest for proper nutrition drives any movement to improve access to and consumption of healthy foods, this understanding can provide a critical context for understanding how food systems and human health are so intimately intertwined. For the most part in this chapter, we leave it to the reader to draw the links between this information and potential food system interventions, although we return in the end to a discussion of public health nutrition approaches. Of course, the best nutrition advice will always necessarily be filtered through the lens of consumer needs, desires, attitudes, understanding, and lifestyles. Perspective 16.1 provides some glimpses into such factors.

Perspective 16.1. Consumer Perspectives

Each year the International Food Information Council Foundation commissions a nationally representative survey to learn about US consumer perspectives on food safety, nutrition, and health. Figure 16.1 a through e represents a sampling of the 2013 findings. These communicate that although people know they should be eating healthy foods, there are competing priorities that factor into decision making. Consumers must also sort through confusing and conflicting messages about what they should and should not eat. These barriers are important to consider when conducting education and outreach to the public about nutrition.

FIGURE 16.1   (a) Most People Are Thinking about the Healthfulness of Their Food; (b) Most Are Making Efforts to Improve Their Diets; (c) Taste and Price Lead the List of Reasons for Food Choices, but Healthfulness Is Third; Over One-Third of Respondents Count Sustainability as an Important Factor; (d) Although Consumers Do Take Some Control over Their Weight, They Describe Numerous Barriers, within and outside of Themselves; (e) Consumers Express Confusion about How Best to Eat Healthfully

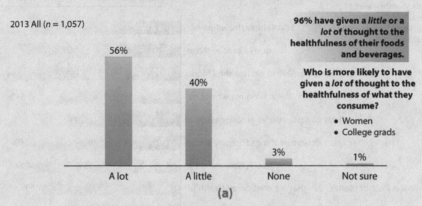

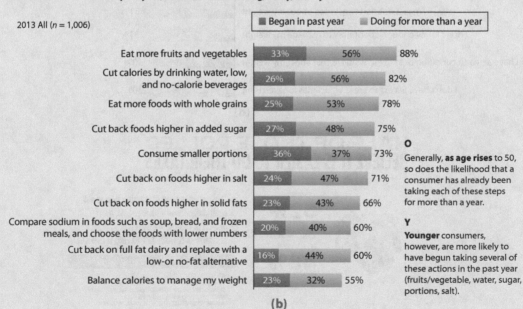

(Continued)

FIGURE 16.1 *(Continued)*

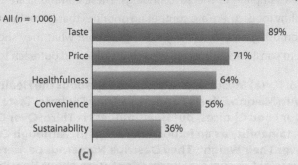

**How much of an impact do the following have
on your decision to buy foods and beverages?**
(% Rating 4 to 5 on 5-point scale, from *No Impact to A Great Impact*)

2013 All (*n* = 1,006)

Taste	89%
Price	71%
Healthfulness	64%
Convenience	56%
Sustainability	36%

(c)

**To what extent, if at all, are the following reasons why you do not try to take more
control over losing/maintaining your weight?**

Base: Trying to
lose/maintain weight
and does not try to take
full control over weight
2013 (*n* = 565)

■ Major reason ■ Minor reason

	Major	Minor	Total
I don't have the willpower	23%	41%	64%
I don't like to exercise	21%	38%	59%
It is too expensive to eat healthful foods	19%	35%	54%
I don't see enough progress when I try	14%	37%	51%
I eat when I'm under emotional strain	21%	29%	50%
I have other, more important things to worry about	12%	38%	50%
I don't have the time	16%	33%	49%
I don't like the taste of many foods that are considered healthful	13%	33%	46%
My genes play too much of a role in my weight	5%	27%	32%
I'm just not that concerned about my weight	4%	27%	31%
I don't know enough about how to manage my weight	5%	26%	31%
I have a health condition or take medications that affect my weight	11%	19%	30%
I don't have access to areas or facilities for exercising	6%	24%	30%

(d)

HALF OF THOSE POLLED
BELIEVE IT IS EASIER TO DO THEIR TAXES
THAN TO FIGURE OUT HOW TO EAT HEALTHFULLLY

THE BREAKDOWN:

52%
OF THOSE POLLED
Think it is harder to figure out what you
should and shouldn't eat to be healthier.

vs.

48%
OF THOSE POLLED
Think it is harder to figure out how to do
your own taxes.

Those most in need of learning how to eat
healthfully, those with high BMI, heart
disease or cholesterol issues, or high blood
pressure – ARE MORE APT TO FIND IT DIFFICULT.

GROUPS MORE LIKELY TO SAY FIGURING OUT WHAT TO EAT IS HARDER:

MEN (55%) vs. 48% of WOMEN
NO COLLEGE DEGREE (56%) vs. 40% of COLLEGE GRADS
BMI in the OBESE (60%) or OVERWEIGHT (54%) range vs. 42% low BMI
HEART DISEASE (59%) or HIGH CHOLESTEROL (54%)
and HIGH BLOOD PRESSURE (57%) vs. 48% NO HEALTH CONDITIONS

(e)

Source: International Food Information Council Foundation (IFIC) (2012).

WHAT IS NUTRITION?

At its simplest, adequate nutrition is composed of sufficient intake of macronutrients and micronutrients, the combination of which provide energy, nutrients, vitamins, and minerals. In individuals, nutrition and dietary patterns affect weight status, health, and lifestyle. The US government makes nutritional recommendations through its Dietary Guidelines for Americans, evidence-based recommendations for dietary habits. In summary, these guidelines promote consuming fewer calories, making informed food choices, and being physically active to attain and maintain a healthy weight and reduce chronic disease.

Energy

Put simply, energy is the "the capacity to do work." Like any machine, the human body needs a regular supply of energy to do its job. In the case of the human body, the "job" is to survive and maintain good health.

The Food and Agriculture Organization (FAO) of the United Nations describes the energy requirement of an individual as the amount of energy intake from food needed to enable the person's energy expenditure (determined by body size and composition)—and to enable a level of physical activity needed for economically necessary and socially desirable activities (The Joint FAO/WHO/UNU Expert Consultation on Energy and Protein Requirements, 1985). The total energy needs of any one body range from one hundred kilocalories to three thousand kilocalories per day. (A **kilocalorie [kcal]**, popularly referred to as a *calorie*, is a unit of energy.)

kilocalorie (kcal)
Formal term for what is commonly referred to as a *calorie*; the amount of energy needed to heat one kilogram of water by one degree Celsius

Total energy needs vary by individual and are determined by factors including the individual's metabolism, energy used to digest foods, and energy expenditure through activities of daily living (including physical activity). Energy balance refers to the balance between calories in and calories out. When more energy is consumed than expended, weight gain may occur, and the reverse. When the food supply (access to and availability of food) and consumption are disproportionate to daily energy requirements, overnutrition or undernutrition (or food waste) may ensue.

macronutrients
Nutrients used in relatively large quantities by the body

micronutrients
Nutrients needed in small amounts; can be found in vitamins, minerals, and trace elements

Essential nutrients are those that need to be consumed through diet because they cannot be produced by the human body. There are two categories of essential nutrients: **macronutrients** and **micronutrients**.

malnutrition
Undernutrition or overnutrition due to obtaining inadequate nutrients or an oversupply

Macronutrients (carbohydrates, fats, and proteins) provide energy the body needs to function and are found in plant and animal structures. These are needed in large amounts (e.g., grams and ounces) and are categorized based on their chemical composition, functions in the body, and food source. Micronutrients, however, are essential dietary elements needed only in very small quantities; they are also known as trace elements. Micronutrients do not provide energy; rather, they ensure that our bodies function properly. Most of us think of **malnutrition** as reflecting inadequate caloric intake. In fact, malnutrition refers to a condition that can develop if a person gets too little *or* too much of any of these essential nutrients. It should be noted that water may also be considered an essential nutrient (Mahan & Escott-Stump, 2003).

NUTRIENTS 101

The foods we consume provide a range of nutrients. Although, as discussed elsewhere in this chapter, there are many benefits to taking a "whole foods" and "whole diet" approach to what we eat, it remains useful to understand the basic evidence describing impacts of the different nutrients.

Macronutrients

FIGURE 16.2   Grains Are a Main Source of Carbohydrates

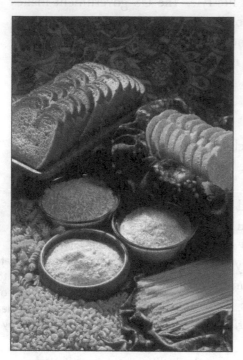

Source: Scott Bauer, USDA. "Grain products."

Carbohydrates   Carbohydrates are plant-based macronutrients that provide four kilocalories of energy per gram. They act as the main source of fuel in the body, are easily used for energy, and provide all the glucose needed for use in all tissues and cells. Carbohydrates are necessary for the central nervous system, kidneys, brain, and muscles (including the heart) to function properly. In addition, carbohydrates can be stored in muscles and liver in the form of glycogen and used later for energy.

The main sources of carbohydrates include grains (see figure 16.2), potatoes, fruits, milk and yogurt, vegetables, beans, nuts, and seeds. As described in table 16.1 and in the following, there are three types: (1) monosaccharides, (2) disaccharides and oligosaccharides, and (3) polysaccharides. The latter two can be broken down in the body to form monosaccharides.

Monosaccharides are the chemically smallest form of carbohydrate, and there are three types commonly found: glucose, galactose, and fructose. Glucose and fructose are the main sugars in fruits and vegetables. The human brain is highly dependent on a steady supply of glucose, and many physiological functions of the body work to provide glucose to the blood stream (glucose in the blood stream is referred to as *blood sugar*).

The second type of carbohydrate—disaccharides and oligosaccharides—is small, water-soluble, and found in foods

TABLE 16.1   Carbohydrate Types

Monosaccharides

Simplest form of sugar and carbohydrate

Glucose	Found in plants. Most widely distributed sugar in nature. Often bound to sucrose or lactose. Absorbed directly into the bloodstream during digestion. The brain depends on a regular, predictable supply of glucose.
Fructose	Fruit sugar is found in honey and fruits. It exists as 1 to 7 percent of the composition of most fruits.

Disaccharides and Oligosaccharides

Simple sugars and carbohydrates found in foods such as sugar beets, legumes, and squash

Sucrose	Table sugar occurs naturally in many foods and is also an additive in commercially processed foods. It's a combination of glucose and fructose molecules.
Lactose	Milk sugar is a combination of glucose and galactose molecules.
Maltose	Malt sugar is most commonly formed as the combination of two glucose molecules. This sweetener is often found in commercial products marketed as "sugar free."

Polysaccharides

Complex carbohydrates, often referred to as *dietary fiber*, digestible and indigestible

Starch	Plant starches are found in grains and vegetables (potatoes, wheat, corn, rice).
Glycogen	Animal starch is a storage form of glucose in the animal (including human) body to ensure maintenance of a regular, predictable supply.

such as beets, legumes, and squash. Along with monosaccharides, these types of carbohydrate are commonly referred to as simple sugars. Some examples of simple sugars are *table sugar* (sucrose), *milk sugar* (lactose), and maltose. Simple sugars are often found in refined foods, providing calories but lacking vitamins, minerals, and fiber. Because they are fermented by gut bacteria, they can cause gas and bloating.

The third type of carbohydrate—polysaccharides—is commonly referred to as a complex carbohydrate. Polysaccharides are composed of starches, which come from grains and vegetables and glycogen, found in animal cells.

Carbohydrate quality is of great importance when considering chronic disease prevention and public health nutrition. High-quality carbohydrates are those that are complex (i.e., polysaccharides), which have a higher number of glucose molecules, and are slower to be digested than simple sugars. By contrast, simple sugars are broken down quickly and used for energy; they spike the insulin response, which sends a message to store excess carbohydrates to fat tissue.

In the following, we discuss three types of sugar and provide examples of how they have played out in public health–public policy debates: table sugar (sucrose), honey, and high fructose corn syrup. All are considered forms of simple carbohydrate, which, when consumed, result in a rapid release of glucose and fructose molecules in the blood stream. Additionally, focus 16.1 discusses food addiction. Among candidates for potentially addictive food ingredients, sugar, as well as fat and salt and their combinations, top the list.

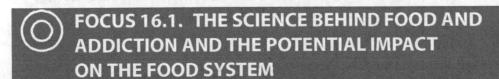

FOCUS 16.1. THE SCIENCE BEHIND FOOD AND ADDICTION AND THE POTENTIAL IMPACT ON THE FOOD SYSTEM

Ashley N. Gearhardt

Evidence has been growing that an addictive response to highly processed foods may be contributing to the obesity epidemic. What is the neurobiological and behavioral evidence for "food addiction"? If food addiction is real, how might it affect the food system and food supply?

Food and Addiction

Much of the initial research on food and addiction emerged from animal models of eating behavior. Rats provided with sugar began to binge on progressively larger quantities, exhibited signs of withdrawal when sugar was removed (or an opioid antagonist was administered) and displayed greater motivation for traditionally addictive substances (e.g., alcohol) (Avena, Rada, & Hoebel, 2008). Neural changes in the dopamine system implicated in addiction were demonstrated in rats maintained on a high-fat diet (e.g., cheesecake) and these animals would continue to seek out high-fat food despite receiving electric shocks (Johnson & Kenny, 2010). Rats (even those exhibiting signs of dependence on drugs of abuse) were more likely to choose saccharin (i.e., a calorie-free sweetener) over traditionally addictive substances (i.e., cocaine), which highlights the high level of reinforcement for sweet ingredients (Lenoir, Serre, Cantin, & Ahmed, 2007).

Neuroimaging and behavioral research in humans also provide support for the addictive potential of certain foods. Palatable foods and drugs of abuse activate similar neural systems (e.g., dopamine and opioid systems) (Volkow, Wang, Fowler, & Telang, 2008). Obese and substance-dependent participants exhibit parallel

(Continued)

(Continued)

patterns of neural response to cues (i.e., increased activation in motivation and reward areas) and consumption (i.e., decreased activation in control and reward areas) (Volkow, Wang, Fowler, Tomasi, & Baler, 2012).

The Yale Food Addiction Scale (YFAS) was developed to measure addictive eating in humans by translating the diagnostic criteria for substance dependence (e.g., withdrawal, loss of control) to relate to food consumption (Gearhardt, Corbin, & Brownell, 2009). Individuals endorsing more symptoms of food addiction on the YFAS (regardless of body mass index) showed a pattern of neural activation in response to cues and consumption that is implicated in other types of addiction (Gearhardt et al., 2011). The similarities identified in the neural system converge with behavioral overlap between addiction and problematic eating. For example, diminished control over consumption, continued use despite negative consequences, elevated levels of craving, and repeated relapse to problematic behavior are key constructs for problematic substance use and eating behavior (Gold, Frost-Pineda, & Jacobs, 2003).

Despite the growing evidence linking addiction and problematic eating, important gaps remain. For example, the degree of overlap between obesity and food addiction is unclear, and the relationship between these constructs deserves further attention. Exploration of what types of foods (or ingredients in these foods) may have the greatest addictive potential is still in its infancy, although ultra-processed foods high in sugar, fat, and salt (e.g., ice cream, pizza) are likely candidates. Finally, the percentage of the population that might be affected by food addiction has not yet been defined. It is likely that only a minority of individuals will have clinically significant food addiction, but addictive substances also trigger widespread subclinical public health problems. Given the easy access, cheap price, and heavy marketing of potentially addictive foods, it is probable that many (if not most) people would experience subclinical addictive eating behaviors (e.g., increased cravings, diminished control) that could result in overeating and weight gain. Thus, assessing the public health impact of potentially addictive foods is of central importance.

The Potential Impact of Addiction on the Food System

If certain foods are addictive, this may affect the food system in meaningful ways. First, ingredients with addictive potential are likely to trigger more cravings and consumption than minimally processed foods for most people (even individuals without food addiction). Increasing the level of addictive ingredients in foods would be expected to enhance the hedonic (pleasurable) response to these foods and increase their market share. Consistent with this idea, the ingredients most likely to be addictive (e.g., sugar, fat, salt) are often added to foods by the industry during processing, and increased consumption of these products has paralleled the rise in obesity rates (Lustig, Schmidt, & Brindis, 2012). Thus, potentially addictive ingredients could be used by the industry to shape increased demand and desire for their products. Second, the elevated reward level of potentially addictive foods may override homeostatic satiety signals and lead to excessive calorie consumption beyond biological requirements (Lutter & Nestler, 2009). Thus, increased demand for addictive foods could lead to more food being produced, transported, and stored than is biologically necessary, which may unnecessarily burden the modern food system. Finally, basic research suggests that consumption of highly processed foods may reduce the brain's sensitivity to reward (Johnson & Kenny, 2010). This could result in an increased preference for ultra-processed foods with artificially high reward levels relative to minimally processed foods (e.g., fruits, vegetables), because foods with lower reward levels would no longer be reinforcing. In sum, the possible implications of addictive foods on physical health, mental well-being, and the food system make this an important area for future research.

Additional Resources

Yale Food Addiction Scale: www.yaleruddcenter.org/resources/upload/docs/what/addiction /FoodAddictionScale09.pdf

Yale Rudd Center for Food Policy and Obesity: www.yaleruddcenter.org

Table sugar initially became widely popular in the eighteenth century as a luxury item. Typically manufactured from sugar cane or sugar beets, it is added not only to cakes, cookies, candies, soft drinks, and other sweets but also is added as a flavor enhancer to items that in the past typically would not have had sugar added (e.g., spaghetti sauce) (see figure 16.3).

Honey, however, although it contains sucrose and starch, is commonly consumed in its natural state with less processing. Honey is made by bees from plant nectar and is calorie dense (sixty-four kcal per tablespoon), but it also contains vitamins, minerals, **flavonoids**, and phytochemicals (described in the following).

High fructose corn syrup (HFCS) is another sweetening product found in many processed foods and used in place of sugar because of its lower cost. HFCS is a manufactured sweetener in which the glucose in cornstarch is enzymatically changed to fructose. It is often added to canned and frozen fruits to preserve the structure, flavor, and color. It is also used in soft drinks and fruit drinks to add body without affecting the flavor. In addition, HFCS is added to a wide variety of foods that aren't necessarily intended to be sweet, such as breads, soups, and condiments.

FIGURE 16.3 Spaghetti Sauce Label Featuring Organic Evaporated Cane Juice (Sugar)

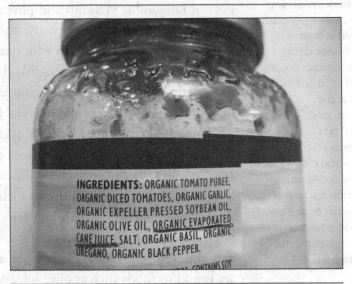

INGREDIENTS: ORGANIC TOMATO PUREE, ORGANIC DICED TOMATOES, ORGANIC GARLIC, ORGANIC EXPELLER PRESSED SOYBEAN OIL, ORGANIC OLIVE OIL, ORGANIC EVAPORATED CANE JUICE, SALT, ORGANIC BASIL, ORGANIC OREGANO, ORGANIC BLACK PEPPER.
CONTAINS SOY

Source: CLF.

flavonoids
Any of a large class of plant pigments that are beneficial to health

There is ongoing debate in the scientific community about whether HFCS is metabolized differently from table sugar and about whether it may be more harmful. Some research indicates that HFCS may play a role in the obesity epidemic (Bray, Nielsen, & Popkin, 2004; Elliott, Keim, Stern, Teff, & Havel, 2002). However, others oppose this view and suggest the evidence does not support the HFCS-obesity link because many of the studies rely on a pure fructose diet using animal models (Forshee et al., 2007; White, 2008). The corn industry is campaigning to protect the public image of HFCS by stating that "your body can't tell the difference" between corn syrup and real sugar. The Corn Refiners Association petitioned the US Food and Drug Administration (FDA) for a name change, replacing "high fructose corn syrup" with "corn sugar" for labeling purposes. In 2012, this petition was denied by the FDA on grounds that HFCS is a liquid, and that because "corn sugar" has long been associated with the sweetener dextrose, the change would cause confusion. The debate on whether HFCS is metabolized differently from table sugar may continue.

More broadly, the typical US diet has shifted to one composed of too many carbohydrates, in particular, simple carbohydrates, which provide an excess of energy. A limited amount of blood glucose is converted to glycogen and stored in the liver and muscles and the remainder is converted to fat. Diets that eliminate or drastically reduce carbohydrate intake, however, also may have harmful effects. With insufficient carbohydrate intake, the body will break down protein for fuel. Further, the body may go into **ketosis**, a state of elevated ketones in the body caused by the breakdown of fatty acids for energy; ketosis stresses the kidneys. Finally, the brain relies on glucose for energy and without it dizziness and weakness may result, negatively affecting physical and mental performance.

ketosis
A state of elevated ketones in the body caused by breakdown of fatty acids for energy

fats (lipids)
Oily substance providing nine kilocalories per gram and stored in human adipose tissue; aid in digestion, absorption, and transport of fat-soluble vitamins and phytochemicals

saturated fats
Triglycerides containing long fatty acid chains that have all available carbon binding sites full with hydrogen bonds and are solid at room temperature; seen as less healthy than unsaturated fats

Fats Dietary **fats (lipids)** provide nine kilocalories per gram and are stored in adipose tissue in the human body. Dietary fat aids in digestion, absorption, and transport of fat-soluble vitamins and phytochemicals. Because the structure of lipids can affect the way they act in the body, understanding these structures is important when considering fats' relationship with health outcomes. Fatty acids are classified by the number of carbons (chain length), the number of double bonds (saturation), and the location of double bonds. Chain length and saturation contribute to the melting temperature of a fat. There are several kinds of fat.

Saturated fats have long fatty acid chains and are solid at room temperature, as is the case with butter and meat (see figure 16.4). There is extensive evidence of their association with cardiovascular disease compared with mono and polyunsaturated fats. These fats are found in foods such as meat, lard, and cream.

Unsaturated fats have shorter fatty acid chains or more double bonds than saturated fats and are liquid at room temperature. They have been shown to decrease the risk of developing heart disease when substituted for saturated fats. Unsaturated fats are found in foods such as olive oil, avocados, nuts, and canola oil.

FIGURE 16.4   Meats and Cheese Contain Saturated Fats

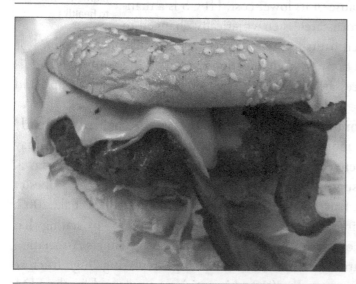

Source: Burger Austin. (2010). Nau's Enfield Drug—Large Bacon Cheeseburger. https://www.flickr.com/photos/burgeraustin/5007282483/

Polyunsaturated fatty acids (PUFAs) have two or more double bonds. They are essential fatty acids, meaning the human body does not make them on their own, and we have to obtain them from our diets. Some commonly known polyunsaturated fatty acids are omega-3 and omega-6. In the typical US diet there are relatively few sources of omega-3 fatty acids, which are found mainly in the fat of cold-water fish such as salmon, sardines, herring, and mackerel, as well as in green vegetables and some eggs. By contrast, sources of omega-6 fatty acids are abundant and include corn, soybeans, seeds, nuts, and the oils extracted from them. Refined vegetable oils, also high in omega-6s, are typically added to snack foods, cookies, crackers, sweets, and fast food.

The body also constructs hormones from fatty acids. In general, hormones derived from the two classes of essential fatty acids have opposite effects. Those from omega-6 fatty acids tend to increase inflammation (an important component of the immune response), blood clotting, and cell proliferation, and those from omega-3 fatty acids decrease those functions. Both families of hormones must be in balance to maintain optimum health. Anthropological research suggests that although our ancestors thrived on diets with omega-6 to omega-3 ratios of approximately 1:1, in the US diet this ratio may be as high as 15:1 or above (Simopoulos, 2008). This low intake of

polyunsaturated fatty acids (PUFAs)
Essential fatty acids that have two or more double bonds; includes omega-3 and omega-6 fatty acids

omega-3 fatty acids affects brain health and functioning because the membranes and signaling use this nutrient.

Trans fats are fats with a certain configuration of bonds between two carbon molecules. Although some trans fats occur naturally during anaerobic fermentation in the rumen of cows and sheep, products made with hydrogenated oils are a major source of trans fats. Hydrogenation is the process of taking a naturally occurring unsaturated fat and adding hydrogen molecules chemically. Hydrogenation can extend the shelf life of foods and replace animal fats such as butter and lard at lower cost, which is why it became popular in the food industry in the 1980s. Trans fats are found in baked goods, snack foods, fried foods, and margarines.

FIGURE 16.5   Trans Fat Levels Decline

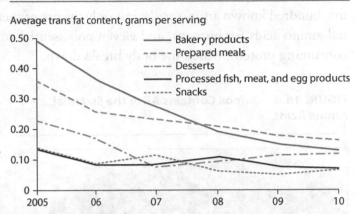

Trans fat levels in new products have dropped dramatically over the last five years.

Source: USDA, Economic Research Service calculations using Mintel Global New Products Database, (2012).

trans fats
Unsaturated fats with bonds added to the fatty acid in processing to make it solid at room temperature and to extend the shelf life of foods; linked to risk of heart disease

Health risks abound with the consumption of trans fats, primarily increased risk for heart disease. For example, a landmark study of 78,778 US women published in 2005 demonstrated increased risk of cardiovascular disease associated with consumption of trans fats (Oh, Hu, Manson, Stampfer, & Willett, 2005). Because of such impacts, regulators have sought to reduce dietary exposures. A 2003 FDA regulation required manufacturers to list trans fat on the Nutrition Facts panel of foods and some dietary supplements; the requirements have been further strengthened since then. A policy evaluation found that blood levels of trans fats dropped 58 percent from 2000 to 2009 in non-Hispanic white adults, demonstrating that the policy has a health-protecting impact (CDC, 2012; Vesper, Kuiper, Mirel, Johnson, & Pirkle, 2012) (see figure 16.5).

Even beyond trans fats, the rise of cardiovascular disease over the past few decades has led to much focus on the issue of overconsumption of fats and the balance of "healthy fat" and "unhealthy fat." For decades, fats as a category were vilified due to their high caloric content, and many Americans avoided them to the extent possible. Low-fat versions of products became popular, even though they typically contain high levels of sugar and salt in the attempt to mask their less appealing tastes. Yet, fats are a necessary nutrient for the human body. They can even play beneficial roles in weight control, due to their impacts on satiety and their ability to enhance appreciation of food. In particular, healthy fats are recommended: an expert panel concluded that risk of cardiovascular disease is reduced when saturated fats are replaced with monounsaturated and polyunsaturated fatty acids (Astrup et al., 2011).

Proteins   Proteins are often referred to as the "building blocks of life." They are responsible for bodily growth, tissue repair, immune function, production of essential hormones and enzymes, preservation of lean muscle mass, and as an energy source when carbohydrates are not available. Also, they are necessary for DNA transcription and RNA translation. Protein consumption has been linked to increased satiety and can assist in weight management.

Proteins are compounds composed of one or more chains of amino acids. Amino acids are organic compounds. The key elements of these are carbon, hydrogen, oxygen, and nitrogen. There are about five hundred known amino acids, but only twenty of them are found in humans. There are nine essential amino acids for humans, and eleven nonessential amino acids. Humans get these amino acids by consuming protein, which the body breaks down.

FIGURE 16.6 Quinoa Contains All of the Essential Amino Acids

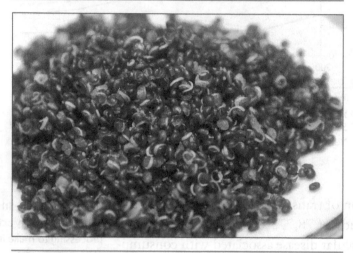

Source: Blairing Media. (2010). Cooked red quinoa. http://en.wikipedia .org/wiki/File:Red_quinoa.png

Plants contain some proteins and amino acids. Animals eat the plants and convert the amino acids to protein. Humans may get their essential amino acids by eating plants or animals, and the human body makes the nonessential amino acids. Animal-derived sources of protein are meats, poultry, fish, eggs, and dairy; plant sources include nuts, legumes, starchy foods, grains, and vegetables. Protein that comes from animal sources, as well as a few nonmeat sources (e.g., quinoa [see figure 16.6], soybeans) are "complete" proteins, meaning they contain all of the essential amino acids. Plant and grain sources of protein that do not contain all of the essential amino acids can be eaten in combinations, such as rice and beans, to obtain a fuller range of amino acids. All essential amino acids should be eaten within approximately the same few days for maximal efficacy in protein synthesis.

Underconsuming protein has widespread implications, because all cells rely on protein and amino acids for repair and building. The side effects of protein deficiency may include weakened immune system, distended stomach, stunted growth, or flaky skin. However, as shown in table 16.2, most Americans consume more than sufficient amounts. Consuming too much protein stresses the kidneys due to a ketogenic state (as with too little carbohydrate).

Micronutrients

Micronutrients, for example, vitamins and minerals, are only needed by humans in small amounts. It is recommended that micronutrients be consumed through whole foods in the diet, with additional supplementation considered if necessary (Institute of Medicine [IOM], 2010). Currently, most Americans are meeting and exceeding their requirements for caloric intake without meeting micronutrient recommendations, because of the consumption of energy-dense, nutrient-poor foods. **Dietary reference intakes (DRIs)** are evidence-based nutrient standards for estimating optimal intakes in healthy individuals, developed by the Institute of Medicine and National Academy of Sciences. The DRI provides broader information than the recommended daily allowance (RDA) and has supplanted it in many places, though the RDA is still listed on nutrition labels and in the tables in this chapter.

dietary reference intakes (DRIs)
Evidence-based nutrient standards set by the Institute of Medicine and the National Academy of Sciences for estimating optimal intakes in healthy individuals

TABLE 16.2 Types of Protein Sources, and Total Fat and Saturated Fat Content

Item	Protein (g/three oz.)	Total Fat (g/three oz.)	Saturated Fat (g/three oz.)
Beef, tenderloin, steak, lean, all grades, cooked, broiled	24.25	6.68	2.55
Chicken, broilers or fryers, breast, skinless, boneless, meat only, enhanced, raw	16.80	2.32	0.55
Fish, salmon, Atlantic, farmed, cooked, dry heat	18.79	10.50	2.13
Egg, whole, raw, fresh	10.68	8.09	2.66
Cheese, cottage, low-fat, 1 percent milk fat	10.54	0.87	0.55
Beans, black, seeds, cooked, boiled	7.54	0.46	0.12
Tofu, raw, regular	6.87	4.07	0.59
Peanuts, all types, raw	21.94	41.88	5.81
Seeds, sunflower seed kernels, dry roasted, without salt	16.44	42.35	4.44
Potatoes, russet, flesh and skin, raw	1.82	0.07	0.02
Broccoli, raw	2.40	0.32	0.039
Quinoa, uncooked	12.01	5.16	0.706
Wheat flour, whole grain	11.24	2.13	0.37
Rice, white, long-grain, regular, cooked	2.29	0.24	0.07

Source: Mahan and Escott-Stump (2003).

Vitamins **Vitamins** are not synthesized in the body in adequate amounts, but they occur naturally in food. Adequate amounts of vitamins are required in order for the body to perform normal physiologic functions, and vitamin deficiencies can cause certain syndromes. Vitamin A, for example, is considered a particularly important nutrient to monitor, because chronic deficiency is the leading cause of blindness in the developing world. Table 16.3 lists physiologic functions of selected vitamins, as well as key food sources and RDA.

vitamins
Naturally occurring compounds essential for normal growth and nutrition and required in small amounts in the diet

Minerals **Minerals** are essential nutrients that mostly exist in the body in their ionic states, either as cations (positively charged ions) or anions (negatively charged ions). Cations are derived from metals, including calcium, copper, iron, magnesium, potassium, sodium, and zinc. Nonmetallic elements yield anions and include iodine as iodide, sulfur as sulfate, phosphorus as phosphate, chlorine as chloride, and fluorine as fluoride. Combinations of anions and cations yield salts such as sodium chloride, calcium phosphate, and sodium iodide. These minerals are grouped into macrominerals (also known as "bulk elements," which are essential in adult humans in amounts of around 100mg/day) and microminerals (elements required in trace amounts for optimal performance of a particular function). Table 16.4 lists selected minerals along with their RDAs, sources, and physiologic functions.

minerals
Essential nutrients that exist mostly in the body in their ionic state, either as cations (positively charged ions) or anions (negatively charged ions)

OTHER NUTRIENTS

The volume, composition, and distribution of body fluids have profound effects on cell function. Water and sodium are two key factors that balance this system. Two other dietary components important for cell function and body growth and maintenance are fiber and phytonutrients.

TABLE 16.3   Vitamins

Vitamin	RDA for Adults	Physiologic Function	Selected Food Sources[a]	Selected Problems Associated with Excess and Deficiencies[*]
Vitamin A	Females: 700 mcg RAE/day Males: 900 mcg RAE/day	• Vision • Bone growth • Reproduction • Cell functions • Immune system	Liver, liver oils, milk fat, eggs, colorful fruits and vegetables, and some cereals	Excess: Liver disease Deficiency: Vision impairment, possible blindness
Vitamin D	5–15 mcg/day	• Calcium absorption • Nerve, muscle, and immune functions	Egg yolks, saltwater fish, liver, some milk and cereal; also synthesized in humans from exposure to sunlight	Excess: Calcification of soft tissues, such as the kidneys, lungs, heart, and tympanic membranes of the ear Deficiency: Rickets in children and osteomalacia in adults, bone pain and muscle weakness, weakened immune system, increased risk for cardiovascular disease, cognitive impairment, asthma, and some cancers
Vitamin E	15 mg α-TE/day	• Antioxidant • Immune system and metabolic processes	Vegetable oils, nuts, seeds, leafy greens, and some cereals	Excess: Impaired bone mineralization, impaired hepatic vitamin A storage, and prolonged blood coagulation Deficiency: Mild anemia, infertility issues, dry hair and loss of hair, muscular weakness, and gastrointestinal diseases
Vitamin K	120 mcg/day	• Creation of proteins, bones, and tissues • Creation of proteins for blood clotting	Green vegetables, dark berries	Excess: Severe jaundice in infants, has produced hemolytic anemia in rats Deficiency: Risk of massive uncontrolled bleeding, stomach pains, cartilage calcification, and severe malformation of developing bone or deposition of insoluble calcium salts in artery walls
Vitamin C	Females: 75 mg/day Males: 90 mg/day	• Antioxidants • Healing • Iron absorption	Citrus, red and green peppers, tomatoes, broccoli, greens, and some juices and fortified cereals	Excess: Gastrointestinal disturbances and diarrhea Deficiency: Impaired wound healing, edema, hemorrhage, fatigue, mood changes, joint and muscle aches, bruising, dental conditions, dry hair and skin, infections

(Continued)

TABLE 16.3 Vitamins *(Continued)*

Vitamin	RDA for Adults	Physiologic Function	Selected Food Sources[a]	Selected Problems Associated with Excess and Deficiencies*
B Vitamins: Vitamin B₁ Vitamin B₂ Vitamin B₆ Vitamin B₁₂ Niacin Biotin Folic Acid Pantothenic Acid	**Vitamin B₁:** Females: 1.1 mg/day Males: 1.2 mg/day **Vitamin B₂:** Females: 1.1 mg/day Males: 1.3 mg/day **Vitamin B₆:** Females: 1.3–1.5 mg/day Males: 1.3–1.7 mg/day **Vitamin B₁₂:** 30 mcg/day **Niacin:** Females: 14 mg NE/day Males: 16 mg NE/day **Biotin:** 30 mcg/day **Folic Acid:** 30 mcg/day **Pantothenic Acid:** 5 mg/day	• Creation of energy from food • Creation of red blood cells	Fish, poultry, meat, eggs, dairy, leafy green vegetables, beans, peas, whole grains, and some fortified cereals and breads	Excess: Very few cases of toxicity associated with B vitamins Deficiency: Weight loss, body weakness and pain, brain damage, irregular heart rate, heart failure, and death if left untreated, depression, reduced cell division

RDA: Recommended dietary allowance
RAE: Retinol activity equivalents
α-TE: α-tocopherol equivalents
NE: Niacin equivalents
[a]Vitamin levels in foods can vary based on cultivar, growing conditions, food processing, and cooking method.
*Mahan and Escott-Stump (2003); US National Library of Medicine (2012); USDA (2010); National Institutes of Health (nd).

Water

An important component of a healthful diet that is often overlooked in health promotion and food systems work is water. The human body is mainly composed of water, approximately 60 to 65 percent for men and 50 to 60 percent for women (Mahan & Escott-Stump, 2003). The human body relies on water for many of its functions, including circulating oxygen, nutrients, hormones, and other substances in the blood, enabling digestion and flushing out waste, and cooling the body via sweat.

Total water intake includes water from fluids (drinking water and other beverages) and the water that is contained in foods. Individual water intake needs vary widely, based in part on level of physical activity and exposure to heat stress.

Unfortunately, for some Americans there is no guarantee of access to clean, safe, and potable drinking water. For example, many schools have antiquated water pipes and fountains, and as a result the water contains lead.

TABLE 16.4 Minerals

Mineral	RDA for Adults	Physiologic Function	Select Food Sources	Selected Problems Associated with Excess and Deficiencies*
Macrominerals				
Calcium	Ages 19–50: 1,000 mg/day Ages 51+: 1,200 mg/day (AI)	• Strong bones and teeth • Healthy muscles and blood vessels • Secrete hormones and enzymes and nervous system functioning	Milk, cheese, yogurt, and leafy, green vegetables such as kale and collard greens	Excess: Excessive calcification in soft tissues, especially in kidneys Deficiency: Low bone mass and osteomalacia
Sodium	1.2–1.5 g/day (AI)	• Function of nerves and muscles • Fluid balance	Table salt and processed foods such as bread, cold cuts, pizza, soups, and cheese	Excess: High blood pressure, buildup of fluid in people with congestive heart failure, cirrhosis, or kidney disease Deficiency: Hyponatremia
Potassium	4.7 g/day (AI)	• Nerve and muscle communication • Elimination of cellular waste	Leafy green vegetables, vine fruits, root vegetables, citrus fruits	Excess: Abnormal and dangerous heart rhythm Deficiency: Muscle weakness, abnormal heart rhythms, raised blood pressure
Microminerals				
Iron	Females: 18 mg/day until menopause, then 8 mg/day Males: 8 mg/day	• Creation of proteins that carry and store oxygen in the body • Creation of many proteins and enzymes in the body	Dried beans, dried fruit, eggs, iron-fortified cereals, liver, lean red meat, oysters, poultry, salmon, tuna, whole grains, and cast iron cookware	Excess: Increased risk of heart disease and cancer in postmenopausal women and older men Deficiency: Iron-deficiency anemia (one of the most common nutritional deficiencies in the United States)
Copper	900 µg/day	• Formation of red blood cells • Healthy blood vessels, nerves, immune system, and bones	Oysters and other shellfish, whole grains, beans, nuts, potatoes, and organ meats	Excess: Liver cirrhosis and abnormal red blood cell formation Deficiency: Anemia, neutropenia, and skeletal abnormalities
Zinc	Females: 8 mg/day Males: 11 mg/day	• Cell division, cell growth, wound healing • Breakdown of carbohydrates	Beef, pork, lamb, dark meat chicken, nuts, whole grains, legumes, and yeast	Excess: Interference with copper absorption Deficiency: Impaired growth, delayed wound healing, immune deficiencies, and impaired appetite

RDA: Recommended dietary allowance
AI: Adequate intake (the consumption and absorption of sufficient food, vitamins, and essential minerals necessary to maintain health)
*Mahan and Escott-Stump (2003); US National Library of Medicine (2012); USDA (2010); National Institutes of Health (nd)

Sodium

In the human body, proper hydration involves a balance of solutes, including sodium and water. Insufficient sodium consumption can lead to a life-threatening emergency called hyponatremia, in which cells swell and heart conditions may ensue. Too much sodium, by contrast, negatively affects blood pressure, buildup of fluid in those with congestive heart failure, cirrhosis, and kidney disease.

There is speculation that an evolutionary need to consume salt may have shaped our innate liking for its taste. Sodium is found in a plethora of foods and is commonly consumed in higher than recommended amounts. Americans consume on average more than 3,400 mg of sodium per day (equivalent to 1.5 teaspoons salt), well above the maximum amounts recommended (2,300 mg/d) (IOM, 2010). Processed foods and menu items prepared outside the home are predominant sources of sodium intake in the United States (IOM, 2010). Chapter 13 discusses sodium in processed foods, with perspectives 16.2 and 13.2 providing critical perspectives on industry usage of sodium. Sensory preferences for salt can be decreased and muted with reduced exposure (IOM, 2010).

Fiber

Dietary fiber is formed from a wide variety of soluble and insoluble monosaccharides other than glucose. It comes from the portion of plants that is not digested by enzymes in the intestinal tract but that may be metabolized by bacteria in the lower gut. Fiber plays an important role in colorectal cancer prevention.

Soluble fibers attract water and form a gel; both of these processes slow digestion. Soluble fiber delays stomach emptying, creates a feeling of satiety (or feeling full), and maintains a steady blood sugar level by increasing insulin sensitivity. Some dietary sources of soluble fiber include cellulose, which comes from whole wheat, bran, and vegetables; hemicellulose, which comes from bran and whole grains; and lignin, which comes from fruits, seeds, and vegetables.

soluble fiber
Indigestible portions of plant foods that attracts water and forms a gel to slow digestion and create a full feeling

Insoluble fibers bind water as they pass through the digestive tract, making stools softer and bulkier. This type of fiber is important to maintaining gut health and helping prevent constipation. In addition, it lowers LDL, or "bad," cholesterol by interfering with the absorption of dietary cholesterol. Fiber consumption helps decrease blood cholesterol levels, maintain bowel integrity and health, control blood sugar levels, increase satiety, and reduce risk for colorectal cancer. Some dietary sources of insoluble fiber include gums, which come from oats, legumes, and barley; and pectin, which comes from apples, citrus fruits, strawberries, and carrots.

insoluble fiber
Indigestible portion of plant food that binds water while passing through the digestive tract, making stools softer and bulkier; important to maintaining gut health and helping prevent constipation

Phytonutrients

Phytonutrients are natural chemicals that occur in plants (e.g., fruits, vegetables, seeds, nuts, and whole grains). Phytonutrients can also be referred to as bioactive phytochemicals and "functional foods." Researchers are actively investigating the health and nutrition implications of these plant-based substances, including carotenoids, phytoestrogens, antioxidants, flavonoids, and resveratrol. The functions of phytonutrients include metabolic alterations, such as increased absorption and in some cases, as with oxalates and phytates, inhibited absorption of vitamins and minerals, detoxification through antioxidants, and anti-inflammatory action. Research has linked

phytonutrients
Compounds in plant foods that have been associated with beneficial functions in the body (e.g., aiding nutrient absorption, inhibiting oxidation, improving cholesterol)

phytonutrients with cancer prevention, as well as improved cholesterol levels, bone health, energy levels, and immune function.

OTHER CONSIDERATIONS: ADDITIVES AND NATURALLY OCCURRING CHEMICALS IN FOOD; ORGANIC FOOD

In addition to the macro- and micronutrients described, various chemicals exist in our food that are either naturally occurring or are added at some point during food production and processing, for purposes including enhancing growth, killing pests, enriching nutrient content, or enhancing flavor, color, texture, or preservation. Chapters 11 and 12 provide insights into food production additives, and chapter 13 discusses the role of additives in food processing. Here, we briefly discuss a few topics relevant to understanding dietary consumption of additives and agricultural chemicals at a population level: enrichment and fortification, and foods produced without chemical fertilizers and pesticides, that is: organically produced foods. Perspective 16.2 also discusses the fact that some food additives remain unresearched or unreported (Willett, 1998).

Enrichment and Fortification

The current food supply includes many processed and semiprocessed food items that are fortified or enriched. **Enrichment** is the addition of nutrients to *restore* the nutritional value lost in processing, for

enrichment
Addition of nutrients to restore nutritional value lost in processing

example, adding iron and certain B vitamins lost while milling grains. **Fortification** is the addition of nutrients to enhance a food's nutritional value, such as adding folate to flour and grain products and iodine to salt.

Some would consider enrichment and fortification to be a beneficial harm-reduction strategy: given that many people are likely to eat processed foods anyway, at least eating such products will give them some nutritional value. Others note that the fortification and enrichment enable marketers to sell these products as healthful, even when their other ingredients are anything but. By misleading consumers, such marketing could lead to overall less healthful diets.

fortification
Addition of nutrients to enhance a food's nutritional value

Perspective 16.2. Reasonable Certainty of No Harm?
Michael F. Jacobson

Many food labels read like the contents of a chemistry set, not a cracker or beverage: sodium stearoyl lactylate, acesulfame potassium, sucrose acetate isobutyrate (Center for Science in the Public Interest [CSPI], 2013a). But the real issue is not the complexity of the ingredients' names, but whether the ingredients are safe.

The Food and Drug Administration, the agency charged with ensuring that food ingredients are safe, requires that they pose a "reasonable certainty of no harm." That standard recognizes that it's not possible to prove that a chemical will be absolutely safe to every individual in every circumstance. Instead, the FDA requires a *reasonable certainty* that a substance won't harm the vast majority of consumers.

Unfortunately, the FDA has ignored that standard time and time again. As a result of FDA's continued inaction, each year tens of thousands of people unnecessarily get sick or die.

The biggest problem is a category of food ingredients that the law calls "generally recognized as safe," or GRAS. When the law went into effect half a century ago, Congress assumed that only substances that were assuredly safe, such as vinegar or citric acid, would be considered GRAS, so it didn't even require companies to inform the FDA that they were introducing such chemicals into the food supply. Congress mandated that other substances be regulated more tightly as "food additives," with FDA preapproval required before they could be used.

Ironically, the FDA has accepted three of the most harmful ingredients in our food supply as being generally recognized as safe, even though public health officials consider them to be "generally recognized as dangerous" at the high levels consumed: partially hydrogenated oil, salt, and sugar.

Partially hydrogenated oil—used for over a century to make shortenings and margarines—is the source of artificial trans fat. Trans fat was long thought to be harmless, but beginning in 1990, careful clinical studies demonstrated that trans fat increases the "bad" cholesterol and reduces the "good" cholesterol in blood. Epidemiology studies then associated trans fat with upwards of fifty thousand premature deaths annually.

Following a decade-long rulemaking, in 2006 the FDA required food labels to list trans fat content. The labeling, together with massive publicity and several lawsuits, persuaded many manufacturers and restaurants to switch to healthier vegetable oils. But meanwhile the evidence that trans fat was the most dangerous fat in our food supply became as solid as the Ivory-soap-like shortenings in which it was abundant. Beginning in 2003, Denmark and several other countries virtually banned partially hydrogenated oils. But since 2006 the FDA has done nothing. As a result, Pop Secret popcorn, Long John Silver's fried foods in most of the country, Marie Callender pies, and other popular products (CSPI, 2013b) still contain the nasty fat, and thousands of people are still dying prematurely.

Salt has been a subject of controversy for well over three decades because excess consumption boosts blood pressure and the risk of heart attacks and strokes. Some meals at Denny's, Olive Garden, and other restaurants have two or three times as much sodium as adults should eat in a single day (CSPI, 2009).

In 1979, the FDA's own advisory committee said there was insufficient evidence to consider salt to be GRAS. The FDA's response was to ask industry to reduce sodium levels. But in 2010, the Institute of Medicine concluded that forty years of voluntary "action" achieved nothing and that it was time for the FDA to regulate. The FDA's response? So far it's only more appeals to industry to voluntarily cut salt.

Sugar and high fructose corn syrup are other biggies on the GRAS list. The average American consumes about eighty pounds of the sweet stuff a year. Long known to promote tooth decay, recent research has found that refined sugars, at least when consumed in beverages, promote overweight and obesity and possibly heart disease. Researchers at the Harvard School of Public Health have estimated that one major source—sugar drinks—of refined sugars has been causing about twenty-five thousand deaths per year from diabetes, heart disease, and cancer (Wade, 2013). FDA's response? Don't even bother asking.

The list of questionable GRAS substances and food additives goes on: the artificial sweetener aspartame has caused cancer in three animal studies (CSPI, 2013a). Mycoprotein, a fungus-based ingredient in Quornbrand imitation meats, causes violent vomiting and anaphylactic reactions, including at least one recent death (CSPI, 2012). Butylated hydroxyanisole (BHA), according to the Department of Health and Human Services, is "reasonably anticipated to be a human carcinogen" (CSPI, 2013a). Red 3 is a food dye that in 1984 FDA said should be (but wasn't) banned because it caused thyroid tumors in animals (CSPI, 2013a). The deceptively named "caramel coloring" long used in soft drinks has been contaminated with dangerous levels of a carcinogen until California—notwithstanding the FDA's pooh-poohing of any risk—forced companies to improve the manufacturing process (CSPI, 2013a).

The FDA could easily ban unnecessary ingredients such as partially hydrogenated vegetable oil, mycoprotein, Red 3, and BHA. And it could set safe conditions of use—limits, warning labels, or other approaches—on substances such as sugar and salt. But the FDA has done nothing about, or has even defended, each of those unsavory substances.

(Continued)

> *(Continued)*
>
> The FDA is hardly the aggressive public-health watchdog that Americans expect and need. What's needed is aggressive oversight by Congress, adequate funding, and a wholesale renovation of the FDA's division that is supposed to be ensuring the safety of food additives.
>
> *Source*: Jacobson (2013). Originally published at: http://thehill.com/blogs/congress-blog/healthcare/316175-reasonable-certainty-of-no-harm)

Organically Grown Food

Organic agriculture is defined as "an ecological production management system that promotes and enhances biodiversity, biological cycles and soil biological activity. It is based on minimal use of off-farm inputs and on management practices that restore, maintain and enhance ecological harmony" (Gold, 2007).Organic production also avoids genetically modified organisms (GMOs), hormones, and antibiotics (Gold, 2007). Organic products are now available in many grocery stores, often with substantial price premiums over conventional products.

Consumers may believe that there are nutritional benefits to eating organic foods; however, most evidence suggests that organic and nonorganic foods are nutritionally similar (Dangour, Lock, Hayter, Aikenhead, Allen, & Uauy, 2010). There may be exceptions; one review of studies suggested that there may be a slight trend toward higher vitamin C content in organically grown leafy vegetables and potatoes than nonorganic (Benbrook, Zhao, Yáñez, Davies, & Andrews, 2008).

There are a multitude of reasons beyond nutrition for why individuals may choose organic food, including supporting production methods and farmers that respect the environment and avoiding food additives (Gold, 2007). The environmental benefits of organically grown foods are clear. Organic diets are lower in pesticides than conventional ones, and because manufactured pesticides are not used in production, workers and the environment also are not exposed (Baker, Benbrook, Growth, & Benbrook, 2002). Further, some people believe that organically produced foods taste better than conventionally produced foods. That perception could lead to increased produce consumption.

PUBLIC HEALTH NUTRITION APPROACHES

In this chapter we have described the "nuts and bolts" of nutrition. How do we use these concepts to promote improved nutrition at the population level? Before concluding, we turn once again to public health nutrition.

An important public health goal is optimum nutrition for everyone, meaning that individuals are food secure with adequate, balanced diets leading to health, well-being, healthy development, and high quality of life. Cultural factors, media and advertising, food access and availability, and social factors all affect food choices at the individual and population levels. For example, although genetic factors and individual-level behaviors can contribute to obesity, the current epidemic is in large part attributed to environmental factors. Maintaining a healthy energy balance is difficult in part because food environments increasingly promote the availability, access, and allure of less healthful foods, contributing to an "obesogenic" environment. On the other side of the energy balance equation, physical activity environments and ultimately individual physical activity behaviors are important to consider.

Although this chapter has broken the diet into its component elements so as to explain basic nutritional concepts, it is important to recognize that public health nutritionists do not recommend that we construct our diets one nutrient or even one meal at a time. Rather, a total diet, as defined by the US Dietary Guidelines Advisory Committee, reflects the combination of foods and beverages that provide energy and nutrients and constitute an individual's complete dietary intake on average over time. The Academy of Nutrition and Dietetics (AND, formerly American Dietetic Association) promotes the total diet or overall pattern of foods eaten as the most important focus of a healthful eating style. In addition, obtaining nutrition via a whole foods approach (versus from supplements, enriched, or fortified foods) exposes the body not only to well-studied nutrients but also to others we may yet know little about, and also to the interactive effects of different nutrients in combination.

As will be described in chapters 17 and 18, actions to help support healthy diets can occur at several different levels: the individual level (e.g., preferences), the social environment (e.g., social support), the physical environment (e.g., retail and food service opportunities in settings such as schools, work sites, early care and education, and the broader community), and the macro-level environment (e.g., systems-level influences such as social norms, food marketing, and food production) (Story, Kaphingst, Robinson-O'Brien, & Glanz, 2008). Although individual dietary interventions and health promotion programs can be effective in situations such as clinical interventions and counseling and nutrition education, these are resource intensive and depend on individual motivation through the short and long term. By contrast, public health nutrition interventions at the population level can be far less expensive and can be effective even for individuals who do not consciously choose to change their behavior. Both national agencies such as the CDC and private organizations such as the Robert Wood Johnson Foundation (with obesity prevention efforts focused on environment and policy) have increasingly supported population-level public health interventions.

Overall, coordinated, multilevel, systems-wide approaches that engage multiple stakeholders may hold the greatest potential for improving population nutritional status. By focusing on a systemic approach, we are better able to identify and repair broken parts of the food system. There is a need for theoretically driven research and practice that uses models of population health behavior change that better integrate individual-level with broader environmental and macro-level policy influences. Figure 16.7 describes the food supply chain and potential points of intervention along it to promote a healthier and more sustainable food system. For example, at or near the point of consumption, we can address issues that are more individual based (e.g., where to shop, foods to purchase, etc.). Further upstream, we can use more environmental and policy-level approaches such as efforts to change healthy food availability and cost, or federal policies to support sustainable food production and more regional and local food distribution systems.

FIGURE 16.7   Supply Chain: Production to Consumption and Potential Points of Intervention

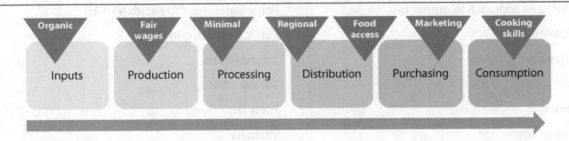

Source: Gretchen Swanson Center.

CONCLUSION

Consumers have grown increasingly concerned about where their food comes from and how it is produced. This curiosity trickles down into the area of nutrition knowledge as well. It is important that those working to improve food systems are equipped with basic nutrition knowledge, such as is presented in this chapter, and an understanding of how nutrition fits into the context of the overall food system. This background enables us to be clear about what types of food should be made available and about recognizing the diversity of ways to meet an individual's food needs—and it helps us to "talk the talk" when bringing in evidence to support such efforts.

Although nutrition is a science, it is also an art. The ways in which food is produced, distributed, and consumed, and the nuances involved in food decision making, cooking, and food's sociocultural associations, are all part of nutrition. These elements can be molded to provide a food system that makes the healthy choice the easy choice.

SUMMARY

It is important for health promotion and food system professionals to understand the basics of nutrition. This chapter summarizes the nutrients, including macro- and micronutrients, and describes their role in the human body, what foods are good sources for specific nutrients, and the consequences of deficiencies or excesses. Use of ingredients with addictive potential in food processing could lead to increased demand, and thus more food being produced, transported, and stored than is biologically necessary. To improve nutrition at a population level, efforts such as the Dietary Guidelines for Americans and policies across various settings need to be employed. A traditional nutrition approach focuses on the components of a healthy diet; a public health nutrition approach seeks to ensure that the *conditions* under which individuals can be healthy are optimized; and a food systems approach to nutrition examines how individual needs for nutrients and energy are being met by the food system. Incorporating public health nutrition and food systems approaches together with traditional nutrition is important for promoting healthy and sustainable diets for all Americans.

KEY TERMS

Dietary reference intakes (DRIs)	Malnutrition
Enrichment	Micronutrients
Fats (lipids)	Minerals
Flavonoids	Phytonutrients
Food systems approach to nutrition	Polyunsaturated fatty acids (PUFAs)
Fortification	Public health nutrition
Insoluble fiber	Saturated fats
Ketosis	Soluble fiber
Kilocalorie	Trans fats
Macronutrients	Vitamins

DISCUSSION QUESTIONS

1. In what ways are a public health nutrition and a food systems approach to nutrition similar? Different? Take a nutritional problem (for example, the imbalance of omega-3 and omega-6 fatty acids in the US diet) and discuss how it would be approached differently by each of these and by traditional nutrition.

2. In perspective 16.1, nearly one-quarter of Americans indicated that they have extremely or very healthful diets. Why do these perceptions differ so greatly from those of nutritionists? What are the implications of these differing perceptions for diet and health?

3. Why is it important for the US Departments of Health and Human Services and Agriculture to update the Dietary Guidelines for Americans every five years?

4. Give some examples of nutritional messages you have heard that conflict with one another. What do you think of the relative benefits and drawbacks of focusing on a whole foods approach rather than focusing on specific messages?

5. The evaluation of the FDA's trans fat labeling regulation suggested dramatic impacts on blood trans fat levels across the population. How do you think labeling affected the change?

6. If some foods or ingredients are deemed addictive, and if food manufacturers who sell those products are aware of those findings, should they be held liable for costs associated with obesity? Why or why not?

7. Why does the current state of the food system lead to Americans overconsuming sodium? What can be done about it?

8. The conclusion states that, "although nutrition is a science, it is also an art." Do you agree? Why or why not?

REFERENCES

Astrup, A., Dyerberg, J., Elwood, P., Hermansen, K., Hu, F. B., Jakobsen, M. U., ... & Willett, W. C. (2011). The role of reducing intakes of saturated fat in the prevention of cardiovascular disease: Where does the evidence stand in 2010? *The American Journal of Clinical Nutrition, 93*(4), 684–688.

Avena, N. M., Rada, P., & Hoebel, B. G. (2008). Evidence for sugar addiction: Behavioral and neurochemical effects of intermittent, excessive sugar intake. *Neuroscience & Biobehavioral Reviews, 32*(1), 20–39.

Baker, B. P., Benbrook, C. M., Growth III,, E., & Benbrook, K. L. (2002). Pesticide residues in conventional, integrated pest management (IPM)-grown and organic foods: Insights from three US data sets. *Food Additives and Contaminants, 19*(5), 427–446.

Benbrook, C., Zhao, X., Yáñez, J., Davies, N., & Andrews, P. (2008). *New evidence confirms the nutritional superiority of plant-based organic foods.* The Organic Center. Retrieved from www.organic-center.org/reportfiles/5367_Nutrient _Content_SSR_FINAL_V2.pdf

Bray, G. A., Nielsen, S. J., & Popkin, B. M. (2004). Consumption of high-fructose corn syrup in beverages may play a role in the epidemic of obesity. *The American Journal of Clinical Nutrition, 79*(4), 537–543.

Center for Science in the Public Interest. (2009). *Heart attack entrées and side orders of stroke.* Retrieved from www.cspinet.org/new/200905111.html

Center for Science in the Public Interest. (2012). *Quorn complaints.* Retrieved from www.cspinet.org/quorn

Center for Science in the Public Interest. (2013a). *Chemical cuisine: Learn about food additives*. Retrieved from www.cspinet.org/reports/chemcuisine.htm#caramel

Center for Science in the Public Interest. (2013b). *Trans fat wall of shame*. Retrieved from www.pinterest.com/cspinutrition /trans-fat-wall-of-shame

Centers for Disease Control and Prevention. (2012). *CDC study finds levels of trans-fatty acids in blood of U.S. white adults has decreased*. Retrieved from www.cdc.gov/media/releases/2012/p0208_trans-fatty_acids.html

Dangour, A., Lock, K., Hayter, A., Aikenhead, A., Allen, E., & Uauy, R. (2010). Nutrition-related health effects of organic foods: A systematic review. *American Journal of Clinical Nutrition, 92*(1), 203–210.

Elliott, S. S., Keim, N. L., Stern, J. S., Teff, K., & Havel, P. J. (2002). Fructose, weight gain, and the insulin resistance syndrome. *The American Journal of Clinical Nutrition, 76*(5), 911–922.

Forshee, R. A., Storey, M. L., Allison, D. B., Glinsmann, W. H., Hein, G. L., Lineback, D. R., ... & White, J. S. (2007). A critical examination of the evidence relating high fructose corn syrup and weight gain. *Critical Reviews in Food Science and Nutrition, 47*(6), 561–582.

Gearhardt, A. N., Corbin, W. R., & Brownell, K. D. (2009). Preliminary validation of the Yale food addiction scale. *Appetite, 52*(2), 430–436.

Gearhardt, A. N., Corbin, W. R., & Brownell, K. D. (2009). Yale Food Addiction Scale. Retrieved from www.yale ruddcenter.org/resources/upload/docs/what/addiction/FoodAddictionScale09.pdf

Gearhardt, A. N., Yokum, S., Orr, P. T., Stice, E., Corbin, W. R., & Brownell, K. D. (2011). Neural correlates of food addiction. *Archives of General Psychiatry, 68*(8), 808–816.

Gold, M. (2007). *Sustainable agriculture: Definitions and terms*. Washington, DC: US Department of Agriculture. Retrieved from www.nal.usda.gov/afsic/pubs/terms/srb9902terms.shtml

Gold, M. S., Frost-Pineda, K., & Jacobs, W. S. (2003). Overeating, binge eating, and eating disorders as addictions. *Psychiatric Annals*.

Institute of Medicine. (2010). *Strategies to reduce sodium intake in the United States*. Washington, DC: The National Academies Press. Retrieved from www.nap.edu/openbook.php?record_id=12818

International Food Information Council Foundation. (2012). *Food & health survey*. Retrieved from www.foodinsight.org /Content/5519/IFICF_2012_FoodHealthSurvey.pdf

Jacobson, M. F. (2013, August 8). Reasonable certainty of no harm? *The Hill*. Retrieved from http://thehill.com/blogs /congress-blog/healthcare/316175-reasonable-certainty-of-no-harm

Johnson, P. M., & Kenny, P. J. (2010). Dopamine D2 receptors in addiction-like reward dysfunction and compulsive eating in obese rats. *Nature Neuroscience, 13*(5), 635–641.

The Joint FAO/WHO/UNU Expert Consultation on Energy and Protein Requirements. (1985). *Energy and protein requirements*. Retrieved from http://www.fao.org/docrep/003/aa040e/aa040e00.htm

Lenoir, M., Serre, F., Cantin, L., & Ahmed, S. H. (2007). Intense sweetness surpasses cocaine reward. *PloS One, 2*(8), e698.

Lustig, R. H., Schmidt, L. A., & Brindis, C. D. (2012). Public health: The toxic truth about sugar. *Nature, 482*(7383), 27–29.

Lutter, M., & Nestler, E. J. (2009). Homeostatic and hedonic signals interact in the regulation of food intake. *The Journal of Nutrition, 139*(3), 629–632.

Mahan, L. K., & Escott-Stump, S. (2003). *Krause's food, nutrition and diet therapy*. Philadelphia: Saunders.

National Institutes of Health. Office of Dietary Supplements (ODS). (nd). *Dietary supplement fact sheets*. Retrieved from http://ods.od.nih.gov

Oh, K., Hu, F. B., Manson, J. E., Stampfer, M. J., Willett, W. C. (2005). Dietary fat intake and risk of coronary heart disease in women: 20 years of follow-up of the nurses' health study. *American Journal of Epidemiology, 161*(7), 672–679.

Simopoulos, A. P. (2008). The importance of the omega-6/omega-3 fatty acid ratio in cardiovascular disease and other chronic diseases. *Experimental Medicine and Biology, 233*(6), 674–88.

Story, M., Kaphingst, K. M., Robinson-O'Brien, R., & Glanz, K. (2008). Creating healthy food and eating environments: Policy and environmental approaches. *Annual Review of Public Health, 29*, 253–272.

US Department of Agriculture. (2010). *DRI tables*. Food and Nutrition Information Center. Retrieved from http://fnic.nal.usda.gov/dietary-guidance/dietary-reference-intakes/dri-tables

US Department of Agriculture Economic Research Service. (2012). http://www.ers.usda.gov/amber-waves/2012-september/trans-fats.aspx#.U8XpJqhupVs

US National Library of Medicine, US Department of Health and Human Services, National Institutes of Health, FOIA, USA.gov. MedlinePlus. (2012). Health Information from the National Library of Medicine [Internet]. Retrieved from www.nlm.nih.gov/hinfo.html

Vesper, H. W., Kuiper, H. C., Mirel, L. B., Johnson, C. L., & Pirkle, J. L. (2012). Levels of plasma trans-fatty acids in non-Hispanic white adults in the United States in 2000 and 2009. *JAMA, 307*, 562–563.

Volkow, N. D., Wang, G. J., Fowler, J. S., & Telang, F. (2008). Overlapping neuronal circuits in addiction and obesity: Evidence of systems pathology. *Philosophical Transactions of the Royal Society B: Biological Sciences, 363*(1507), 3191–3200.

Volkow, N. D., Wang, G. J., Fowler, J. S., Tomasi, D., & Baler, R. (2012). Food and drug reward: Overlapping circuits in human obesity and addiction. In *Brain Imaging in Behavioral Neuroscience* (pp. 1–24). Berlin: Springer.

Wade, L. (2013). *Sugary drinks linked to 180,000 deaths worldwide*. CNN. Retrieved from www.cnn.com/2013/03/19/health/sugary-drinks-deaths

White, J. S. (2008). Straight talk about high-fructose corn syrup: What it is and what it ain't. *The American Journal of Clinical Nutrition, 88*(6), 1716S-1721S.

Willett, W. (1998). *Nutritional epidemiology* (2nd ed.). New York: Oxford University Press.

Yale Food Addiction Scale: www.yaleruddcenter.org/resources/upload/docs/what/addiction/FoodAddictionScale09.pdf

Yale Rudd Center for Food Policy and Obesity: Retrieved from www.yaleruddcenter.org

Healthy Food Environments

Patricia L. Truant and Roni A. Neff

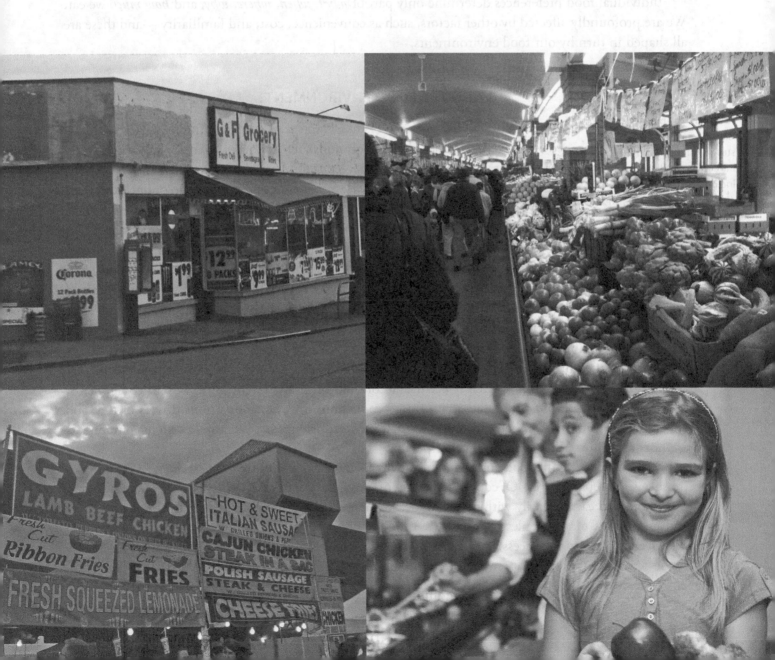

> **Learning Objectives**
>
> - Describe evidence regarding the structure and health impacts of food environments in homes, schools, work sites, stores, and restaurants.
>
> - Discuss strategies for measuring food environments.
>
> - List factors that shape the food environment from geography to within-site characteristics to societal structures.
>
> - Describe intervention strategies to improve home, school, work, retail, restaurant, and other community food environments.
>
> - Understand the nuances and limitations in food environment research, theory, and terminology.

Individual food preferences determine only part of *what, when, where, why,* and *how much* we eat. We are profoundly affected by other factors, such as convenience, cost, and familiarity—and these are all shaped in turn by our food environments.

WHAT IS A FOOD ENVIRONMENT?

food environment
All aspects of our surroundings that may influence our diets, including physical locations and marketing, media, and online exposures

The term **food environment** refers to all aspects of our surroundings that may influence our diets. It includes physical locations such as homes, schools, workplaces, food stores, restaurants, gardens, and emergency food assistance sites. It also includes the neighborhoods surrounding these places and marketing, media, and online exposures. Food environments are also shaped by available transportation, physical and social boundaries, and land use: residential, business, agricultural, or mixed-use. Figure 17.1 provides a model of food environment influences from individual to macro-level factors. In this chapter we focus on the third ring, the physical environment—recognizing that, more broadly, food environments are also affected by an area's economic development, social factors such as inequalities and segregation, ethnicity and culture—and more broadly still by distribution systems and food and agriculture policy. This model is structured differently from the broad food system model presented in chapter 1 (see figure 1.1) in order to focus in on how food environment factors can affect diet. Figure 1.1 contributes complementary perspectives by helping us consider food acquisition within the broader context of the system within which it occurs. Accordingly, it draws attention to system components, including resource inputs, the food chain from production to waste, and various drivers of the food system. Most important, it helps us recognize that the relationships between these system components are not static, but rather, in constant interplay.

When discussing the food environment, the focus is generally on proximate influences rather than those several steps removed. Of course, meanings of "proximate" can differ. In a city, someone may work, live, shop, and eat primarily within a few blocks, whereas in suburban or rural areas, the closest stores and restaurants may be miles from home. And, our perceptions of the food environment, including perceived proximity and access, familiarity, and comfort, are at least as important in determining choices as the actual contours of that environment (Caspi, Kawachi, Subramanian, Adamkiewicz, & Sorensen, 2012).

FIGURE 17.1   Socioecological Model

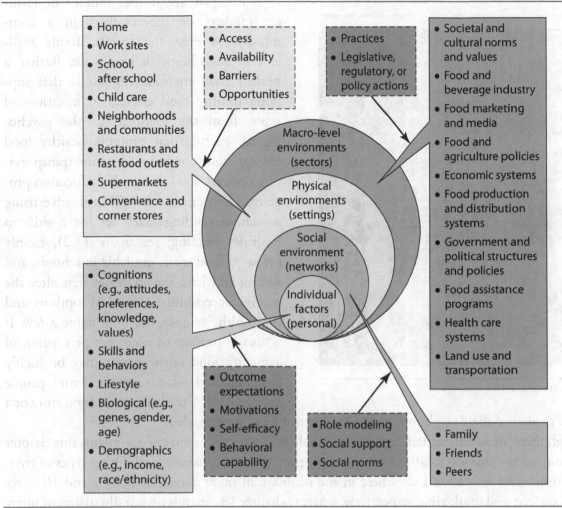

- Home
- Work sites
- School, after school
- Child care
- Neighborhoods and communities
- Restaurants and fast food outlets
- Supermarkets
- Convenience and corner stores

- Access
- Availability
- Barriers
- Opportunities

- Practices
- Legislative, regulatory, or policy actions

- Societal and cultural norms and values
- Food and beverage industry
- Food marketing and media
- Food and agriculture policies
- Economic systems
- Food production and distribution systems
- Government and political structures and policies
- Food assistance programs
- Health care systems
- Land use and transportation

Macro-level environments (sectors)

Physical environments (settings)

Social environment (networks)

Individual factors (personal)

- Cognitions (e.g., attitudes, preferences, knowledge, values)
- Skills and behaviors
- Lifestyle
- Biological (e.g., genes, gender, age)
- Demographics (e.g., income, race/ethnicity)

- Outcome expectations
- Motivations
- Self-efficacy
- Behavioral capability

- Role modeling
- Social support
- Social norms

- Family
- Friends
- Peers

Source: Story, Kaphingst, Robinson-O'Brien, and Glanz (2008).

The food environment includes not only where food is located but also the specific options and the experience of acquiring food there—the number of different ice creams in a supermarket freezer, the attractiveness of product packaging, the color and freshness of produce on a farmers market table, handicap accessibility, or even the way a store's staff treats its customers. In processing those experiences, we are far less rational and more impulsive than we believe ourselves to be, as shown in the behavioral economics literature (chapter 7). For example, the greater the portion size, the more we will consume. The greater the variety of offerings, the more of them the consumer will want. People are also more likely to stick with the default option presented—that is, accepting fries with their burgers instead of requesting salads (Just, Mancino, & Wansink, 2007). Food purveyors routinely use insights such as these to create ambiance within stores and restaurants enticing us to buy their products. Increasingly, public health interventionists are catching on, too, using these same approaches to promote healthier choices (Cohen & Babey, 2012; Gittelsohn & Lee, 2013). For example, **healthy defaults** (such as an automatic vegetable with your meal, or milk or water instead of soda) can help tip the balance toward better nutrition.

healthy defaults
Options provided that make the healthy choice the easy choice

FIGURE 17.2   Farmer's Fridge Healthy Vending Kiosks

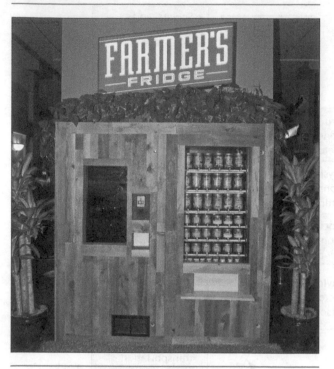

Source: Farmer's Fridge. Used with permission.

So what is a *healthy* food environment? It is not just about the number of farmers markets or supermarkets in a community, or even the specific foods available in one's home or workplace. Rather, a healthy food environment is one that supports healthy food choices in a variety of ways, from the logistical to the psychological. Factors that promote healthy food environments include adequate transportation options, food and garden education programs, restrictions on billboard advertising or school vending machines (or a shift to healthier vending; see figure 17.2), freshly prepared food made available in schools, and zoning and land-use strategies that alter the relative accessibility of healthy options and less-healthy temptations—to name a few. It is also important to note that perception of a quality food environment may be highly individualized—for example, some people may consider having an ethnic food store or a community garden in their neighborhood preferable to a large supermarket.

Although there are social, virtual, and even psychological aspects of food environments, this chapter focuses on important physical locations where people purchase and consume food. Other types of environmental influences are covered elsewhere in the textbook in more detail; chapters 9 and 10 cover culture and society, and marketing, respectively, whereas chapter 18 expands on our discussion of interventions.

Environment is not destiny. Those with high motivation to eat healthfully can manage to do so even in environments with limited options and plentiful temptations. Conversely, people with the resources and geographical opportunities to eat fresh produce and other healthy foods morning, noon, and night may still choose to consume unhealthy food, for many reasons. Nonetheless, food environments shape what choices will be most feasible, and likely, and they subconsciously alter preferences and consumption patterns.

The US diet has changed dramatically since the middle of the twentieth century, partly because of technological advances; consumer preferences for convenience food; economic, social, and lifestyle changes; and food and agricultural policies. The physical food environment has simultaneously reflected and helped drive these changes. Today we can find food almost everywhere we look (for example, see figure 17.3). Gas stations and big-box stores are among the fastest growing food sources, whereas nonfood retailers sell candy and soda in the checkout line. Theaters, cafes, food trucks, and supermarket sections pump out aromas to tempt us. Schools, workplaces, and hospitals provide convenient access to unhealthy foods in vending machines, snack stands, and cafes. Processed convenience foods and sugar-sweetened beverages (SSBs) are also often sold in extra-large portion sizes and at low prices. Eating out

FIGURE 17.3   The Contiguous United States as Visualized by Distance to Nearest McDonald's

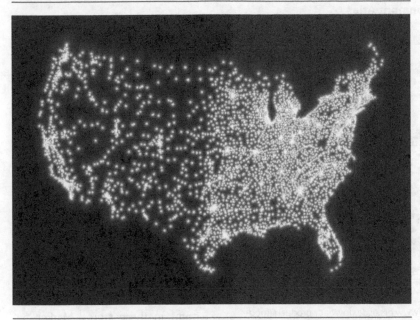

Source: Stephen Van Worley. (September 2010). Data Pointed datapointed.net. Used with permission.

has become more frequent over the last several decades, and customers get more calories and fat when they eat out compared to when they prepare meals at home, as described in perspective 15.1.

At the same time, some aspects of our food environment are improving. Increased awareness of nutrition and food environments has led to great creativity and effort invested in interventions, particularly those addressing underserved areas. Additionally, many efforts are underway to make locally produced food more available in all types of food environments. For example, farmers market numbers more than quadrupled nationwide from 1,755 markets in 1994 to 8,144 in 2013 (US Department of Agriculture Agricultural Marketing Service, 2013).

How do we track food environment changes, and how do we understand their impacts, for communities, for people, and for health? To address such questions empirically (via research), it is valuable to condense the food environment's complexity into simplified measures. Focus 17.1 describes ways to do that.

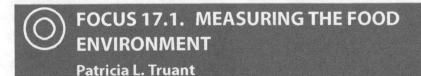

FOCUS 17.1. MEASURING THE FOOD ENVIRONMENT
Patricia L. Truant

It is often necessary to characterize food environments quantitatively or spatially for purposes of research, planning, policy, and practice. In these measures, the presence of supermarkets is most commonly used as an indicator of healthfulness. As the field has developed, broader metrics have become more common, including those characterizing the variety of restaurants and small stores, and transportation (Wang, Gonzalez, Ritchie, & Winkleby, 2006).

A variety of data sources exist for assessing food retail environments. The US Department of Agriculture [USDA] Food Environment Atlas is an interactive web tool presenting county-level data on 168 indicators, including retail food locations, food prices, community characteristics, and nutrition assistance programs. The visual interface enables users to create specialized maps highlighting factors and regions of interest. Figure 17.4 shows the county-level percentage of households without cars and more than one mile from grocery stores.

(Continued)

(Continued)

FIGURE 17.4   USDA Food Environment Atlas

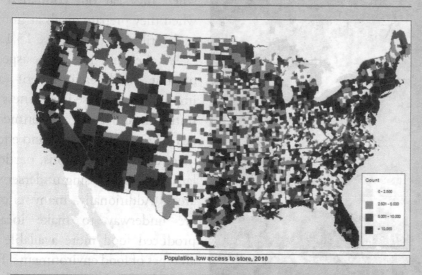

Population, low access to store, 2010

Source: USDA (2014). Public domain. http://www.ers.usda.gov/data-products/food-environment-atlas/.aspx

More localized measures can be especially useful in determining how best to breach food access gaps. For example, the Centers for Disease Control and Prevention's (CDC) *Healthier Food Retail* (CDC, nd) provides information on available resources for assessing local food environments.

Although food environment maps can document presence or absence of certain types of stores, often we want to know about the quality of items in these stores. Market basket audits or healthy food availability indexes (HFAI), which quantify the types of foods for sale in stores, are often used in conjunction with mapping to get a broad and nuanced description of an area's food availability. The USDA Economic Research Service Food Store Survey Instrument and the Nutrition Environment Measures Survey (NEMS) (with versions for stores and restaurants) are two common tools; both can be modified to meet communities' needs.

The NEMS retail food store tool, for example, measures availability and pricing of eleven foods of varying types and nutritional quality:

- Milk

- Fruits

- Vegetables

- Ground beef

- Hot dogs

- Frozen dinners

- Baked goods

- Beverages

- Whole grain bread

- Baked chips

- Cereal

Other approaches to measuring the food environment include quantifying store shelf space for various items, conducting interviews or surveys with store owners, or analyzing sales data, receipts, and nutrient content of restaurant menus, school lunches, vending machines, or other food retailers (National Cancer Institute, 2013).

A comprehensive food environment assessment can be helpful for understanding factors beyond the retail sector, including production, transportation, food security, consumer perception, and public policies. Guides for conducting these assessments have been compiled by the USDA and the Community Food Security Coalition (Pothukuchi, Joseph, Burton, & Fisher, 2002; USDA, 2012).

Researchers studying the food environment (similar to all researchers) must ensure their data are valid and reliable. Data quality in public records, web searches, and other secondary data sources may be questionable at best, including because businesses frequently start up and shut down. Ground-truthing, or direct observation of stores by visiting mapped locations, can be time-intensive but it is the best way to verify location information (Sharkey, 2009).

EQUITY

There are clear inequities in food environment quality, especially across racial, ethnic, and income groups. Areas with fewer resources and those with higher minority populations tend to have fewer options for buying healthy foods than wealthier and predominantly Caucasian areas; often, these same areas have relatively abundant options for purchasing unhealthy foods in restaurants, carry-outs, convenience stores and small grocery stores like the one in figure 17.5.

Inequities may be entrenched in the day-to-day experiences of individuals and communities, and even accepted as a fact of life. These inequities can translate to differences in diet quality, and in turn result in health disparities. Multiple studies have found differential retail and restaurant access by neighborhood. For example, in Baltimore, predominantly African American and lower-income neighborhoods were found to have less healthy food availability than predominantly white and higher-income areas, because of different types of stores and different offerings within stores (Franco, Diez Roux, Glass, Caballero, & Brancati, 2008). These differences can be associated with diet healthfulness (Story et al., 2008).

Such areas have been termed, **food deserts** This term has been criticized for its emphasis on a community's deficits and, some would say, subtle racial overtones. Some advocates feel this term stigmatizes residents without encouraging real community-driven solutions, as discussed in perspective 17.1. At the same time, the term *food desert* has been beneficial from a policy standpoint, catalyzing attention to underserved areas and helping officials identify specific areas

FIGURE 17.5 Family Cigarette Grocery Store

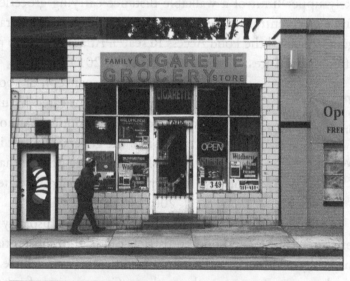

Source: PJ Roldan, Flickr Commons (2011). http://www.flickr.com/photos/26856943@N03/7044377969/

food deserts
Areas with low access to healthy foods, commonly low-income urban or rural areas without nearby supermarkets; there are several specific definitions

in need of focus and resources. Accordingly, some advocates reserve the term for usage in public policy context.

A federal working group defined food deserts as "census tract(s) with a substantial share of residents who live in low-income areas that have low levels of access to a grocery store or healthy, affordable retail outlet" (USDA, nd). They further defined "low income communities" as those with either a poverty rate of 20 percent or higher, or a median family income of 80 percent or less than the area's median family income. "Low-access communities" were defined as those with at least five hundred people or 33 percent of the population residing more than one mile from a supermarket or large grocery store (or ten miles in rural areas). Based on this definition, 23.5 million people in the United States live in food deserts (USDA, nd).

The specific definition of a *food desert* is important because it affects eligibility for grants and other opportunities. Officials in urban areas, including Baltimore, found that the one-mile criterion meant there would be few or no food deserts within their cities, despite the substantial gaps in food access. The City of Baltimore worked with the Johns Hopkins Center for a Livable Future to develop a definition better suited to many urban areas: "An area where the distance to a supermarket is more than 1/4 mile, the median household income is at or below 185% of the Federal Poverty Level, over 40% of households have no vehicle available, and the average Healthy Food Availability Index score for supermarkets, convenience and corner stores is low" (Baltimore Food Policy Initiative, 2010) (shown in figure 17.6). This definition recognizes that for families without their own transportation, one-quarter mile is a likely upper limit of a walkable distance carrying groceries. The city is now using this definition to target interventions. The USDA also recognizes the federal definition is not one-size-fits-all, and the agency released the Food Access Research Atlas in 2013 to provide an updated mapping resource using different measures of food access (USDA, 2013b).

food swamps
Areas where food options are predominantly relatively unhealthy foods at locations such as convenience stores and fast food outlets

To complement the concept of food deserts, a new term has arisen—**food swamps**, meaning areas permeated by unhealthy foods at locations such as convenience stores and fast food outlets. Although this term may be equally distasteful as *food deserts* to some, the general concept is useful and may be at least as important in shaping health. Indeed, a perspective that jointly characterizes gaps and oversaturation of a food environment may ultimately be most valuable (Rose et al., 2009; Ver Ploeg et al., 2009).

Other factors beyond retail food environments also play a role. Heterogeneity in school food policies between wealthier and poorer districts can lead to substantial differences in exposure to SSBs and other unhealthy products. Socioeconomic differences in vehicle ownership can make it far easier for some people to travel to stores than others. Communities further differ in transportation connectivity and enforcement of handicap accessibility laws. And, employees in higher-wage jobs are more likely to have longer maternity leaves and the flexibility and space to pump breast milk for their babies than those in lower-wage jobs, thus increasing the likelihood of longer duration breastfeeding, with its documented health benefits. Different communities may have different access to safety nets such as emergency food assistance programs. These inequities are problematic not only because of the health outcomes that could result but also because they reflect injustices.

FIGURE 17.6 2012 Baltimore City Food Environment Map

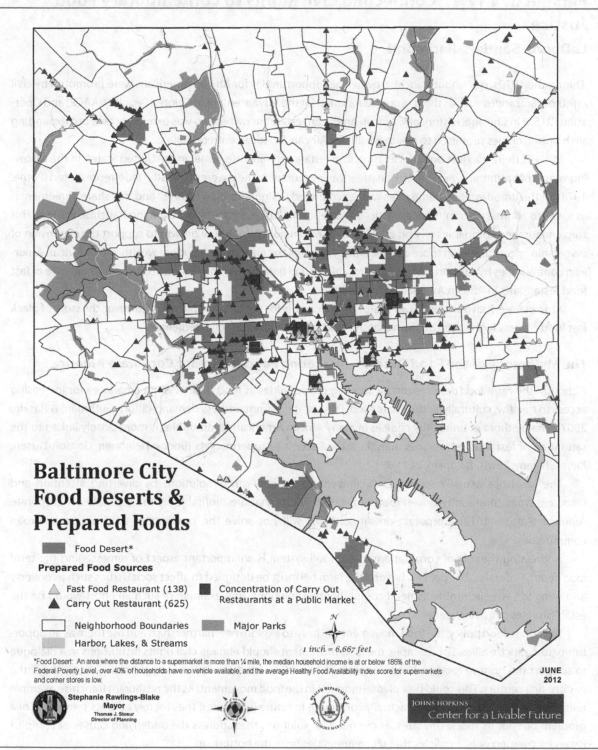

Baltimore City Food Deserts & Prepared Foods

Food Desert*

Prepared Food Sources

△ Fast Food Restaurant (138)
▲ Carry Out Restaurant (625)

■ Concentration of Carry Out Restaurants at a Public Market

☐ Neighborhood Boundaries
Harbor, Lakes, & Streams

Major Parks

N

1 inch = 6,667 feet

*Food Desert: An area where the distance to a supermarket is more than ¼ mile, the median household income is at or below 185% of the Federal Poverty Level, over 40% of households have no vehicle available, and the average Healthy Food Availability Index score for supermarkets and corner stores is low.

JUNE 2012

Stephanie Rawlings-Blake
Mayor
Thomas J. Stosur
Director of Planning

JOHNS HOPKINS
Center for a Livable Future

Source: CLF.

Perspective 17.1. Connecting Civil Rights to Contemporary Food Justice

LaDonna Sanders-Redmond

During the 1970s, restaurant franchise ownership opportunities for African Americans were promoted by civil rights organizations such as the National Association for the Advancement of Colored People (NAACP) and Operation P.U.S.H in Chicago. Historically, African American restaurant ownership was extremely rare, but expanding such opportunities promised to create wealth for African American entrepreneurs.

In 1967, there was just one African American restaurant franchise owner in the United States. In the following years, that number grew, but African American restaurant owners were still vastly underrepresented (Petrie, 1978). At the time, fast food companies were encouraged to sign "moral covenants" and "fair share agreements" as a way to address discriminatory practices that kept African Americans from becoming franchise owners. This step encouraged companies relying on African American dollars for future growth to support the expansion of ownership opportunities in those communities. However, the effort to create more wealth within African American communities by supporting fast food franchising had unintended consequences: an overabundance of fast food restaurants in African American communities.

African American franchise owners are not responsible for the obesity epidemic. However, the story of black fast food owners highlights the ways that the food system makes strange bedfellows.

The Mythology of the Food Desert—Marketing Food Justice for Corporate America

Although the term *food desert* is catchy, labeling communities as food deserts is not a panacea for increasing access to healthy, culturally appropriate food. Further, it does not address demand (Short, Guthman, & Raskin, 2007). The plethora of unhealthy choices in many African American communities is more closely linked to the saturation of fast food restaurants than the lack of access to supermarkets (Boone-Heinonen, Gordon-Larsen, Kiefe, Shikany, Lewis, & Popkin, 2011).

The label has actually served to circumvent community-driven solutions by diverting attention and resources from community-driven food projects to efforts that are profitable by the standards of corporate America (Patton, 2012). Corporate-driven solutions will not solve the problem of food access in urban communities.

Addressing the role of corporations in our food system is an important aspect of remessaging the term *food desert*. Federal public policies beyond the farm bill must be designed to affect social issues such as poverty and hunger. Systemic problems need comprehensive solutions; one example of such an effort would be the establishment of a living wage.

To change food policy, the food movement will have to explore new partnerships and use them as an opportunity to politicize allies. For example, the food movement should engage civil rights institutions in a dialogue to support the right to food and encourage them to address food access issues as *the* civil rights issue of the twenty-first century. This could be a pivotal moment in the food movement. As the restaurant franchise example tells us, steps toward equality can actually contribute to future injustices if they merely address symptoms of a problem but not its roots. This stresses our need for solutions that address the underlying causes of complex issues by creating public policies that lift communities from the bottom up.

HOMES, SCHOOLS, WORKPLACES

This section focuses on locations important to the daily food environment: home, schools, and workplaces. The next section discusses the built food environment, namely, restaurants and stores. Following discussion of each environment is an overview of relevant intervention strategies.

Homes

Americans consume about two-thirds of their calories (Guthrie, Lin, & Frazao, 2002) and spend about half their food budgets on foods prepared in the home (Hayden, Blissard, Bhuyan, & Nayga, 2004). Meals eaten at home tend to have fewer calories, less fat and saturated fat, and more fiber, calcium, and iron than meals eaten away from home (Guthrie et al., 2002). For children, adults typically act as "nutritional gatekeepers" by deciding what foods are available in the home, how they are served, and in what quantities. Parents' fruit and vegetable intake is a strong predictor of fruit and vegetable consumption among their children (Cooke, Wardle, Gibson, Sapochnik, Sheiham, & Lawson, 2004). Sitting down at the family dinner table on a regular basis has also been linked to children and adolescents eating more vitamins and minerals, fruits, vegetables, grains, and calcium—and less fried food, SSBs, and trans fats (Neumark-Sztainer, Larson, Fulkerson, Eisenberg, & Story, 2010).

FIGURE 17.7 Bowl of Fruit on the Counter

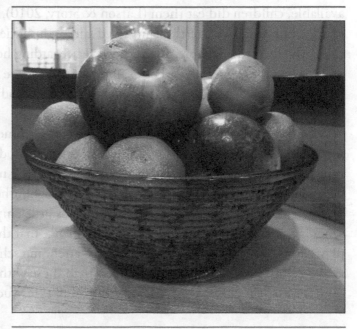

Source: CLF/Neff.

Although it sounds obvious, keeping healthy foods in the home makes it more likely that adults and children alike will eat them. Nutritious choices can be encouraged by keeping them accessible (i.e., placing a bowl of fruit on the counter [see figure 17.7] or cut-up vegetables in the refrigerator). Conversely, when high-calorie snack food is purchased in bulk and stored in visible locations, consumption rates increase (Chandon & Wansink, 2002).

Schools

Many students spend the majority of weekday waking hours at school during the academic year. They may consume up to 50 percent of their daily calories at school (Larsen & Gilliland, 2009; Larson & Story, 2009). Although federal school breakfast and lunch programs now must adhere to national nutrition standards, the food environment at many schools also includes **competitive foods**—mostly high-fat or high-sugar snacks or beverages—in vending machines, cafeteria á la carte lines, and school stores. These "compete" with the federal school meals. In 2010–2011,

competitive foods
The mostly high-fat or high-sugar snacks or beverages in vending machines, cafeteria á la carte lines, and school stores that compete with the federal school meal offerings and are outside the scope of national school nutrition guidelines

80 percent of public elementary schools, 96 percent of public middle schools, and 98 percent of public high schools lacked policies on competitive food and beverages. A small percentage (13 percent, 4 percent, and 2 percent, respectively) had weak policies (Chriqui et al., 2013). Competitive foods were outside the scope of federal requirements for nutrition until the passage of the Healthy Hunger-Free Kids Act of 2010, which required USDA to set standards for all school foods. In June 2013, USDA finalized these new standards, called the "Smart Snacks in Schools" program (USDA, 2013a). For more details on the new standards, see www.fns.usda.gov/cnd/governance/legislation/allfoods.htm.

One review of multiple studies found clear evidence that children ate more healthfully when competitive foods were not available in their schools; and further, that when healthier foods were made available, children did eat them (Larson & Story, 2010). Although some of the reviewed studies found a lack of impact, most of these involved adding healthier options without subtracting the less healthy ones. The literature is more mixed, however, regarding how changing competitive food regulations will affect students' overall diets. For example, there is some evidence that dissatisfaction with school food may encourage adolescents to skip lunch and buy food from nearby convenience stores or take-outs (Dammann & Smith, 2010).

The food environment surrounding schools also merits attention. About one-third of US public secondary schools nationwide have at least one fast food restaurant or convenience store within a half mile, and in the largest cities that figure is higher. The numbers of restaurants and convenience stores near schools vary by SES, with lower-income neighborhoods having more outlets than higher-income ones (Zenk & Powell, 2008). Although there is little empirical data linking proximity of food stores to schools and students' diets, there is some evidence that the food environment surrounding schools does play a role. One study found that students attending schools over one kilometer from the nearest convenience store had healthier overall diets than those with closer stores. Further, the density of fast food outlets near schools affected diet quality as well (He, Tucker, Irwin, Gilliland, Larsen, & Hess, 2012).

Workplaces

Most US adults spend about half their waking hours at work, and thus many of their daily calories are consumed in and around work settings. There is much diversity in workplaces, from the traditional large office or factory setting on which most workplace food environment research is based, to smaller offices, to mobile and home-based work sites. Sources of food vary across these workplace types, but can include company cafeterias, office building food courts, vending machines, meetings or events, fund-raisers, and food in shared office and kitchen space. Employees may also patronize nearby stores, snack stands, and restaurants.

Employee dietary choices are also influenced by environmental factors such as employer policies, social and organizational support for healthy behaviors, workplace wellness programs, and social norms about meals, including eating at one's desk (Larson & Story, 2009). Workplace infrastructure (such as availability of refrigerators and microwaves) and policies structuring the length and timing of breaks contribute to the food environment and shape opportunities to eat healthfully (Sorensen, Linnan, & Hunt, 2004).

Homes, Schools, and Workplace Interventions

Homes, schools, and workplaces have been settings for a variety of food environment interventions, described in the following and summarized in table 17.1. Among the environments covered in this

TABLE 17.1 Examples of Interventions in Home, School, and Workplace Environments

	Objective	Intervention	Results	Reference
Home	Reduce sugar-sweetened beverage consumption in overweight, obese teens	Make calorie-free beverages available in home via delivery Regular check-ins with participants, parents One-year intervention, second-year follow-up	Reduced SSB consumption during and post intervention Reduced increases in BMI after intervention, but not at follow-up	Ebbeling et al. (2012)
	Replace calorie-dense snacks with nutritious alternatives; increase fruit and vegetable consumption	Make fresh-cut fruits and vegetables readily available in home	Parents, children with higher reported availability at home consumed 1.2 (fruit) and 0.7 (vegetable) more servings per day.	Kratt, Reynolds, and Shewchuk (2000)
School	Reduce consumption of high-fat, high-sugar snacks	Remove unhealthy competitive foods from school environment in á la carte lines, school stores, and vending machines	Review article found children's diets were healthier when competitive foods were not available. One study found reduced intake of SSBs when no snack bar was present; another study reported higher fruit and vegetable intake when no unhealthy competitive foods were available.	Larson and Story (2010)
	Increase fresh produce consumption	Change school environment by adding salad bars to cafeterias	Cross-sectional study of elementary students found increased fruit and vegetable consumption, and lower calorie, cholesterol, and fat intake after salad bar was introduced.	Slusser, Cumberland, Browdy, Lange, and Neumann (2007)
		USDA Fresh Fruit and Vegetable Program adds fruits and vegetables into outside-meal environment in low-income elementary schools by providing them for free	A 2011 interim evaluation found a 15 percent increase in produce consumption; overall calorie intake was not significantly increased.	Olsho, Klerman, and Bartlett (2011)
	Support positive attitudes toward gardening and fresh produce	Add garden into school environment along with garden-based nutrition education	Review article describes anecdotal reports of positive outcomes such as nutritional attitudes, leadership skills, and academic achievement.	Robinson-O'Brien, Story, and Heim (2009)

(Continued)

TABLE 17.1 *(Continued)*

	Objective	Intervention	Results	Reference
Work sites	Reduce cancer and cardiovascular risks and promote a healthy lifestyle	Point-of-purchase food labeling in cafeteria environment, more healthy options in cafeterias and vending machines, increased communications surrounding health	Systematic review of work-site health promotion programs found evidence that these programs can effectively modify fruit and vegetable and fat intake.	Engbers, van Poppel, Chin, Paw, and van Mechelen (2005)
	Increase fresh produce consumption	Subsidizing fruit and vegetables and making more produce options available in work environment	Sales of fruit and salads tripled during a three-week cafeteria intervention providing increased fruit and salad options and prices discounted by 50 percent.	Jeffery, French, Raether, and Baxter (1994)
	Prevent obesity	On-site farmers markets, free healthy snacks and water; office food policies; promotion of nearby healthy restaurant options	A review of workplace interventions found that a variety of environmental approaches on diet and physical activity can positively influence healthy behaviors and help address obesity.	Pratt et al. (2007)

chapter, interventions in homes have been least studied (Knowlden & Sharma, 2012). The most common type of intervention uses parent education on home food environment as one element of a multipronged approach, making it difficult to separate out each component's unique effect. An alternate type of intervention that may improve home food environments is improving access to federal nutrition assistance programs. SNAP increases the likelihood there is adequate food in the home and may encourage home cooking in order to stretch the available dollars, whereas the WIC program goes farther by only allowing purchasing of designated healthier foods.

Schools are a popular site for intervention because of the captive audience and students' formative age. States may set school food regulations going beyond federal rules, and in many cases states have taken the lead on innovative policy. An increasingly popular type of school food intervention seeks to modify the available foods by providing increased produce, often accompanied by educational programs. Unfortunately, it has been difficult for many low-income school districts to take advantage of some of these food environment interventions because of cost. They are also often limited by physical facilities, such as availability of cooking kitchens.

Employers also have an incentive to invest in improving employee nutrition, because such efforts can pay off in lower absenteeism and chronic disease, increased productivity, and enhanced employee satisfaction (Jensen, 2011). At least as important for many employers, improved employee health can mean reduced health insurance premiums. Most large employers offer some health promotion interventions addressing individual behavior including diet. A small but growing number of workplace food environment interventions also target environmental concerns alongside nutrition. For example, perspective 17.2 describes the efforts of one food service company to provide more sustainably produced food to its patrons. Regardless of the specific workplace intervention, effectiveness increases with management commitment, supervisor support, worker representative engagement, and development of supportive organizational structures; as well as taking a multilevel approach and taking into account workers' lives outside the workplace (Sorensen et al., 2004).

Perspective 17.2. Striving for "Food Service for a Sustainable Future"
Fedele Bauccio

In 1987, when I cofounded Bon Appétit Management Company, you rarely saw fresh produce in food service. It was canned and served with mystery meat. I thought America's college students and corporate employees deserved better than that. So I hired professional chefs to cook fresh, flavorful food from scratch. It was a revolutionary thing to do.

Clients appreciated that focus: we now operate more than five hundred cafés for corporations, universities, and specialty venues in thirty-two states. The simple act of cooking from scratch also started us down a path toward what eventually became our mission: "food service for a sustainable future." It includes sourcing local food, from animals raised humanely, and looking at how farmworkers are treated. Although it sounds like a straightforward concept, none of these efforts were easy. And for some of them, we still have a long way to go. It wasn't originally all about sustainability. For our chefs, it came down to taste. They wanted the best ingredients, and that quest for flavor eventually led us, in the mid- to late 1990s, to want to buy fresh-picked produce straight from the farm.

Strangely enough, we weren't greeted with open arms. Kimberly Triplett, then our executive chef at American University in Washington, DC, remembers approaching a local farmer, Brett Grohsgal, about buying his beautiful melons. He turned her down, saying, "You don't deserve my melons!" He just couldn't believe that a food service company would treat his produce with the proper respect.

So Kimberly went to visit Brett at Even' Star Organic Farm. She walked through the fields with him and told him how Bon Appétit was different. She convinced him to sell his produce to us—and he still does to this day. We formally launched our Farm to Fork preferred purchasing program in 1999, requiring all of our chefs to buy at least 20 percent of their ingredients from small, owner-operated farms, fishers, and artisan producers within 150 miles of their kitchens. Thanks to efforts like Kimberly's, we've registered more than 1,400 folks like Brett with the Farm to Fork program—and we spend tens of millions of dollars on their products every year.

Our Farm to Fork producers, however, can't supply us with anywhere near the amount of meat, poultry, and eggs we go through. We have to buy from large producers, but we've made it our mission to work with them to change their practices.

In 2003, we committed to poultry raised without routine nontherapeutic antibiotics in their feed or water (and later, to ground beef as well). I am concerned about how the abuse of antibiotics in agriculture—it's put in feed to make animals grow faster and to try and stave off illness from overcrowding—is making the drugs less effective for humans. And inspired by a question asked by one of our student diners, we partnered with The Humane Society of the United States in 2005 to commit to sourcing all of our shell eggs from cage-free sources. Improving how the animals in our supply chain are treated has not gone as smoothly as local purchasing, however. The supply of humanely raised meat is not keeping pace with demand, and we've had to make incremental commitments. In August 2012 we were able to line up a national supplier and make certified humane ground beef a companywide requirement, which was a major victory. (Ground beef accounts for half

(Continued)

(Continued)

of our beef purchases.) We also committed to switching all our pork to come from pigs raised without the cruel practice of gestation crates by 2015. We were the first food service company to make such a commitment and we've set a deadline at least two years sooner than any other company has. It took us 'til 2014 to line up a source for bacon, and I don't actually know how we're going to make that aggressive deadline for the rest of our pork. The major producers seem to be in no hurry to scrap their millions of tiny metal cages for sows and build more humane group housing. Our biggest sustainable sourcing challenge so far has been about farm labor. In 2009 I was contacted by the Coalition of Immokalee Workers (CIW), a community-based organization of immigrants working in low-wage jobs throughout the state of Florida. Immokalee is where 90 percent of the tomatoes sold east of the Mississippi in winter months are grown. I went down there, and the conditions I saw for those farm-workers were appalling. We had no hesitation joining the CIW's campaign to improve the pickers' wages and working conditions—the first food service company to do so.

That experience opened our eyes to the plight of farmworkers. All over America they are routinely exploited, cheated out of the legal minimum wage for their hours worked, and subject to sexual and other forms of harassment. Through Bon Appétit's foundation arm, we partnered with United Farm Workers (with support from Oxfam America) to author a comprehensive report that detailed how few rights they enjoy compared to other workers.

What remains unclear is how we can best help. Sourcing local food and humanely raised meat is a cake-walk compared to figuring out who picked our food—and whether they were treated fairly. But we're working on it. We're a founding member of a groundbreaking, multi-stakeholder partnership called the Equitable Food Initiative that's developed a program that will improve the lives of farmworkers, the safety of the food being grown, and the stewardship of the land. As I write this, those worker-empowering standards are being tested on several large produce farms with hundreds of employees.

Farmworkers don't seem too much on consumers' radar yet, but I think that will change. Back when Kimberly was trying to persuade Brett to sell us his melons, "locavore" wasn't yet a mainstream concept, let alone a word. I'm proud that we've consistently been ahead of the curve in trying to source as sustainably as we can while still growing as a company. We have been excited to see issues we care about move into the mainstream, with the rise of the food movement. The more companies—and consumers—who care about these issues, the more leverage we have.

THE BUILT FOOD ENVIRONMENT

The built food environment includes retail food stores and restaurants, gardens, streets, transportation, visible advertising; and intangibles such as community safety and the cultural experience of obtaining food in existing venues. We focus particularly on retail food outlets and restaurants, whereas focus 17.3, at the end of the section, discusses the role of gardens in the food environment. Most analyses consider an individual's built food environment to be defined by an area proximal to the home; however, as will be discussed, the evidence is clear that people routinely travel outside their neighborhoods for preferred stores and restaurants, desired products, and, especially, low prices. Areas along transportation routes to school and work and areas near those sites also particularly merit further study (Kerr, Frank, Sallis, Saelens, Glanz, & Chapman, 2012). One of the important tools for studying retail food environments, and food environments more broadly, is mapping—discussed in focus 17.2.

FOCUS 17.2. IS THERE A MAP FOR THAT? USING GIS MAPS TO UNDERSTAND OUR FOOD SYSTEMS

Amanda Behrens

Faced with soaring rates of obesity and chronic disease, the City of Baltimore decided in 2008 that it needed to do something to increase residents' access to healthy, affordable food. City leaders convened a food policy task force charged with making recommendations to improve Baltimore's food environment. One recommendation was to support research on food deserts.

As described in the text, the Center for a Livable Future (CLF)'s Food System Mapping team worked with the city to create the Baltimore City Food Environment Map, including developing a new *food desert* definition (see figure 17.6). More than simply depicting food deserts in the city, the map helped the city prioritize areas for intervention.

People have been layering data over maps to analyze spatial relationships since well before the advent of computers, but a project such as the Baltimore City Food Environment Map illustrates how far the field has come. Geographic information systems (GIS) were first developed in North America in the 1960s, initially to inventory land and natural resources or plot demographics. As technology improved, more institutions and organizations began using GISs for a wider variety of applications, including national defense, urban planning, archeology, real estate, and public health. A modern GIS integrates hardware, software, and data for capturing, managing, analyzing, and displaying location-based information. Today, health practitioners and academics use GIS to identify causal relationships, increase the accuracy of their own data, improve their research, and drive policies.

GIS as a Visual Tool

Some maps are strictly visual and do not use analysis, such as maps helping consumers locate types of food and interactive, crowdsourced maps that let users add data and create their own displays. GIS maps can also elevate interest in an issue, help identify areas of concern for policy makers, and help communities characterize and communicate about their own situations. For example, food maps can bring together data on food production, processing, distribution, and consumption, along with social, economic, demographic, and environmental data, to improve understanding of complex relationships within the food environment. Visually presenting information can enable interpretations that would not be possible by looking only at tables and raw data.

GIS as an Analytical Tool

Mapping can also serve as an analytical tool. GIS can calculate distances and can identify areas of varying density, such as areas with a high density of fast food or of poultry farming (one example is Food & Water Watch's Factory Farm Map at factoryfarmmap.org). Geographic data analysis using statistical tools can quantify relationships between spatial variables. For example, to understand the relationship between county-level food insecurity rates and number of emergency food sites, we could input site addresses into a GIS program, and use the software to map the sites and link them with counties. Then, the data could be exported to statistical software for analysis. Note that in analyzing spatial data, special statistical methods such as multilevel modeling are required to account for the fact that nearby areas are more likely to be more similar to each other than areas farther away, and thus that data are not independent.

(Continued)

(Continued)

Another analytic use for mapping is to examine foodsheds—regions around metropolitan areas that could, theoretically, produce the food consumed by that population (Hedden, 1929). Typical foodshed analyses consider residents' caloric intake and the amount of food produced. Then, various scenarios of consumption, land use, or foodshed size can be manipulated and explored. For example, one 2008 study at Cornell University examined the capacity for New York State to supply its own food needs and found that even considering *potential* agricultural land area, New York State is insufficient to provide the state's food needs, when New York City is included (Peters, Wilkins, & Fick, 2007). Not surprising, considering the size of the population, but important because the study indicates that certain population centers must consider a broader region for their food needs.

GIS Limitations

Although we highlight many benefits to using GIS, the technology also has limitations. GIS is only as good as the data added to it, and it can be misused and therefore lead to misinformation. Different mapping choices can dramatically affect the messages conveyed. Imagine a high-income neighborhood situated next to a low-income neighborhood, in the same zip code. Demographics and health indicators may be quite different in these two areas, however, a zip code–based analysis would mask these. Mappers also often define geographic areas based on size or distance; small changes in these choices can result in dramatically different results. Another challenge is that we tend to trust what our eyes see more than we might if the same scenario were laid out in text; we may not recognize that there could be alternate explanations for the evidence. Thus, data portrayal and presentation choices must be carefully considered. Solid documentation and notes regarding limitations should always accompany GIS products. Researchers studying the food environment (similar to all researchers) must ensure their data are valid and reliable.

In the context of food environment research, GIS has become an effective tool for mapping and measurement. It is significant to note the far-reaching effects of GIS technology and how maps can build understanding, influence perspectives, and inform policy.

Retail Food Stores

People purchase food from a wide variety of retail outlets, including traditional sites such as supermarkets, grocery stores, and convenience stores; and increasingly, from alternative sites including gas stations, specialty food stores, farmers markets and farm stands, food trucks, and superstores such as Costco and Walmart. Larger retailers such as supermarkets, superstores, and warehouse clubs accounted for 75 percent of US food sales in 2008 (Ver Ploeg et al., 2009).

Of the traditional store types (supermarkets, grocery stores, convenience stores, and corner stores), supermarkets generally have the largest selection of products, including relatively healthy and relatively unhealthy items, and their prices tend to be lower because of superior wholesale purchasing power. Grocery stores—smaller than supermarkets but offering products in most departments—stock dry and canned goods, and typically have smaller selections of perishable items than supermarkets. Convenience stores and corner stores have limited shelf space and tend to stock primarily staple foods and snacks, with little or no fresh produce (although some, particularly in immigrant neighborhoods, do stock significant quantities of produce). See chapter 14 for more details on the food distribution system. The existence of a supermarket in a community—with its fresh produce and wide variety—is often used as an indicator of community access to healthy food (Harries, Kim, & Treering, 2011). This is an imperfect proxy, however, because supermarket quality varies.

Since the 1970s (and earlier), supermarkets have proliferated in sprawling suburban areas, thanks in part to ample land for building stores and parking lots (see figure 17.8), and to mergers and buyouts, and the exodus of wealthier residents from urban centers. At the same time, many urban supermarkets have closed their doors and have not been replaced, for reasons including real estate and wage costs, zoning issues, and theft (Eisenhauer, 2001). Competition from chain supermarkets has also been blamed for putting smaller, independent grocers out of business and resulting in poorer access for people without reliable and affordable transportation (Walker, Keane, & Burke, 2010).

Low-income neighborhoods have significantly fewer supermarkets—25 percent fewer—than middle-income neighborhoods, according to one national study that linked food stores in 28,050 zip codes to census data (Powell, Slater, Mirtcheva, Bao, & Chaloupka, 2007). Studies have also found racial disparities in supermarket availability even after accounting for differences in income. In Detroit, the availability of supermarkets was just 52 percent that of similar white neighborhoods (Powell et al., 2007). Some urban residents may rely on convenience stores to stock up on necessities in between supermarket trips, which can pose a different access issue: lack of affordability. Prices at convenience stores are typically higher than at other stores (Larson & Story, 2009). SNAP participants who live far from supermarkets might conduct only one major shopping trip per month, after funds are disbursed. To avoid spoilage, they may not be able to buy fresh produce lasting the entire month. And, the local convenience or corner store may have few healthy options for shoppers in between supermarket trips.

Rural areas too may suffer from low supermarket access. The addition of a superstore into an area can make it difficult for smaller grocers to survive, limiting the options to the one superstore and potentially increasing the often already-long distance traveled (see figure 17.9). It is not uncommon for a rural consumer to drive fifteen or twenty miles to a supermarket—a hardship in time and gasoline costs.

There is debate about how disparate access to healthy food may affect health. During the 1990s and early 2000s, multiple studies and reviews (Larson, Story, & Nelson, 2009; Story et al., 2008) indicated that those who live near supermarkets tend to have healthier diets, greater fruit and vegetable intakes,

FIGURE 17.8 Newer Supermarkets with Parking Areas Gained in Popularity Compared to Older, More Urban Ones without Them

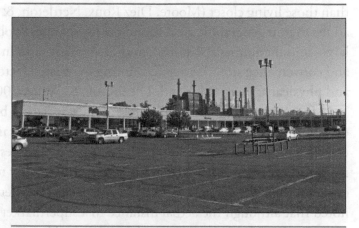

Source: John Donges (2012). Flickr Commons.

FIGURE 17.9 Shuttered Supermarket in a Small Town

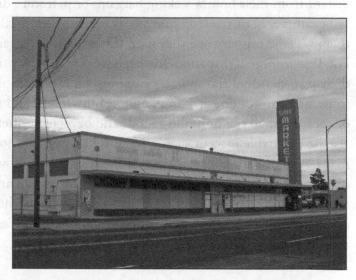

Source: Dvortygirl (2012). Shuttered supermarket. Flickr Commons.

and possibly, lower rates of obesity and diet-related disease, compared to those living farther away. For example, one study found that adults living more than a mile from supermarkets in Forsyth County, North Carolina, Baltimore, and New York City were 25 to 46 percent less likely to eat healthy diets than those living closer (Moore, Diez Roux, Nettleton, & Jacobs, 2008). Another study of ten thousand adults in four geographic areas found the lowest rates of obesity in census tracts with large food stores (or large- and medium-sized stores), and the highest rates in areas with only smaller stores (medium-sized and convenience stores), after accounting for related factors including income, race, gender, education, and physical activity (Morland, Diez Roux, & Wing, 2006).

More recently, several studies found no association between some measures of low access and diet quality or BMI (Block, Christakis, O'Malley, & Subramanian, 2011; Caspi et al, 2012; Shier, An, & Sturm, 2012). Overall, comparison across food access studies is difficult because of the variety of methods, measures, and geographic scales; data quality regarding retail locations is also mixed. As the evidence evolves, nuances emerge as discussed elsewhere and summarized here. Caspi et al. (2012) noted that although the actual distance to a supermarket said little about a person's fruit and vegetable consumption, those who *perceived* that they had better access actually ate more produce. Further, there were substantial levels of mismatch between consumers' perceptions and the mapped distance. Additionally, a distance-from-home model may be inappropriate because consumers may travel to stores distant from their homes seeking bargains or patronize different stores on their way to work or school. For example, in one Seattle study, only one in seven participants reported that the supermarket nearest them was the primary one they used (Drewnowski, Aggarwal, Hurvitz, Monsivais, & Moudon, 2012). Food environment disparities further have very different significance depending on whether people have their own personal transportation. Using supermarket presence as a proxy for access is flawed in that some small stores do carry fresh and healthy foods, and some supermarkets have low-quality produce or meats and all sell unhealthy foods and beverages, often at lower prices than small stores. There will also be inevitable inaccuracies in identifying store locations because of data errors and lack of updated maps. And, for simplicity these measures use "as the crow flies" distance, however, in some cases those distances differ markedly from actual distance on roads and do not take into account public transportation routes. Last, a variety of factors affect individuals' shopping decisions, including affordability, time cost, convenience, information, appeal, and comfort (Caspi et al., 2012). These findings underline the need to approach interventions broadly.

Restaurants

Americans are dining out more frequently than in previous decades (Story et al., 2008). Forty-eight cents of every dollar spent on food is spent at a restaurant, making restaurants a $632-billion-dollar-a-year industry (National Restaurant Association, 2012). "Away-from-home" food comes in many shapes and sizes—from fast food chains to small carry-out restaurants to mobile trucks; cafeterias to snack bars to family-style dining to fine dining. We often choose these venues for reasons such as food preference, convenience, atmosphere, or price (see figure 17.10). The food environments approach suggests that distance and exposure also matter, contributing to convenience and the desire to go to a particular restaurant.

Frequent fast food consumption is linked to obesity, higher-calorie diets, and lower consumption of fruit, nonstarchy vegetables, milk, and important micronutrients (Larson & Story, 2009). The evidence is less clear regarding how much living near fast food affects food choices and obesity risk;

for example, in one review, seven studies supported that association but eight did not (Fleischhacker, Evenson, Rodriguez, & Ammerman, 2011). The relationship may also differ by sex, income, and age (Boone-Heinone et al., 2011). In Fleischhacker's review, only one out of five studies of children supported an association between fast food environment and BMI (2011), although other studies do find neighborhood linkages to purchasing frequency and diet quality (He et al., 2012; Boone-Heinone et al., 2011).

Fast food restaurants are ubiquitous, but they are particularly prevalent in low-income and minority neighborhoods. Neighborhood racial composition seems to be an even stronger predictor of location than SES (Hilmers, Hilmers, & Dave, 2011). Some argue that the racial segregation of African American neighborhoods is the reason behind disproportionately high fast food density in those areas because of economic and population characteristics, physical infrastructure, and social factors that

FIGURE 17.10   The Type and Quality of Food, the Atmosphere, and the Convenience of a Restaurant May Entice a Family to Eat out Instead of Eating In

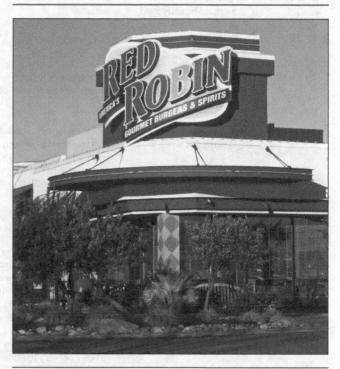

Source: J. Winters (2008). Wikimedia Commons.

encourage their development (Kwate, 2008). Beyond chain restaurants, many low-income and African American neighborhoods are also dotted with independent carry-out restaurants, including those serving Chinese food, buffets, and deep-fried meals.

Although most research attention has focused on fast food, food at nearly all restaurants is higher in calories, fat, sodium, and cholesterol than food we might eat at home; and portion sizes are considerably in excess of USDA recommendations. The nonprofit Center for Science in the Public Interest has detailed some of the most unhealthy restaurant meals, including the Fried Cheese Melt with fries at Denny's: 1,260 calories; Applebee's provolone stuffed meatballs with fettuccine: 1,520 calories; and the Cheesecake Factory's Farmhouse Burger, weighing in at 1,530 calories plus 460 calories for the French fries. More pricey restaurants are not exempt—Morton's Steakhouse's porterhouse steak and mashed potatoes provide 2,240 calories, 70 grams of saturated fat, and more than a day's supply of sodium (Hurley & Liebman, 2011). Large portion sizes at all restaurant types encourage overeating and can also influence our perceptions of "normal" portions to serve at home.

Retail and Restaurant Interventions

Creative approaches have proliferated for addressing retail food environments, as shown in table 17.2 and in the following. Approaches include supporting supermarket development in underserved areas, bringing healthier items into existing stores, and bringing food delivery into underserved areas (see figure 17.11), as well as mandating offerings via federal programs such as WIC. In 2010, the WIC program required that all stores accepting WIC stock certain healthier items. Because most supermarkets

TABLE 17.2   Examples of Food Environment Interventions in Retail and Restaurants

	Objective	Intervention	Results	Reference
Retail	Incentivize new stores to increase healthy food access in underserved areas	Healthy Food Financing Initiative	Program addresses access inequalities, but evidence on health improvements remains scant and mixed. Additional studies are ongoing.	Cummins, Petticrew, Higgins, Findlay, and Sparks (2005); Flint, Cummins, and Matthews (2012)
	Improving healthy options at existing stores	Small store healthy food environment interventions	Demonstrated short-term success at changing store inventory, purchasing, and food behaviors	Gittlesohn, Rowan, and Gadhoke (2012)
	Increase access to healthy, local produce	Establishing farmers markets and community gardens; distributing food at community-based sites such as churches or clinics	Evidence suggests consumers of all SES and ethnic backgrounds tend to prefer fresh, local, and organic produce, so efforts to improve access and affordability may help increase fruit and vegetable consumption.	Bellows, Alcaraz, and Hallman (2010)
	Link residents to healthy food via transportation and mobile services	Approaches include selling fresh produce from mobile produce trucks (New York City Green Carts); store-operated shuttle services; and Baltimore's Virtual Supermarket, allowing customers to use SNAP benefits and receive free grocery delivery to libraries and other sites.	Evaluation of Green Carts found opportunities for improved placement of carts and inventory; however, no information is available on sales. Evaluations of other transportation and mobile service interventions are scarce.	Lucan, Maroko, Shanker, and Jordan (2011)
Restaurants	Encourage healthier choices at restaurants by displaying nutritional information	Menu labeling adds nutrition information to restaurant menus and enables motivated consumers to compare products and make informed decisions. This encourages restaurants to develop healthier recipes. Cities and states around the country began implementing menu labeling in the late 2000s but the Affordable Care Act of 2010 made menu labeling national law.	Several studies have suggested that exposure to menu labeling in restaurants reduces calorie intake in a subset of patrons and increases awareness of nutritional content. Other studies find no significant impacts; for example, one reported no changes in purchasing, although interestingly people who noticed and used menu labels ate fewer fast food meals.	Auchincloss, Mallya, Leonberg, Ricchezza, Glanz, and Schwarz (2013); Hammond, Goodman, Hanning, and Daniel (2013); Pulos and Leng (2010); Vadiveloo, Dixon, and Elbel (2011)
	Changing zoning codes to limit density of fast food restaurants	Some municipalities have restaurant-related zoning regulations, often primarily for reasons other than health. Policies range from outright bans of certain types of restaurants, to bans within specific areas, to limiting the number or density of fast food restaurants. Detroit restricts fast food within five hundred feet of a school. These regulations have been controversial because of concerns including equity and fairness to businesses.	Little evidence of changing food consumption. Most regulations focus on fast food and do not restrict other restaurants and stores that sell less-healthy foods, thus diluting potential impacts.	Mair, Pierce, and Teret (2005)

already have such items, this successful regulation had the greatest impact on offerings at the many smaller stores distributed throughout communities (Hillier, McLaughlin, Cannuscio, Chilton, Krasny, & Karpyn, 2012).

To obtain sustainable change in food environments, these supply-side strategies must be complemented with efforts to build demand for the healthier products. An explosion of new interventions aims to do that. Price manipulation strategies, as described in chapter 7, are particularly popular and hold strong promise.

Another common demand-side approach is modifying the in-store food environment with shelf labels characterizing product healthfulness (see focus 10.1). Such "point-of-choice nutrition information" is premised on the idea that if consumers knew which items were healthier, they would choose them. Unfortunately, in some cases consumers also associate "better for you" labels with "worse tasting" and purposely avoid such products. Effective marketing may help overcome such biases.

Two main types of food environment interventions for restaurants include **menu labeling** and zoning to restrict locations. Other valuable restaurant interventions have addressed issues including portion size (see perspective 15.1), restricting provision of toys to children, healthier default options (such as apples instead of French fries), posting signs or menu cues encouraging healthier options, banning food components such as trans fats, and changing the in-restaurant atmosphere to create subconscious cues that reduce consumption while increasing satisfaction. Additionally, an increasingly active movement has sought to improve the health, wages, and treatment of workers in restaurants (see perspective 4.3).

FIGURE 17.11 Baltimore's Virtual Supermarket Program Delivers Groceries to Libraries, Senior Centers, and Other Community Sites

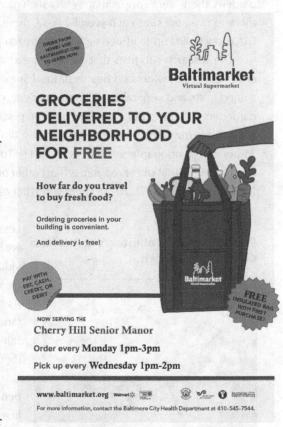

Source: Baltimarket.

menu labeling
Altering within-restaurant food environment by adding nutrition information and calorie counts to restaurant menus and menu boards; enables motivated consumers to compare products and make informed decisions about their food choices

FOCUS 17.3. CONNECTING PEOPLE AND THEIR FOOD SYSTEMS: WHY GARDENS MATTER
Jill S. Litt, James Hale, and Michael Buchenau

When you look around Denver these days, there is more food being grown, whether in front yards or community gardens, public or private spaces, schools or churches. In a population-based survey in Denver, 57 percent of residents across Denver's neighborhoods self-identified as gardeners. Even more surprising, 13 percent of

(Continued)

(Continued)

residents indicated they currently gardened in one of Denver's community gardens (Litt, Soobader, Turbin, Hale, Buchenau, & Marshall, 2011). In 2005, when we began studying the health and social benefits of community gardens, there were approximately fifty such gardens in the city, and Denver Urban Gardens (DUG) established three to five new sites each year. By 2012, there were 125 DUG gardens throughout the city, and on average DUG now builds up to fifteen new gardens each year and has dozens of proposed projects in its queue.

Our research suggests that gardens are associated with health-promoting processes and that they influence health behaviors and health status. For example, our research showed that community gardeners consumed fruits and vegetables 5.7 times per day, compared with home gardeners (4.6 times per day) and nongardeners (3.9 times per day). Moreover, 56 percent of community gardeners met national recommendations to consume fruits and vegetables at least five times per day, compared with 37 percent of home gardeners and 25 percent of nongardeners (Litt et al., 2011). This observed difference in fruit and vegetable consumption is almost double that observed across most other published interventions (Ammerman, Lindquist, Lohr, & Hersey, 2002; Thomson & Ravia, 2011), suggesting that gardening is a viable way to increase fruit and vegetable intake.

FIGURE 17.12   Volunteers at Atlantis Community Garden

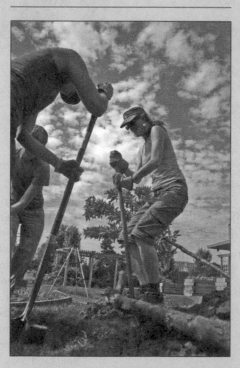

Source: Denver Urban Gardens (2009). http://dug .org/photo-gallery/

Our research inquired about the emotional and social processes that may explain these observed differences. For example, we learned that participation in community gardens enables individuals to connect with their everyday landscapes in a way that generates healthy sensory, emotional, and spiritual experiences. As one gardener framed it, "You're here in the middle of the city, (and you) look around and see all the buildings and everything, but then yet when you're in this garden, it just all goes away" (figure 17.12).

We found that most gardeners participate in community gardens because of an enthusiasm for growing their own food, "I just like digging in the dirt and watching things grow and … eating my own vegetables."

Beyond a place to experience growing food, gardeners gain sensitivity to natural processes. Scores of gardeners stated things such as, "It's a different time. Sense of time I think, you know, versus when you're a kid and you don't have any involvement with nature, it's hard to get the sense of that, you know, tempo." This "tempo" implies an embodied aesthetic understanding and response to the processes and rhythms of nature within the garden such as seasonal changes, water use, harvesting, growing techniques, in other words—the ebb and flow of working in a garden.

Such aesthetic experiences influence the relationship between humans and their natural, social, and built environments (Foster, 2009) by fostering social involvement, social connections with others, and triggering emotional experiences such as how people feel about where they live (neighborhood attachment). As one gardener related, "If it hadn't been for the garden I don't know how I would have made it through the first year [after the spouse's death]. So that gives you an idea of the connections, the value, and what that garden means to people. [It is] a place of healing, refuge, and connection" (Hale, Knapp, Bardwell, Buchenau, Marshall, Sancar, & Litt, 2011).

Many gardeners explain the social experience as being one of the primary benefits of participating in a community garden. One gardener expressed, "The things that grow out of (gardening), you know, kids learning, our neighbors socializing and becoming comfortable and feeling they have a real community, those things are the products in addition to whatever is grown. But, I mean, the social products of the garden are really the results and the garden itself is simply infrastructure."

Gardens show us a way to reconnect people to their landscapes and create a healthy relationship with food and supporting food systems. Such settings enable residents to think not only about what they are planting in the ground but also how they will nurture relationships with fellow gardeners and their broader community. Importantly, many gardeners report that they develop their garden-based values and aesthetics from a young age. It is therefore important to expose people to gardens when they're young—particularly in urban settings where such opportunities are typically rarer (figure 17.13).

At the neighborhood level, gardens have the potential to simultaneously address many individual- and community-level factors, such as food security, the availability of healthy food, safety, and social capital. Their reach extends beyond gardeners to include residents who are not directly involved but who benefit indirectly from donated produce, social activities, and garden-sponsored farmers markets. Thus, gardens have the potential to play a very real part in fortifying the foundation for improved and lasting neighborhood health and well-being.

FIGURE 17.13   Mentors and Youth at Youth Farmers Market

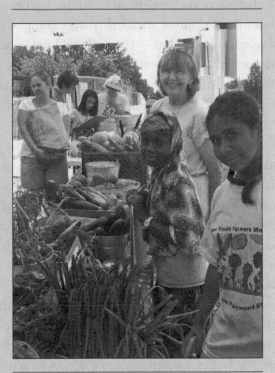

Source: Denver Urban Gardens (2009). Connecting generations mentors and youth at Fairview youth farmers market. http://dug.org/photo-gallery/

CONCLUSION

For those seeking to change eating behaviors, food environments are a valuable target for several reasons. First, as described throughout this chapter, environmental exposures help determine our routine eating behaviors and the level of challenge we face in making change. Providing healthy environments supports individuals' decisions to eat healthfully. Second, the many inequities in environmental exposures to food represent an injustice and contribute to health disparities. Third, targeting environments focuses attention on structural factors that affect diet, including business and governmental practices, and avoids "blaming the victim"—placing the onus on individuals to overcome these challenges alone. Fourth, environmental changes can have lasting effects and can bring about change without individual effort, because they become incorporated into structures, systems, policies, and sociocultural norms; most do not need to be continually renewed. Last, addressing the environment can make change for many people at once, rather than one by one, reducing costs and extending the reach of interventions.

There are drawbacks as well to focusing on environmental changes. Although they can have meaningful effects across whole populations, their effects on any one individual are often limited. For example, shifting the average BMI across a city by one-half point can have significant public health benefits and lead to real health care cost savings—but for any individual, that BMI reduction may be far less meaningful. Although in some ways food environment interventions might be "too macro," in other ways they might actually be "too micro." In fact, strong interventions to improve an area's economy or address social disparities might do more to change food environments—and people's vulnerability to them—than direct food-centric interventions. Finally, although food environment interventions have been linked to changes in preferences and diets, it has been more challenging to link them with concrete health benefits, in part because this is an emerging area of research (Lytle, 2009) and because the impacts are diffuse, with many factors contributing to food consumption and health status.

A systems approach to food environments means seeing those environments as embedded within, and constantly interacting with, broader factors in the macro environment, nonfood factors in the proximal environment, and numerous other factors inside and around us. A food environment intervention ideally should be presented as one component of a multipronged approach. Ultimately, most experts agree that the most effective way to bring about change is intervening at many different levels at once, including environmental, policy, and individual factors on the supply and demand side, treating the environment as a complex system. Community engagement and outreach are indispensable for building awareness and interest in any intervention.

Through the 1990s and the early part of the 2000s, the base of evidence continued to build indicating access disparities and affirming the impacts of food environments, particularly retail. A round of more recent studies, however, indicates a need for a more nuanced approach. They highlight the need for better measurement of access as actually experienced by consumers and clearer understanding of the determinants of consumer choice given various levels of access. Additionally, some studies find no association between various food environment variables and diet. The proper interpretation of these findings remains unclear. Further research will help clarify the questions, improve methods, and deepen insights into relevant interactions and confounding factors, and into the nuances of these contrasting findings and how they may interrelate. Ultimately this research will yield fresh ideas about how to encourage effective interventions.

There has been an unusual level of local, state, and federal policy-maker support for retail and restaurant interventions, including experimental approaches. Contributing to this support is a strong desire to do *something* about obesity, the upward percolation of research on food environments and food deserts, and the growing food movement. Some of the new interventions will be threatened as budgets grow tighter, but others will be seen as relatively cost-effective approaches to costly problems. There is great need for additional and more rigorous evaluation. Further, there is a need to analyze the role of local food environments in the context of national and global food system dynamics, including those addressed in chapters 7, 8, 11, 12, and 14. As we gain more sophisticated perspectives on the mechanisms by which food environments affect behavior, intervention developers will gain fresh ideas and new tools. There are many opportunities to participate in the effort to understand and create healthier food environments.

SUMMARY

This chapter described food environments and their importance to population health. Food environments are the surroundings and settings that influence people's food choices and diets. Physical aspects of the food environment include homes, schools, workplaces, restaurants, retailers, and gardens. Some interventions to improve the food environment include improving school food, advocating for more full-service supermarkets, increasing healthy options at existing stores, providing nutrition information at the point of purchase, addressing affordability of healthy foods, building community gardens, and making healthier choices the default option at restaurants.

We provided an overview of the major research findings, ongoing uncertainties, and the increasingly nuanced perspective emerging as the study of food environments evolves and matures. Key challenges include measuring the physical environment, designing studies to produce valid conclusions absent of confounding results, determining long-term impacts, and characterizing interactions among individual, social, and environmental factors. Despite the challenges, there is much interest in food environment interventions to create healthy defaults, improve access, and address equity issues and health disparities. Interventionists should work with communities to increase the likelihood that interventions will meet community needs.

KEY TERMS

Competitive foods

Food deserts

Food environment

Food swamps

Healthy defaults

Menu labeling

DISCUSSION QUESTIONS

1. Think about your own food environment and how your food choices are affected by the options around you. How would you change your food environment to a "healthy default" that would affect your own choices?

2. Should cities and states help establish supermarkets and other fresh food retailers (similar to the HFFI approach)? Is the argument for this intervention stronger from an equity perspective, a health perspective, or are both equally compelling? Is there a way to mesh this approach with the concerns raised in perspective 17.1?

3. Should cities consider zoning restrictions to limit fast food locations near schools? Why or why not?

4. How can food environment interventions be simultaneously "too micro" and "too macro"?

5. Do you think researchers will eventually be able to prove the extent to which the food environment influences obesity, diabetes, and other diet-related diseases? Why or why not?

REFERENCES

Ammerman, A. S., Lindquist, C. H., Lohr, K. N., & Hersey, J. (2002). The efficacy of behavioral interventions to modify dietary fat and fruit and vegetable intake: A review of the evidence. *Preventive Medicine*, *35*(1), 25–41.

Auchincloss, A. H., Mallya, G. G., Leonberg, B. L., Ricchezza, A., Glanz, K., & Schwarz, D. F. (2013). Customer responses to mandatory menu labeling at full-service restaurants. *American Journal of Preventive Medicine*, *45*(6), 710–719.

Baltimore Food Policy Initiative. (2010). *Food deserts*. Retrieved from www.baltimorecity.gov/Government/Agencies Departments/Planning/BaltimoreFoodPolicyInitiative/FoodDeserts.aspx

Bellows, A. C., Alcaraz V. G., & Hallman, W. K. (2010). Gender and food: A study of attitudes in the USA towards organic, local, U.S. grown, and GM-free foods. *Appetite, 55*(3), 540–550.

Block, J. P., Christakis, N. A., O'Malley, A. J., & Subramanian, S. V. (2011). Proximity to food establishments and body mass index in the Framingham heart study offspring cohort over 30 years. *American Journal of Epidemiology, 174*(10), 1108–1114.

Boone-Heinone, J., Gordon-Larsen, P., Kiefe, C. I., Shikany, J. M., Lewis, C. E., & Popkin, B. M. (2011). Fast food restaurants and food stores: Longitudinal associations with diet in young to middle-aged adults; The CARDIA study. *Archives of Internal Medicine, 171*(13), 1162–1170.

Caspi, C. E., Kawachi, I., Subramanian, S. V., Adamkiewicz, G., & Sorensen, G. (2012). The relationship between diet and perceived and objective access to supermarkets among low-income housing residents. *Social Science & Medicine, 75*(7), 1254–1262.

Centers for Disease Control. (nd). *Healthier food retail: Beginning the assessment process in your state or community.* Retrieved from www.cdc.gov/obesity/downloads/hfrassessment.pdf

Chandon, P., & Wansink, B. (2002). When are stockpiled products consumed faster? A convenience-salience framework of postpurchase consumption incidence and quantity. *Journal of Marketing Research, 39*(3), 321–335.

Chriqui, J. F., Resnick, E. A., Schneider, L., Schermbeck, R., Adcock, T., Carrion, V., & Chaloupka, F. J. (2013). *School district wellness policies: Evaluating progress and potential for improving children's health five years after the federal mandate; school years 2006–07 through 2010–11 (Vol. 3). Bridging the Gap Program, Health Policy Center, Institute for Health Research and Policy.* Chicago: University of Illinois at Chicago.

Cohen, D. A., & Babey, S. H. (2012). Contextual influences on eating behaviours: Heuristic processing and dietary choices. *Obesity Reviews, 13*(9), 766–779.

Cooke, L. J., Wardle, J., Gibson, E., Sapochnik, M., Sheiham, A., & Lawson, M. (2004). Demographic, familial and trait predictors of fruit and vegetable consumption by pre-school children. *Public Health Nutrition, 7*(2), 295–302.

Cummins, S., Petticrew, M., Higgins, C., Findlay, A., & Sparks, A. (2005). Large scale food retailing as an intervention for diet and health: Quasi-experimental evaluation of a natural experiment. *Journal of Epidemiology and Community Health, 59*(12), 1035–1040.

Dammann, K., & Smith, C. (2010). Food-related attitudes and behaviors at home, school, and restaurants: Perspectives from racially diverse, urban, low-income 9- to 13-year-old children in Minnesota. *Journal of Nutrition Education and Behavior, 42*(6), 389–397.

Drewnowski, A., Aggarwal, A., Hurvitz, P. M., Monsivais, P., & Moudon, A. V. (2012). Obesity and supermarket access: Proximity or price? *American Journal of Public Health, 102*(8), e74–e80.

Ebbeling, C. B., Feldman, H. A., Chomitz, V. R., Antonelli, T. A., Gortmaker, S. L., Osganian, S. K., & Ludwig, D. S. (2012). A randomized trial of sugar-sweetened beverages and adolescent body weight. *New England Journal of Medicine, 367*(15), 1407–1416.

Eisenhauer, E. (2001). In poor health: Supermarket redlining and urban nutrition. *GeoJournal, 53*(2), 125–133.

Engbers, L. H., van Poppel, M.N.M., Chin, A., Paw, M.J.M., & van Mechelen, W. (2005). Worksite health promotion programs with environmental changes: A systematic review. *American Journal of Preventive Medicine, 29*(1), 61–70.

Fleischhacker, S. E., Evenson, K. R., Rodriguez, D. A., & Ammerman, A. S. (2011). A systematic review of fast food access studies. *Obesity Reviews, 12*(5), e460–e471.

Flint, E., Cummins, S., & Matthews, S. (2012). OP84 Do supermarket interventions improve food access, fruit and vegetable intake and BMI? Evaluation of the Philadelphia fresh food financing initiative. *Journal of Epidemiology and Community Health, 66*(Suppl. 1), A33.

Foster, J. (2009). Environmental aesthetics, ecological action and social justice. In M. Smith, J. Davidson, L. Cameron & L. Bondi (Eds.), *Emotion, place and culture* (pp. 97–114). Burlington, VT: Ashgate.

Franco, M., Diez Roux, A. V., Glass, T. A., Caballero, B., & Brancati, F. L. (2008). Neighborhood characteristics and availability of healthy foods in Baltimore. *American Journal of Preventive Medicine, 35*(6), 561–567.

Gittelsohn, J., & Lee, K. (2013). Integrating educational, environmental, and behavioral economic strategies may improve the effectiveness of obesity interventions. *Applied Economic Perspectives and Policy*, *35*(1), 52–68.

Gittelsohn, J., Rowan, M., & Gadhoke, P. (2012). Interventions in small food stores to change the food environment, improve diet, and reduce risk of chronic disease. *Preventing Chronic Disease*, *9*, E59.

Guthrie, J. F., Lin, B. H., & Frazao, E. (2002). Role of food prepared away from home in the American diet, 1977–78 versus 1994–96: Changes and consequences. *Journal of Nutrition Education and Behavior*, *34*(3), 140–150.

Hale, J., Knapp, C., Bardwell, L., Buchenau, M., Marshall, J. A., Sancar, F., & Litt, J. S. (2011). Connecting food environments and health through the relational nature of aesthetics: Gaining insight through the community gardening experience. *Social Science & Medicine*, *72*, 1853–1863.

Hammond, D., Goodman, S., Hanning, R., & Daniel, S. (2013). A randomized trial of calorie labeling on menus. *Preventive Medicine*, *57*(6), 860–866.

Harries, C., Kim, E., & Treering, D. (2011). *Food for every child: The need for more supermarkets in Maryland*. Philadelphia: The Food Trust.

Hayden, S., Blissard, N., Bhuyan, S., & Nayga, R.M.J. (2004). *The demand for food away from home: Full-service or fast food?* Washington, DC: US Department of Agriculture Economic Research Service.

He, M., Tucker, P., Irwin, J. D., Gilliland, J., Larsen, K., & Hess, P. (2012). Obesogenic neighbourhoods: The impact of neighbourhood restaurants and convenience stores on adolescents' food consumption behaviours. *Public Health Nutrition*, *15*(12), 2331.

Hedden, W. P. (1929). *How great cities are fed*. New York: D. C. Heath and Company.

Hillier, A., McLaughlin, J., Cannuscio, C. C., Chilton, M., Krasny, S., & Karpyn, A. (2012). The impact of WIC food package changes on access to healthful food in 2 low-income urban neighborhoods. *Journal of Nutrition Education and Behavior*, *44*(3), 210–216.

Hilmers, A., Hilmers, D. C., & and Dave, J. (2011). Neighborhood disparities in access to healthy foods and their effects on environmental justice. *American Journal of Public Health*, *9*, 1644.

Hurley, J., & Liebman, B. (2011). *Xtreme eating 2011*. Washington, DC: Nutrition Action Healthletter.

Jeffery, R. W., French, S. A., Raether, C., & Baxter, J. E. (1994). An environmental intervention to increase fruit and salad purchases in a cafeteria. *Preventive Medicine*, *23*(6), 788–792.

Jensen, J. D. (2011). Can worksite nutritional interventions improve productivity and firm profitability? A literature review. *Perspectives in Public Health*, *131*(4), 184–192.

Just, D. R., Mancino, L., & Wansink, B. (2007). *Could behavioral economics help improve diet quality for nutrition assistance program participants?* (No. 43). Washington, DC: US Department of Agriculture Economic Research Service.

Kerr, J., Frank, L., Sallis, J. F., Saelens, B., Glanz, K., & Chapman, J. (2012). Predictors of trips to food destinations. *International Journal of Behavioral Nutrition & Physical Activity*, *9*(1), 58–67.

Knowlden, A., & Sharma, M. (2012). Systematic review of family and home-based interventions targeting paediatric overweight and obesity. *Obesity Reviews*, *13*(6), 499–508.

Kratt, P., Reynolds, K., & Shewchuk, R. (2000). The role of availability as a moderator of family fruit and vegetable consumption. *Health Education & Behavior*, *27*(4), 471–482.

Kwate, N.O.A. (2008). Fried chicken and fresh apples: Racial segregation as a fundamental cause of fast food density in black neighborhoods. *Health & Place*, *14*(1), 32–44.

Larsen, K., & Gilliland, J. (2009). A farmers' market in a food desert: Evaluating impacts on the price and availability of healthy food. *Health & Place*, *15*(4), 1158–1162.

Larson, N., & Story, M. (2009). A review of environmental influences on food choices. *Annals of Behavioral Medicine*, *38*, 56–73.

Larson, N., & Story, M. (2010). Are "competitive foods" sold at school making our children fat? *Health Affairs*, *29*(3), 430–435.

Larson, N., Story, M., & Nelson, M. (2009). Neighborhood environments: Disparities in access to healthy foods in the U.S. *American Journal of Preventive Medicine, 36*(1), 74–81.

Litt, J. S., Soobader, M., Turbin, M. S., Hale, J., Buchenau, M., & Marshall, J. A. (2011). The influences of social involvement, neighborhood aesthetics and community garden participation on fruit and vegetable consumption. *The American Journal of Public Health, 101,* 1466–1473.

Lucan, S. C., Maroko, A., Shanker, R., & Jordan, W. B. (2011). Green carts (mobile produce vendors) in the Bronx—optimally positioned to meet neighborhood fruit-and-vegetable needs? *Journal of Urban Health: Bulletin of the New York Academy of Medicine, 88*(5), 977–981.

Lytle, L. A. (2009). Measuring the food environment: State of the science. *American Journal of Preventive Medicine, 36*(4, Suppl.), S134–S144. doi:10.1016/j.amepre.2009.01.018

Mair, J. S., Pierce, M. W., & Teret, S. P. (2005). *The city planner's guide to the obesity epidemic: Zoning and fast food.* Washington, DC: Center for Law and the Public's Health at Johns Hopkins and Georgetown Universities.

Moore, L. V., Diez Roux, A. V., Nettleton, J. A., & Jacobs, D. R., Jr., (2008). Associations of the local food environment with diet quality—a comparison of assessments based on surveys and geographic information systems: The multi-ethnic study of atherosclerosis. *American Journal of Epidemiology, 167*(8), 917–924.

Morland, K., Diez Roux, A. V., & Wing, S. (2006). Supermarkets, other food stores, and obesity: The atherosclerosis risk in communities study. *American Journal of Preventive Medicine, 30*(4), 333–339.

National Cancer Institute. (2013). *Measures of the food environment: Defining measures (instruments and methodologies).* Retrieved from https://riskfactor.cancer.gov/mfe/defining-measures-instruments-and-methodologies

National Restaurant Association. (2012). *National restaurant association 2012 restaurant industry overview.* Retrieved from www.restaurant.org/research/facts

Neumark-Sztainer, D., Larson, N. I., Fulkerson, J. A., Eisenberg, M. E., & Story, M. (2010). Family meals and adolescents: What have we learned from project EAT (eating among teens)? *Public Health Nutrition, 13*(07), 1113.

Olsho, L., Klerman, J., & Bartlett, S. (2011). *Food and nutrition service evaluation of the fresh fruit and vegetable program (FFVP): Interim evaluation report.* Cambridge, MA: Abt Associates.

Patton, L. (2012). Michelle Obama's food desert plan yields few new stores: Retail. *Bloomberg News,* May 7.

Peters, C. J., Wilkins, J. L., & Fick, G. W. (2007). Testing a complete-diet model for estimating the land resource requirements of food consumption and agricultural carrying capacity: The New York State example. *Renewable Agriculture and Food Systems, 22,* 145–153.

Petrie, P. W. (1978). Fast food and quick bucks. *Black Enterprise, pp. 28–30.*

Pothukuchi, K., Joseph, H., Burton, H., & Fisher, A. (2002). *What's cooking in your food system: A guide to community food assessment.* Community Food Security Coalition. Retrieved from www.foodsecurity.org/CFAguide-whatscookin.pdf

Powell, L. M., Slater, S., Mirtcheva, D., Bao, Y., & Chaloupka, F. J. (2007). Food store availability and neighborhood characteristics in the United States. *Preventive Medicine, 44*(3), 189–195.

Pratt, C. A., Lemon, S. C., Fernandez, I. D., Goetzel, R., Beresford, S. A., French, S. A., . . . Webber, L. S. (2007). Design characteristics of worksite environmental interventions for obesity prevention. *Obesity, 15*(9), 2171–2180.

Pulos, E., & Leng, K. (2010). Evaluation of a voluntary menu-labeling program in full-service restaurants. *American Journal of Public Health, 100*(6), 1035–1039.

Robinson-O'Brien, R., Story, M., & Heim, S. (2009). Impact of garden-based youth nutrition intervention programs: A review. *Journal of the American Dietetic Association, 109*(2), 273–280.

Rose, D., Hutchinson, P. L., Bodor, J. N., Swalm, C. M., Farley, T. A., Cohen, D. A., & Rice, J. C. (2009). Neighborhood food environments and body mass index: The importance of in-store contents. *American Journal of Preventive Medicine, 37*(3), 214–219.

Sharkey, J. R. (2009). Measuring potential access to food stores and food-service places in rural areas in the U.S. *American Journal of Preventive Medicine, 36*(4 Suppl.), S151–S155.

Shier, V., An, R., & Sturm, R. (2012). Is there a robust relationship between neighbourhood food environment and childhood obesity in the USA? *Public Health, 126*(9), 723–730.

Short, A., Guthman, G., & Raskin, S. (2007). Food deserts, oases, or mirages? Small markets and community food security in the San Francisco Bay Area. *Journal of Planning Education and Research, 26*(3), 352–364.

Slusser, W. M., Cumberland, W. G., Browdy, B. L., Lange, L., & Neumann, C. (2007). A school salad bar increases frequency of fruit and vegetable consumption among children living in low-income households. *Public Health Nutrition, 10*(12), 1490–1496.

Sorensen, G., Linnan, L., & Hunt, M. K. (2004). Worksite-based research and initiatives to increase fruit and vegetable consumption. *Preventive Medicine, 39*(Suppl. 2), 94–100.

Story, M., Kaphingst, K. M., Robinson-O'Brien, R., & Glanz, K. (2008). Creating healthy food and eating environments: Policy and environmental approaches. *Annual Review of Public Health, 29*, 253–272.

Thomson, C. A., & Ravia, J. (2011). A systematic review of behavioral interventions to promote intake of fruit and vegetables. *Journal of the American Dietetic Association, 111*(10), 1523–1535. US Department of Agriculture. (nd). *Food deserts*. Retrieved from http://apps.ams.usda.gov/fooddeserts/foodDeserts.aspx

US Department of Agriculture. (2012). *Community food security assessment toolkit*. Retrieved from www.ers.usda.gov/Publications/EFAN02013

US Department of Agriculture. (2013a). *Agriculture secretary Vilsack highlights new "smart snacks in school" standards; will ensure school vending machines, snack bars include healthy choices*. Retrieved from www.usda.gov/wps/portal/usda/usdahome?contentid=2013/06/0134.xml

US Department of Agriculture. (2013b). *Food access research atlas*. Retrieved from www.ers.usda.gov/data-products/food-access-research-atlas.aspx#.UVIHeFtAR30

US Department of Agriculture Agricultural Marketing Service. *Food Deserts*. Retrieved August 7, (2014) from http://apps.ams.usda.gov/fooddeserts/foodDeserts.aspx

US Department of Agriculture Agricultural Marketing Service. (2013). *Farmers market growth: 1994–2013; National count of farmers market directory listings*. Retrieved from www.ams.usda.gov/AMSv1.0/ams.fetchTemplateData.do?template=TemplateS&leftNav=WholesaleandFarmersMarkets&page=WFMFarmersMarketGrowth&description=Farmers%20Market%20Growth&acct=frmrdirmkt

Vadiveloo, M. K., Dixon, L. B., & Elbel, B. (2011). Consumer purchasing patterns in response to calorie labeling legislation in New York City. *The International Journal of Behavioral Nutrition and Physical Activity, 8*, 51.

Ver Ploeg, M., Breneman V., Farrigan T., et al. (2009). *Access to affordable and nutritious food: Measuring and understanding food deserts and their consequences; Report to Congress*. Washington, DC: US Department of Agriculture Economic Research Service.

Walker, R. E., Keane, C. R., & Burke, J. G. (2010). Disparities and access to healthy food in the United States: A review of food deserts literature. *Health & Place, 16*(5), 876–884.

Wang, M. C., Gonzalez, A. A., Ritchie, L. D., & Winkleby, M. A. (2006). The neighborhood food environment: Sources of historical data on retail food stores. *The International Journal of Behavioral Nutrition and Physical Activity, 3*, 15.

Zenk, S. N., & Powell, L. M. (2008). US secondary schools and food outlets. *Health & Place, 14*(2), 336–346.

Chapter 18

Intervening to Change Eating Patterns

How Can Individuals and Societies Effect Lasting Change through Their Eating Patterns?

Linden Thayer, Molly DeMarco, Larissa Calancie, Melissa Cunningham Kay,
and Alice Ammerman

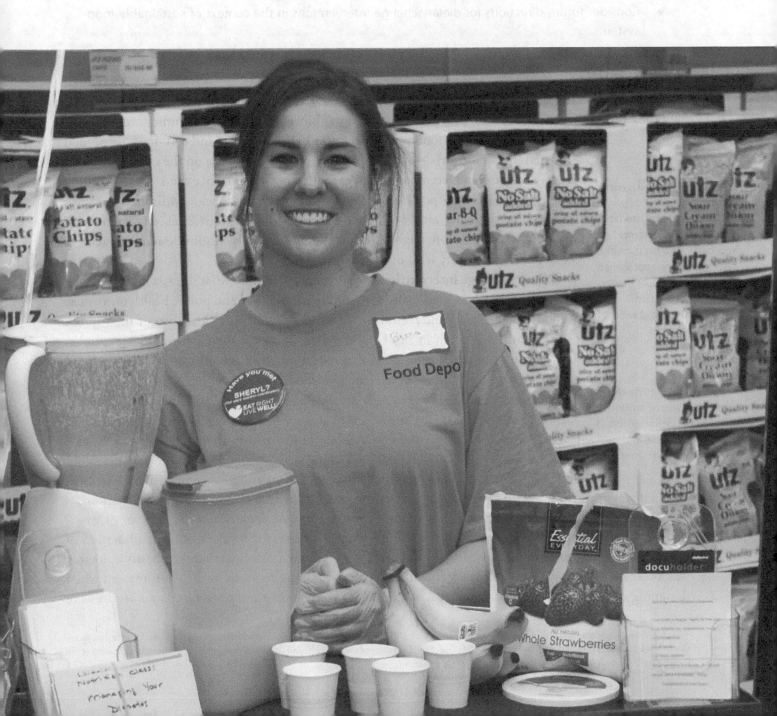

Learning Objectives

- Define *dietary change intervention* and what dietary changes may improve public health.

- Understand the socioecological model (SEM) as it relates to dietary change.

- Understand why theories of change are used to design dietary change interventions and describe key theories of change.

- Review examples of dietary change interventions at the individual, interpersonal, organizational, community, and policy levels, and compare the reach and effectiveness of intervening at different levels of the SEM.

- Recognize strategies that can improve intervention effectiveness.

- Consider future directions for dietary change interventions in the context of sustainable food systems.

Eating is a personal as well as a social and cultural activity. Eating patterns are shaped by individual tastes and micro-environments, as well as broad geographic, cultural, and economic forces. Eating patterns in turn shape food **systems** because consumers demand certain types of food prepared in specific ways—quick convenient meals for people on the go or nectarines in New England in December. Changes in dietary patterns since the 1940s, including consumption of larger portion sizes and more processed foods and limited access to more wholesome and local foods, have taken a toll on individual, environmental, and public health. Improving public health requires interventions designed to achieve dietary change at every level of the food system.

systems
Complex networks of relationships in which each component proceeds independently and under its own logic; also, systems approach, systems thinking, systems theory: approaches, thought patterns, or theory that focus on systems; typically contrasted with linear approaches

dietary change intervention
Program or plan to modify what, how, where, and why individuals consume food to improve individual and public health outcomes

Dietary change interventions are attempts to modify what, how, where, and why individuals consume food in order to improve individual and public health outcomes. Why conduct dietary interventions? As of January 2012, at least five of the top ten leading causes of death in the United States are diet related. Heart disease, stroke, and diabetes account for more than seven hundred thousand deaths each year and are intimately linked with overweight and obesity, which now affects more than two in three American adults (Flegal, Carroll, Kit, & Ogden, 2012; Minino, Murphy, Xu, & Kochanek, 2011). Until recently, dietary interventions focused primarily on teaching *individuals* to make better food choices within their homes, schools, and work environments. Guidance about making wiser selections from vending machines and restaurants, packing healthier lunches, and offering more nutritious snacks to children was and still is a part of counseling and print materials intended to improve eating patterns.

But when the medical community had to abandon the term *adult onset diabetes* in favor of *type 2* diabetes because children were increasingly suffering from a disease that results from a combination of poor diet, too little physical activity, and excess body fat, and when it was clear that the obesity epidemic was a real and growing global threat, interventionists began looking seriously at the environment when designing dietary interventions. Phrases such as *toxic food environment* and *perfect storm for obesity* were

This chapter was supported by Cooperative Agreement Number U48-DP001944 from the Prevention Research Center Program at the Centers for Disease Control and Prevention. The findings and conclusions in this chapter are those of the author(s) and do not necessarily represent the official position of the Centers for Disease Control and Prevention.

coined to describe the fact that teaching people to make good choices was not enough. When immersed in an environment constantly tempting us with too much food of poor nutritional quality, making good choices is often not an option or requires heroic levels of restraint and self-discipline.

The recognition that individual decision making alone is not the answer to a healthy diet prompted a shift upstream in the approach to changing eating patterns—greater emphasis is now placed on how family, community, and policy affect individual eating patterns in addition to personal behavior. The **socioecological model (SEM)**, also described in chapter 17, provides a useful framework. Because of its centrality to this chapter, we show the model here as well; figure 18.1 shows how individual level influences (food-related behaviors, preferences, beliefs) are surrounded by larger forces, such as family, workplace, school, and community. In turn, these environments are affected by organizational- and systems-level policies that can add or remove barriers to healthy eating and dictate the frequency, volume, and types of food available. Current dietary intervention research focuses increasingly on policy and environmental change (the outer rings of the SEM) in the hope of making individual-level decisions healthier by default—making the healthy choice the easy choice.

socioecological model (SEM)
Framework for comparing the effects of nested spheres of influence on a behavior change intervention (individual, interpersonal, organizational, community, policy)

FIGURE 18.1   Diagram of the Socioecological Model

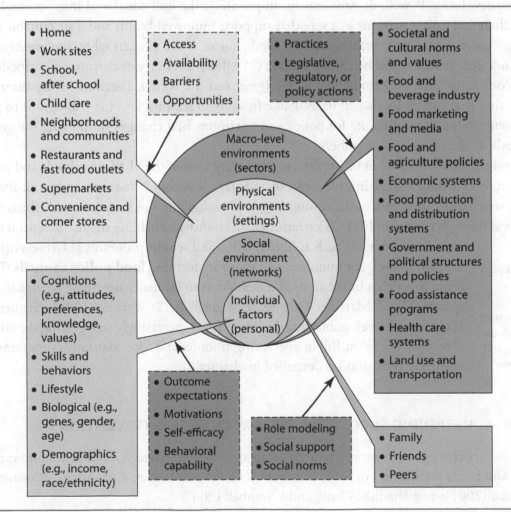

Source: Story, Kaphingst, Robinson-O'Brien, and Glanz (2008).

But even this focus on policy and environmental change may not be enough in the face of a food system based on a business model that relies in part on excess consumption at the individual level. The explosion of prepared food product availability is associated with excess calorie intake (Guthrie, Lin, & Frazao, 2002), as is the increasing shift toward food dollars spent away from home and the decline in home food preparation skills (Jabs & Devine, 2006; Nielsen, Siega-Riz, & Popkin, 2002). As discussed in other chapters, our more centralized and vertically integrated food system, along with other factors, has resulted in excess availability of highly processed food products of limited nutritional value. This food system has also moved many of us away from the sociocultural aspects of food and eating that have sustained us for centuries: families coming together for home-prepared meals lasting long enough to share meaningful conversation; sharing the harvest from home gardens, fresh and preserved; valuing culinary skills outside of reality TV shows; and taking time to simply savor good food.

Dietary change is increasingly motivated by goals beyond nutrition and obesity, including social goals such as seeking a more environmentally sustainable food system, supporting local farmers, or ensuring better treatment for workers or animals. Of late, there is much interest in interventions that address nutritional and food system goals jointly. Research has demonstrated that children who participate in school or community gardens and in preparing their own food are more likely to try new foods and to eat more produce. For example, one study suggests that children of parents who prioritize locally grown food show a higher intake of fruits and vegetables, even after controlling for family income, education, household size, race, gender, SNAP use, and health insurance status (Smith, De Marco, Kearney, Jones, Powell, & Ammerman, in press). At the individual and interpersonal levels of the SEM, changing eating patterns in a way that supports improved health and a sustainable food system requires more than simply making healthy food choices at the kitchen table, the grocery store, or in restaurants. Key attitudes and behaviors include (1) willingness to try or consume new foods; (2) the ability to cook with what is seasonally available (greens in the winter, zucchini in the summer) and the expectation that not all foods will be available fresh in all seasons; and (3) willingness to purchase locally grown foods and to advocate for policy and environmental changes supporting the availability of such foods to all community members.

Food system interventions can be implemented at every level of the SEM. In schools and work sites, organization-level dietary change interventions include farm-to-school programs and work-site farmers markets. A step further upstream to the community level includes farmers markets and efforts to ensure access to food through the use of EBT (electronic benefits transfer), enabling the use of federal nutrition assistance programs such as SNAP, WIC, and seniors programs at farmers markets. At the policy level, communities and states are forming **food policy councils (FPCs)** to bring together a broad array of stakeholders to influence upstream change in the food system (Hood, Martinez-Donate, & Meinen, 2012; Wekerle, 2004) (chapter 6). And at the federal level, public health advocates are increasingly recognizing the critical role played by the Farm Bill in everything from federal food assistance programs to food industry regulation (as described in chapter 8).

food policy councils (FPCs) Group of stakeholders representing various segments of the food system and organized with the goal of addressing strengths and limitations in that system

DESIGNING SUCCESSFUL DIETARY CHANGE INTERVENTIONS

Successful dietary change interventions tend to use evidence-based strategies, have clear and measurable outcomes, and be theory based. For more on research design, see Hulley, Cummings, Browner, Grady, and Newman (2007); and Shadish, Cook, and Campbell (2002).

Why Use Theory to Guide Dietary Change Interventions?

A **theory** "presents a systematic way of understanding events or situations. It is a set of concepts, definitions, and propositions that explain or predict these events or situations by illustrating the relationships between variables" (Glanz & Rimer, 1997, p. 4). The key concepts that make up a theory are known as **constructs**. Theory guides research into why people do or do not engage in healthy behaviors and helps identify what should be measured during a dietary change intervention program. Review of the literature suggests that theory-based dietary change interventions can result in greater effects than interventions developed without theory guidance (Samuel-Hodge et al., 2009). The multilevel constructs contributing to the complexity of our current food system can be best understood using theories, or combinations of theories and constructs, that span the socioecological model.

Key Theories of Behavior Change

Improving the public health impacts of food systems involves behavior changes of individuals, organizations, *and* communities. Many theories are described in the literature and applied in public health research. Here we highlight a few of the most common theories and how they can be applied to changing eating patterns at different levels of the SEM. For additional information about behavior change theories, refer to Glanz and Rimer (1997); and Glanz, Rimer, and Viswanathan (2008).

Individual-Level Theories   Individual-level theories include the **health belief model (HBM)**, the **theory of planned behavior (TPB)**, and the **transtheoretical model (TTM)**. See table 18.1 for more information on each theory and its constructs. The HBM addresses individuals' perceptions of a health threat, the benefits of avoiding the threat, and influences on a decision to act to avoid or mitigate the threat. Key constructs of the HBM include perceived susceptibility, perceived severity, perceived benefits, perceived barriers, cues to action, and self-efficacy. The TPB focuses on individuals' attitudes toward a health behavior, perceived norms, and beliefs about the difficulty or ease of behavior change. Key constructs of TPB are behavioral intention, attitude, subjective norms, and perceived behavioral control. The TTM suggests that behavior change happens as a process over time (six stages: precontemplation, contemplation, preparation, action, maintenance, termination). The process is not linear, but rather people move between stages as they change behavior, relapse, and change again.

These individual-level theories can be applied in new ways, incorporating behaviors and attitudes that relate to not just improving one's personal eating patterns but also to creating a more sustainable food system. For example, the health threat construct of the HBM could be framed in terms of threats to the health of our ecosystem and food justice, as well as threats to one's personal risk for cancer or cardiovascular disease.

theory
A systematic way of understanding events or situations; a set of concepts, definitions, and propositions that explain or predict events or situations by illustrating the relationships between variables

constructs
Key concepts that make up a theory

health belief model (HBM)
Individual-level behavior change theory addressing perceptions of a health threat, benefits of avoiding the threat, and influences on a decision to act to avoid or mitigate the threat; key constructs include perceived susceptibility, perceived severity, perceived benefits, perceived barriers, cues to action, and self-efficacy

theory of planned behavior (TPB)
An individual-level behavior change theory that focuses on individuals' attitudes toward a health behavior, perceived norms, and beliefs about the difficulty or ease of behavior change; key constructs are behavioral intention, attitude, subjective norms, and perceived behavioral control

transtheoretical model (TTM)
An individual-level behavior change theory that suggests that behavior change happens as a process over time (six stages: precontemplation, contemplation, preparation, action, maintenance, termination); the process is not linear; people move between stages as they change behavior, relapse, and change again

TABLE 18.1   Individual-Level Health Behavior Theories

Theory	Constructs	Explanation
Health belief model (HBM)		*Why do/do not people participate in prevention behaviors?*
	Perceived susceptibility	Beliefs about the chances of getting a condition
	Perceived severity	Beliefs about the seriousness of a condition and its consequences
	Perceived benefits	Beliefs about the effectiveness of taking action to reduce risk or seriousness
	Perceived barriers	Beliefs about the material and psychological costs of taking action
	Cues to action	Factors that activate "readiness to change"
	Self-efficacy	Confidence in one's ability to take action
Theory of planned behavior (TPB)		*Explore the relationship between attitude and beliefs and intentions; behavioral intention is the most important determinant of behavior*
	Behavioral intention	Perceived likelihood of performing behavior
	Attitude	Personal evaluation of the behavior
	Subjective norms	Beliefs about whether key people approve or disapprove of the behavior
	Perceived behavioral control	Belief that one has and can exercise control over performing the behavior
Transtheoretical model (TTM)	*Stages of change*	*Behavior change is a process, not an event*
	Precontemplation	Has no intention of taking action (behavior change) within the next six months
	Contemplation	Intends to take action in the next six months
	Preparation	Intends to take action within the next thirty days and has taken some behavioral steps in that direction
	Action	Has changed behavior for less than six months
	Maintenance	Has changed behavior for more than six months

Source: Adapted from Glanz et al. (2008).

social cognitive theory (SCT)
Interpersonal-level behavior change theory that explores how personal and environmental factors work individually and in concert to affect health behavior; key constructs include reciprocal determinism, self-efficacy, observational learning, expectations, reinforcements, and facilitation

Interpersonal-Level Theory   Interpersonal-level theory includes **social cognitive theory (SCT)**, which explores how personal and environmental factors work individually and in concert to affect health behavior. Key constructs of SCT include reciprocal determinism, self-efficacy, observational learning, expectations, reinforcements, and facilitation. See table 18.2 for definitions and more information. SCT is often applied at the organizational and community levels, and SCT-based programs can also inform policy-level changes because this theory highlights person-environment interactions.

One application of the SCT is recognizing how intervention content and interventionists' attitudes toward program participants may affect efficacy. Focus 18.1 describes the issue of weight stigma and provides recommendations for preventing and addressing it.

TABLE 18.2   Interpersonal-Level Theory

Theory	Constructs	Explanation
Social cognitive theory (SCT)	Reciprocal determinism	The dynamic interaction of the person, behavior, and environment in which the behavior is performed
	Self-efficacy	Confidence in one's ability to take action and overcome barriers
	Observational learning	Behavioral acquisition that occurs by watching the actions and outcomes of others' behavior
	Expectations	Anticipated outcomes of a behavior
	Reinforcements	Responses to a person's behavior that increase or decrease the likelihood of reoccurrence
	Facilitation	Providing structures and resources that enable behavior

Source: Adapted from Glanz et al. (2008).

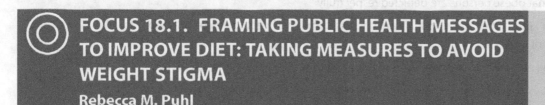

FOCUS 18.1. FRAMING PUBLIC HEALTH MESSAGES TO IMPROVE DIET: TAKING MEASURES TO AVOID WEIGHT STIGMA

Rebecca M. Puhl

With the increase in overweight and obesity prevalence, numerous public health campaigns have surfaced to improve nutrition and eating behaviors. These have targeted weight-related health behaviors through approaches such as promoting fruit and vegetable intake, reducing portion sizes and sugar-sweetened beverage consumption, and increasing physical activity. Although these efforts aim to promote healthy behaviors, some public health messages are framed in ways that inadvertently stigmatize the individuals they intend to help. Thus, it is important to examine stigma in the context of weight-related public health messages. Although there has been attention to how stigma creates barriers to prevention and treatment for other conditions, such as HIV/AIDS, cancer, mental illness, and sexually transmitted diseases, to date this topic has mostly been ignored for obesity.

This absence of attention to weight stigma in public health communication is concerning because individuals who are overweight and obese are vulnerable to pervasive societal stigmatization and prejudice. Stigmatization of obese children and adults has been consistently documented in domains including health care, employment, education, interpersonal relationships, and the media (Puhl & Heuer, 2009). This form of stigma remains largely socially acceptable and is present in some public health campaigns.

For example, a 2011 Children's Health Care of Atlanta campaign to address childhood obesity involved billboards and commercials portraying obese youth with captions such as "Stocky, Chubby, and Chunky are Still Fat" and "Big Bones Didn't Make Me This Way, Big Meals Did" (Crary, 2011). In 2012, Disney's Epcot Center launched an exhibit called "Habit Heroes" to address childhood obesity and promote healthy eating and exercise behaviors in children, which featured animated obese villains named "Lead Bottom" and "The Glutton" (Hubbard, 2012). Although both of these campaigns were stopped following public criticism, they serve as examples of how easily messages intended to promote health behaviors can instead reinforce stigma and blame toward the very people their messages intend to help. Misguided messages have even surfaced among leading public health officials. In 2010, the British Public Health Minister urged health care providers in Britain to call their obese patients "fat" in order to motivate them to lose weight, because calling them "obese" would not provide sufficient motivation to become healthier (Martin, 2010).These examples may reflect unintentional consequences of well-meaning efforts or may stem from perceptions that stigmatization is necessary to provide incentive or motivation for individuals to engage in healthy behaviors to prevent and reduce obesity. Evidence, however,

(Continued)

(Continued)

suggests that exposure to weight stigmatization can increase risk of unhealthy eating behaviors (Schvey, Puhl, & Brownell, 2011) and avoidance of physical activity (Vartanian &Novak, 2010). In addition, weight stigmatization increases vulnerability to a range of negative psychological health consequences, such as depression, anxiety, low self-esteem, poor body image, and suicidal thoughts and behaviors (see review by Puhl & Heuer, 2009), as well as avoidance of health care services (Amy, Aalborg, Lyons, & Keranen, 2006). Thus, stigmatizing messages pertaining to obesity and eating behaviors in public health efforts could potentially contribute to weight gain, increase societal weight bias, and deliver the opposite of the intended effect.

To address this problem, recommendations include:

- Monitoring of message content to avoid pejorative language, weight-based stereotypes, and blaming obese persons for excess weight
- Ensuring that obese persons are depicted respectfully
- Promoting specific health behaviors (e.g., increased fruit and vegetable consumption) for all individuals regardless of body size
- Shifting the emphasis of messages from a focus on appearance (e.g., thinness) to health behaviors
- Consistent evaluation of public responses to message content
- Provision of training in stigma reduction for health educators and public health professionals (Puhl & Heuer, 2010)

Although weight stigmatization is often addressed as an issue of social injustice, it is also an issue central to public health. Weight stigmatization contributes to health disparities, compromises prevention and treatment efforts, leads to unfair treatment of overweight and obese persons, and reduces quality of life for children and adults who are targeted. Attention to weight bias and its significant consequences must be prioritized in the national public health discourse to help ensure that health messages promote optimal lifestyle behavior change without instilling shame or stigma toward those most in need of support.

Beyond obesity stigma, it is important to address and reduce any stigmatization that may be present in other food system interventions. For example, some efforts to promote diets that are local, plant-based, have less environmental impact, or address concerns for animal welfare might inadvertently stigmatize conventional diets and individuals who eat them. Thus, avoiding unintentional stigma requires ongoing attention to the range of factors that contribute to an individual's dietary choices, such as price, preferences, cultural influences, and access to foods.

outcome measures
The standard against which the end result of the intervention is assessed

body mass index (BMI)
A measure based on an individual's weight and height (weight in kilograms divided by height squared), commonly used to determine overweight and obesity status BMI: <18.5 = underweight; 18.5–24.9 = normal weight; 25–29.9 = overweight; ≥30 = obese; alternative measures are used in children

How Do We Know That a Dietary Change Intervention Worked?

Dietary change interventions at any level of the SEM should ideally demonstrate effectiveness before they are disseminated to the wider public health community for implementation. Researchers studying dietary change interventions must select **outcome measures** to evaluate the impact of a particular intervention or program on individual and public health. Outcome measures such as **body mass index (BMI)** (a proxy for body fatness), waist circumference, insulin resistance, and high blood pressure are the preferred determinants of dietary intervention success because these variables are correlated with health outcomes such as diabetes and cardiovascular disease (the number one cause of death in the United States) (Hoyert & Xu, 2012). Dietary intervention studies often lack resources and time to study long-term outcomes such as change in BMI, however, so researchers may instead use more proximal measures such as change in fruit and vegetable consumption or self-reported change in perceived ability to cook healthy meals as evidence for intervention effectiveness. These more proximal measures can demonstrate short-term behavior change, but do not guarantee long-term behavior change or improvements in individual or population health.

Where in the SEM Should We Intervene?

The **RE-AIM framework**, originally developed as a dietary intervention evaluation tool, can help researchers determine at what level of the SEM to intervene by highlighting challenges presented when intervening at a given level (see table 18.3) (Virginia Tech College of Agriculture and Science, 2012). The RE-AIM framework pushes researchers and practitioners to think beyond individual impact to consider program *reach* (who and how many does the intervention reach); *efficacy* (does the intervention work?); *adoption* (ease of use by individuals and organizations); *implementation* (consistency of use and ability to replicate); and *maintenance* (of intervention effects in individuals over time). For example, social cognitive theory might indicate that a particular dietary counseling intervention would have a positive impact on individual behavior, but if the program implementation is too costly, time-consuming, or only reaches a fraction of the intended audience, it would behoove the research team to

RE-AIM framework
Intervention evaluation framework focusing on program reach, efficacy, adoption, implementation, and maintenance

TABLE 18.3   Comparing Impact of Interventions Targeted to Different Levels of the Socioecological Model (SEM)

		Individual	Interpersonal	Organizational	Community	Policy
R	Reach	Small	Small	Moderate	Moderate–Large	Large
E	Efficacy	Successful interventions will show positive change in **individual behavior**	Successful interventions will show positive change in **individual behavior**	Successful interventions will show positive change in **organization-level outcomes and or individual behavior**	Successful interventions will show positive change at the **community level**	Successful interventions will show positive change at the **level on which the policy is implemented** (e.g., local, regional, or federal)
A	Adoption	(Depends on the intervention); relatively easy				(Depends on the intervention); relatively difficult to implement
I	Implementation	Usually designed for narrow section of the population (less applicable to other populations without testing modifications)				Usually designed for a broad section of the population
M	Maintenance	Relatively difficult to sustain over time				Relatively easy to sustain over time

consider intervening at a different level of the SEM or to use a different intervention. A less expensive program may achieve smaller individual behavior change, but if it reaches one hundred times more people the program may have significant population-level health benefits.

CASE STUDIES

The following case studies illustrate programs and policies at each level of the SEM associated with dietary change interventions, discuss intervention associations with food systems, and highlight the benefits and barriers to intervening at each level. As you will see, none of these interventions focus solely on diet change for the sake of diet change alone—the interventionists are interested in improving health for as many people as possible in a sustainable approach that maintains diet change and health for the long term.

Individual-Level Interventions

Successful interventions can address multiple levels of the socioecological model. We begin with traditional individual-level dietary change interventions.

New Leaf: An Individual Dietary Change Intervention   *A New Leaf* is a structured assessment and counseling tool with adaptable strategies to help individuals identify practical strategies to improve health and reduce disease risk through diet and exercise in any adult population (Keyserling et al., 2008). Originally, the *New Leaf* program was designed for low-income women with limited education living in rural communities, many of whom suffer a higher burden of disease compared to regional averages and who have limited access to health care resources. Such health disparities underscore the need for effective interventions designed with the needs and resources of high-risk populations in mind.

The *New Leaf* intervention uses constructs from HBM and TTM to address individual diet behaviors through risk assessment, tailored feedback, goal setting, and follow-up and reinforcement provided by health counselors and community health advisors. Health counselors, who can be health care professionals or **lay health advisors**, are trained to deliver the *New Leaf* counseling tool to intervention participants in accessible settings. Lay health advisors are community volunteers without formal health care training. *A New Leaf* also includes SCT constructs such as social support provided through group sessions led by health counselors and phone calls from lay health advisors.

lay health advisors
Individuals indigenous to a community who serve as a link between community members and traditional health delivery systems

How well does the *New Leaf* intervention work? In one study of 236 women age forty to sixty-four, the *New Leaf* counseling and group-support program increased the aggregate fruit and vegetable intake 2.5 servings per day in the intervention group from baseline to follow up (estimated from changes in serum carotenoid levels). The intervention also increased light and moderate physical activity participation assessed by accelerometers. Dietary risk assessment scores decreased in the intervention group, indicating a reduced risk of diet-related disease relative to controls (Keyserling et al., 2008). In keeping with the RE-AIM framework, researchers designed *A New Leaf* for implementation in a variety of clinical and community settings with little additional cost. *A New Leaf* increases individual demand for healthy food, and so will require the support of healthy food environments to maximize individual diet change success.

Another type of individual-level intervention is the public education campaign, intended to shift population behavior one individual at a time. Meatless Monday, described in focus 18.2, is one such intervention; it includes organizational behavior change components.

FOCUS 18.2. MEATLESS MONDAY: A SIMPLE IDEA THAT SPARKED A MOVEMENT
Allison Righter

Meatless Monday, a growing international movement, communicates a simple public health message: "one day a week, cut out meat" to improve your health and the health of the environment (see figure 18.2).

The Meatless Monday concept can be traced back to rationing programs during WW I and WW II, which urged families to aid the war efforts by reducing consumption of key staple foods. More than sixty years later, the campaign was revived through a unique collaboration between marketing and public health professionals seeking a solution to an important public health issue.

Concerned over the rising prevalence of chronic diseases associated with excessive saturated fat intake (primarily from meat and animal products), former advertising executive Sid Lerner teamed up with the Johns Hopkins Bloomberg School of Public Health in 2003. The school's dean at the time, Alfred Sommer, and professor Robert Lawrence, director of the Johns Hopkins Center for a Livable Future,

FIGURE 18.2   Meatless Monday Encourages Consumers to Cut Out Meat Every Monday

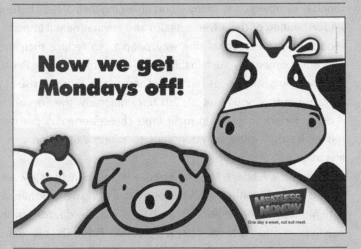

Source: Meatless Monday.

noted that one of the national health objectives in the US Surgeon General's *Healthy People 2010* report called for a 15 percent reduction in dietary saturated fat. Realizing that 15 percent of a typical week's twenty-one meals is about three meals, or just one day's worth, Lerner seized the opportunity to resurrect the Meatless Monday idea as a health behavior change campaign. Reducing the demand for meat would also help alleviate the serious environmental burden and public health impacts associated with industrial food animal production. Moreover, encouraging people to make small changes, starting with just one day a week is a moderate and flexible approach that could make a big collective difference.

In the past ten years, the Meatless Monday campaign has attracted an ever-increasing number of participants and advocates, including leading health professionals, celebrities, chefs, hospitals, schools, restaurants, food companies, and entire communities. By using creative marketing strategies and providing recognition, resources, and an online community for its supporters, the Meatless Monday message reaches and appeals to a diverse population. The campaign has continued to spread in a "viral" manner through a strong social media presence (with over sixty thousand Facebook likes and thirty thousand Twitter followers as of June 2014).

(Continued)

(Continued)

Meatless Monday has caught the attention of prominent thought leaders such as Sir Paul McCartney, who launched a Meat-Free Monday campaign in England in 2009, and Michael Pollan, who endorsed Meatless Monday along with Oprah Winfrey on her show in 2010. Celebrity chefs such as Mario Batali have also publicly endorsed the campaign and introduced it in their restaurants, inspiring hundreds of chefs and restaurant owners to follow suit. In early 2011, Sodexo, one of the largest food services providers in North America, launched a Meatless Monday initiative across the company's network of health care, government, corporate, and school cafeterias as part of their "Better Tomorrow" plan for health and sustainability (Sodexo offers Meatless Monday option to promote health and wellness, 2011). This helped create momentum for more colleges, universities, K–12 schools, hospitals, and other institutions (more than two thousand as of January 2013) to pledge their support for the campaign. Even entire cities, such as Los Angeles, California, have signed Meatless Monday resolutions (Pamer, 2012), and representatives from at least thirty-four countries across the globe have embraced the campaign in some fashion.

According to a 2012 national survey, approximately 43 percent of US adults are aware of the Meatless Monday campaign, and many report changing their dietary behaviors as a result (FGI Research, 2012). As public understanding of the adverse health and environmental impacts of a high-meat diet has increased, Meatless Monday has emerged as one way people can reduce their meat intake and instead fill up on nutritious and environmentally sustainable plant-based alternatives. Replacing meat with whole plant foods such as legumes, nuts, and seeds has been shown to reduce the risk of cardiovascular disease, certain cancers, and all-cause mortality (Pan et al., 2012). Additionally, the Environmental Working Group (2011) estimates that if every American gave up meat (and cheese) one day per week for a year, the reduction in greenhouse gas emissions would be equivalent to taking 7.6 million cars off the road, or driving ninety-one billion less miles.

Among weekdays, Monday offers a unique benefit as a weekly prompt for promoting healthy behaviors. Results of two literature reviews showed that using periodic messaging and leveraging the cultural associations with Monday as the beginning of the week (i.e., the day for a fresh start) can help improve the effectiveness of health promotion strategies (Fry & Neff, 2009, 2010). This research has been the foundation of a larger umbrella organization, the Lerner-founded Monday Campaigns, of which Meatless Monday is now a part. Since 2005, the Monday Campaigns has used this "Monday approach" to health communication messaging surrounding nutrition, physical activity, stress, smoking, and sexual health. According to its president, Peggy Neu, "Monday is an amazingly powerful day of the week to motivate people. It's the January of the week and a good day to pick up a positive action."

With fifty-two Mondays in every year, Meatless Monday offers many chances to start and maintain reduced-meat eating behaviors over time. This campaign is illustrative of how one simple idea can spark a movement that advocates a moderate approach to improve individual health and a more sustainable food system for all.

Interpersonal-Level Interventions

Peers, family, and immediate sources of social influence comprise the interpersonal level in the SEM. Interactions between people inform the way individuals make decisions by establishing norms, shaping identities, and designating roles in specific situations. When considering food choices, norms established between people in close social proximity (i.e., family, peers, friends, etc.) heavily influence decisions, especially in social eating situations.

Weight Wise: Interpersonal Dietary Change Intervention   Weight Wise is based on TTM and SCT and uses group sessions led by a moderator trained in **motivational interviewing (MI)** to leverage the power of social support (a SCT construct) to improve individual weight status, including diet change. Motivational interviewing is a guided conversation that does not aim for behavior change, but rather elicits individuals' own reasons for change over the course of one or several sessions (Miller & Johnson, 2001). Once individuals identify and explore their own reasons for making a healthy change, it is anticipated that this realization will *lead* to behavior change through overcoming identified barriers and use of available resources. Moderators and group participants build norms around healthy choices and support each other in working toward individual goals that participants share in discussions with the group.

> **motivational interviewing (MI)**
> A guided conversation that does not aim for behavior change but rather for individual realization, which may lead to behavior change through overcoming identified barriers and using available resources

At the conclusion of a five-month intervention trial that included 143 women, Weight Wise participants had a greater average weight loss than members of the control group, and those who attended more group counseling sessions lost more weight, providing evidence of a **dose-response effect** (Samuel-Hodge et al., 2009). For example, participants who attended all sixteen group sessions lost an average of 6.7 kg, whereas participants who attended fewer than ten group sessions lost an average of 1.6 kg. A follow-up study showed that Weight Wise is also cost-effective. Participants' abilities to maintain weight loss, more difficult than initial weight loss, will be assessed in future research.

> **dose-response effect**
> The change of strength of effect based on differing levels of exposure

Weight Wise group sessions can increase social support and empowerment, and can be used to leverage advocacy efforts around the community food environment. For example, in the initial Weight Wise study, participants worked with the local farmers market to produce cooking demonstrations using local products to increase their peer groups' exposure to healthy food.

Organizational-Level Interventions

Organizations, such as schools, work sites, churches, and professional or neighborhood groups, may have positive or negative effects on individual dietary behavior. Fairly small changes to an organization's environment can have an immediate impact on a large group of people. Imagine the exercise benefits if everyone in a sixth floor office suddenly has to take the stairs because the company removed the elevator. Organizational change can be difficult if many individuals must reach consensus about that change or resented if a single individual makes the decision. How organizational change is implemented is important for intervention success; organizations present opportunities to build social support for desirable behavior change because they reach many people and are important sources of social norms and values.

Even if not explicitly stated, organizational interventions tend to rely on modifying SCT constructs, such as facilitation, reinforcements, observational learning, self-efficacy, and reciprocal determinism, to alter dietary behaviors. Think about how each of the following interventions addresses these SCT constructs to achieve diet change.

Schools   The school environment can have a significant impact on the quality of children's food choices. More than half of all school children consume the majority of their daily calories through school meal programs, á la carte options, vending machines, and school stores (Story, Kaphingst, &

Farm-to-School (F2S)
Organizational intervention that brings local and regional farm produce to schools, often with the aim of increasing fruit and vegetable consumption and benefit local and regional agriculture

French, 2006). **Farm-to-School (F2S)** programs are organizational interventions that aim to increase children's fruit and vegetable consumption by making produce more accessible, increase student knowledge of nutrition and agriculture, and support local farmers. Emerging research suggests that if a child continuously encounters local apples on her school lunch counter and visits an apple orchard, she is more likely to consume apples (Lakkakula, Geaghan, Wong, Zanovec, Pierce, & Tuuri, 2011; Wang et al., 2010). At the organizational level of the SEM, the interdependence of sustainable food systems and individual health become increasingly clear. Other organizations, including hospitals and large corporations, are establishing farm-to-institution programs, building on the farm-to-school model to increase member, staff, and client access to and appreciation of fresh healthy foods.

FIGURE 18.3   Students Picking Greens from Their School Garden

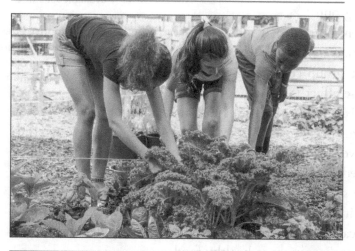

Source: Michael Milli, CLF.

Establishing a school garden (see figure 18.3) can also contribute to healthy eating patterns and willingness to try new foods (Chatzi et al., 2007; Contento, 2008). Studies of school gardens have shown they can significantly increase the number of servings of fruits and vegetables that children consume (Robinson-O'Brien, Story, & Heim, 2009).

Focus 18.3 describes the Real Food Challenge, an organizational-level intervention that challenges institutional food providers to shift their purchasing.

FOCUS 18.3. REAL FOOD CHALLENGE
Anim Steel

When she headed to college, Katie Blanchard wasn't thinking a lot about food. After a few months on a rural campus in Southern Minnesota, however, industrial food and agriculture were hard to avoid. A long-standing interest in the environment prompted her to learn more. Katie did lab projects testing water contaminated by surrounding animal feedlots and got to know immigrants in the community who were seeking opportunities beyond back-breaking days in the local turkey slaughterhouses.

She started to see connections between the food in the cafeteria and many of the social and ecological issues she was learning about from the local community. Though it seemed like the food supply chain should be obvious in an agricultural town, Katie had no idea where almost any of the food in the cafeteria came from, how it got there, or how people and the environment were treated in the process.

Her classes weren't giving her many answers, so Katie turned to an emerging national student organization called the Real Food Challenge (RFC). The RFC had developed a tool to increase transparency in cafeteria food purchasing by assessing the percentage of local, fair, green, and humane food purchased—what they called *real food*. And they declared their challenge: to shift $1 billion of college and university food purchasing to real food within ten years.

With a few others, Katie organized a summit for a hundred students from around the region, who converged on a small town in Iowa to share experiences and ideas on working together. The RFC had organized summits in New England and California, but this was the first in the Midwest. The students discussed how to use the power and stature of their colleges and universities to change the food system that they all agreed was unjust, unhealthy, and unsustainable.

Because young people are inheriting a world in which climate disasters, debt, and diabetes are becoming the norm, students united around food as a tool for social change makes sense. They imagine a "real food" system that truly nourishes producers, consumers, communities, and the earth (see figure 18.4).

FIGURE 18.4   Real Food Wheel

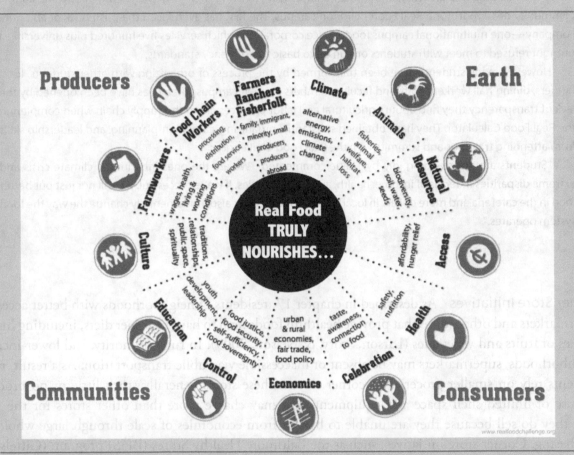

Source: Real Food Challenge.

In just four years, students trained and supported by the RFC had secured nearly $50 million in real food purchasing commitments. More than eighty thousand students on three hundred campuses across the country participated in RFC-affiliated events on Food Day 2012, a national day of action for healthy, just, and sustainable food. On many of those campuses, students launched campaigns for the Real Food Campus Commitment, a pledge to ensure complete transparency in university food supply chains and shift at least 20 percent of the university's food purchasing budget to real food for their campus dining halls.

Becoming one of the first signatories of the Real Food Campus Commitment, University of Vermont president John Bramley commented, "UVM can play an important role not just in educating students or researching

(Continued)

(Continued)

the issues but by actually seeking to be part of the solution, in the way we choose to feed the 15,000 members of our community."

The potential impact of many universities signing on is big. Not only would redirecting dollars create new opportunities for the most socially and environmentally responsible farmers but also it will set a precedent for other institutional buyers, such as hospitals, parks, and museums. Only three companies dominate the contracted cafeteria business in this country, so changes made in the college sector can ripple outward quickly.

Working for this change does not come without challenges. Students have encountered resistance throughout their campaigns. Local dining managers and university administrators are often reluctant to make change. Students are busy, and it takes a lot of work to bring them together to organize a substantial community of support for a Real Food Policy on campus. The RFC has even faced the push back of an entire company—one multinational campus food service corporation (which services five hundred plus universities) outright refused to meet with students or sign on to basic transparency standards.

However, many students have been transformed by the process of organizing with other students, local farmers, dining hall workers, staff, and faculty members on their campus. Their eyes have been opened by the lack of transparency they find about agricultural and labor practices along the supply chain when completing the Real Food Calculator. They have obtained substantial organizing, campaign-planning, and leadership skills from attending trainings and summits with the Real Food Challenge.

"Students are not standing idly by," Katie commented. "We are the ones inheriting a climate crisis and extreme disparities in terms of income, health, and opportunities. If we're successful, we will not just put better food in the cafeteria and more dollars in local farmer's pockets, but also fundamentally change the way the food system operates."

Corner Store Initiatives As described in chapter 17, residents of neighborhoods with better access to supermarkets and other stores that provide healthful foods tend to have healthier diets, including higher intakes of fruits and vegetables (Larson, Story, & Nelson, 2009). In rural, minority, and lower-income neighborhoods, supermarkets may be absent or inaccessible via public transportation. As a result, most residents rely on smaller groceries or corner stores. These stores generally stock little or no produce because of limited shelf space and equipment, and may charge more than other stores for the produce they do sell because they are unable to benefit from economies of scale through large wholesale purchasing. Corner store initiatives, such as the Baltimore Healthy Stores (BHS) program (Gittelsohn & Sharma, 2009; Gittelsohn et al., 2012) have the potential to effect dietary change by increasing access to healthy foods. BHS uses formative research to identify cultural eating and shopping habits, and intervenes to address constructs from the SCT: self-efficacy (educating consumers and owners), observational learning (exposure to fresh produce and preparation methods in corner stores), and reinforcement through health communication and social marketing that target specific audiences identified in formative research (primary shoppers and family food gatekeepers). Labels identifying healthy food and incentives (e.g., coupons) are used to encourage consumption of healthy items such as fruits and vegetables; government incentive programs can help corner store initiatives to ensure that healthy items are stocked without adding an economic burden to store owners. There are also examples of connecting corner stores with small, local farmers and suppliers to strengthen local food systems (The Food Trust, 2012).

Perspective 18.1 provides additional advice from researcher Joel Gittelsohn for promoting the success of organizational- and community-level interventions.

Perspective 18.1. Building a Better Food Environment
Joel Gittelsohn

From 1990 to 2001, I worked on a series of interventions to reduce risk for obesity and future chronic disease in low-income minority populations. These programs had two main features: they were school-based and they were unsuccessful in reducing obesity. In fact, the great majority of community interventions to reduce obesity in children have been school-based, and most have not been successful in affecting obesity. What gives? I have concluded that it doesn't matter what you tell or offer children in the school setting if they then go out into their community and have access to cheap high-sugar and -fat foods, with few healthier options.

Since 2001, I have been working to develop, implement, and evaluate programs to improve the food environment outside of schools—in Baltimore City, American Indian reservations, First Nations reserves, Pacific Islander communities, and other communities. Our programs have taken place in small food stores (see figure 18.5), carryout restaurants, recreation centers, churches, and work sites, and have focused on increasing access to healthier foods and then promoting these foods through culturally appropriate media at the point of purchase (see, for example: Curran, Gittelsohn, Anliker, Ethelbah, Blake, Sharma, & Caballero, 2005; Gittelsohn & Rowan, 2011; Gittelsohn, Rowan, & Gadhoke, 2012; Gittelsohn & Sharma, 2009; Song, Gittelsohn, Anliker, Sharma, Suratkar, Mattingly, & Kim, 2012; Song, Gittelsohn, Kim, Suratkar, Sharma, & Anliker, 2010; Vastine, Gittelsohn, Ethelbah, Anliker, & Caballero, 2005). We commonly work in more than one venue in the same program, including with schools. We use a variety of approaches and materials in each setting, including posters, shelf labels, taste tests, radio announcements, classroom curricula, flyers, brochures, giveaway items, and special events. We've had some success, and some failure. We found that different things work in different places. Here are some general lessons learned:

FIGURE 18.5   Scene from a Corner Store Intervention: Fresh, Healthy Options Next to Snack Foods

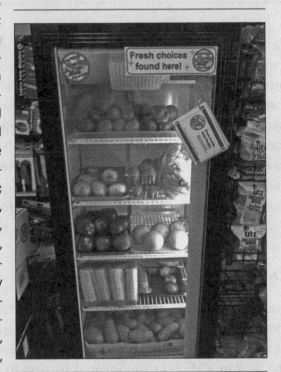

Source: Alison Cuccia, Healthy Corner Stores Project.

1. **Do your homework first.** By this I mean read up on the setting you want to work in. The odds are strong that someone has worked in the same setting you want to work in and may have looked at similar issues.

2. **Conduct formative research to help plan your program.** Formative research can include qualitative (e.g., in-depth interviews, focus groups) and quantitative (e.g., twenty-four-hour dietary recalls) approaches for information gathering. Make sure you include all stakeholders.

(Continued)

(Continued)

3. **Work with the community from the beginning.** Plan workshops and other group activities that will engage community members and all the relevant stakeholders, and make them part of the solution.

4. **Choose a health behavior change conceptual framework (e.g., social cognitive theory, social marketing, health belief model, etc.) or come up with one of your own.** A common error in community food environment improvement programs is taking a simplistic approach—thinking that just increasing people's knowledge will resolve the problem. But this is usually not the case.

5. **Pay attention to culture.** In every setting, people work within different value systems. The kinds of messaging and communications that work with one segment of the population will not work with another. Choose messaging and approaches that resonate with the community you are working in.

6. **Work with retailers.** First realize that small food retailers work within a food environment of their own, which can limit the sorts of foods they can sell. In some areas, there are only one to two wholesalers who supply food for these stores. Work in stages with retailers to build rapport. Promote the healthier foods they already sell first. Make sure you meet some of their needs first—such as helping them with signage.

Faith Communities Faith communities are often concerned about the physical health of their congregants, and these organizations are ripe for intervention because many people turn to their faith-based institution for advice and establishment of social norms (see focus 9.1). Tools such as *Faithful Families Eating Smart and Moving More* help faith communities to think through policy changes they can make within their congregation to create an environment supporting and encouraging healthy eating behaviors (Eat Smart, Move More, 2011). One faith community in rural North Carolina is using the church as an incubator space to teach young people how to garden and farm in an effort to improve local diets and increase the community's economic and environmental sustainability; larger studies are needed to determine efficacy and effectiveness of such programs (UNC Center for Health Promotion and Disease Prevention, 2011; Smith et al., in press).

Community-Level Interventions

Public health practitioners often choose to target the collective well-being of a community to promote behavior change. Community-level interventions can support systems and policies that promote healthy eating or redress systems and policies that create barriers to healthy eating. Community-level change can address environmental barriers to health and affect a large population, but it is not easy to successfully navigate a community from identifying a health problem to implementing and sustaining solutions. Several studies have aimed to address diet at the community level, but evaluation is difficult because so many factors influence individual and collective behavior. The potential for community-level interventions to inspire positive, lasting change, however, is appealing to researchers and policy makers alike.

community-based participatory research (CBPR)
Research in partnership with community members and with community participation in all aspects of the research

An increasingly popular strategy underlying multilevel dietary interventions is **community-based participatory research (CBPR)**, in which researchers partner with community members to address the problems most important to the community, and in the process, help leverage community support and expertise (Viswanathan et al., 2004; Wieland et al., 2012; Zoellner, Motley, Wilkinson, Jackman, Barlow, &

Hill, 2012). Better outcomes are expected when more of the community—including local government, schools, academics, community organizations, businesses, and individuals—support the initiative.

Shape Up Somerville Shape Up Somerville (SUS) is a community-wide intervention addressing childhood obesity in Somerville, Massachusetts (Economos et al., 2007, Shape Up Somerville, 2012). Local government, academia, schools, health care providers, and businesses formed a partnership and made changes in many of the places that touch children's lives. For example, the project changed school food by removing processed foods such as chips and eliminating high calorie–high fat items from fundraisers, implemented nutrition education during and after school, increased school-based physical activity, added nutrient labels to menu items in local restaurants, addressed parent knowledge through outreach and education, implemented a farmers market initiative, and hosted healthy community events. SUS engaged in CBPR and maintained a community advisory council to initiate and maintain the community's engagement with the project. SUS's success is due in no small part to the efforts of Somerville's mayor, who championed the cause and facilitated community engagement. SUS is an ongoing project, but data from the first year suggest that this holistic approach to dietary change resulted in a significant decrease in BMI z-score (a measurement that reflects a percentile relative to a specified distribution of BMI for age) in children at high risk for obesity (Economos et al., 2007).

Heart Healthy Lenoir The Heart Healthy Lenoir (HHL) Project is another example of a community-level dietary change intervention (UNC Center for Health Promotion and Disease Prevention, 2012). Whereas SUS addresses childhood obesity, HHL is designed to develop and test better ways to reduce heart disease in a rural county in North Carolina. Similar to SUS, HHL addresses dietary change from a number of angles, guided by a coalition of community members, academic researchers, and strategic organizational partners poised to make healthy environmental changes throughout the community from hospitals to restaurants. A high blood pressure study group works with local health care providers to improve individual blood pressure management, a lifestyle change study is testing the effects of individual versus group counseling on diet and physical activity change, and a genetics study is exploring the effects of interactions among genes, family history, and the environment on cardiovascular disease risk.

The project's CBPR roots provide the research team and community advisors flexibility to address community concerns as they arise. For example, when residents noted during project planning that it was hard to eat healthfully when dining out in the community, study staff developed information on healthy restaurant offerings. Community- and policy-level interventions are selected and implemented using a structured stakeholder interview process that assesses what community members perceive as the most "winnable" policy changes (Jilcott Pitts, Whetstone, Wilkerson, Smith, & Ammerman, 2012). Some of these policies include supporting local farmers, farmers markets, and increasing access to healthy food. By building grassroots community support, these initiatives have a better chance of success. HHL is ongoing and results are not yet available.

Policy-Level Interventions

Policy-level changes often complement organizational- and community-level change. Policy activities and strategies can shape food environments that help make the healthy choice the easy choice. They codify changes in systems and social structures to foster positive changes in healthy eating behaviors. Intervening at the policy level can affect the greatest number of people, and should be based on rigorous research and theory-driven programming. Developing policy based on theory, however, is often not feasible or of interest to those setting policy. At the same time, some policy changes face opposition from policymakers and stakeholders with vested interest in the status quo. Similar to community change, the support of government, academics, industry, nonprofits, and individuals is important to achieving successful dietary change policy. For a comprehensive framework to guide public health policy development and implementation, refer to Hendriks, Jansen, Gubbels, De Vries, Paulussen, and Kremers (2013).

Food Policy Councils   As described in chapter 6, food policy councils draw together stakeholders representing various segments of the food system with the goal of addressing strengths and limitations in that system, including access to healthy foods for low-income households and potential opportunities for low-wealth agricultural communities (Scherb, Palmer, Frattaroli, & Pollack, 2012). Food policy councils have crafted or promoted numerous programs and policies to change eating habits through direct and indirect means, particularly by supporting healthy food environments that facilitate individual and collective diet change.

Electronic Benefits Transfer Use at Farmers Markets   SNAP in the late 1990s switched from paper vouchers to the use of debit cards electronically loaded with SNAP benefits or **electronic benefit transfer (EBT)**. Farmers markets and farm stands that formerly accepted paper vouchers can now accept SNAP only if they purchase EBT terminals that can swipe and debit these cards. This challenge has limited access to locally grown fresh fruits, vegetables, eggs, dairy, and meats for low-income households. Policies that provide funds to assist farmers markets and farm stands to purchase these terminals and support related costs such as staffing and outreach to potential customers can remove this barrier to access (Farmers Market Coalition, 2012). In North Carolina, a pilot program was initiated in 2011 to enable farmers markets to accept EBT benefits from three different nutrition assistance programs: SNAP, WIC, and the Senior Farmers' Market Nutrition Program (North Carolina Sustainable Local Food Advisory Council, 2011). Another innovative strategy to change eating behaviors using EBT is the Market Match program run by the Crescent City Farmers Market in New Orleans and now replicated in a number of other markets (Crescent City Farmers Market, nd). Using private donations, Crescent City Farmers' Market matches SNAP benefits up to $25 per market visit while supplies last. These efforts can contribute to positive dietary change for low-income groups (while increasing revenue for farmers); Health Bucks, for example, another market match program in New York City, resulted in increased produce consumption among Health Bucks users (Center for Training and Research Translation, 2010). The economic sustainability of grant-based or privately funding market match programs can be tenuous, so institutionalization of EBT programs and universal access are important concerns for promoters of healthy and local food systems.

USDA-funded Child Nutrition Programs   The US Department of Agriculture administers a number of school nutrition programs, including the National School Lunch, National School Breakfast, and Summer Food Service program. Meals must meet the **Dietary Guidelines for Americans (DGAs)**, though specific menus are set locally. The new meal pattern for the National School Lunch Program went into effect in School Year 2012–2013 and increases availability of fruit, vegetables, and whole

electronic benefit transfer (EBT)
Debit cards electronically loaded with SNAP benefits (formerly known as Food Stamps)

Dietary Guidelines for Americans (DGAs)
The health and nutrition guidelines reviewed by an expert panel and produced by the US Department of Agriculture and US Department of Health and Human Services that govern all federal nutrition policy and programs

grains, sets more specific calorie requirements, and further reduces sodium in school meals (US Department of Agriculture, nd). These programs provide the majority of meals for many low-income children and the opportunity to improve child dietary intake and support for sustainable food systems (Campbell, Nayga, Park, & Silva, 2011; Suitor & Gleason, 2002).

FUTURE DIRECTIONS FOR DIETARY CHANGE INTERVENTIONS

Poor diet and unhealthy food systems play an enormous role in the rise of crippling, costly chronic diseases, including obesity, diabetes, and heart disease. Evidence suggests that primary prevention of these conditions, especially through diet change, is the best way to improve individual and population health. As our understanding of individual-environment interactions expands, dietary change interventions continue to evolve from the traditional individual-level counseling session. Although the possible levels of the SEM on which to intervene remain constant, the types of interventions, and the methods of delivery continue to change. Social media and social networking offer potential for dietary change interventions based on strategies such as social support, education, or the motivation derived from public declarations of commitment. New online and mobile technologies provide additional tools, including periodic messaging and reminders, options to obtain recipes and shopping lists, and the opportunity to track behaviors and progress toward goals. There are hundreds of diet-related smartphone apps available, for example, although researchers have yet to test many theory-based mobile phone interventions and equitable technology access must always be a concern.

The power of community champions, individuals such as the mayor of Somerville, Massachusetts who encourage community engagement and community change, may also have an important role in dietary change interventions. Trusted leaders who have the support of the community should be leveraged in future efforts to garner the collaboration needed for healthy, sustainable change.

Sustainable dietary change is supported at the individual level when all levels of the food system are brought into line with individuals' needs. And the food system will not change unless individuals, organizations, communities, and government demand changes that will facilitate improvements in dietary behavior.

We started this chapter with the question, "How can individuals and societies effect lasting change through their eating patterns?" We have discussed how engaging individuals in the broader system of food production and distribution can have a positive impact on their own eating habits by enhancing access to and appreciation for healthy local options. Engaging adults and children in gardening, visiting farms, and cooking can increase their interest in and consumption of fresh produce, and provide a better understanding of the environmental, economic, and social costs of the current food system. We also described how individual food purchasing habits that prioritize local, sustainably grown food can contribute to more economically viable communities that foster respect and appreciation for food producers and distributors, casting a vote for a future food system that is truly sustainable.

SUMMARY

Chronic diseases, such as obesity and diabetes, are on the rise in the United States, and experts are seeking many ways to improve public health. Dietary change interventions are attempts to modify what, how, where, and why individuals consume food in order to improve individual and public health outcomes. Changes can be made at many levels of the socioecological model (SEM), and changes to dietary habits and food systems simultaneously have the potential to improve public health more dramatically than changes in either sphere of influence alone (Huang, Drewnosksi, Kumanyika, & Glass, 2009).

Successful dietary change interventions use valid research methods, have clear and measurable outcomes, and are theory-based. Behavior change theories can address individual-, interpersonal-, or systems-level change. RE-AIM (reach, efficacy, adoption, implementation, maintenance) is a useful tool to help researchers consider the impact of a given dietary and food system intervention. Intervening at different levels of the SEM has pros and cons (targeted individual-level impact versus broad population-level impact). In addition to the interventions highlighted in the chapter text, several other approaches are presented in focus and perspective boxes.

Dietary change efforts that incorporate interventions at multiple levels of the SEM within the context of building healthier food systems have the greatest potential to improve human, environmental, and social health.

KEY TERMS

Body mass index (BMI)

Community-based participatory research (CBPR)

Constructs

Dietary change intervention

Dietary Guidelines for Americans (DGA)

Dose-response effect

Electronic benefit transfer (EBT)

Farm-to-School (F2S)

Food policy councils (FPCs)

Health belief model (HBM)

Lay health advisors

Motivational interviewing (MI)

Outcome measures

RE-AIM framework

Social cognitive theory (SCT)

Socioecological model (SEM)

Systems

Theory

Theory of planned behavior (TPB)

Transtheoretical model (TTM)

DISCUSSION QUESTIONS

1. What is an example of a dietary change intervention in your community? At what level of the socioecological model (SEM) is this program intervening? What are the pros and cons of this intervention for human health and food system sustainability? How would you change this intervention and why?

2. How could the National School Lunch and Breakfast Programs support a sustainable food system? What needs to change in order to accomplish this goal? What support is needed to make this change?

3. How can individual-level dietary change interventions support broader food system change?

4. Some interventions aimed at achieving dietary change have drawn accusations of paternalism (taking away individual liberty based on the idea that the policy maker knows best) or advancing weight stigma. What are some examples of such interventions? To what extent do you agree or disagree with this criticism? When do the potential positive effects of an intervention outweigh the potential harms?

5. Do you have a chapter of the Real Food Challenge on your own campus? If so or if not, what sorts of interventions would be most helpful for improving your campus's food environment?

REFERENCES

Amy, N. K., Aalborg, A., & Lyons, P., & Keranen, L. (2006). Barriers to routine gynecological cancer screening for White and African-American obese women. *International Journal of Obesity*, *30*, 147–155.

Campbell, B., Nayga, R. M., Park, J. L., & Silva, A. (2011). Does the national school lunch program improve children's dietary outcomes? *American Journal of Agricultural Economics*, *93*(4), 1099–1130.

Center for Training and Research Translation. (2010). *Health bucks*. Retrieved from www.center-trt.org/?p=intervention& id=1109

Chatzi, L., Apostolaki, G., Bibakis, I., Skypala, I., Bibaki-Liakou, V., Tzanakis, N., … Cullinan, P. (2007). Protective effect of fruits, vegetables and the Mediterranean diet on asthma and allergies among children in Crete. *Thorax*, *62*(8), 677–683.

Contento, I. R. (2008). Nutrition education: Linking research, theory, and practice. *Asia Pacific Journal of Clinical Nutrition*, *17*(Suppl. 1), 176–179.

Crary, D. (2011). *Do Georgia's child obesity ads go too far? Huffington Post*. Retrieved from www.huffingtonpost.com/2011/05/02/georgia-child-obesity-ads_n_856255.html

Crescent City Farmers Market. (nd). *Market match: Meeting shoppers halfway*. Retrieved from www.crescentcityfarmers market.org/index.php?page=market-match

Curran, S., Gittelsohn, J., Anliker, J. A., Ethelbah, B., Blake, K., Sharma, S., & Caballero, B. (2005). Process evaluation of a store-based environmental obesity intervention on two American Indian reservations. *Health Education Research*, *20*(6), 719–729.

Eat Smart, Move More. (2011). *Faithful families eating smart and moving more*. Retrieved from www.eatsmartmovemorenc .com/FaithfulFamilies/FaithfulFamilies.html

Economos, C. D., Hyatt, R. R., Goldberg, J. P., Must, A., Naumova, E. N., Collins, J. J., & Nelson, M. E. (2007). A community intervention reduces BMI z-score in children: Shape Up Somerville first year results. *Obesity*, *15*(5), 1325–1336.

Environmental Working Group. (2011). *Meat eater's guide to climate change and health*. Retrieved from www.ewg.org/ meateatersguide/at-a-glance-brochure

Farmers Market Coalition. (2012). *Farmers' market coalition*. Retrieved from http://farmersmarketcoalition.org/programs

FGI Research. (2012). *FGI survey report 2012: Meatless Monday online panel results*. Retrieved from www.meatlessmonday .com/images/photos/2012/10/FGI-Survey-Report.pdf

Flegal, K. M., Carroll, M. D., Kit, B. K., & Ogden, C. L. (2012). Prevalence of obesity and trends in the distribution of body mass index among US adults, 1999–2010. *JAMA*, *307*(5), 491–497.

The Food Trust. (2012). *Healthy Corner Stores issue brief*, pp. 1–6.

Fry, J. P., & Neff, R. A. (2009). Periodic prompts and reminders in health promotion and health behavior interventions: Systematic review. *Journal of Medical Internet Research*, *11*(2), e16.

Fry, J. P., & Neff, R. A. (2010). *Healthy Monday: Two literature reviews*. The Johns Hopkins Center for a Livable Future. Retrieved from www.jhsph.edu/research/centers-and-institutes/johns-hopkins-center-for-a-livable-future/_pdf/pro jects/HM/healthymondayreport.pdf

Gittelsohn, J., & Rowan, M. (2011). Preventing diabetes and obesity in American Indian communities: The potential of environmental interventions. *American Journal of Clinical Nutrition*, *93*(5), 1179S–1183S.

Gittelsohn, J., Rowan, M., & Gadhoke, P. (2012). Intervening in small food stores to change the food environment, improve diet and reduce risk from chronic disease. *Preventing Chronic Disease*, *9*, E59.

Gittelsohn, J., & Sharma, S. (2009). Physical, consumer and social aspects of measuring the food environment among diverse low-income populations. *American Journal of Preventive Medicine*, *36*(4S), S1.

Glanz, K., & Rimer, B.K. (1997). *Theory at a glance: A guide for health promotion practice*. Retrieved from www.cancer.gov/cancertopics/cancerlibrary/theory.pdf

Glanz, K., Rimer, B. K., & Viswanathan, K. (2008). *Health behavior and health education: Theory, research, and practice* (4th ed). San Francisco: Jossey-Bass.

Guthrie, J. F., Lin, B. H., & Frazao, E. (2002). Role of food prepared away from home in the American diet, 1977–78 versus 1994–96: Changes and consequences. *Journal of Nutrition Education and Behavior*, *34*(3), 140–150.

Hendriks, A.-M., Jansen, M.W.J., Gubbels, J. S., De Vries, N. K., Paulussen, T., & Kremers, S.P.J. (2013). Proposing a conceptual framework for integrating local public health policy, applied to childhood obesity—the behavior change ball. *Implementation Science*, *8*(45), 16.

Hood, C., Martinez-Donate, A., & Meinen, A. (2012). Promoting healthy food consumption: A review of state-level policies to improve access to fruits and vegetables. *WMJ*, *111*(6), 283–288.

Hoyert, D. L., & Xu, J. (2012). Deaths: Preliminary data for 2011. *National Vital Statistics Reports*, *61*(6), 1–51.

Huang, T. T., Drewnosksi, A., Kumanyika, S., & Glass, T. A. (2009). A systems-oriented multilevel framework for addressing obesity in the 21st century. *Preventing Chronic Disease*, *6*(3), A82.

Hubbard, A. (2012). *Disney World shuts obesity exhibit after criticism*. Retrieved from www.latimes.com/news/nation/nationnow/la-na-nn-disney-obesity-exhibit-20120302,0,4947393.story

Hulley, S. B., Cummings, S. R., Browner, W. S., Grady, D. G., & Newman, T. B. (2007). *Designing clinical research* (3rd ed). Philadelphia: Lippincott Williams & Wilkins.

Jabs, J., & Devine, C. M. (2006). Time scarcity and food choices: An overview. *Appetite*, *47*(2), 196–204.

Jilcott Pitts, S. B., Whetstone, L. M., Wilkerson, J. R., Smith, T. W., & Ammerman, A. S. (2012). A community-driven approach to identifying "winnable" policies using the Centers for Disease Control and Prevention's Common Community Measures for Obesity Prevention. *Preventing Chronic Disease*, *9*, E79.

Keyserling, T. C., Samuel-Hodge, C. D., Jilcott, S. B., Johnston, L. F., Garcia, B. A., Gizlice, Z., ... Ammerman, A. S. (2008). Randomized trial of a clinic-based, community-supported, lifestyle intervention to improve physical activity and diet: The North Carolina enhanced WISEWOMAN project. *Preventive Medicine*, *46*(6), 499–510.

Lakkakula, A., Geaghan, J. P., Wong, W. P., Zanovec, M., Pierce, S. H., & Tuuri, G. (2011). A cafeteria-based tasting program increased liking of fruits and vegetables by lower, middle and upper elementary school-age children. *Appetite*, *57*(1), 299–302.

Larson, N. I., Story, M. T., & Nelson, M. C. (2009). Neighborhood environments: Disparities in access to healthy foods in the U.S. *American Journal of Preventive Medicine*, *36*(1), 74–81.

Martin, D. (2010). *Obese? Just call them fat: Plain-speaking doctors will jolt people into losing weight, says minister*. Retrieved from www.dailymail.co.uk/news/article-1298394/Call-overweight-people-fat-instead-obese-says-health-minister.html

Miller, C. E., & Johnson, J. L. (2001). Motivational interviewing. *Canadian Nurse*, *97*(7), 32–33.

Minino, A. M., Murphy, S. L., Xu, J., & Kochanek, K. D. (2011). Deaths: Final data for 2008. *National Vital Statistics Reports*, *59*(10), 1–126.

Nielsen, S. J., Siega-Riz, A. M., & Popkin, B. M. (2002). Trends in energy intake in U.S. between 1977 and 1996: Similar shifts seen across age groups. *Obesity Research*, *10*(5), 370–378.

North Carolina Sustainable Local Food Advisory Council. (2011). *Annual report*. Retrieved from www.ncagr.gov/localfood/documents/2011_NCSLFAC_Annual_Report.pdf

Pamer, M. (2012). *Los Angeles City Council embraces "Meatless Mondays."* NBC Los Angeles, November 9. Retrieved from www.nbclosangeles.com/news/local/Los-Angeles-City-Council-Embraces-Meatless-Mondays-Vegetarian-178244541.html

Pan, A., Sun, Q., Bernstein, A M., Schulze, M. B., Manson, J. E., Stampfer, M. J., Willet, W. C., & Hu, F. B. (2012). Red meat consumption and mortality: Results from 2 prospective cohort studies. *Archives of Internal Medicine*, *127*(7), 555–563.

Puhl, R. M., Andreyeva, T., & Brownell, K. D. (2008). Perceptions of weight discrimination: prevalence and comparison to race and gender discrimination in America. *International Journal of Obesity, 32,* 992–1000.

Puhl, R. M., & Heuer, C. A. (2009). The stigma of obesity: A review and update. *Obesity, 17*(5), 941–964.

Puhl, R. M., & Heuer, C. A. (2010). Obesity stigma: Important considerations for public health. *American Journal of Public Health, 100,* 1019—1028.

Robinson-O'Brien, R., Story, M., & Heim, S. (2009). Impact of garden-based youth nutrition intervention programs: A review. *Journal of American Dietetic Association, 109*(2), 273–280.

Samuel-Hodge, C. D., Johnston, L. F., Gizlice, Z., Garcia, B. A., Lindsley, S. C., Bramble, K. P., ... Keyserling, T. C. (2009). Randomized trial of a behavioral weight loss intervention for low-income women: The Weight Wise Program. *Obesity, 17*(10), 1891–1899.

Schvey, N., Puhl, R. M., & Brownell, K. D. (2011). The impact of weight stigma on caloric consumption. *Obesity, 19,* 1957–1962.

Shadish, W. R., Cook, T. D., & Campbell, D. T. (2002). *Experimental and quasi-experimental designs for causal inference.* Boston: Houghton Mifflin.

Shape Up Somerville. (2012). Retrieved from www.somervillema.gov/departments/health/sus

Scherb, A., Palmer, A., Frattaroli, S., & Pollack, K. (2012). Exploring food system policy: A survey of food policy councils in the United States. *Journal of Agriculture, Food Systems, and Community Development,* pp. 1–12.

Smith, T. W., De Marco, M., Kearney, W., Jones, C., Powell, A., & Ammerman, A. (in press). *Growing partners: Building a community-academic partnership to address health disparities in rural North Carolina.* Progress in Community Health Partnerships: Research, Education, and Action.

Sodexo offers Meatless Monday option to promote health and wellness. (2011). *PR Newswire,* January 20. Retrieved from www.prnewswire.com/news-releases/sodexo-offers-meatless-monday-option-to-promote-health-and-wellness-114290119.html

Song, H. J., Gittelsohn, J., Anliker, J., Sharma, S., Suratkar, S., Mattingly, M., & Kim, M. (2012). Understanding a key feature of urban food stores to develop nutrition intervention. *Journal of Hunger and Environmental Nutrition, 58,* 396–399.

Song, H. J., Gittelsohn, J., Kim, M., Suratkar, S., Sharma, S., & Anliker, J. A., (2010). Korean-American storeowners' perceived barriers and motivators for implementing a corner store-based nutrition program. *Health Promotion Practice, 12*(3), 472–482.

Story, M., Kaphingst, K. M., & French, S. (2006). The role of schools in obesity prevention. *Future Child, 16*(1), 109–142.

Story, M., Kaphingst, K. M., Robinson-O'Brien, R., & Glanz, K. (2008). Creating healthy food and eating environments: Policy and environmental approaches. *Annual Review of Public Health, 29,* 253–272.

Suitor, C. W., & Gleason, P. M. (2002). Using dietary reference intake-based methods to estimate the prevalence of inadequate nutrient intake among school-aged children. *Journal of the American Dietetic Association, 102*(4), 530–536.

UNC Center for Health Promotion and Disease Prevention. (2011). *Harvest of hope.* Retrieved from www.hpdp.unc.edu/research/current-projects/harvest-of-hope

UNC Center for Health Promotion and Disease Prevention. (2012). *Heart healthy Lenoir.* Retrieved from http://hearthealthylenoir.com

US Department of Agriculture. (nd). *National school lunch program.* Retrieved from www.fns.usda.gov/cnd/lunch

Vartanian, L. R., & Novak, S. A. (2010). Internalized societal attitudes moderate the impact of weight stigma on avoidance of exercise. *Obesity, 19*(4), 757–762.

Vastine, A. E., Gittelsohn, J., Ethelbah, B., Anliker, J., & Caballero, B. (2005). Formative research and stakeholder participation in intervention development. *American Journal of Health Behavior, 29*(1), 57–69.

Virginia Tech College of Agriculture and Science. (2012). *RE-AIM: Reach efficacy adoption implementation maintenance.* Retrieved from www.re-aim.org

Viswanathan, M., Ammerman, A., Eng, E., Garlehner, G., Lohr, K. N., Griffith, D., ... Whitener, L. (2004). Community-based participatory research: Assessing the evidence. *Evidence Report/Technology Assessment (Summary)*, 99, 1 –8.

Wang, M. C., Rauzon, S., Studer, N., Martin, A. C., Craig, L., Merlo, C., ... Crawford, P. (2010). Exposure to a comprehensive school intervention increases vegetable consumption. *Journal of Adolescent Health*, 47(1), 74–82.

Wekerle, G. R. (2004). Food justice movements: Policy, planning, and networks. *Journal of Planning Education and Research*, 23, 378–386.

Wieland, M. L., Weis, J. A., Palmer, T., Goodson, M., Loth, S., Omer, F., ... Sia, I. G. (2012). Physical activity and nutrition among immigrant and refugee women: A community-based participatory research approach. *Women's Health Issues*, 22(2), e225–e232.

Zoellner, J., Motley, M., Wilkinson, M. E., Jackman, B., Barlow, M. L., & Hill, J. L. (2012). Engaging the Dan River Region to reduce obesity: Application of the comprehensive participatory planning and evaluation process. *Family Community Health*, 35(1), 44–56.

Glossary

Accumulation Aggregation of a product to make transportation and other functions economical (14)

Acute pesticide poisoning Any illness or health effect resulting from suspected or confirmed exposure to a pesticide within forty-eight hours (2)

Additives Ingredients used in formulation to perform desired functions, such as emulsifiers, flavors, and colorants (13)

Adulterants Compounds that contaminate food (13)

Advanced meat recovery Automated method for removing small pieces of meat left behind during deboning (13)

Agenda setting Process by which problems and alternative solutions to address them rise to the attention of the public and policy makers (8)

Agent-based modeling (ABM) A quantitative systems modeling technique in which complex dynamics are modeled by constructing "artificial societies" on computers (1)

Agrobiodiversity Genetic diversity of domesticated plants and animals (3)

Agroecology The science and practice of applying ecological principles to agriculture to develop practices that work with nature to mimic natural processes and conserve ecological integrity; other labels for ecological approaches to agriculture include *ecological agriculture, agricultural ecology, sustainable agriculture, permaculture* (1, 3, 11, 12)

Agroecosystems Communities of organisms in an agricultural setting (e.g., plants, animals, fungi, bacteria), their environment (e.g., soil, water), and the interactions among them (12)

Agroforestry Combining tree production with crops or grazing; the latter is sometimes called *silvopastoralism* (3)

Algal bloom A rapid accumulation of algae (12)

Allocation Rerouting the product supply to various segments of the distribution system (primarily to wholesalers and retailers) (14)

Animal husbandry The branch of agriculture concerned with the care and breeding of domestic animals (9)

Animal waste Feces, urine, or soiled bedding (e.g., poultry litter) (12)

Anthropogenic Human-caused (3)

Appropriations bills Legislation that sets money aside for specific spending (8)

Aquaculture Farm-raising fish, crustaceans, shellfish, or aquatic plants, either inland in tanks or ponds, or in enclosures in lakes, rivers, or oceans (3, 12)

Aquifers Underground water basins (3)

Arsenical drugs Drugs containing the element arsenic; added to some animal feeds to increase feed efficiency, promote weight gain, and prevent infection (12)

Assorting Combining products from different sources to supply a customer that requires a variety of products (e.g., wholesalers combine foods from different sources to supply a supermarket's produce department) (14)

Authorizing legislation Bill that creates a new federal program, extends the life of an existing program, or repeals existing law, though it does not provide program funding (8)

Behavioral economics Subfield of economics that assumes consumers do not make perfectly rational decisions; incorporates theories and models from psychology and other adjacent fields (7)

Beneficial insects Insects that eat crop pests or provide other ecosystem services, such as pollination (3)

Benefit-cost analysis Method of analysis that estimates total social benefits and costs of a project; used to provide insight into whether an initiative will be a net winner or loser to society (7)

Best management practices (BMPs) Agricultural practices designed to minimize adverse environmental effects (12)

Biocapacity The area of productive land and water available to produce resources or absorb carbon dioxide waste, given current management practices (3)

Biological controls Use of natural predators or diseases to control pests (3)

Body mass index (BMI) A measure based on an individual's weight and height (weight in kilograms divided by height squared), commonly used to determine overweight and obesity status BMI: < 18.5 = underweight; 18.5–24.9 = normal weight; 25–29.9 = overweight; ≥ 30 = obese; alternative measures are used in children (18)

Breaking down a heterogeneous supply A sorting function of the distribution system that separates products with different prices or for different buyers (e.g., a citrus packing plant sorts oranges by grade and size) (14)

Buffer zones Strips of vegetation along streams and rivers that prevent stream bank erosion and may provide habitat for wildlife species (3)

CAFOs See **Concentrated animal feeding operations** (3)

Cancer A group of diseases characterized by uncontrolled division of abnormal body cells (2)

Cap-and-trade systems Systems by which a government entity sets an upper limit on total pollution in a particular industry or economy sector, and each firm in that sector is allotted pollution credits (7)

Cardiovascular disease (CVD) A group of diseases that affect the heart or blood vessels (2)

Cerebrovascular disease Disease affecting blood flow to the brain (2)

Chairman's mark Draft bill that the chairperson of a committee or subcommittee uses as the starting point for developing legislation (8)

Checkoff Commodity checkoff programs are funds collected through small fees placed on farmers producing commodities such as corn, milk, or beef; checkoff programs fund research and promotion for their specific commodities (8)

ChooseMyPlate An educational program and visual "plate" developed by the US Department of Agriculture to promote healthy eating to consumers based on the 2010 Dietary Guidelines for Americans (15)

Chronic diseases Diseases that progress slowly and persist for many years (2)

Colonized People can carry a pathogenic organism on or inside their body, but show no signs of illness or infection (12)

Commodity(ies) Agricultural crop(s) produced at a large scale; commonly refers to corn, soybeans, wheat, rice, cotton, and animal products (8, 11)

Communication channels Media and venues through which marketing is conducted, such as television, the Internet, print, radio, video games, schools, stores, or restaurants (10)

Community The unit of analysis in community food security; as defined by stakeholders, may refer to a neighborhood, town, county, or even a region (6)

Community-based participatory research (CBPR) Research in partnership with community members and with community participation in all aspects of the research (18)

Community food assessment (CFA) The main tool and process used to measure a local food system (6)

Community food security (CFS) A condition in which all community residents obtain a safe, culturally acceptable, nutritionally adequate diet through a sustainable system that maximizes community self-reliance, social justice, and democratic decision making (6)

Community-supported agriculture (CSA) Program in which consumers and farmers share the risks and benefits of agriculture; there are many models, but most commonly consumers pay a farmer at the beginning of a season and receive weekly produce distributions (9)

Comparative advantage The climatic, labor, or geographic advantage of one area to produce a product more efficiently and at cheaper cost than another (7, 11)

Competitive foods The mostly high-fat or high-sugar snacks or beverages in vending machines, cafeteria, á la carte lines, and school stores that compete with the federal school meal offerings and are outside the scope of national school nutrition guidelines (17)

Complementary good A good, *a*, whose demand decreases when the price of a good, *b*, decreases, all else being equal (7)

Concentrated animal feeding operations (CAFOs) Environmental Protection Agency category for large facility in which animals are confined and fed or maintained for at least forty-five days out of the year, the operation does not produce crops or vegetation, and it meets size thresholds (e.g., 1,000 cattle, 10,000 swine, or 125,000 chickens may classify as a "large CAFO," depending on how animal waste is managed); also feedlots, confinement facilities (12)

Conservation practices Farming practices that reduce loss of soil and water and often improve their quality (8)

Consolidation The shift toward fewer and larger operations in an industry (12, 14)

Constant exposure Marketing approach in which advertisements for a product are found in many media such as billboards, newspapers, and magazines, and as samples on doorsteps (10)

Constructs Key concepts that make up a theory (18)

Coronary artery disease Disease involving reduced blood flow to the heart muscle (2)

Cover cropping Planting crops aimed at preventing erosion, building soil fertility, and suppressing weeds when soil would otherwise be vacant (3)

Credence attributes Food attributes, such as nutritional quality, that cannot readily be ascertained by the consumer even after consuming a product (7)

Crop rotations Sequencing different crops on the same field to use nutrients effectively and avoid pest outbreaks (3)

Cultivars Plant varieties produced by breeding (4)

Cultural service A type of ecosystem service; psychological and emotional benefits from human relations with ecosystems (e.g., recreational, aesthetic, and spiritual experiences) (3)

Culture Beliefs, behaviors, traditions, customs, and other ways of being that are consciously and unconsciously learned and transmitted among individuals and populations (9)

Dead zone Area of water with insufficient oxygen to support most organisms (3, 12)

Deadweight loss Loss when some external force causes a market to move away from its free market equilibrium; takes form of decreased revenues, increased prices, and reduced quantity produced versus what would happen in a free market (7)

Demand expansion A government policy that increases demand for a particular good or service (7)

Diabetes A chronic health condition in which the body's cells do not adequately take in blood glucose (2)

Diet history method Information collection, usually by a trained interviewer, about frequencies of intake of various foods and the typical makeup of meals (15)

Diet-related diseases Diseases associated with certain dietary patterns (2)

Dietary change interventions Programs or plans to modify what, how, where, and why individuals consume food to improve individual and public health outcomes (18)

Dietary Guidelines for Americans (DGA) The health and nutrition guidelines reviewed by an expert panel and produced by the US Department of Agriculture and US Department of Health and Human Services that govern all federal nutrition policy and programs (15, 18)

Dietary reference intakes (DRIs) Evidence-based nutrient standards set by the Institute of Medicine and the National Academy of Sciences for estimating optimal intakes in healthy individuals (15, 16)

Dietary supplements Products intended to supplement the diet by providing vitamins, minerals, herbs, or other substances (15)

Differentiated products Products that differ from those of competitors, such as based on quality, cultivar, or production method, and thus typically can be sold for higher prices (11)

Distribution channel Path through which food products travel from farm to consumer; the food distribution system is composed of various channels, such as the supermarket channel and the food service channel (14)

Diverse farming systems Planting patterns that include two or more species interplanted together, fields that are planted in rotation of different crops, and crop-livestock integration on the farm (11)

Dose-response effect The change of strength of effect based on differing levels of exposure (18)

Drivers Trends, events, or entities that have a large influence on a process (e.g., a political process) (1)

Ecological approach Framework rooted in the notion that multiple factors such as economic, social, cultural, political, and institutional structures shape outcomes such as food insecurity or public health (5)

Ecological footprinting A measure of human demand on ecosystems, typically expressed in hectares of biologically productive land (3)

Ecological integrity Ability of an ecosystem to maintain normal functions (3)

Economic concentration Extent to which a market is dominated by relatively few firms (14)

Economies of scale The advantages occurring when quantity of production becomes large and a firm has lower total costs than at lower levels of output; can level off or be reduced after a certain size (7, 11)

Ecosystem services Benefits that humans derive from ecosystems (1, 3)

Elasticity The degree to which consumers are responsive to price changes (7)

Electronic benefit transfer (EBT) Debit cards electronically loaded with SNAP benefits (formerly known as Food Stamps) (18)

Endocrine disruption Chemical interference with the body's endocrine system, which may result in adverse developmental, reproductive, neurological, and immune effects in humans and wildlife (2)

Endotoxin Toxin present in outer membrane of certain bacteria (whether the bacteria are alive or dead); released when bacterium dies; human exposure has been associated with adverse health effects including inflammation and fever (12)

Energy density Amount of calories provided by a food, relative to its mass or volume; in contrast with nutrient-dense foods, energy dense foods have high calories relative to volume (2)

Enrichment Addition of nutrients to restore nutritional value lost in processing (16)

Entitlement program Program that guarantees access to certain benefits for all who qualify (e.g., Social Security benefits) (5, 8)

Environmental determinants of health Factors in the biophysical environment, including the built environment, that affect health (1)

Epidemiologic transition A shift in the patterns of disease among a population, whereby infectious diseases are gradually surpassed by chronic illness as the primary cause of morbidity (illness) and death (2)

Equilibrium The balance achieved when many optimizing individuals interact with one another in markets (7)

Erosion Washing or blowing away of topsoil (3)

Eutrophication Abnormal increases in nutrient levels (particularly nitrogen and phosphorus) in waterways, often due to runoff from excessive application of nutrients to crops (3)

Externality A cost of providing a product or service that is imposed on people who were not involved in the transaction, including future generations; also called *external cost*; can be negative (costs imposed on others) or positive (7)

Farm state States that have commodity agriculture as an important part of their rural economy, usually referring to states in the Midwest and southeast United States (8)

Farm-to-school (F2S) Organizational intervention that brings local and regional farm produce to schools, often with the aim of increasing fruit and vegetable consumption and benefit local and regional agriculture (18)

Fats (lipids) Oily substance providing nine kilocalories per gram and stored in human adipose tissue; aid in digestion, absorption, and transport of fat-soluble vitamins and phytochemicals; see also **Saturated fat, Trans fat** (16)

Feedlots Confinement facilities, usually outdoors, where animals (typically cattle) are fed for the purpose of rapid weight gain prior to slaughter (12)

Fish stocks Amounts of commercially desirable fish (3)

Fixed costs Costs of production that do not vary depending on the number of units produced (7)

Flavonoids Any of a large class of plant pigments that are beneficial to health (16)

Folk traditions Informal beliefs or customs that are usually handed down orally from one generation to the next (9)

Food availability assessment Assessment measuring use of basic commodities, such as wheat, beef, and eggs at the farm level or an early stage of processing (15)

Food availability data series Time series data measuring food supplies available for domestic consumption (USDA Economic Research Service) (15)

Food balance sheets Provide a comprehensive picture of a country's food supply patterns by showing availability of food items for human consumption for a specified time period (Food and Agriculture Organization) (15)

Food-borne illness Illness resulting from recent ingestion of contaminated food (e.g., with microbial pathogens or toxins) (2)

Food deserts Areas with low access to healthy foods, commonly low-income urban or rural areas without nearby supermarkets; there are several specific definitions (17)

Food distribution system System that brings food from farms to tables (14)

Food environments All aspects of our surroundings that may influence our diets, including physical locations and marketing, media, and online exposures (4, 17)

Food frequency questionnaire Assessment tool asking about usual frequency of consumption of a select group of foods for a specific period of time (15)

Food insecurity Having inadequate economic resources to enable consistent access to safe, adequate, and nutritious food to support an active and healthy life for all household members (low food security: reduced quality, variety, desirability of diet; very low food security: multiple indications of disrupted eating patterns and reduced food intake) (2, 5, 6)

Food justice Movement seeking to address ways in which racial and economic inequalities pervade food system practices and processes from production to consumption (6)

Food policy councils (FPCs) Group of stakeholders representing various segments of the food system and organized with the goal of addressing strengths and limitations in that system (18)

Food record Detailed record of foods and beverages an individual consumes over a given period of time (15)

Food retail format Type of retail outlet, in terms of range of products and services, pricing, promotional programs, operating style, or store design and visual merchandising (e.g., traditional supermarkets, specialty food shops) (14)

Food safety Prevention of health risks associated with contaminated food (2)

Food security "Access by all people at all times to enough food for an active, healthy life" (Coleman-Jensen, Nord, Andrews, & Carlson, 2012, p. 2) (5)

Food supply chain People, activities, and resources involved in getting food from farms, ranches, waters, and other sources to consumers; major stages include production, processing, distribution, retail (2)

Food swamps Areas where food options are predominantly relatively unhealthy foods at locations such as convenience stores and fast food outlets (17)

Food system A system encompassing all the activities and resources that go into producing, distributing, and consuming food; the drivers and outcomes of those processes; and all the relationships and feedback loops between system components (1).

Food systems approach to nutrition Approach that considers the impacts of food on human health and the processes involved in producing, transforming, distributing, accessing, consuming, and disposing of food (16)

Foodways An individual's or group's culturally based food preparation and consumption behaviors and traditions, including the material production of food (9)

Fortification Addition of nutrients to enhance a food's nutritional value (16)

Four-firm concentration ratio (CR4) Represents level of concentration (i.e., the number of sellers) in a market for a good or service (e.g., if the CR4 score = 65 that means 65 percent of the market is controlled by only four firms) (7)

Front groups Organizations with neutral-sounding names and objective-seeming spokespeople who are actually funded by corporations and work for their interests (10)

Front of package A location for placing labeling messages (10)

Gastroenteritis Inflammation of the intestinal lining (e.g., as a result of Norovirus infection) (2)

Global supply chain Interconnected system of food exports and imports bringing crops and products to major marketing outlets (11)

Green manure Legumes that fix nitrogen (3)

Green Revolution A foundation-funded initiative between the 1940s and 1970s to introduce new hybrids and agricultural technology including synthetic fertilizers, pesticides, and irrigation to developing countries, primarily in Latin America and Asia (3)

Greenwashing Exaggerated claims of environmental benefits (3)

Growers In hog and poultry industries, refers to those contracting with a vertically integrated company to raise animals until they are ready for slaughter (12)

Health "A state of complete physical, mental and social well-being and not merely the absence of disease or infirmity" (World Health Organization, 1946) (1)

Health and human rights framework A lens through which public health is understood to be shaped by how well a government respects, protects, and fulfills its people's human rights (5)

Health belief model (HBM) Individual-level behavior change theory addressing perceptions of a health threat, benefits of avoiding the threat, and influences on a decision to act to avoid or mitigate the threat; key constructs include perceived susceptibility, perceived severity, perceived benefits, perceived barriers, cues to action, and self-efficacy (18)

Health claims Claims used in marketing, indicating that a food or diet will benefit health (10)

Health disparities Differences in health status among groups of people based on factors such as socioeconomic status (SES), race, ethnicity, immigration status, environmental exposures, gender, education, disability, geographic location, or sexual orientation (1, 4)

Health inequities Health disparities resulting from systemic, avoidable, unfair, and unjust practices and policies (4)

Health promotion The optimization of the body's systems and building reserves against forces averse to good health; education and other activities aimed at promoting health (2)

Healthy defaults Options provided that make the healthy choice the easy choice (17)

Healthy foods "Foods that provide essential nutrients and energy to sustain growth, health and life while satiating hunger; usually fresh or minimally processed foods, naturally dense in nutrients, that when eaten in moderation and in combination with other foods, sustain growth, repair and maintain vital processes, promote longevity, reduce disease, and strengthen and maintain the body and its functions. Healthy foods do not contain ingredients that contribute to disease or impede recovery when consumed at normal levels. Options provided that make the healthy choice the easy choice" (University of Washington, 2013) (1)

Healthy People 2020 The US ten-year goals and objectives that guide national health promotion and disease prevention efforts (US Department of Health and Human Services) (15)

Heart disease Disease affecting the heart, such as coronary artery disease and congestive heart failure (2)

Hedgerows Dense hedges between fields or along streams (3)

Heuristics Rules of thumb consumers use to make choices (7)

Horizontal Integration When companies take over or merge with other companies competing in the same enterprise (12)

Household Food Security Survey Module (HFSSM) Eighteen-item survey from the US Department of Agriculture Economic Research Service that is considered the gold standard measure of severity and depth of food insecurity in the United States (5)

Human right to adequate food Realized when every man, woman, and child, alone or in community with others, has physical and economic access at all times to adequate food or means for its procurement, according to the United Nations (United Nations Economic and Social Council, 1999) (1, 5)

Hypertension High blood pressure (2)

Impulse buys Unplanned purchases (10)

Industrial food animal production (IFAP) An approach to meat, dairy, and egg production characterized by specialized operations designed for a high rate of production, large numbers of animals confined at high density, large quantities of localized animal waste, and substantial inputs of financial capital, fossil fuel, feed, pharmaceuticals, and indirect inputs embodied in feed (e.g., fuel and freshwater) (1, 2, 12)

Inelastic Consumers not being relatively responsive to price changes (7)

Information asymmetries When buyers in a market have less information about goods or services than the sellers or the reverse (7)

Input firms Firms selling inputs to farmers (14)

Inputs Resources and materials entering a production system, such as feed, drugs, energy, water, and labor (1)

Insoluble fibers Indigestible portions of plant foods that binds water while passing through the digestive tract, making stools softer and bulkier; important to maintaining gut health and helping prevent constipation (16)

Integrated Different channels and techniques being used together (10)

Integrated pest management (IPM) A system of controlling pests using least toxic pesticides applied only when necessary to avoid economic loss (3)

Integrators In the hog and poultry industries, refers to the vertically integrated companies that coordinates multiple successive stages of the supply chain (12)

Jurisdiction The subjects and functions assigned to a committee of Congress (8)

Ketosis A state of elevated ketones in the body caused by breakdown of fatty acids for energy (16)

Kilocalorie (kcal) Formal term for what is commonly referred to as a *calorie*; the amount of energy needed to heat one kilogram of water by one degree Celsius (16)

Lagoons Cesspits used to store liquid cattle or swine waste (12)

Law of demand Refers to the marketing concept that when the price of a (normal) good rises, the quantity demanded will decline (7)

Lay health advisors Individuals indigenous to a community who serve as a link between community members and traditional health delivery systems (18)

Legumes Members of the pea family of plants (*Leguminaceae*) (3)

Life-course perspective A framework that incorporates analysis of the relationship among social, behavioral, and biological factors as they develop throughout an individual's life and social context (5)

Macronutrients Nutrients used in relatively large quantities by the body (16)

Malnutrition Undernutrition or overnutrition due to obtaining inadequate nutrients or an oversupply (16)

Mandates Policies that use incentives or penalties to encourage certain actions across an industry, such as the renewable fuels standard, which requires a certain level of renewable fuel use in the United States (8)

Manure Animal waste intended for use as fertilizer (12)

Market concentration The extent to which market shares in an industry are owned by a small number of companies (7, 12)

Market failure Economic concept describing the occurrence of an inefficient market outcome (7)

Marketing "The activity, set of institutions, and processes for creating, communicating, delivering, and exchanging offerings that have value for customers, clients, partners, and society at large" (AMA, 2007) (10)

Marketing channel intermediaries Businesses that participate in the food distribution channel beyond the farm gate (14)

Measured media "Above-the-line" or "traditional" media, such as television, cinema, radio, and print press, which are tracked by media research companies (10)

Mechanization In agriculture, generally refers to replacement of human and animal labor with machinery (12)

Menu labeling Altering within-restaurant food environment by adding nutrition information and common calorie counts to restaurant menus and menu boards; enables motivated consumers to compare products and make informed decisions about their food choices (17)

Merchant wholesaler(s) A type of wholesaler who typically buys and resells food, assembles it for distribution, loads it for transport, and delivers it to an array of customers (e.g., supermarkets, food service establishments, or the export market) (14)

Micronutrients Nutrients needed in small amounts and can be found in vitamins, minerals, and trace elements (16)

Minerals Essential nutrients that exist mostly in the body in their ionic state, either as cations (positively charged ions) or anions (negatively charged ions) (16)

Monocultures Large plantings of a single variety of a single crop (3)

Monopoly Market characterized by one seller and many buyers (7)

Morbidity Illness or symptom; alternately, disease incidence rate (2)

Motivational interviewing (MI) A guided conversation that does not aim for behavior change but rather for individual realization, which may lead to behavior change through overcoming identified barriers and using available resources (18)

National School Lunch Program (NSLP) Federally assisted meal program operating in public and nonprofit private schools and residential care institutions to provide nutritious meals to children at low or no cost (5)

Naturally occurring compounds Chemical compounds that occur naturally in plants (in contrast to those that are manufactured) (13)

Natural capital Living organisms and natural environments that provide goods and services imperative for human survival and well-being; forms the foundation for all economic activity (12)

Nitrates Naturally occurring form of nitrogen, essential for plant growth; formed when microorganisms break down manure, decaying plants, or other organic matter (12)

Nitrogen cycle Transformation of nitrogen from elemental N to nitrate, nitrite, and other nitrogen compounds and back to N, affected by natural and human processes (3)

Nonmeasured media "Below-the-line" or "nontraditional" media, such as the Internet, stores, or schools (10)

Nontherapeutic antibiotic use Antibiotic use in the absence of clinical disease, as diagnosed by a licensed veterinarian (e.g., for growth promotion or disease prevention) (12)

No-till farming Planting crops directly into the residue of the former crop without plowing (1)

Nutrient claims Claims about the level of a nutrient in a food; used in marketing (10)

Nutrient density In food, refers to the levels of key nutrients, such as fiber and vitamins, relative to the amount of calories; commonly used to describe foods considered to be healthy (10)

Obese Adults are considered obese if their body mass index (BMI) is 30 or higher, that is, if they are over 20 percent heavier than what is considered a healthy weight range for someone of their height (1, 2)

Omnibus bills Legislation covering multiple diverse or unrelated topics (8)

Open ocean aquaculture Offshore (as opposed to inland) fish farms; fish typically raised in netted enclosures or cages anchored to the sea floor or floating on the surface (12)

Opportunity cost What one must give up in order to get something else (4)

Optimization Doing the best one can with available resources (7)

Organic farming Farming system that eschews use of synthetic pesticides and fertilizers and emphasizes building soil quality (3)

Outcome measures The standard against which the end result of the intervention is assessed (18)

Overexploitation Excessive harvesting of a population (e.g., fish) such that the population cannot recover to its previous size (3)

Overweight Adults are considered overweight if their body mass index (BMI) is 25.0 or higher, that is, if they are up to 20 percent heavier than what is considered a healthy weight range for someone of their height (1)

Own-price elasticity of demand A measure of consumer responsiveness to price changes for a particular good (7)

Pastoralists Traditional livestock herders (3)

Pasture-based system A model of food animal production in which animals are primarily raised outdoors for all or most of the year, and are free to graze or forage (even if diets are supplemented with feed, as is common with hogs and poultry) (12)

Pathogens Disease-causing organisms (e.g., *Staphylococcus aureus* [bacteria], Influenza [virus], and *Cryptosporidium* [parasite]) (2, 12)

Perennial polycultures Systems of mixed crop species that complement each other in the field, exploit natural resources through the entire soil profile, and produce edible grains and forage for livestock; promote their own fertility and pest management and maintain a healthy farm ecosystem (11)

Permaculture The permanent agriculture and stable culture that comes from careful design of integrated annual and perennial crops, livestock, and production practices that contribute to healthy soils, crops, animals, and people (11)

Pesticides Natural or synthetic chemicals used with the intent of killing, repelling, or controlling populations of target organisms ("pests") that interfere with human interests; includes insecticides (targeted to insects), herbicides (targeted to plants), and fungicides (targeted to fungi) (2)

Phytochemicals See **Phytonutrients**

Phytonutrients Compounds in plant foods that have been associated with beneficial functions in the body (e.g., aiding nutrient absorption, inhibiting oxidation, improving cholesterol) (2, 16)

Point of sale (POS) The place where purchases are made; can be specific to the register or refer more broadly to within a store (10)

Political economy Generally refers to study of social relations, particularly the power relations that mutually constitute the production, distribution, and consumption of resources; in the context of CFS, refers to how political and policy processes shape the way food is produced, distributed, and consumed (6)

Polycultures Planting multiple crops close together in ways that maximize beneficial interactions between species (3)

Polyunsaturated fatty acids (PUFAs) Essential fatty acids that have two or more double bonds; includes omega-3 and omega-6 fatty acids (16)

Population-based approach Approach or intervention aimed at changing factors affecting the entire population; see **Targeted approach** (1, 4)

Precautionary approach (or principle) Approach based on the idea that if an activity raises significant threat of harm to human health or the environment, it should be stopped or slowed (e.g., precautionary measures should be taken) even if the cause-and-effect relationships are not fully established by scientific evidence; places the burden of proof that the activity is not harmful on the activity's proponent (e.g., a manufacturer); also precautionary principle (2)

Prediabetes A condition in which blood glucose levels are elevated, but not high enough to be classified as diabetes (2)

Preemption Limitation by a higher level of government on what actions can be taken by a lower level of government (8)

Price ceilings Price levels used in supply management policies that designate the price at which an agricultural commodity should not go above (8)

Price floors Price levels used in supply management policies that designate the price at which an agricultural commodity should not go below (8)

Primary prevention Approach that addresses root causes and tries to stop harmful exposures before they happen; secondary prevention involves treating early stage conditions to prevent worsening; tertiary prevention involves mitigating the effects of disease (1)

Product traceability The ability to track a food product back through the distribution system to the farm from which it came (6)

Promotion "Any form of commercial communication or message that is designed to, or has the effect of, increasing the recognition, appeal and/or consumption of particular products and services" (World Health Organization, 2010. p.7) (10)

Provisioning services A type of ecosystem service; direct provision from ecosystems of goods (e.g., food, medicine, timber, fiber, biofuels) valuable to humans (3)

Psychographic Similar to a demographic group, but based instead on lifestyles and values, which may be shared regardless of demography, geography, or behaviors (10)

Public goods Benefits, such as clean air and public libraries, for which it is not possible to exclude only some people and for which one person's usage does not reduce availability for others (8)

Public health "The science and art of preventing disease, prolonging life and promoting … health … through organized community efforts" (Winslow, 1920, p. 30) (1)

Public health nutrition An approach to nutrition emphasizing the application of food and nutrition knowledge, policy, and research to the improvement of the health of populations (16)

Quota Government policy mandating level of production for a good or service, typically above what would be produced in a free market (7)

RE-AIM framework Intervention evaluation framework focusing on program reach, efficacy, adoption, implementation, and maintenance (18)

Real consumer prices Prices as paid by consumers that have been adjusted to account for the changing value of currency (e.g., inflation) (12)

Reauthorization The legislative process by which Congress renews, amends, or terminates existing programs (8)

Recirculating aquaculture systems Indoor or outdoor production systems in which fish are raised in tanks and water is continuously filtered (to remove fish waste) and recirculated through the system (12)

Regulating services A type of ecosystem service; control of the rate and extent of natural processes (e.g., water filtration, waste decomposition, climate regulation, crop pollination, regulation of some human diseases) (3)

Regulatory body An agency or other government entity mandated under the terms of a legislative act to ensure compliance with its provisions (8)

Renewal cycles Length of time before a piece of legislation expires and requires new authorization; the Farm Bill is expected to be renewed every five years (8)

Reporting out Act of finalizing a committee's drafting of legislation and bringing it to the attention of the broader Congressional body (8)

Resilience Ability to recover from perturbations, adapt so as to reduce harm from future perturbations, or learn to avoid perturbations (1, 3)

Rotational grazing Practice of regularly moving animals to new areas of pasture (12)

Routinizing To standardize procedures and transactions in order to minimize costs in the food distribution system (14)

Runoff The flow of water from rain, irrigation water, and other sources over land; often carries topsoil and contaminants into bodies of water (3, 12)

Salinization A process in which salts accumulate in upper layers of soil, often from improper irrigation techniques, although sometimes because of naturally occurring concentrations of salt (3)

Satiety Feeling of fullness (2)

Saturated fats Triglycerides containing long fatty acid chains that have all available carbon binding sites full with hydrogen bonds and are solid at room temperature; seen as less healthy than unsaturated fats (16)

School Breakfast Program Federal program providing cash assistance to states to operate nonprofit breakfast programs in schools and residential child-care institutions (5)

Segmentation The process of dividing consumers into groups who are likely to respond in the same way to products and promotional (marketing) activity (10, 14)

Seniors Farmers' Market Nutrition Program Provides grants to states, territories, and tribes to provide coupons to seniors for food at farmers markets, roadside stands, and from community-supported agriculture (8)

Shelf life The length of time a food takes to become undesirable (13)

Signposts Indications such as green flags on the front of food packages to show that a product is "better for you" (10)

Siltation Accumulation of soil particles in bodies of water (3)

Slow food An international food movement in which supporters promote local production and preparation of food for individual health, creating community, and enjoyment (9)

Social cognitive theory (SCT) Interpersonal-level behavior change theory that explores how personal and environmental factors work individually and in concert to affect health behavior; key constructs include reciprocal determinism, self-efficacy, observational learning, expectations, reinforcements, and facilitation (18)

Social determinants of health Social and economic conditions that affect human health, such as where a person lives (1)

Social marketing Application of marketing methods developed by the commercial sector to campaigns that promote social benefits including health; does not refer to marketing using social media (10)

Socioecological model (SEM) Framework for comparing the effects of nested spheres of influence on a behavior change intervention (individual, interpersonal, organizational, community, policy) (18)

Soil fertility Capacity of soil to support plant growth; affected by microbial activity, contamination, organic matter, soil type, and other factors (3)

Soluble fibers Indigestible portions of plant foods that attracts water and forms a gel to slow digestion and create a full feeling (16)

Special interests A group of people acting together to influence the legislative process (8)

Special Supplemental Nutrition Program for Women, Infants, and Children (WIC) Federal program for eligible pregnant, breastfeeding, postpartum women, and young children who are living at or below 185 percent of the federal poverty line (5)

Specialty crops Fruits and vegetables, tree nuts, dried fruits, and other crops that are intensely cultivated and generally demand higher prices in the market than commodity crops (11)

Species richness Number of species per unit of area (3)

Standard American Diet (SAD) Diet common to US citizens, characterized by excess caloric intake of refined grains, added sugars, added fats, meats, total calories, and sodium, and inadequate intake of fruits and vegetables (2)

Standard systems Sets of production criteria that farmers or businesses meet to provide buyers (another business or the end consumer) with a guarantee of qualities important to them

Strip cropping Planting crops with different structural characteristics in rows to minimize wind erosion (3)

Structural determinants of health Factors related to the economic, political, and social hierarchal issues (e.g., level of power and privilege) that affect health (1)

Subsidies Government policy providing consumers or producers with a per-unit discount on consumption or production of a good or service (7)

Subsistence Growing food solely for household use (in contrast to commercial sales) (3)

Substitute goods Goods whose demand increases when the price of another good increases, all else being equal (7)

Subsystem A system that is also a component of a broader system (e.g., the food production system is a subsystem of the food system) (1)

Superfoods Foods promoted as having unusually high nutritional or health values (9)

Supplemental Nutrition Assistance Program (SNAP) Federal food assistance for qualifying low-income households; formerly known as the Food Stamp Program and also referred to as EBT (electronic benefits transfer) (5)

Supply management policies Policies that use incentives, taxes, and regulation to affect the available supply of an agricultural commodity; most often used as a mechanism for reducing large fluctuations in commodity prices; less common than in the past (8)

Supporting services A type of ecosystem service; functions provided by ecosystems that are necessary for the provision of all other ecosystem services (e.g., the cycling of nutrients through an ecosystem and breakdown of waste) (3)

Sustainable harvest levels For wild-capture fisheries: maximum amount of fish that can be harvested without depleting fish populations below levels necessary to sustain harvests over the long term (12)

Systems Complex networks of relationships in which each component proceeds independently and under its own logic; also, systems approach, systems thinking, systems theory: approaches, thought patterns, or theory that focus on systems; typically contrasted with linear approaches (1, 18)

Targeted approach Approach to intervention that targets activities to a specific segment of the population; see **Population-based approach** (4)

Tariffs Taxes levied on goods as they enter a country (8)

Taxes Government policy charging a per-unit fee on the consumption or production of a good or service (7)

Tax incentives Policies that aim to incentivize behavior change by reducing the amount of taxes paid (or providing exemptions) for those who make change (8)

The Emergency Food Assistance Program (TEFAP) Program that provides US Department of Agriculture commodities to states, which distribute the food through local emergency food providers (5)

Theory A systematic way of understanding events or situations; a set of concepts, definitions, and propositions that explain or predict events or situations by illustrating the relationships between variables (18)

Theory of planned behavior (TPB) An individual-level behavior change theory that focuses on individuals' attitudes toward a health behavior, perceived norms, and beliefs about the difficulty or ease of behavior change; key constructs are behavioral intention, attitude, subjective norms, and perceived behavioral control (18)

Thrifty Food Plan (TFP) Low-cost food plan providing adequate nutrition, used as the basis for USDA calculations of SNAP allotments (5)

Titles Similar to book chapters, but for legislation: breaking a bill into topics (8)

Total average cost Total cost divided by the number of units produced (7)

Total costs Sum of fixed and variable costs (7)

Total diet approach Dietary pattern that focuses on the combination of foods and beverages that comprise people's total diets on average over time (15)

Trade promotion Producers marketing to other actors in the food system, such as primary producers marketing their products to manufacturers or manufacturers promoting their products to retailers (10)

Trans fats Unsaturated fats with bonds added to the fatty acid in processing to make it solid at room temperature and to extend the shelf life of foods; linked to risk of heart disease (16)

Transtheoretical model (TTM) An individual-level behavior change theory that suggests that behavior change happens as a process over time (six stages: precontemplation, contemplation, preparation, action, maintenance, termination); the process is not linear; people move between stages as they change behavior, relapse, and change again (18)

Twenty-four-hour dietary recall A quantitative research method in which individuals are asked to recall types and amounts of all foods and beverages eaten in the prior twenty-four hours (15)

Type 2 diabetes The most common form of diabetes; the body either resists the effects of insulin—a hormone that regulates the uptake of glucose into cells—or does not produce enough insulin to maintain a normal glucose level (2)

Unit elastic Consumer demand responds proportionally to price changes (7)

Unit operations Steps within processes; used to describe the tasks involved in food processing (13)

Variable costs Costs of production that vary with number of units produced (7)

Veganism Diet that includes no foodstuffs with animal origins, including animal meat, fish, dairy, eggs, and honey (9)

Vegetarianism Diet that includes no animal meat or fish, but may include eggs and dairy (9)

Vertical integration The merging of two or more businesses involved in different stages of the supply chain for the same product(s) (e.g., the distribution and sales of supermarket goods) (12, 14)

Viral reassortment The exchange of genetic material between different viral strains within the same host (12)

Vitamins Naturally occurring compounds essential for normal growth and nutrition and required in small amounts in the diet (16)

Volatilized Changed from a liquid to a gaseous state (3)

Water activity Measure of the amount of water in a food available to participate in chemical reactions and microbial growth; influences food texture (13)

Wetlands Marshy areas where water remains close to the surface for all or most of the year (3)

What We Eat in America (WWEIA) Two-day dietary intake interview component of the annual National Health and Nutrition Examination Survey; the only nationally representative dietary survey in the United States (US Department of Agriculture and US Department of Health and Human Services) (15)

Wicked problems Problems for which stakeholders do not agree on the problem or its causes; each attempt to create a solution changes the problem; solutions are not right or wrong, just better or worse; solutions must be tailored to the situation; and they cannot be solved by people from any one discipline alone; multidisciplinary approaches are required (1)

Wild-capture fisheries Area of water designated for harvesting fish (12)

Wild-caught seafood Fish or other aquatic animals that are caught in the wild as opposed to farm raised (12)

Wild (natural) biodiversity The genetic diversity of ecosystems not managed by humans (3)

Window of opportunity Time-limited opportunity for taking action, when chances of success are relatively high (8)

Photo Credits

INTRODUCTION

Figure I.3
Source: Shydi Griffin, Baltimore City. Child's Poster about Healthy Food Placed on City Buses. Used with permission.

Figure I.4
Source: Local Food Hub. Used with permission.

Figure I.5
Source: Mia Cellucci, CLF.

Figure I.6
Source: Johns Hopkins Diversity Leadership Council. Used with permission.

Figure I.7
Source: Michael Milli, CLF..

Figure I.8
Source: istock photo.

Figure I.9
Source: USDA.

Figure I.10
Source: Local Food Hub. Used with permission.

CHAPTER 1

Cover photos
Source: Michael Milli, CLF
Source: Shutterstock. 140295688.

Figure 1.2
Source: USDA.

Figure 1.3
Source: chichacha. (2008). Apple.
https://www.flickr.com/photos/10673045@N04/2387957261/in/photolist-4D1UuV-4R5YRW

Figure 1.4
Source: CLF.

Figure 1.5
Source: Nicholas Lampert. Used with permission.

Figure 1.6
Source: Jim Weber, The Commercial Appeal. Used with permission.

Figure 1.8a
Source: istockphoto 20863061

Figure 1.8b
Source: istockphoto 6218137

Figure 1.8c
Source: istockphoto 33603160

Figure 1.8d
Source: USDA. (2013). FoodCorps Dennis and kids w kale.
https://www.flickr.com/photos/usdagov/10691922064

CHAPTER 2

Cover photo (collage)
Source: Alisha Vargas. (2009). 100_8967.
https://www.flickr.com/photos/alishav/3534215167/
Source: CDC. (2012). Patient having blood pressure taken by nurse.
http://commons.wikimedia.org/wiki/File:Patient_having_blood_pressure_taken_by_nurse.tiff
Source: O'Dea. (2012). Chest x-ray – postanterior view.
http://commons.wikimedia.org/wiki/File:Chest_x-ray_-_posteroanterior_view.jpg

Figure 2.4
Source: Tim McCabe, USDA NRCS.

Figure 2.5
Source: Industrial butcher. Corespics Vof | Dreamstime.com.

Figure 2.6
Source: CDC 10993, Janice Haney Carr. Salmonella.

CHAPTER 3

Cover photo
Source: Lynn Betts, USDA. Soil erosion.

Figure 3.1
Source: John Flannery. (2013). Bee on Zinnea.
https://www.flickr.com/photos/drphotomoto/9417297659/

Figure 3.2
Source: Kenn Hammond. Wikimedia commons.

CHAPTER 4

Cover photo
Source: Migrant Justice. Used with permission.

Figure 4.5
Source: Ruth Burrows, CLF.

Figure 4.6
Source: ROC. Restaurant Opportunities Center Protest. Used with permission.

Figure 4.7
Source: Carole Morison. Used with permission.

CHAPTER 5

Cover photo
Source: Michael Milli, CLF.

Figure 5.1
Source: Kevin Dooley. (2011). Read.
https://www.flickr.com/photos/pagedooley/5926270312/.

Figure 5.2
Source: Taina P., Witnesses to Hunger Boston. Restaurant. Used with permission.

Figure 5.3
Source: Crystal S., Witnesses to Hunger Philadelphia. Breakfast. Used with permission.

Figure 5.4
Source: Bonita C., Witnesses to Hunger Boston. Deep Freezer. Used with permission.

Figure 5.5
Source: Barbara I., Witnesses to Hunger Philadelphia. My Neighbor's Kitchen. Used with permission.

Figure 5.6
Source: Shaunte B., Witnesses to Hunger Baltimore. Number 9,584. Used with permission.

Figure 5.7
Source: Imani S., Witnesses to Hunger Philadelphia. Hungry Child Asking Caseworker for Something to Eat. Used with permission.

Figure 5.8
Source: Erica S., Witnesses to Hunger Philadelphia. Oodles of Noodles. Used with permission.

Figure 5.9
Source: USDA. (2011). Amboy 3.
https://www.flickr.com/photos/usdagov/6057054938/

CHAPTER 6

Cover photo
Source: Mark Dennis. Used with permission.

Figure 6.1
Source: Ruth Burrows, CLF. Mobile Produce Truck.

Figure 6.2
Source: Local Food Hub. "Farm to School Week Madness at the Warehouse." Used with permission.

Figure 6.3
Source: USDA. "20120708-OSEC-LSC-0074."
http://www.flickr.com/photos/usdagov/7531863328/in/set-72157630487867390/

Figure 6.6
Source: Brent Kim, CLF. Rose Street Garden, Baltimore.

Figure 6.7
Source: Leah Rimkus. ABC Bulk Produce Markets Stock the Items the City Determines Will Be Sold at a Fixed Price, 13 Cents per Pound. Used with permission.

Figure 6.8
Source: Leah Rimkus. The Line for One of Three "People's Restaurants" a Half Hour Before Opening Time; Meals Cost about 50 Cents; Diners Come from All Socioeconomic Groups. Used with permission.

CHAPTER 7

Cover photo
Source: Figure created by Rebecca Boehm.
Source: Gary Yost. Man selling oranges.
http://flic.kr/p/ejo2Zz
Source: Ron Nichols. Red barn and farm field.
http://flic.kr/p/fzbrUG

Figure 7.1
Source: A Healthier Michigan. (2003). Whole Foods. Flickr commons.
https://www.flickr.com/photos/healthiermi/5592358753

Figure 7.2
Source: Kathleen M. Rownland, 2011, USGS. Cropped.
http://gallery.usgs.gov/photos/07_14_2011_m52Tkw7JJe_07_14_2011_3#.U3JXuSgWl0o

Figure 7.3
Source: Pacific Coast Producers. Rominger Brothers Farm. Used with permission.

Figure 7.4
Source: South Dakota Corn. Corn Production. Used with permission.

Figure 7.6
Source: Poolie. (2008). American Soda.
https://www.flickr.com/photos/poolie/2474643298/

CHAPTER 8

Cover photo
Source: Architect of the Capitol. (1997). United States Capitol.
http://en.wikipedia.org/wiki/File:United_States_Capitol_-_west_front.jpg

Figure 8.2
Source: USDA Natural Resources Conservation Service. NRCSDC01001.

Figure 8.4
Source: National Archives. "Inspection of Carcasses, 1910."

Figure 8.8
Source: USDA, Natural Resource Conservation Service. NRCSAZ02083. 2011.

CHAPTER 9

Cover photo
Source: istockphoto

Figure 9.1
Source: istolethetv. (2006). "Mostly scorpions." Flickr commons.
https://www.flickr.com/photos/istolethetv/3189658885 Cropped.

Figure 9.3
Source: Rashida S. Mar B. (2010). Steamed Crabs.
https://www.flickr.com/photos/rashidasimmons/4923676817/

Figure 9.4
Source: Ed Kohler. (2009). Halal meat and grocery.
https://www.flickr.com/photos/edkohler/4169867343/in/set-72157613846391752/

Figure 9.5
Source: Edsel Little. (2011). Passover Seder Plate.
http://www.flickr.com/photos/edsel_/5638974836/

Figure 9.6
Source: Franciscan Center. Used with permission.

Figure 9.7
Source: Justin Marty. (2007). Danger—Men Cooking.
https://www.flickr.com/photos/jmarty/418854968/..

Figure 9.8
Source: Bob Jagendorf. (2007). Zombie girl having a snack, Zombiewalk, Asbury Park NJ.
https://www.flickr.com/photos/bobjagendorf/3978897574/.

Figure 9.9
Source: Michael Milli, CLF. Waverly Farmers Market.

CHAPTER 10

Cover photo
Source: Graphic created by Michael Milli, CLF.

Figure 10.1
Source: Mike Mozart. (2014). "Mikaela Shiffrin Wheaties Cereal Box US Ski Team Olympics General Mills Breakfast Cereal Box."
https://www.flickr.com/photos/jeepersmedia/14091279907/

Figure 10.2
Source: Freewheeling daredevil. (2008). "Brian Vickers Red Bull Toyota Camry."
https://www.flickr.com/photos/daredevil26/2264564102/

Figure 10.3
Source: Michael Milli, CLF.

Figure 10.4
Source: Michael Milli, CLF.

Figure 10.7
Source: Pamela Berg, CLF.

Figure 10.8
Source: Seth Anderson. (2012). Bloomberg as The Nanny.
https://www.flickr.com/photos/swanksalot/7320906998

CHAPTER 11

Cover photo
Source: Nicholas A. Tonelli. (2010). Monoculture.
https://www.flickr.com/photos/nicholas_t/4719020153/.

Figure 11.1
Source: USDA. http://www.flickr.com/photos/41284017@N08/6303010576

Figure 11.2
Source: USDA. http://www.flickr.com/photos/41284017@N08/6302886826

Figure 11.7
Source: Local Food Hub. (2013). Locally Grown Romanesco Broccoli from Malcolm's Market Garden in Augusta County, VA. Used with permission.

Figure 11.8
Source: USDA NRCS. http://www.nrcs.usda.gov/wps/portal/nrcs/photogallery/ia/newsroom/gallery/?cid=1716&position=Promo#1

Figure 11.9
Source: US Fish and Wildlife Service. https://www.flickr.com/photos/usfwshq/10820402344/in/set-72157637382485506

CHAPTER 12

COVER PHOTO
Source: Tim McCabe, NRCS
Source: Lynn Betts, NRCS
Source: StevenW. (2011). Cow.
https://www.flickr.com/photos/helloeveryone123/5962090641/.
Source: Bob Nichols, NRCS.

Figure 12.4
Source: Michael Milli, CLF. Aquaponics.

Figure 12.6
Source: NRCS
Source: Mercy for Animals MFA. (2011).
http://www.flickr.com/photos/mercyforanimals/6556759163/in/set-72157628531396063
Source: iStockphoto
Source: Jeff Vanuga, NRCS.

Figure 12.9
Source: Jeff Vanuga, USDA Natural Resources Conservation Service.

Figure 12.10
Source: Christopher Stevens, CLF.

CHAPTER 13

Cover photo
Source: Michael Milli, CLF.

Figure 13.1
Source: José Cruz, ABr. (2008). Embrapa news sp of cassava.
http://commons.wikimedia.org/wiki/File:Embrapa_news_sp_of_cassava_%28José_Cruz_ABr%29
   _25jan2008.jpg.

Figure 13.3
Source: Andreas Praefcke. (2008). Texas State Fair honey.
http://en.wikipedia.org/wiki/File:Texas_State_Fair_honey.jpg.

Figure 13.4
Source: Hiperbaric. High-Pressure Processing Apparatus. Used with permission.

Figure 13.5
Source: David Kamm, US Army. Food Retort.

Figure 13.7
Source: KVDP. (2008).
http://en.wikipedia.org/wiki/File:Healthy_Snacks.JPG

Figure 13.8
Source: David Falconer, US EPA. Old Soda Cans.

Figure 13.10
Source: Paul Wilkinson. (2012). Frozen Peas.
https://www.flickr.com/photos/eepaul/8042533270/

CHAPTER 14

Cover photo
Source: Roy Luck. (2011). Stacked containers at Bayport container terminal.
https://www.flickr.com/photos/royluck/5647125141/

Figure 14.2
Source: Soil-Science.info. (2000).Germination of Winter Wheat..
http://en.wikipedia.org/wiki/File:Veranotrigo.jpg.

Figure 14.3
Source: Nick Saltmarsh. Distribution center, J. Sainsburys.

Figure 14.4
Source: Dwight Burdette. (2011). Subway restaurant Pittsfield Township Michigan.
http://en.wikipedia.org/wiki/File:Subway_restaurant_Pittsfield_Township_Michigan.JPG

Figure 14.5
Source: Maryland Pride. (2010). Laurel Walmart Produce Section.
http://commons.wikimedia.org/wiki/File:Laurel_Walmart_Produce_Section.jpg

Figure 14.6
Source: Brave New Films. (2005). 001_1.
https://www.flickr.com/photos/walmartmovie/25962894/.

Figure 14.11
Source: Michael Milli, CLF.

Figure 14.16
Source: Infrogmation of New Orleans. (2010). Loxley Farm Market interior.
http://commons.wikimedia.org/wiki/File:Loxley_Farm_Market_interior.JPG

Figure 14.17
Source: CLF. CSA Weekly Share Items.

CHAPTER 15

Cover photo
Source: istockphoto

Figure 15.1
Source: (rinse). (2009). bananas.
https://www.flickr.com/photos/rinses/3602799397/

Figure 15.3
Source: Dale Frost. Port of San Diego. (2008). Dole Honduras in San Diego.
http://commons.wikimedia.org/wiki/File:Dole_Honduras_in_San_Diego.jpg

Figure 15.7
Source: Evan-Amos. (2011). McD-Bacon-Egg-Cheese-McGriddle.
http://commons.wikimedia.org/wiki/User:Evan-Amos/Food#mediaviewer/File:McD-Bacon-Egg-
Cheese-McGriddle.jpg

Figure 15.8
Source: CLF.

Figure 15.9
Source: Nenyedi. (2007). Snack machine 3538.
http://en.wikipedia.org/wiki/File:Snack_machine_3538.JPG.

CHAPTER 16

Cover photo
Source: istockphoto

Figure 16.2.
Source: Scott Bauer, USDA. Grain products.
http://commons.wikimedia.org/wiki/File:GrainProducts.jpg

Figure 16.3
Source: CLF.

Figure 16.4
Source: Burger Austin. (2010). Nau's Enfield Drug – Large Bacon Cheeseburger.
https://www.flickr.com/photos/burgeraustin/5007282483/.

Figure 16.6.
Source: Blairing Media. (2010). Cooked red quinoa.
http://en.wikipedia.org/wiki/File:Red_quinoa.png..

CHAPTER 17

Cover photo
Sources: Jessie Hirsch. (2008). G&F Grocery. https://www.flickr.com/photos/jhirsch/2182835511/
Source: Brian Zim. (2010). West Side Market, Cleveland, OH.
Source: Paulo Ordoveza (2009). County fair food banners.
https://www.flickr.com/photos/brownpau/3843529497/
Source: istockphoto

Figure 17.2
Source: Farmer's Fridge. Used with permission.

Figure 17.3
Source: Stephen Van Worley. (September 2010). Data Pointed datapointed.net. Used with permission.

Figure 17.5
Source: PJ Roldan. (2011). Family Cigarette Grocery Store.
https://www.flickr.com/photos/26856943@N03/7044377969/

Figure 17.7
Source: CLF.

Figure 17.8
Source: John Donges (2012). 574.
https://www.flickr.com/photos/mendrakis/8132483865. Used with permission.

Figure 17.9
Source: Dvortygirl (2012). Shuttered supermarket.
https://www.flickr.com/photos/dvortygirl/7156304688/

Figure 17.10
Source: J. Winters (2008).
http://commons.wikimedia.org/wiki/File:Red_Robin_in_Tukwila,_Washington.jpg

Figure 17.12
Source: Denver Urban Gardens (2009). Volunteers at Atlantis Community Garden. http://dug.org
/photo-gallery.

Figure 17.13
Source: Denver Urban Gardens (2009). Connecting generations mentors and youth at Fairview youth
farmers market. http://dug.org/photo-gallery.

CHAPTER 18

Cover photo
Source: Michael Milli, CLF.

Figure 18.3
Source: Michael Milli, CLF.

Figure 18.5
Source: Alison Cuccia, Healthy Corner Stores Project. Used with permission.

Index

Eisenhauer, E., 443
Eitzer, B. D., 271
El-Ansary, A. I., 360
Elbel, B., 383, 446
Elder, R. O., 308
Electronic benefits transfer (EBT), 460, 476, 487
Elgethun, K., 35
Elitzak, H., 249–250, 292
Elliott, S. S., 407
Elwood, P., 409
Emberson, J., 30
Emborg, H.-D., 301
Emes, Y., 318
Endo, G., 43
Endocrine disruption, 42, 487
Endotoxin, 303, 487
Energy, 63–64; density, 31, 487
Eng, E., 474–475
Engbers, L.H., 438
Enrichment, 416
Enterline, K., 139
Entitlement program, 190, 487
Enver, A., 176
Environmental health, 33
Environmental Protection Agency (EPA), 43, 164, 165, 206, 340
Environmental Working Group, 45, 468
EPA. See Environmental Protection Agency (EPA)
Epcot Center (Disney), 463
Epidemic of Absence (Velasquez), 30
Epidemiologic transition, 27, 487
Epode, 177
Epp, M. D., 268
Epstein, J. M., 6
Equilibrium, 161, 488
Ericksen, P., 64
Eriksen, M., 42, 43
Erinosho, T. O., 255
Ervin, R. B., 86
Escott-Stump, S., 403, 411, 413
Eslami, E., 119, 120
ETC Group, 69, 71
Ethanol, 167
Ethelbah, B., 473
Ettinger de Cuba, S., 78, 108
European Union (EU), 393
Eutrophication, 66, 488
Evans, A., 250
Evansville, Indiana, 220

Even' Star Organic Farm, 439
Evenson, K. R., 445
Externality, 162, 488
Ezekowitz, M. D., 33
Ezzati, M., 28

F

Fabry, V. J., 64, 65
Fact-based labels, 244
Facts Up Front, 245
Fahs, M. C., 111
Faith, J. J., 28
Faithful Families Eating Smart and Moving More, 474
Falkenmark, M., 64
Famous Amos Chocolate Chip Cookies (NuVal LLC), 244
Fan, Z. J., 40
FAO. See Food and Agriculture Organization (FAO; United Nations)
Farbman, J., 139–140
Farley, T. A., 432
Farm Bill. See US Farm Bill (1995)
Farm state, 193, 488
Farmer, P., 83
Farmers' Market Coalition, 141, 476
Farming, economic viability of, 1840s to 1990s, 195–197
Farming systems: and agroecology and organic farming, 277–278; and bright future for farmers in middle?, 274–276; and emergence of industrial agriculture, 267–271; environmental impacts of, 279–280; and farms producing for local and regional markets, 274–277; and food security, 280; history of: from local to industrial, 266–267; and overview of industrial crop farming, 271–274; public health impacts of, 280–281; social impacts of, 281–282; traditional systems (United States), 267
Farmland protection, 57–59
Farm-to-School (F2S) programs, 470, 488
Farrell, T. J., 226, 227
Farrigan, T., 432
Fast Food Nation (Schlosser), 94, 229
Fats (lipids), 408, 488
Faucher, J., 249
Fausti, S. W., 270–271
FDA. See US Food and Drug Administration (FDA)
Fecondo, G., 268
Federal Poverty Level, 432
Feeding America, 138

Hayden, S., 435

Hayes-Conroy, J., 84

Hays, C. L., 356

Hayter, A., 418

Hazen, S. L., 31

He, M., 436, 445

Health and human rights framework, 126, 490

Health belief model (HBM), 461, 462, 490

Health Bucks, 476

Health disparities, 80, 490

Health inequities, 80, 490; ecological approach to, 82–83; model, 82 Fig. 4.2

Healthier Food Retail (Centers for Disease Control), 430

Healthy defaults, 427, 490

Healthy Food Availability Index, 432

Healthy Food Financing Initiative, 208

Healthy Hunger-Free Kids Act (2010), 436

Healthy Incentives Pilot (HIP), 175, 176

Healthy People 2020 (Department of Health and Human Services), 376

Healthy Student Act (Mississippi), 145

Healthy Weight Commitment Foundation (HWFC), 177

Heart Healthy Lenoir (HHL), 475

Heathcote, S., 302

Heckman, J. J., 114

Hedden, W. P., 442

Hedgerows, 71, 72, 491

Heidenreich, P. A., 33

Heim, S., 470

Hcin, G. L., 407

Heinberg, R., 55, 63

Heinemann, J. A., 270

Heinz, 246

Heinz Center, 55

Heisey, P. W., 274

Heller, M. C., 70, 75

Henderson, V. R., 88

Hendricks, A.-M., 476

Hendrickson, M., 273, 282

Hendrickson, M. K., 298

Henson, S. J., 248

Herath, D., 298

Hermansen, K., 409

Hernández, A. F., 36

Hernandez-Pelletier, M., 110

Herren, H. R., 54, 271

Hersey, J., 448

Hess, P., 436

Heterogeneous supply, breaking down, 484

Heuer, C. A., 30, 445, 463, 464

Heuristics, 491

Higgins, C., 446

Higginson, C. S., 244

High fructose corn syrup (HFCS), 407

Hilbeck, A., 270

Hill, J. D., 71–72, 270

Hill, J. L., 474–475

Hillier, A., 88, 446–447

Hilmers, A., 445

Hilmers, D., 445

Himes, J. H., 110

Ho, L. S., 83

Ho, P., 270–271

Hodge, J. G., 209

Hodgson, E., 271

Hodkin, 271

Hodne, C., 301, 302

Hoebel, B. G., 281, 405

Hoeft, B., 381

Hoekstra, A. Y., 60, 61

Hoekstra, R. M., 41

Hoerrner, K., 250

Hofferth, S. L., 121

Hoffmann, A. M., 270–271

Hoisington, D., 270

Holbem, D. H., 143

Holcomb, J. P., 143

Holland, J. H., 5

Hollenbeck, A., 231

Holtcamp, W., 36

Holt-Giménez, E., 149, 150

Homestead Act, 191, 195, 197

Hong, S. C., 177

Hood, C., 460

Hoppe, R. A., 167, 348

Horovitz, B., 88

Horowitz, A., 114

Horowitz, J., 272

Horrigan, L., 34, 289, 304

Horton, M. K., 35

Horton, R. A., 302

Horwath, W. R., 69

Horwitz, S., 354

Hota, B., 301

Hotchkiss, A. K., 336

Hotchkiss, J. H., 336, 337, 341